Pearson Custom **HEALTH PROFESSIONS**

Community College of Baltimore County
OFAD 141
Medical Terminology

PEARSON

Senior Vice President, Editorial: Patrick F. Boles
Senior Acquisitions Editor: Debbie Coniglio
Development Editor: Abbey Lee Briggs
Editorial Assistant: Jeanne Martin
Operations Manager: Eric M. Kenney
Production Manager: Jennifer Berry
Rights Manager: Michael E. Mushlitz
Art Director: Renée Sartell
Cover Designer: Tess Mattern

Cover Art: "Red Sticking Plasters" courtesy of Yasuhide Fumoto/Getty Images, Inc. "Doctor Sewing Heart Back Together" courtesy of Jonathan Evans/Getty Images, Inc.

Printed in the United States of America.

Please visit our website at *www.pearsonlearningsolutions.com.*

Attention bookstores: For permission to return any unsold stock, contact us at *pe-uscustomreturns@pearson.com.*

Pearson Learning Solutions, 501 Boylston Street, Suite 900, Boston, MA 02116
A Pearson Education Company
www.pearsoned.com

ISBN 10: 1-256-54876-6
ISBN 13: 978-1-256-54876-8

Table of Contents

Introduction to Medical Terminology

Learning Objectives

Upon completion of this chapter, you will be able to:

- Discuss the four parts of medical terms.
- Recognize word roots and combining forms.
- Identify the most common prefixes and suffixes.
- Define word building and describe a strategy for translating medical terms.
- State the importance of correct spelling of medical terms.
- State the rules for determining singular and plural endings.
- Discuss the importance of using caution with abbreviations.
- Recognize the documents found in a medical record.
- Recognize the different healthcare settings.
- Understand the importance of confidentiality.

From Chapter 1 of *Medical Terminology: A Living Language*, 4/e. Bonnie F. Fremgen. Suzanne S. Frucht.

Medical Terminology at a Glance

Learning medical terminology can initially seem like studying a strange new language. However, once you understand some of the basic rules as to how medical terms are formed using word building, it will become much like piecing together a puzzle. The general guidelines for forming words; an understanding of word roots, combining forms, prefixes, and suffixes; pronunciation; and spelling are discussed in this chapter. In addition, "Med Term Tips" are sprinkled throughout the text to assist in clarifying some of the material. New medical terms discussed in each section are listed separately at the beginning of the section, and the chapter contains pathological, diagnostic, treatment, and surgical terms. You can use these lists as an additional study tool for previewing and reviewing terms.

Understanding medical terms requires you to be able to put words together or build words from their parts. It is impossible to memorize thousands of medical terms; however, once you understand the basics, you can distinguish the meaning of medical terms by analyzing their prefixes, suffixes, and word roots. Remember that there will always be some exceptions to every rule, and medical terminology is no different. We will attempt to point out these exceptions where they exist. Most medical terms, however, do follow the general rule that there is a **word root** or fundamental meaning for the word, a **prefix** and a **suffix** that modify the meaning of the word root, and sometimes a **combining vowel** to connect other word parts. You will be amazed at the seemingly difficult words you will be able to build and understand when you follow the simple steps in word building (see Figure 1 ■).

■ **Figure 1** Nurse completing a patient report. Healthcare workers use medical terminology in order to accurately and efficiently communicate patient information to each other.

Building Medical Terms from Word Parts

Four different word parts or elements can be used to construct medical terms:

1. The **word root** is the foundation of the word.

   cardiogram = record of the heart

2. A **prefix** is at the beginning of the word.

   pericardium = around the heart

3. A **suffix** is at the end of the word.

   card**itis** = inflammation of the heart

4. The **combining vowel** is a vowel (usually o) that links the word root to another word root or a suffix.

   cardi**o**my**o**pathy = disease of the heart muscle[1]

The following sections on word roots, combining vowels and forms, prefixes, and suffixes will consider each of these word parts in more detail and present examples of some of those most commonly used.

Word Roots

The word root is the foundation of a medical term and provides us with the general meaning of the word. The word root often indicates the body system or part of the body that is being discussed, such as *cardi* for heart. At other times the word root may be an action. For example, the word root *cis* means to cut (as in incision).

A term may have more than one word root. For example, **osteoarthritis** (oss tee oh ar THRY tis) combines the word root *oste* meaning bone and *arthr* meaning the joints. When the suffix *-itis*, meaning inflammation, is added, we have the entire word, meaning an inflammation involving bone at the joints.

Combining Vowel/Form

To make it possible to pronounce long medical terms with ease and to combine several word parts, a combining vowel is used. This is most often the vowel *o*. Combining vowels are utilized in two places: between a word root and a suffix or between two word roots.

To decide whether to use a combining vowel between a word root and suffix, first look at the suffix. If it begins with a vowel, do not use the combining vowel. If, however, the suffix begins with a consonant, then use a combining vowel. For example: To combine *arthr* with *-scope* will require a combining vowel: **arthroscope** (AR throh scope). But to combine *arthr* with *-itis* does not require a combining vowel: **arthritis** (ar THRY tis).

The combining vowel is typically kept between two word roots, even if the second word root begins with a vowel. For example, in forming the term **gastroenteritis** (gas troh en ter EYE tis) the combining vowel is kept between the two word roots *gastr* and *enter* (gastrenteritis is incorrect). As you can tell from pronouncing these two terms, the combining vowel makes the pronunciation easier.

When writing a word root by itself, its **combining form** is typically used. This consists of the word root and its combining vowel written in a word root/vowel form, for example, *cardi/o*. Since it is often simpler to pronounce word roots when they appear in their combining form, this format is used throughout this book.

Med Term Tip

Medical terms are built from word parts:

Word Building Part	Example (Meaning)
1. Word root	*cardi* (heart)
2. Prefix	*peri-* (around)
3. Suffix	*-itis* (inflammation)

When these components are put together, the word *pericarditis* is formed, meaning inflammation around the heart.

Med Term Tip

Remember to break down every word into its components (prefix, word root/combining form, and suffix) when learning medical terminology. Do not try to memorize every medical term. Instead, figure out how the word is formed from its components. In a short time you will be able to do this automatically when seeing a new term.

Common Combining Forms

Some commonly used word roots in their combining form, their meaning, and examples of their use follow. Review the examples to observe when a combining vowel was kept and when it was dropped according to the rules presented on the preceding page.

Combining Form	Meaning	Example (Definition)
aden/o	gland	adenopathy (gland disease)
carcin/o	cancer	carcinoma (cancerous tumor)
cardi/o	heart	cardiac (pertaining to the heart)
chem/o	chemical	chemotherapy (treatment with chemicals)
cis/o	to cut	incision (process of cutting into)
dermat/o	skin	dermatology (study of the skin)
enter/o	small intestine	enteric (pertaining to the small intestine)
gastr/o	stomach	gastric (pertaining to the stomach)
gynec/o	female	gynecology (study of females)
hemat/o	blood	hematic (pertaining to the blood)
hydr/o	water	hydrocele (protrusion of water [in the scrotum])
immun/o	immune	immunology (study of immunity)
laryng/o	voice box	laryngeal (pertaining to the voice box)
morph/o	shape	morphology (study of shape)
nephr/o	kidney	nephromegaly (enlarged kidney)
neur/o	nerve	neural (pertaining to a nerve)
ophthalm/o	eye	ophthalmic (pertaining to the eye)
ot/o	ear	otic (pertaining to the ear)
path/o	disease	pathology (study of disease)
pulmon/o	lung	pulmonary (pertaining to the lungs)
rhin/o	nose	rhinoplasty (surgical repair of the nose)
ur/o	urine, urinary tract	urology (study of the urinary tract)

mast/o – breast

Prefixes

A new medical term is formed when a prefix is added to the front of the term. Prefixes frequently give information about the location of an organ, the number of parts, or the time (frequency). For example, the prefix *bi-* stands for two of something, such as **bilateral** (bye LAH ter al), which means having two sides. However, not every term will have a prefix.

Common Prefixes

Some of the more common prefixes, their meanings, and examples of their use follow. When written by themselves, prefixes are followed by a hyphen.

Prefix	Meaning	Example (Definition)
a-	without, away from	aphasia (without speech)
an-	without	anoxia (without oxygen)
ante-	before, in front of	antepartum (before birth)

anti-	against	antibiotic (against life)
auto-	self	autograft (a graft from one's own body)
brady-	slow	bradycardia (slow heartbeat)
dys-	painful, difficult	dyspnea (difficulty breathing)
endo-	within, inner	endoscope (instrument to view within)
epi-	upon, over	epigastric (upon or over the stomach)
eu-	normal, good	eupnea (normal breathing)
hetero-	different	heterograft (a graft from another person's body)
homo-	same	homozygous (having two identical genes)
hyper-	over, above	hypertrophy (overdevelopment)
hypo-	under, below	hypoglossal (under the tongue)
infra-	under, beneath, below	infraorbital (below, under the eye socket)
inter-	among, between	intervertebral (between the vertebrae)
intra-	within, inside	intravenous (inside, within a vein)
macro-	large	macrocephalic (having a large head)
micro-	small	microcephalic (having a small head)
neo-	new	neonate (newborn)
pan-	all	pancarditis (inflammation of all the heart)
para-	beside, beyond, near	paranasal (near or alongside the nose)
per-	through	percutaneous (through the skin)
peri-	around	pericardial (around the heart)
post-	after	postpartum (after birth)
pre-	before, in front of	prefrontal (in front of the frontal bone)
pseudo-	false	pseudocyesis (false pregnancy)
retro-	backward, behind	retrograde (movement in a backward direction)
sub-	below, under	subcutaneous (under, below the skin)
super-	above, excess	supernumerary (above the normal number)
supra-	above	suprapubic (above the pubic bone)
tachy-	rapid, fast	tachycardia (fast heartbeat)
trans-	through, across	transurethral (across the urethra)
ultra-	beyond, excess	ultrasound (high-frequency sound waves)

Med Term Tip

Be very careful with prefixes; many have similar spellings but very different meanings. For example:

anti- means "against"; *ante-* means "before"

inter- means "between"; *intra-* means "inside"

per- means "through"; *peri-* means "around"

Number Prefixes

Some common prefixes pertaining to the number of items or measurement, their meanings, and examples of their use follow.

Prefix	Meaning	Example (Definition)
bi-	two	bilateral (two sides)
hemi-	half	hemiplegia (paralysis of one side/half of the body)
mono-	one	monoplegia (paralysis of one extremity)
multi-	many	multigravida (woman pregnant more than once)
nulli-	none	nulligravida (woman with no pregnancies)
poly-	many	polyuria (large amounts of urine)

quad-	four	quadriplegia (paralysis of all four extremities)
semi-	partial, half	semiconscious (partially conscious)
tri-	three	triceps (muscle with three heads)
uni-	one	unilateral (one side)

Suffixes

A suffix is attached to the end of a word to add meaning, such as a condition, disease, or procedure. For example, the suffix *-itis*, which means inflammation, when added to *cardi-* forms the new word **carditis** (car DYE tis), which means inflammation of the heart. Every medical term *must* have a suffix. The majority of the time, the suffix is added to a word root, as in carditis above. However, terms can also be built from a suffix added directly to a prefix, without a word root. For example, the term **dystrophy** (DIS troh fee), which means abnormal development, is built from the prefix *dys-* (meaning abnormal) and the suffix *-trophy* (meaning development).

Med Term Tip

Remember, if a suffix begins with a vowel, the combining vowel is dropped: for example, *mastitis* rather than *mastoitis*.

Common Suffixes

Some common suffixes, their meanings, and examples of their use follow. When written by themselves, suffixes are preceded by a hyphen.

Suffix	Meaning	Example (Definition)
-algia	pain	gastralgia (stomach pain)
-cele	hernia, protrusion	cystocele (protrusion of the bladder)
-cise	cut	excise (to cut out)
-cyte	cell	erythrocyte (red cell)
-dynia	pain	cardiodynia (heart pain)
-ectasis	dilation	bronchiectasis (dilated bronchi)
-gen	that which produces	mutagen (that which produces mutations)
-genesis	produces, generates	osteogenesis (produces bone)
-genic	producing, produced by	carcinogenic (producing cancer)
-ia	state, condition	hemiplegia (condition of being half paralyzed)
-iasis	abnormal condition	lithiasis (abnormal condition of stones)
-ism	state of	hypothyroidism (state of low thyroid)
-itis	inflammation	cellulitis (inflammation of cells)
-logist	one who studies	cardiologist (one who studies the heart)
-logy	study of	cardiology (study of the heart)
-lysis	destruction	osteolysis (bone destruction)
-malacia	abnormal softening	chondromalacia (abnormal cartilage softening)
-megaly	enlargement, large	cardiomegaly (enlarged heart)
-oma	tumor, mass	carcinoma (cancerous tumor)
-osis	abnormal condition	cyanosis (abnormal condition of being blue)
-pathy	disease	myopathy (muscle disease)
-plasia	development, growth	dysplasia (abnormal development)
-plasm	formation, development	neoplasm (new formation)
-ptosis	drooping	proctoptosis (drooping rectum)

-rrhage	excessive, abnormal flow	hemorrhage (excessive bleeding)
-rrhea	discharge, flow	rhinorrhea (discharge from the nose)
-rrhexis	rupture	hysterorrhexis (ruptured uterus)
-sclerosis	hardening	arteriosclerosis (hardening of an artery)
-stenosis	narrowing	angiostenosis (narrowing of a vessel)
-therapy	treatment	chemotherapy (treatment with chemicals)
-trophy	nourishment, development	hypertrophy (excessive development)

Adjective Suffixes

The following suffixes are used to convert a word root into an adjective. These suffixes usually are translated as *pertaining to*.

Suffix	Meaning	Example (Definition)
-ac	pertaining to	cardiac (pertaining to the heart)
-al	pertaining to	duodenal (pertaining to the duodenum)
-an	pertaining to	ovarian (pertaining to the ovary)
-ar	pertaining to	ventricular (pertaining to a ventricle)
-ary	pertaining to	pulmonary (pertaining to the lungs)
-eal	pertaining to	esophageal (pertaining to the esophagus)
-iac	pertaining to	chondriac (pertaining to cartilage)
-ic	pertaining to	gastric (pertaining to the stomach)
-ical	pertaining to	neurological (pertaining to the study of the nerves)
-ile	pertaining to	penile (pertaining to the penis)
-ior	pertaining to	superior (pertaining to above)
-ory	pertaining to	auditory (pertaining to hearing)
-ose	pertaining to	adipose (pertaining to fat)
-ous	pertaining to	intravenous (pertaining to within a vein)
-tic	pertaining to	acoustic (pertaining to hearing)

Surgical Suffixes

The following suffixes indicate surgical procedures.

Suffix	Meaning	Example (Definition)
-centesis	puncture to withdraw fluid	arthrocentesis (puncture to withdraw fluid from a joint)
-ectomy	surgical removal	gastrectomy (surgically remove the stomach)
-ostomy	surgically create an opening	colostomy (surgically create an opening for the colon through the abdominal wall)
-otomy	cutting into	thoracotomy (cutting into the chest)
-pexy	surgical fixation	nephropexy (surgical fixation of a kidney)
-plasty	surgical repair	dermatoplasty (surgical repair of the skin)
-rrhaphy	suture	myorrhaphy (suture together muscle)

Med Term Tip

Surgical suffixes have very specific meanings:

-otomy means "to cut into"
-ostomy means "to create a new opening"
-ectomy means "to cut out" or "remove"

Procedural Suffixes

The following suffixes indicate procedural processes or instruments.

Suffix	Meaning	Example (Definition)
-gram	record or picture	electrocardiogram (record of heart's electricity)
-graph	instrument for recording	electrocardiograph (instrument for recording the heart's electrical activity)
-graphy	process of recording	electrocardiography (process of recording the heart's electrical activity)
-meter	instrument for measuring	audiometer (instrument to measure hearing)
-metry	process of measuring	audiometry (process of measuring hearing)
-scope	instrument for viewing	gastroscope (instrument to view stomach)
-scopy	process of visually examining	gastroscopy (process of visually examining the stomach)

Word Building

Word building consists of putting together several word elements to form a variety of terms. The combining form of a word may be added to another combining form along with a suffix to create a new descriptive term. For example, adding *hyster/o* (meaning uterus) to *salping/o* (meaning fallopian tubes) along with the suffix *-ectomy* (meaning surgical removal of) forms **hysterosalpingectomy** (hiss-ter-oh-sal-pin-JEK-toh-mee), the removal of both the uterus and the fallopian tubes. You will note that the combining vowel *o* is dropped when adding the suffix *-ectomy* since two vowels are not necessary.

Interpreting Medical Terms

The following strategy is a reliable method for puzzling out the meaning of an unfamiliar medical term.

Med Term Tip

To gain a quick understanding of a term, it may be helpful to you to read from the end of the word (or the suffix) back to the beginning (the prefix), and then pick up the word root. For example, *pericarditis* reads inflammation (*-itis*) surrounding (*peri-*) the heart (*cardi/o*).

Step
1. Divide the term into its word parts.
2. Define each word part.

3. Combine the meaning of the word parts.

Example
gastr/o/enter/o/logy
gastr = stomach
o = combining vowel, no meaning
enter = small intestine
o = combining vowel, no meaning
-logy = study
stomach, small intestine, study of

Pronunciation

You will hear different pronunciations for the same terms depending on where people were born or educated. As long as it is clear which term people are discussing, differing pronunciations are acceptable. Some people are difficult to understand over the telephone or on a transcription tape. If you have any doubt about a term being discussed, ask for the term to be spelled. For example, it is often difficult to hear the difference between the terms **abduction** and **adduction**. However, since the terms refer to opposite directions of movement, it is very important to double check if there is any question about which term was used.

Each new term is introduced in boldface type, with the phonetic or "sounds like" pronunciation in parentheses immediately following. The part of the word that should receive the greatest emphasis during pronunciation appears in capital letters: for example, **pericarditis** (per ih car DYE tis).

Spelling

Although you will hear differing pronunciations of the same term, there will be only one correct spelling. If you have any doubt about the spelling of a term or of its meaning, always look it up in a medical dictionary. If only one letter of the word is changed, it could make a critical difference for the patient. For example, imagine the problem that could arise if you note for insurance purposes that a portion of a patient's **ileum**, or small intestine, was removed when in reality he had surgery for removal of a piece of his **ilium**, or hip bone.

Some words have the same beginning sounds but are spelled differently. Examples include the following:

Med Term Tip

If you have any doubt about the meaning or spelling of a word, look it up in your medical dictionary. Even experienced medical personnel still need to look up a few words.

Sounds like *si*

psy	**psychiatry** (sigh-KIGH-ah-tree)
cy	**cytology** (sigh-TALL-oh-gee)

Sounds like *dis*

dys	**dyspepsia** (dis-PEP-see-ah)
dis	**dislocation** (dis-low-KAY-shun)

Singular and Plural Endings

Many medical terms originate from Greek and Latin words. The rules for forming the singular and plural forms of some words follow the rules of these languages rather than English. For example, the heart has a left atrium and a right atrium for a total of two *atria*, not two *atriums*. Other words, such as *virus* and *viruses*, are changed from singular to plural by following English rules. Each medical term needs to be considered individually when changing from the singular to the plural form. The following examples illustrate how to form plurals.

Words ending in	Singular	Plural
-a	vertebra	vertebrae
-ax	thorax	thoraces
-ex or -ix	appendix	appendices
-is	metastasis	metastases
-ma	sarcoma	sarcomata
-nx	phalanx	phalanges
-on	ganglion	ganglia
-us	nucleus	nuclei
-um	ovum	ova
-y	biopsy	biopsies

Abbreviations

Abbreviations are commonly used in the medical profession as a way of saving time. However, some abbreviations can be confusing, such as *SM* for simple mastectomy and *sm* for small. Use of the incorrect abbreviation can result in problems for a patient, as well as with insurance records and processing. If you have any concern that you will confuse someone by using an abbreviation, spell out the word instead. It is never acceptable to use one's own abbreviations. All types of healthcare facilities will have a list of approved abbreviations, and it is extremely important that you become familiar with this list and follow it closely.

The Medical Record

The **medical record** or chart documents the details of a patient's hospital stay. Each healthcare professional who has contact with the patient in any capacity completes the appropriate report of that contact and adds it to the medical chart. This results in a permanent physical record of the patient's day-to-day condition, when and what services he or she received, and the response to treatment. Each institution adopts a specific format for each document and its location within the chart. This is necessary because each healthcare professional must be able to locate quickly and efficiently the information he or she needs in order to provide proper care for the patient. The medical record is also a legal document. Therefore, it is essential that all chart components be completely filled out and signed. Each page must contain the proper patient identification information: the patient's name, age, gender, physician, admission date, and identification number.

While the patient is still in the hospital, a unit clerk is usually responsible for placing documents in the proper place. After discharge, the medical records department ensures that all documents are present, complete, signed, and in the correct order. If a person is readmitted, especially for the same diagnosis, parts of this previous chart can be pulled and added to the current chart for reference (see Figure 2 ■). Physicians' offices and other outpatient care providers such as clinics and therapists also maintain a medical record detailing each patient's visit to their facility.

A list of the most common elements of a hospital chart with a brief description of each follows.

History and Physical—Written or dictated by the admitting physician; details the patient's history, results of the physician's examination, initial diagnoses, and physician's plan of treatment

Physician's Orders—Complete list of the care, medications, tests, and treatments the physician orders for the patient

Nurse's Notes—Record of the patient's care throughout the day; includes vital signs, treatment specifics, patient's response to treatment, and patient's condition

■ **Figure 2** Health information professionals maintain accurate, orderly, and permanent patient records. Medical records are securely stored and available for future reference.

Physician's Progress Notes—Physician's daily record of the patient's condition, results of the physician's examinations, summary of test results, updated assessment and diagnoses, and further plans for the patient's care

Consultation Reports—Reports given by specialists whom the physician has asked to evaluate the patient

Ancillary Reports—Reports from various treatments and therapies the patient has received, such as rehabilitation, social services, or respiratory therapy

Diagnostic Reports—Results of diagnostic tests performed on the patient, principally from the clinical lab (for example, blood tests) and medical imaging (for example, X-rays and ultrasound)

Informed Consent—Document voluntarily signed by the patient or a responsible party that clearly describes the purpose, methods, procedures, benefits, and risks of a diagnostic or treatment procedure

Operative Report—Report from the surgeon detailing an operation; includes a pre- and postoperative diagnosis, specific details of the surgical procedure itself, and how the patient tolerated the procedure

Anesthesiologist's Report—Relates the details regarding the substances (such as medications and fluids) given to a patient, the patient's response to anesthesia, and vital signs during surgery

Pathologist's Report—Report given by a pathologist who studies tissue removed from the patient (for example, bone marrow, blood, or tissue biopsy)

Discharge Summary—Comprehensive outline of the patient's entire hospital stay; includes condition at time of admission, admitting diagnosis, test results, treatments and patient's response, final diagnosis, and follow-up plans

Healthcare Settings

The use of medical terminology is widespread. It provides healthcare professionals with a precise and efficient method of communicating very specific patient information to one another, regardless of whether they are in the same type of facility (see Figure 3 ■). Descriptions follow of the different types of settings where medical terminology is used.

Acute Care or General Hospitals—Provide services to diagnose (laboratory, diagnostic imaging) and treat (surgery, medications, therapy) diseases for a short period of time; in addition, they usually provide emergency and obstetrical care

Specialty Care Hospitals—Provide care for very specific types of diseases; for example, a psychiatric hospital

Nursing Homes or Long-Term Care Facilities—Provide long-term care for patients who need extra time to recover from an illness or injury before returning home, or for persons who can no longer care for themselves

Ambulatory Care, Surgical Centers, or Outpatient Clinics—Provide services that do not require overnight hospitalization; the services range from simple surgeries to diagnostic testing or therapy

Figure 3 A nurse and medical assistant review a patient's chart and plan his or her daily care.

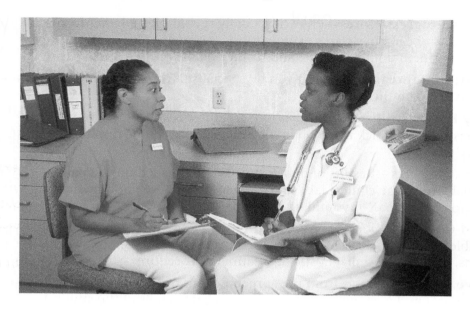

Physicians' Offices—Provide diagnostic and treatment services in a private office setting

Health Maintenance Organization (HMO)—Provides a wide range of services by a group of primary-care physicians, specialists, and other healthcare professionals in a prepaid system

Home Health Care—Provides nursing, therapy, personal care, or housekeeping services in the patient's own home

Rehabilitation Centers—Provide intensive physical and occupational therapy; they include inpatient and outpatient treatment

Hospice—Provides supportive treatment to terminally ill patients and their families

Confidentiality

Anyone who works with medical terminology and is involved in the medical profession must have a firm understanding of confidentiality. Any information or record relating to a patient must be considered privileged. This means that you have a moral and legal responsibility to keep all information about the patient confidential. If you are asked to supply documentation relating to a patient, the proper authorization form must be signed by the patient. Give only the specific information that the patient has authorized. The Health Insurance Portability and Accountability Act of 1996 (HIPAA) set federal standards that provide patients with more protection of their medical records and health information, better access to their own records, and greater control over how their health information is used and to whom it is disclosed.

Chapter Review

Terminology Checklist

Below are all key terms presented in this chapter. Use this list as a study tool by placing a check in the box in front of each term as you master its meaning.

- ☐ acute care hospitals
- ☐ ambulatory care centers
- ☐ ancillary reports
- ☐ anesthesiologist's report
- ☐ combining form
- ☐ combining vowel
- ☐ consultation report
- ☐ diagnostic reports
- ☐ discharge summary
- ☐ general hospitals
- ☐ health maintenance organization (HMO)

- ☐ history and physical
- ☐ home health care
- ☐ hospices
- ☐ informed consent
- ☐ long-term care facilities
- ☐ medical record
- ☐ nurse's notes
- ☐ nursing homes
- ☐ operative report
- ☐ outpatient clinics
- ☐ pathologist's report

- ☐ physicians' offices
- ☐ physician's orders
- ☐ physician's progress notes
- ☐ prefix
- ☐ rehabilitation centers
- ☐ specialty care hospitals
- ☐ suffix
- ☐ surgical centers
- ☐ word root

Practice Exercises

A. Complete the following statements.

1. The combination of a word root and the combining vowel is called a(n) __combining-form__

2. The vowel that connects two word roots or a suffix with a word root is usually a(n) __O__.

3. A word part used at the end of a word root to change the meaning of the word is called a(n) __suffix__.

4. A(n) __prefix__ is used at the beginning of a word to indicate number, location, or time.

5. Although the pronunciation of medical terms may differ slightly from one person to another, the __spelling__ must never change.

6. The four components of a medical term are __word root__, __prefix__, __suffix__, and __combining vowel__.

B. Define the following combining forms.

1. aden/o __gland__
2. carcin/o __cancer__
3. cardi/o __heart__
4. chem/o __chemical__
5. cis/o __to cut__
6. dermat/o __skin__
7. enter/o __small intestine__

8. gastr/o __stomach__
9. gynec/o __female__
10. hemat/o __blood__
11. hydr/o __water__
12. immun/o __immune__
13. laryng/o __voice box__
14. morph/o __shape__

Introduction to Medical Terminology

15. nephr/o _kidney_

16. neur/o _nerve_

17. ophthalm/o _eye_

18. ot/o _ear_

19. pulmon/o _lung_

20. rhin/o _nose_

21. ur/o _urine, urinary tract_

C. Define the following suffixes.

1. -plasty _surgical repair_

2. -stenosis _narrowing_

3. -itis _inflammation_

4. -al _pertaining to_

5. -algia _pain_

6. -otomy _cutting into_

7. -megaly _enlargement, large_

8. -ectomy _surgical removal_

9. -rrhage _(excessive) abnormal flow_

10. -centesis _puncture to withdraw fluid_

11. -gram _record or picture_

12. -ac _pertaining to_

13. -malacia _abnormal softening_

14. -ism _state of_

15. -rrhaphy _suture_

16. -ostomy _surgically create an opening_

17. -pexy _surgical fixation_

18. -rrhea _discharge, flow_

19. -scopy _process of visually examining_

20. -oma _tumor, mass_

D. Join a combining form and a suffix to form words with the following meanings.

1. study of lungs _pulmonology_

2. pain relating to a nerve _neuralgia_

3. nose discharge or flow _rhinorrhea_

4. abnormal softening of a kidney __nephromalacia__

5. enlarged heart __cardiomegaly__

6. cutting into the stomach __gastrotomy__

7. inflammation of the skin __dermatitis__

8. surgical removal of the voice box __laryngectomy__

9. surgical repair of a joint __arthroplasty__

10. gland disease __adenopathy__

E. Write a prefix for each of the following expressions.

1. within, inside __intra-__

2. large __macro-__

3. before, in front of __ante-__

4. around __peri-__

5. new __neo-__

6. without __an-__

7. half __hemi-__

8. painful, difficult __dys-__

9. above __supra-__

10. over, above __hyper-__

11. many __multi-, poly-__

12. slow __brady-__

13. self __auto-__

14. across __trans-__

15. two __bi-__

F. Circle the prefixes in the following terms and define in the space provided.

1. (tachy)cardia __rapid, fast__

2. (pseudo)cyesis __false__

3. (hypo)glycemia __under, below__

4. (inter)costal __among, between__

5. (eu)pnea __normal, good__

6. (post)operative __after__

7. (mono)plegia __one__

8. (sub)cutaneous __below, under__

G. Change the following singular terms to plural terms.

1. metastasis __metastases__

2. ovum __ova__

3. diverticulum __diverticula__

4. atrium __atria__

5. diagnosis __diagnoses__

6. vertebra __vertebrae__

Introduction to Medical Terminology

H. Use the suffix -ology, meaning *the study of*, to write a term for each medical specialty.

1. heart _cardiology_
2. stomach _gastrology_
3. skin _dermatology_
4. eye _opthalmology_
5. urinary tract _urology_

6. kidney _naphrology_
7. blood _hematology_
8. female _gynecology_
9. nerve _neurology_
10. disease _pathology_

I. Build a medical term by combining the word parts requested in each question.

For example, use the combining form for *spleen* with the suffix meaning *enlargement* to form a word meaning *enlargement of the spleen* (answer: *splenomegaly*).

1. combining form for *heart* _cardi/o_
   suffix meaning *abnormal softening* _-malacia_
   cardiomalacia
   term meaning *softening of the heart*

2. word root form for *stomach* _gastr/o_
   suffix meaning *to surgically create an opening* _-ostomy_
   gastrostomy
   term meaning *creating an opening into the stomach*

3. combining form for *nose* _rhin/o_
   suffix meaning *surgical repair* _-plasty_
   rhinoplasty
   term meaning *surgical repair of the nose*

4. prefix meaning *over, above* _hyper-_
   suffix meaning *nourishment, development* _-trophy_
   hyper-trophy
   term meaning *overdevelopment*

5. combining form meaning *disease* _path/o_
   suffix meaning *the study of* _-ology_
   pathology
   term meaning *the study of disease*

6. word root meaning *gland* _aden/o_
   suffix for *tumor/mass* _-oma_
   adenoma
   term meaning *gland tumor or mass*

7. combining form meaning *stomach* _gastr/o_
   combining form meaning *small intestine* _anter/o_
   suffix meaning *study of* _-ology_
   gastroenterology
   term meaning *study of stomach and small intestine*

8. word root meaning *ear* _ot/o_
   suffix meaning *inflammation* _-itis_
   otitis
   term meaning *ear inflammation*

9. prefix meaning *water* _hydro-_
   suffix meaning *treatment* _-therapy_
   hydrotherapy
   term meaning *water treatment*

10. combining form meaning *cancer* _carcin/o_
    suffix meaning *that which produces* _-gen_
    carcinogen
    term meaning *that which produces cancer*

Introduction to Medical Terminology

J. Match each definition to its term.

1. _l_ Provides services for a short period of time
2. _e_ Complete outline of a patient's entire hospital stay
3. _j_ Describes purpose, methods, benefits, and risks of procedure
4. _f_ Contains updated assessment, diagnoses, and further plans for care
5. _d_ Provides supportive care to terminally ill patients and families
6. _k_ Written by the admitting physician
7. _m_ Reports results from study of tissue removed from the patient
8. _o_ Written by the surgeon
9. _g_ Provides services not requiring overnight hospital stay
10. _n_ Report given by a specialist
11. _b_ Record of a patient's care through the day
12. _h_ Clinical lab and medical imaging reports
13. _a_ Provides intensive physical and occupational therapy
14. _c_ Report of treatment/therapy the patient received
15. _i_ Provides care for patients who need more time to recover

a. rehabilitation center
b. nurse's notes
c. ancillary report
d. hospice
e. discharge summary
f. physician's progress notes
g. ambulatory care center
h. diagnostic report
i. long-term care facility
j. informed consent
k. history and physical
l. acute care hospital
m. pathologist's report
n. consultation report
o. operative report

Multimedia Preview

Additional interactive resources and activities for this chapter can be found on the Companion Website.

Website Highlights—www.prenhall.com/fremgen

MULTIPLE CHOICE QUIZ

Take advantage of the free-access on-line study guide that accompanies your textbook. You'll find a multiple-choice quiz that provides instant feedback that allows you to check your score and see what you got right or wrong. By clicking on this URL you'll also access links to download mp3 audio reviews, current news articles, and an audio glossary.

Body Organization

Learning Objectives

Upon completion of this chapter, you will be able to:

- Recognize the combining forms introduced in this chapter.
- Correctly spell and pronounce medical terms and anatomical structures relating to body structure.
- Discuss the organization of the body in terms of cells, tissues, organs, and systems.
- Describe the common features of cells.
- Define the four types of tissues.
- List the major organs found in the twelve organ systems.
- Describe the anatomical position.
- Define the body planes.
- Identify regions of the body.
- Define directional and positional terms.
- List the body cavities and their contents.
- Locate and describe the nine anatomical and four clinical divisions of the abdomen.
- Build body organization medical terms from word parts.
- Interpret abbreviations associated with body organization.

From Chapter 2 of *Medical Terminology: A Living Language*, 4/e. Bonnie F. Fremgen. Suzanne S. Frucht.

Body Organization at a Glance

Arrangement

The body is organized into levels. Each level is built from the one below it. In other words, the body as a whole is composed of systems, a system is composed of organs, an organ is composed of tissues, and tissues are composed of cells.

Levels

cells   tissues   organs   systems   body

Combining Forms

abdomin/o	abdomen	muscul/o	muscle
adip/o	fat	neur/o	nerve
anter/o	front	organ/o	organ
brachi/o	arm	oste/o	bone
caud/o	tail	pelv/o	pelvis
cephal/o	head	peritone/o	peritoneum
cervic/o	neck	pleur/o	pleura
chondr/o	cartilage	poster/o	back
crani/o	skull	proxim/o	near to
crur/o	leg	pub/o	genital region
cyt/o	cell	somat/o	body
dist/o	away from	spin/o	spine
dors/o	back of body	super/o	above
epitheli/o	epithelium	system/o	system
glute/o	buttock	thorac/o	chest
hist/o	tissue	ventr/o	belly
infer/o	below	vertebr/o	vertebra
later/o	side	viscer/o	internal organ
medi/o	middle		

Med Term Tip

Prefixes and suffixes will be used over and over again in your medical terminology course, making it easier to recognize new terms more quickly. New combining forms, prefixes, and suffixes are at the beginning the chapter.

Body Organization Illustrated

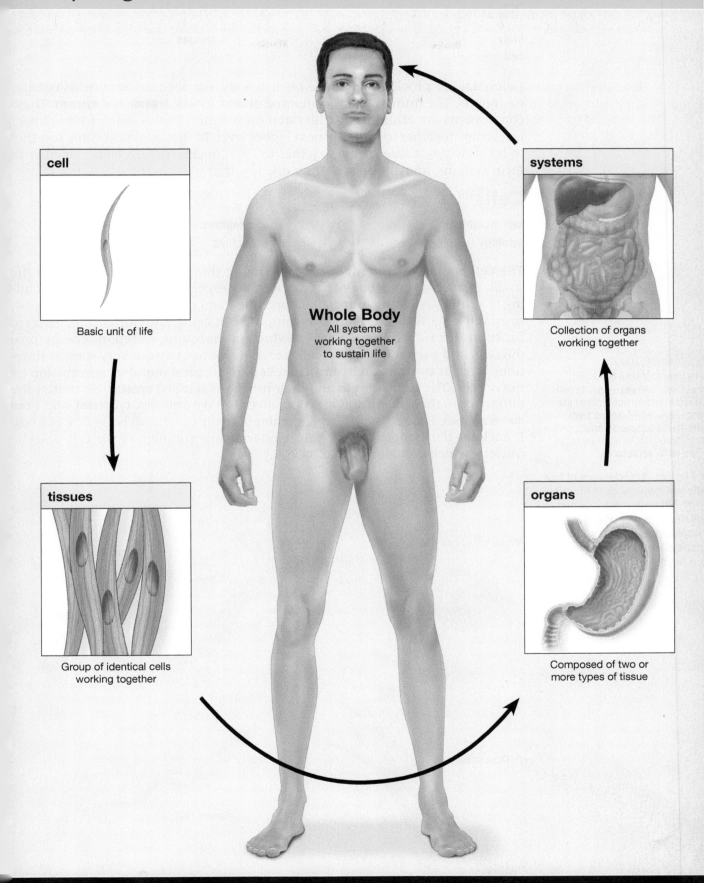

cell

Basic unit of life

tissues

Group of identical cells
working together

Whole Body
All systems
working together
to sustain life

systems

Collection of organs
working together

organs

Composed of two or
more types of tissue

1

Levels of Body Organization

body	organs	tissues
cell	systems	

Before taking a look at the whole human body, we need to examine its component parts. The human **body** is composed of **cells**, **tissues**, **organs**, and **systems**. These components are arranged in a hierarchical manner. That is, parts from a lower level come together to form the next higher level. In that way, cells come together to form tissues, tissues come together to form organs, organs come together to form systems, and all the systems come together to form the whole body.

Cells

cell membrane	cytoplasm (SIGH-toh-plazm)
cytology (sigh-TALL-oh-jee)	nucleus

The cell is the fundamental unit of all living things. In other words, it is the smallest structure of a body that has all the properties of being alive: responding to stimuli, engaging in metabolic activities, and reproducing itself. All the tissues and organs in the body are composed of cells. Individual cells perform functions for the body such as reproduction, hormone secretion, energy production, and excretion. Special cells are also able to carry out very specific functions, such as contraction by muscle cells and electrical impulse transmission by nerve cells. The study of cells and their functions is called **cytology**. No matter the difference in their shape and function, all cells have a **nucleus**, **cytoplasm**, and a **cell membrane** (see Figure 1 ■). The cell membrane is the outermost boundary of a cell. It encloses the cytoplasm, the watery internal environment of the cell, and the nucleus which contains the cell's DNA.

Med Term Tip

Cells were first seen by Robert Hooke over 300 years ago. To him, the rectangular shapes looked like prison cells, so he named them cells. It was a common practice for early anatomists to name an organ solely on its appearance.

■ **Figure 1** Examples of four different types of cells from the body. Although each cell has a cell membrane, nucleus, and cytoplasm, each has a unique shape depending on its location and function.

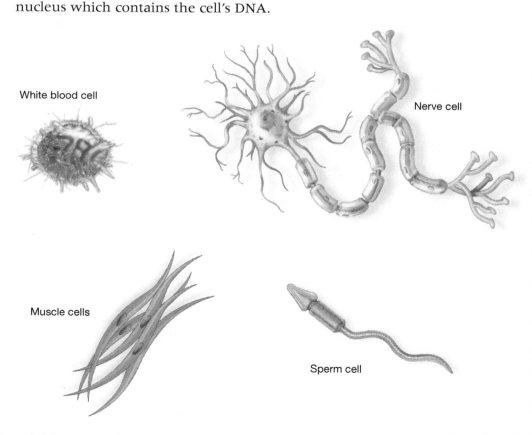

White blood cell

Nerve cell

Muscle cells

Sperm cell

Tissues

connective tissue
epithelial tissue (ep-ih-THEE-lee-al)
histology (hiss-TALL-oh-jee)

muscle tissue
nervous tissue

Histology is the study of tissue. A tissue is formed when like cells are grouped together and function together to perform a specific activity. The body has four types of tissue: **muscle tissue**, **epithelial tissue**, **connective tissue**, and **nervous tissue**.

Muscle Tissue

cardiac muscle
muscle fibers

skeletal muscle
smooth muscle

Muscle tissue produces movement in the body through contraction, or shortening in length, and is composed of individual muscle cells called **muscle fibers** (see Figure 2 ■). Muscle tissue forms one of three basic types of muscles: **skeletal muscle**, **smooth muscle**, or **cardiac muscle**. Skeletal muscle is attached to bone. Smooth muscle is found in internal organs such as the intestine, uterus, and blood vessels. Cardiac muscle is found only in the heart.

Epithelial Tissue

epithelium (ep-ih-THEE-lee-um)

Epithelial tissue, or **epithelium**, is found throughout the body and is composed of close-packed cells that form the covering for and lining of body structures. For example, both the top layer of skin and the lining of the stomach are epithelial tissue (see Figure 2). In addition to forming a protective barrier, epithelial tissue may be specialized to absorb substances (such as nutrients from the intestine), secrete substances (such as sweat glands), or excrete wastes (such as the kidney tubules).

Connective Tissue

adipose (ADD-ih-pohs)
bone

cartilage (CAR-tih-lij)
tendons

Connective tissue is the supporting and protecting tissue in body structures. Because connective tissue performs many different functions depending on its location, it appears in many different forms so that each is able to perform the task required at that location. For example, **bone** provides structural support for the whole body. **Cartilage** is the shock absorber in joints. **Tendons** tightly connect skeletal muscles to bones. **Adipose** provides protective padding around body structures (see Figure 2).

Nervous Tissue

brain
nerves

neurons
spinal cord

Nervous tissue is composed of cells called **neurons** (see Figure 2). This tissue forms the **brain**, **spinal cord**, and a network of **nerves** throughout the entire body. This allows for the conduction of electrical impulses to send information between the brain and the rest of the body.

Med Term Tip

The term *epithelium* comes from the prefix *epi-* meaning "on top of" and the combining form *theli/o* meaning "nipple" (referring to any projection from the surface).

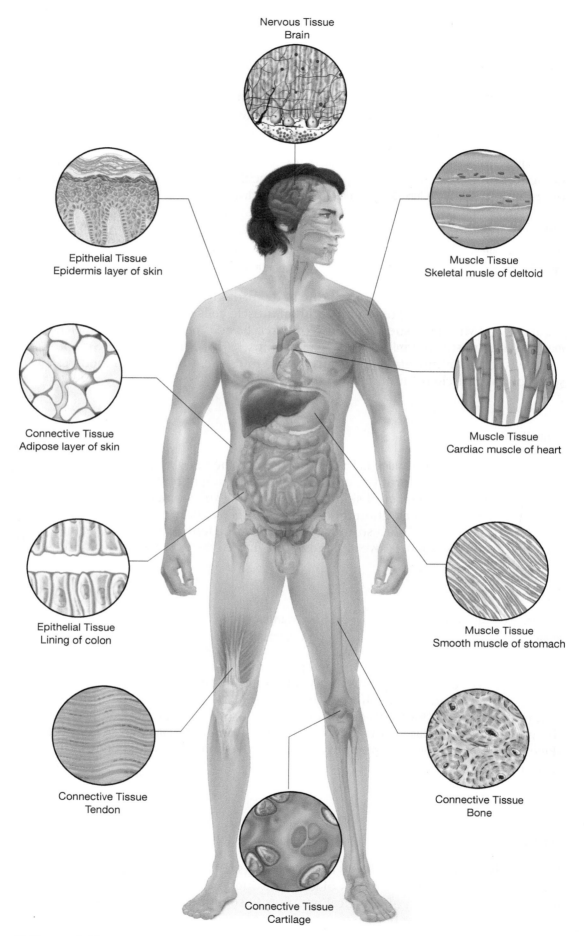

Nervous Tissue
Brain

Epithelial Tissue
Epidermis layer of skin

Muscle Tissue
Skeletal musle of deltoid

Connective Tissue
Adipose layer of skin

Muscle Tissue
Cardiac muscle of heart

Epithelial Tissue
Lining of colon

Muscle Tissue
Smooth muscle of stomach

Connective Tissue
Tendon

Connective Tissue
Bone

Connective Tissue
Cartilage

■ **Figure 2** The appearance of different types of tissues—muscle, epithelial, nervous, connective— and their location within the body.

Organs and Systems

Organs are composed of several different types of tissue that work as a unit to perform special functions. For example, the stomach contains smooth muscle tissue, nervous tissue, and epithelial tissue that allow it to contract to mix food with digestive juices.

A system is composed of several organs working in a coordinated manner to perform a complex function or functions. To continue our example, the stomach plus the other digestive system organs—the oral cavity, esophagus, liver, pancreas, small intestine, and colon—work together to ingest, digest, and absorb our food.

Table 1 ■ presents the organ systems that will be studied in this text along with the major organs found in each system, the system functions, and the medical specialties that treat conditions of that system.

Table 1	Organ Systems of the Human Body	
SYSTEM/MEDICAL SPECIALTY	**STRUCTURES**	**FUNCTIONS**
Integumentary (in-teg-you-MEN-tah-ree) **dermatology** (der-mah-TALL-oh-jee)	• skin • hair • nails • sweat glands • sebaceous glands	Forms protective two-way barrier and aids in temperature regulation.
Musculoskeletal (MS) (mus-qu-low-SKEL-et-all) **orthopedics** (or-thoh-PEE-diks) **orthopedic surgery** (or-the-PEE-dik)	• bones • joints • muscles	Skeleton supports and protects the body, forms blood cells, and stores minerals. Muscles produce movement.

Table 1	Organ Systems of the Human Body (continued)	
SYSTEM/MEDICAL SPECIALTY	**STRUCTURES**	**FUNCTIONS**
Cardiovascular (CV) (car-dee-oh-VAS-kew-lar) **cardiology** (car-dee-ALL-oh-jee)	• heart • arteries • veins	Pumps blood throughout the entire body to transport nutrients, oxygen, and wastes.
Blood (**Hematic** System) (he-MAT-tik) **hematology** (hee-mah-TALL-oh-jee)	• plasma • erythrocytes • leukocytes • platelets	Transports oxygen, protects against pathogens, and controls bleeding.
Lymphatic (lim-FAT-ik) **immunology** (im-yoo-NALL-oh-jee)	• lymph nodes • lymphatic vessels • spleen • thymus gland • tonsils	Protects the body from disease and invasion from pathogens.

Table 1   Organ Systems of the Human Body (continued)

SYSTEM/MEDICAL SPECIALTY	STRUCTURES	FUNCTIONS
Respiratory **otorhinolaryngology** (ENT) (oh-toh-rye-noh-lair-ing-GALL-oh-jee) **pulmonology** (pull-mon-ALL-oh-jee) **thoracic surgery** (tho-RASS-ik)	• nasal cavity • pharynx • larynx • trachea • bronchial tubes • lungs	Obtains oxygen and removes carbon dioxide from the body.
Digestive or **Gastrointestinal** (GI) **gastroenterology** (gas-troh-en-ter-ALL-oh-jee) **proctology** (prok-TOL-oh-jee)	• oral cavity • pharynx • esophagus • stomach • small intestine • colon • liver • gallbladder • pancreas • salivary glands	Ingests, digests, and absorbs nutrients for the body.
Urinary (YOO-rih-nair-ee) **nephrology** (neh-FROL-oh-jee) **urology** (yoo-RALL-oh-jee)	• kidneys • ureters • urinary bladder • urethra	Filters waste products out of the blood and removes them from the body.

Table 1 — Organ Systems of the Human Body (continued)

SYSTEM/MEDICAL SPECIALTY	STRUCTURES	FUNCTIONS
Female reproductive **gynecology** (GYN) (gigh-neh-KOL-oh-jee) **obstetrics** (OB) (ob-STET-riks)	• ovary • fallopian tubes • uterus • vagina • vulva • breasts	Produces eggs for reproduction and provides place for growing baby.
Male reproductive **urology** (yoo-RALL-oh-jee)	• testes • epididymis • vas deferens • penis • seminal vesicles • prostate gland • bulbourethral gland	Produces sperm for reproduction.
Endocrine (EN-doh-krin) **endocrinology** (en-doh-krin-ALL-oh-jee)	• pituitary gland • pineal gland • thyroid gland • parathyroid glands • thymus gland • adrenal glands • pancreas • ovaries • testes	Regulates metabolic activities of the body.

Table 1	Organ Systems of the Human Body	
SYSTEM/MEDICAL SPECIALTY	**STRUCTURES**	**FUNCTIONS**
Nervous **neurology** (noo-RAL-oh-jee) **neurosurgery** (noo-roh-SIR-jer-ee)	• brain • spinal cord • nerves	Receives sensory information and coordinates the body's response.
Special senses **ophthalmology** (off-thal-MALL-oh-jee)	• eye	Vision
otorhinolaryngology (ENT) (oh-toh-rye-noh-lair- ing-GALL-oh-jee)	• ear	Hearing and balance

Body

anatomical position

As seen from the previous sections, the body is the sum of all the systems, organs, tissues, and cells found in it. It is important to learn the anatomical terminology that applies to the body as a whole in order to correctly identify specific locations and directions when dealing with patients. The **anatomical position** is used when describing the positions and relationships of structures in the human body. A body in the anatomical position is standing erect with the arms at the side of the body, the palms of the hands facing forward, and the eyes looking straight ahead. In addition, the legs are parallel with the feet, and the toes are pointing forward (see Figure 3 ■). For descriptive purposes the assumption is always that the person is in the anatomical position even if the body or parts of the body are in any other position.

Body Planes

coronal plane (kor-RONE-al)

coronal section

cross-section

frontal plane

frontal section

horizontal plane

longitudinal section

median plane

sagittal plane (SAJ-ih-tal)

sagittal section

transverse plane

transverse section

The terminology for body planes is used to assist medical personnel in describing the body and its parts. To understand body planes, imagine cuts slicing through the body at various angles. This imaginary slicing allows us to use more specific language when describing parts of the body. These body planes, illustrated in Figure 4 ■, include the following:

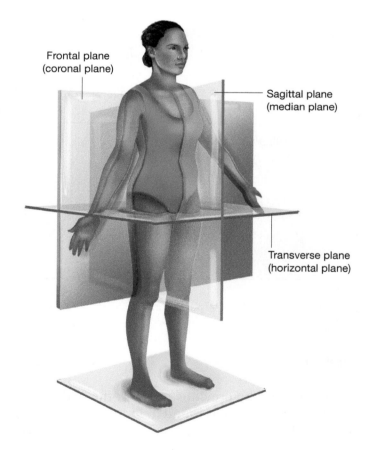

■ **Figure 3** The anatomical position: standing erect, gazing straight ahead, arms down at sides, palms facing forward, fingers extended, legs together, and toes pointing forward.

■ **Figure 4** The planes of the body. The sagittal plane is vertical from front to back, the frontal plane is vertical from left to right, and the transverse plane is horizontal.

1. **Sagittal plane:** This vertical plane, also called the **median plane**, runs lengthwise from front to back and divides the body or any of its parts into right and left portions. The right and left sides do not have to be equal. A cut along the sagittal plane yields a **sagittal section** view of the inside of the body.
2. **Frontal plane:** The frontal, or **coronal plane**, divides the body into front and back portions. In other words, this is a vertical lengthwise plane running from side to side. A cut along the frontal plane yields a **frontal** or **coronal section** view of the inside of the body.
3. **Transverse plane:** The transverse, or **horizontal plane**, is a crosswise plane that runs parallel to the ground. This imaginary cut would divide the body or its parts into upper and lower portions. A cut along the transverse plane yields a **transverse section** view of the inside of the body.

The terms **cross-section** and **longitudinal section** are frequently used to describe internal views of structures. A longitudinal section is a produced by a lengthwise slice along the long axis of a structure. A cross-section view is produced by a slice perpendicular to the long axis of the structure.

Body Regions

abdominal region (ab-DOM-ih-nal)

brachial region (BRAY-kee-all)

cephalic region (she-FAL-ik)

cervical region (SER-vih-kal)

crural region (KREW-ral)

dorsum (DOOR-sum)

gluteal region (GLOO-tee-all)

lower extremities

pelvic region (PELL-vik)

pubic region (PEW-bik)

thoracic region (tho-RASS-ik)

trunk

upper extremities

vertebral region (VER-tee-bral)

The body is divided into large regions that can easily be identified externally. The **cephalic region** is the entire head. The neck is the **cervical region** and connects the head to the **trunk** (the torso). The trunk is further subdivided into different anterior and posterior regions. The anterior side consists of the **thoracic** (the chest), **abdominal, pelvic,** and **pubic** (genital) **regions**. The posterior side consists of the **dorsum** (the back), **vertebral region,** and **gluteal** (buttock) **region**. The **upper extremities** (UE) and **lower extremities** (LE) are attached to the trunk. The upper extremities or **brachial regions** are the arms. The lower extremities or **crural regions** are the legs. See Figure 5 ■ to locate each region on the body.

Med Term Tip

As you learn medical terminology, it is important that you remember not to use common phrases and terms any longer. Many people commonly use the term *stomach* (an organ) when they actually mean *abdomen* (a body region).

Body Cavities

abdominal cavity

abdominopelvic cavity
(ab-dom-ih-noh-PELL-vik)

cranial cavity (KRAY-nee-al)

diaphragm (DYE-ah-fram)

mediastinum (mee-dee-ass-TYE-num)

parietal layer (pah-RYE-eh-tal)

parietal peritoneum

parietal pleura

pelvic cavity

pericardial cavity (pair-ih-CAR-dee-al)

peritoneum (pair-ih-toh-NEE-um)

pleura (PLOO-rah)

pleural cavity (PLOO-ral)

spinal cavity

thoracic cavity

viscera (VISS-er-ah)

visceral layer (VISS-er-al)

visceral peritoneum

visceral pleura

The body is not a solid structure; it has many open spaces or cavities. The cavities are part of the normal body structure and are illustrated in Figure 6 ■. We

Figure 5 Anterior and posterior views of the body illustrating the location of various body regions.

Figure 5 Anterior and posterior views of the body illustrating the location of various body regions.

can divide the body into four major cavities—two dorsal cavities and two ventral cavities.

The dorsal cavities include the **cranial cavity**, containing the brain, and the **spinal cavity**, containing the spinal cord.

The ventral cavities include the **thoracic cavity** and the **abdominopelvic cavity**. The thoracic cavity contains the two lungs and a central region between them called the **mediastinum**. The heart, aorta, esophagus, trachea, and thymus gland are located in the mediastinum. There is an actual physical wall between the thoracic cavity and the abdominopelvic cavity called the **diaphragm**. The diaphragm is a muscle used for breathing. The abdominopelvic cavity is generally subdivided into a superior **abdominal cavity** and an inferior **pelvic cavity**. The organs of the digestive, excretory, and reproductive systems are located in these cavities. The organs

Figure 6 The dorsal (red) and ventral (blue) body cavities.

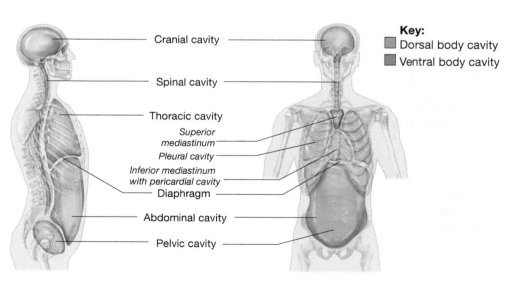

Lateral view　　　　　**Anterior view**

within the ventral cavities are referred to as a group as the internal organs or **viscera**. Table 2 ■ describes the body cavities and their major organs.

All of the cavities are lined by, and the viscera are encased in, a two-layer membrane called the **pleura** in the thoracic cavity and the **peritoneum** in the abdominopelvic cavity. The outer layer that lines the cavities is called the **parietal layer** (i.e., **parietal pleura** and **parietal peritoneum**), and the inner layer that encases the viscera is called the **visceral layer** (i.e., **visceral pleura** and **visceral peritoneum**).

Within the thoracic cavity, the pleura is subdivided, forming the **pleural cavity**, containing the lungs, and the **pericardial cavity**, containing the heart. The larger abdominopelvic cavity is usually subdivided into regions so different areas can be precisely referred to. Two different methods of subdividing this cavity are used: the anatomical divisions and the clinical divisions. Choose a method partly on personal preference and partly on which system best describes the patient's condition. See Table 3 ■ for a description of these methods for dividing the abdominopelvic cavity.

Directional and Positional Terms

Directional terms assist medical personnel in discussing the position or location of a patient's complaint. Directional or positional terms also help to describe one process, organ, or system as it relates to another. Table 4 ■ presents commonly used terms for describing the position of the body or its parts. They are listed in pairs that have opposite meanings: for example, superior versus inferior, anterior versus posterior, medial versus lateral, proximal versus distal, superficial versus deep, and supine versus prone. Directional terms are illustrated in Figure 7 ■.

Med Term Tip

The kidneys are the only major abdominopelvic organ located outside the sac formed by the peritoneum. Because they are found behind this sac, their position is referred to as *retroperitoneal*.

Med Term Tip

Remember when using location or direction terms, it is assumed that the patient is in the anatomical position unless otherwise noted.

Table 2	Body Cavities and Their Major Organs
CAVITY	**MAJOR ORGANS**

Dorsal cavities
  Cranial cavity
  Spinal cavity
	
	Brain
	Spinal cord

Ventral cavities Thoracic cavity	 Pleural cavity: lungs Pericardial cavity: heart Mediastinum: heart, esophagus, trachea, thymus gland, aorta
Abdominopelvic cavity Abdominal cavity	 Stomach, spleen, liver, gallbladder, pancreas, and portions of the small intestines and colon
Pelvic cavity	Urinary bladder, ureters, urethra, and portions of the small intestines and colon *Female:* uterus, ovaries, fallopian tubes, vagina *Male:* prostate gland, seminal vesicles, portion of the vas deferens

Table 3 — Methods of Subdividing the Abdominopelvic Cavity

Anatomical Divisions of the Abdomen

- **Right hypochondriac** (high-poh-KON-dree-ak): Right lateral region of upper row beneath the lower ribs.

- **Epigastric** (ep-ih-GAS-trik): Middle area of upper row above the stomach.

- **Left hypochondriac:** Left lateral region of the upper row beneath the lower ribs.

- **Right lumbar:** Right lateral region of the middle row at the waist.

- **Umbilical** (um-BILL-ih-kal): Central area over the navel.

- **Left lumbar:** Left lateral region of the middle row at the waist.

- **Right iliac** (ILL-ee-ak): Right lateral region of the lower row at the groin.

- **Hypogastric** (high-poh-GAS-trik): Middle region of the lower row beneath the navel.

- **Left iliac:** Left lateral region of the lower row at the groin.

Right hypochondriac region | Epigastric region | Left hypochondriac region
Right lumbar region | Umbilical region | Left lumbar region
Right iliac region | Hypogastric region | Left iliac region

Med Term Tip

To visualize the nine anatomical divisions, imagine a tic-tac-toe diagram over this region.

Med Term Tip

The term *hypochondriac*, literally meaning "under the cartilage" (of the ribs), has come to refer to a person who believes he or she is sick when there is no obvious cause for illness. These patients commonly complain of aches and pains in the hypochondriac region.

Clinical Divisions of the Abdomen

- **Right upper quadrant (RUQ):** Contains majority of liver, gallbladder, small portion of pancreas, right kidney, small intestines, and colon.

- **Right lower quadrant (RLQ):** Contains small intestines and colon, right ovary and fallopian tube, appendix, and right ureter.

- **Left upper quadrant (LUQ):** Contains small portion of liver, spleen, stomach, majority of pancreas, left kidney, small intestines, and colon.

- **Left lower quadrant (LLQ):** Contains small intestines and colon, left ovary and fallopian tube, and left ureter.

- **Midline organs:** uterus, bladder, prostate gland.

Liver (majority)
Right kidney
Colon
Pancreas (small portion)
Gallbladder
Small intestines

RIGHT UPPER QUADRANT

Liver (small portion)
Spleen
Left kidney
Stomach
Colon
Pancreas (majority)
Small intestines

LEFT UPPER QUADRANT

RIGHT LOWER QUADRANT

Colon
Small intestines
Right ureter
Appendix
Right ovary (female)
Right fallopian tube (female)

LEFT LOWER QUADRANT

Colon
Small intestines
Left ureter
Left ovary (female)
Left fallopian tube (female)

MIDLINE AREA
Bladder - Uterus (female) - Prostate (male)

Body Organization

Figure 7 Anterior and lateral views of the body illustrating directional terms.

Table 4	Terms for Describing Body Position
superior (soo-PEE-ree-or) or **cephalic** (seh-FAL-ik)	More toward the head, or above another structure. (see Figure 7 ■). *Example:* The adrenal glands are superior to the kidneys.
inferior (in-FEE-ree-or) or **caudal** (KAWD-al)	More toward the feet or tail, or below another structure. (see Figure 7). *Example:* The intestine is inferior to the heart.
anterior (an-TEE-ree-or) or **ventral** (VEN-tral)	More toward the front or belly-side of the body. (see Figure 7). *Example:* The navel is located on the anterior surface of the body.
posterior (poss-TEE-ree-or) or **dorsal** (DOR-sal)	More toward the back or spinal cord side of the body. (see Figure 7). *Example:* The posterior wall of the right kidney was excised.
medial (MEE-dee-al)	Refers to the middle or near the middle of the body or the structure. (see Figure 7). *Example:* The heart is medially located in the chest cavity.
lateral (lat) (LAT-er-al)	Refers to the side. (see Figure 7). *Example:* The ovaries are located lateral to the uterus.
proximal (PROK-sim-al)	Located nearer to the point of attachment to the body. (see Figure 7). *Example:* In the anatomical position, the elbow is proximal to the hand.
distal (DISS-tal)	Located farther away from the point of attachment to the body. (see Figure 7). *Example:* The hand is distal to the elbow.
apex (AY-peks)	Tip or summit of an organ. *Example:* We hear the heart beat by listening over the apex of the heart.

Table 4	Terms for Describing Body Position
base	Bottom or lower part of an organ. *Example:* On the X-ray, a fracture was noted at the base of the skull.
superficial	More toward the surface of the body. *Example:* The cut was superficial.
deep	Further away from the surface of the body. *Example:* An incision into an abdominal organ is a deep incision.
supine (soo-PINE)	The body lying horizontally and facing upward (see Figure 8A ▇). *Example:* The patient is in the supine position for abdominal surgery.
prone (PROHN)	The body lying horizontally and facing downward (see Figure 8B ▇). *Example:* The patient is placed in the prone position for spinal surgery.

■ **Figure 8A** The supine position.

■ **Figure 8B** The prone position.

Word Building

When using medical terms to indicate different areas of the body or organs, it is usually necessary to turn the combining form into an adjective. For example, *gastr/o* becomes *gastric* or *ventr/o* becomes *ventral*. This is done by adding an adjective suffix to the combining form that translates as *pertaining to*. The following list contains examples of frequently used medical terms relating to body structure that are built directly from word parts. It is important to study this list because there are no rules about which of the several *pertaining to* suffixes to use.

COMBINING FORM	SUFFIX	MEDICAL TERM	DEFINITION
abdomin/o	-al	**abdominal** (ab-DOM-ih-nal)	pertaining to the abdomen
anter/o	-ior	**anterior** (an-TEE-ree-or)	pertaining to the front
brachi/o	-al	**brachial** (BRAY-kee-all)	pertaining to the arm
caud/o	-al	**caudal** (KAWD-al)	pertaining to the tail
cephal/o	-ic	**cephalic** (she-FAL-ik)	pertaining to the head
cervic/o	-al	**cervical** (SER-vih-kal)	pertaining to the neck
crani/o	-al	**cranial** (KRAY-nee-al)	pertaining to the skull
crur/o	-al	**crural** (KREW-ral)	pertaining to the leg
dist/o	-al	**distal** (DISS-tal)	pertaining to away
dors/o	-al	**dorsal** (DOR-sal)	pertaining to the back of body
epitheli/o	-al	**epithelial** (ep-ih-THEE-lee-al)	pertaining to the epithelium
glute/o	-al	**gluteal** (GLOO-tee-all)	pertaining to the buttocks
infer/o	-ior	**inferior** (in-FEE-ree-or)	pertaining to below

Word Building *(continued)*

COMBINING FORM	SUFFIX	MEDICAL TERM	DEFINITION
later/o	-al	**lateral** (LAT-er-al)	pertaining to the side
medi/o	-al	**medial** (MEE-dee-al)	pertaining to the middle
muscul/o	-ar	**muscular** (MUSS-kew-lar)	pertaining to muscles
neur/o	-al	**neural** (NOO-ral)	pertaining to nerves
organ/o	-ic	**organic** (or-GAN-ik)	pertaining to organs
pelv/o	-ic	**pelvic** (PELL-vik)	pertaining to the pelvis
peritone/o	-al	**peritoneal** (pair-ih-toe-NEE-all)	pertaining to the peritoneum
pleur/o	-al	**pleural** (PLOO-ral)	pertaining to the pleura
poster/o	-ior	**posterior** (poss-TEE-ree-or)	pertaining to the back
proxim/o	-al	**proximal** (PROK-sim-al)	pertaining to near
pub/o	-ic	**pubic** (PEW-bik)	pertaining to the genital region
somat/o	-ic	**somatic** (so-MAT-ik)	pertaining to the body
spin/o	-al	**spinal**	pertaining to the spine
super/o	-ior	**superior** (soo-PEE-ree-or)	pertaining to above
system/o	-ic	**systemic** (sis-TEM-ik)	pertaining to systems
thorac/o	-ic	**thoracic** (tho-RASS-ik)	pertaining to the chest
ventr/o	-al	**ventral** (VEN-tral)	pertaining to the belly side
vertebr/o	-al	**vertebral** (VER-the-bral)	pertaining to the vertebrae
viscer/o	-al	**visceral** (VISS-er-al)	pertaining to internal organs

Abbreviations

AP	anteroposterior	**lat**	lateral	**OB**	obstetrics
CV	cardiovascular	**LE**	lower extremity	**PA**	posteroanterior
ENT	ear, nose, and throat	**LLQ**	left lower quadrant	**RLQ**	right lower quadrant
GI	gastrointestinal	**LUQ**	left upper quadrant	**RUQ**	right upper quadrant
GYN	gynecology	**MS**	musculoskeletal	**UE**	upper extremity

Chapter Review

Terminology Checklist

Below are all Body Organization key terms presented in this chapter. Use this list as a study tool by placing a check in the box in front of each term as you master its meaning.

- ☐ abdominal
- ☐ abdominal cavity
- ☐ abdominal region
- ☐ abdominopelvic cavity
- ☐ adipose
- ☐ anatomical position
- ☐ anterior
- ☐ apex
- ☐ base
- ☐ blood
- ☐ body
- ☐ bone
- ☐ brachial
- ☐ brachial region
- ☐ brain
- ☐ cardiac muscle
- ☐ cardiology
- ☐ cardiovascular system
- ☐ cartilage
- ☐ caudal
- ☐ cell
- ☐ cell membrane
- ☐ cephalic
- ☐ cephalic region
- ☐ cervical
- ☐ cervical region
- ☐ connective tissue
- ☐ coronal plane
- ☐ coronal section
- ☐ cranial
- ☐ cranial cavity
- ☐ cross-section
- ☐ crural
- ☐ crural region
- ☐ cytology
- ☐ cytoplasm
- ☐ deep
- ☐ dermatology
- ☐ diaphragm

- ☐ digestive system
- ☐ distal
- ☐ dorsal
- ☐ dorsum
- ☐ endocrine system
- ☐ endocrinology
- ☐ epigastric
- ☐ epithelial
- ☐ epithelial tissue
- ☐ epithelium
- ☐ female reproductive system
- ☐ frontal plane
- ☐ frontal section
- ☐ gastroenterology
- ☐ gastrointestinal system
- ☐ gluteal
- ☐ gluteal region
- ☐ gynecology
- ☐ hematic system
- ☐ hematology
- ☐ histology
- ☐ horizontal plane
- ☐ hypogastric
- ☐ immunology
- ☐ inferior
- ☐ integumentary system
- ☐ lateral
- ☐ left hypochondriac
- ☐ left iliac
- ☐ left lower quadrant
- ☐ left lumbar
- ☐ left upper quadrant
- ☐ longitudinal section
- ☐ lower extremities
- ☐ lymphatic system
- ☐ male reproductive system
- ☐ medial
- ☐ median plane
- ☐ mediastinum

- ☐ muscle fibers
- ☐ muscle tissue
- ☐ muscular
- ☐ musculoskeletal system
- ☐ nephrology
- ☐ nerves
- ☐ nervous system
- ☐ nervous tissue
- ☐ neural
- ☐ neurology
- ☐ neurons
- ☐ neurosurgery
- ☐ nucleus
- ☐ obstetrics
- ☐ ophthalmology
- ☐ organic
- ☐ organs
- ☐ orthopedic surgery
- ☐ orthopedics
- ☐ otorhinolaryngology
- ☐ parietal layer
- ☐ parietal peritoneum
- ☐ parietal pleura
- ☐ pelvic
- ☐ pelvic cavity
- ☐ pelvic region
- ☐ pericardial cavity
- ☐ peritoneal
- ☐ peritoneum
- ☐ pleura
- ☐ pleural
- ☐ pleural cavity
- ☐ posterior
- ☐ proctology
- ☐ prone
- ☐ proximal
- ☐ pubic
- ☐ pubic region
- ☐ pulmonology

- ☐ respiratory system
- ☐ right hypochondriac
- ☐ right iliac
- ☐ right lower quadrant
- ☐ right lumbar
- ☐ right upper quadrant
- ☐ sagittal plane
- ☐ sagittal section
- ☐ skeletal muscle
- ☐ smooth muscle
- ☐ somatic
- ☐ special senses
- ☐ spinal
- ☐ spinal cavity

- ☐ spinal cord
- ☐ superficial
- ☐ superior
- ☐ supine
- ☐ systemic
- ☐ systems
- ☐ tendons
- ☐ thoracic
- ☐ thoracic cavity
- ☐ thoracic region
- ☐ thoracic surgery
- ☐ tissues
- ☐ transverse plane
- ☐ transverse section

- ☐ trunk
- ☐ umbilical
- ☐ upper extremities
- ☐ urinary system
- ☐ urology
- ☐ ventral
- ☐ vertebral
- ☐ vertebral region
- ☐ viscera
- ☐ visceral
- ☐ visceral layer
- ☐ visceral peritoneum
- ☐ visceral pleura

Practice Exercises

A. Complete the following statements.

1. The levels of organization of the body in order from smallest to largest are: __cells__, __tissues__, __organs__, __systems__, __whole body__.

2. No matter its shape, all cells have a __nucleus__, __cytoplasm__, and __cell membrane__.

3. __Histology__ is the study of tissue.

4. __Epithelial__ tissue lines internal organs and serves as a covering for the skin.

5. In the __anatomical__ position the body is standing erect with arms at sides and palms facing forward.

6. The __right lower__ quadrant of the abdomen contains the appendix.

7. The dorsal cavities are the __cranial__ cavity and the __spinal__ cavity.

8. There are __nine__ anatomical divisions in the abdominal cavity.

9. The __right iliac__ region of the abdominal cavity is located in the right lower lateral region near the groin.

10. Within the thoracic cavity the lungs are found in the __pleural__ cavity and the heart is found in the __pericardial__ cavity.

B. Match each body plane to its definition.

1. __C__ frontal plane   a. divides the body into right and left

2. __a__ sagittal plane   b. divides the body into upper and lower

3. __b__ transverse plane   c. divides the body into anterior and posterior

C. Match each term to its definition.

1. n distal
2. f prone
3. k lateral
4. d inferior
5. a deep
6. e apex
7. m base
8. i posterior
9. b superficial
10. j supine
11. h anterior
12. l medial
13. c proximal
14. g superior

a. away from the surface
b. toward the surface
c. located closer to point of attachment to the body
d. caudal
e. tip or summit of an organ
f. lying face down
g. cephalic
h. ventral
i. dorsal
j. lying face up
k. to the side
l. middle
m. bottom or lower part of an organ
n. located further away from point of attachment to the body

D. Circle the prefixes in the following terms and define in the space provided.

1. epigastric ___ upon, over
2. intervertebral ___ among, between
3. intramuscular ___ within, inside
4. pericardium ___ around
5. hypochondriac ___ under, below
6. retroperitoneal ___ backward, behind
7. substernal ___ below, under
8. transurethral ___ through, across

E. Build terms for each expression using the correct prefixes, suffixes, and combining forms.

1. pertaining to spinal cord side ___ spinal
2. pertaining to the chest ___ thoracic
3. pertaining to above ___ superior
4. pertaining to the tail ___ caudal

Body Organization

5. pertaining to internal organs __viscaral__
6. pertaining to the side __lateral__
7. pertaining to away from __distal__
8. pertaining to nerves __neural__
9. pertaining to systems __systemic__
10. pertaining to the muscles __muscular__
11. pertaining to the belly side __ventral__
12. pertaining to the front __anterior__
13. pertaining to the head __cephalic__
14. pertaining to middle __medial__

F. Write the abbreviations for the following terms.

1. musculoskeletal __MS__
2. lateral __lat__
3. right upper quadrant __RUQ__
4. cardiovascular __CV__

5. gastrointestinal __GI__
6. anteroposterior __AP__
7. obstetrics __OB__
8. left lower quadrant __LLQ__

G. Define the following combining forms.

1. viscer/o __pertaining to internal organs__
2. poster/o __back__
3. abdomin/o __abdomen__
4. thorac/o __chest__
5. medi/o __middle__
6. ventr/o __belly__
7. anter/o __front__

8. hist/o __tissue__
9. epitheli/o __epithelium__
10. crani/o __skull__
11. somat/o __body__
12. proxim/o __near to__
13. cephal/o __head__

H. For each organ listed below, identify the name of the system it belongs to and then match it to its function.

	Organ	System		Function
1.	d skin	Integumentary	a.	supports the body
2.	i heart	Cardiovascular	b.	provides place for growing baby
3.	g stomach	Digestive	c.	filters waste products from blood
4.	b uterus	Female Reproductive	d.	provides two-way barrier
5.	a bones	Musculoskeletal	e.	produces movement
6.	j lungs	Respiratory	f.	produces sperm
7.	c kidney	Urinary	g.	ingest, digest, absorb nutrients
8.	f testes	Male Reproductive	h.	coordinates body's response
9.	h brain	Nervous	i.	pumps blood through blood vessels
10.	e muscles	Musculoskeletal	j.	obtains oxygen

I. Match each organ to its body cavity.

1. a gallbladder   a. right upper quadrant

2. c appendix   b. left upper quadrant

3. f urinary bladder   c. right lower quadrant

4. e small intestines   d. left lower quadrant

5. a right kidney   e. all quadrants

6. d left ovary   f. midline structure

7. b stomach

8. e colon

9. c right ureter

10. b pancreas (majority)

J. For each term below, write the corresponding body region.

1. head   Cephalic   5. neck   cervical

2. genitals   pubic   6. arm   brachial

3. leg   crural   7. back   dorsum

4. buttocks   gluteal   8. leg   crural

K. Use the following terms in the sentences that follow.

cardiology   otorhinolaryngology   urology   gynecology
ophthalmology   gastroenterology   dermatology   orthopedics

1. John is a musician who plays an electric bass guitar and is experiencing difficulty in hearing soft voices. He would consult a physician in _Otorhinolaryngology_

2. Ruth is a stock trader with the Chicago Board of Trade. She has had a pounding and racing heartbeat. She would consult a physician specializing in _cardiology_.

3. Mary Ann is experiencing excessive bleeding from the uterus. She would consult a _gynecology_ doctor.

4. Jose has fractured his wrist in a fall. He would be seen for an examination by a physician in _orthopedics_.

5. A physician who performs eye exams specializes in the field of _opthalmology_

6. When her daughter had repeated bladder infections, Mrs. Cortez sought the opinion of a specialist in _urology_.

7. Martha could not get rid of a persistent skin rash with over-the-counter creams. She decided to make an appointment with a specialist in _dermatology_

8. After reviewing his X-ray, the specialist in _gastroenterology_ informed Mr. Sparks that he had a stomach ulcer.

Labeling Exercise

A. Body Organization Review

Write the labels for this figure on the numbered lines provided.

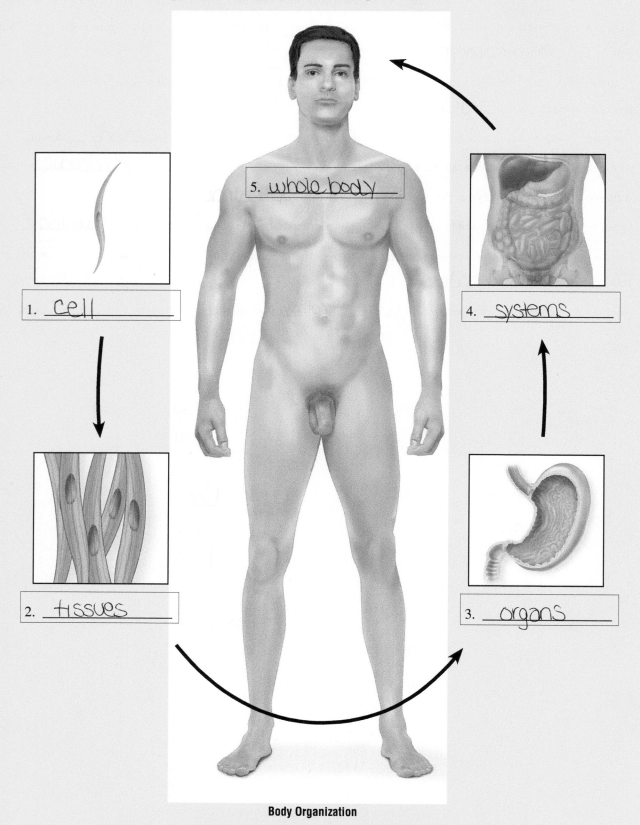

1. cell

2. tissues

3. organs

4. systems

5. whole body

Body Organization

B. Anatomy Challenge

1. Write the labels for this figure on the numbered lines provided.

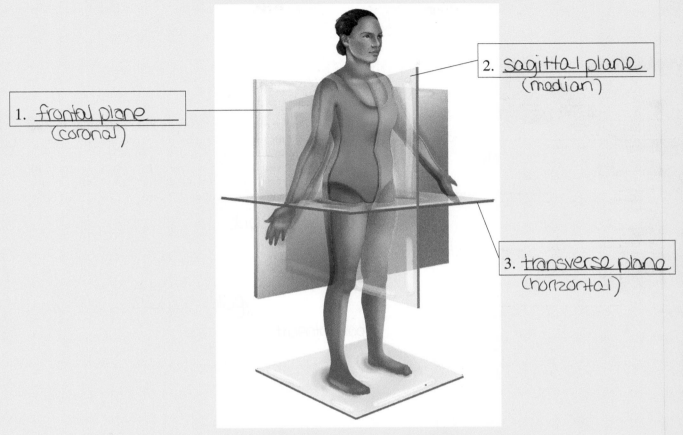

1. frontal plane (coronal)

2. sagittal plane (median)

3. transverse plane (horizontal)

2. Write the labels for this figure on the numbered lines provided.

1. cephalic
2. cervical
3. thoracic
4. brachial
5. abdominal
6. pelvic
7. pubic
8. crural
9. trunk
10. vertebral
11. dorsum
12. gluteal

Body Organization

Multimedia Preview

Additional interactive resources and activities for this chapter can be found on the Companion Website.

Website Highlights—www.prenhall.com/fremgen

TRUE/FALSE QUIZ

Take advantage of the free-access on-line study guide that accompanies your textbook. You'll find a true/false quiz that provides instant feedback that allows you to check your score and see what you got right or wrong. By clicking on this URL you'll also access links to download mp3 audio reviews, current news articles, and an audio glossary.

Integumentary System

Learning Objectives

Upon completion of this chapter, you will be able to:

- Identify and define the combining forms, prefixes, and suffixes introduced in this chapter.
- Correctly spell and pronounce medical terms and major anatomical structures relating to the integumentary system.
- List and describe the three layers of skin and their functions.
- List and describe the four purposes of the skin.
- List and describe the accessory organs of the skin.
- Build and define integumentary system medical terms from word parts.
- Identify and define integumentary system vocabulary terms.
- Identify and define selected integumentary system pathology terms.
- Identify and define selected integumentary system diagnostic procedures.
- Identify and define selected integumentary system therapeutic procedures.
- Identify and define selected medications relating to the integumentary system.
- Define selected abbreviations associated with the integumentary system.

From Chapter 3 of *Medical Terminology: A Living Language*, 4/e. Bonnie F. Fremgen. Suzanne S. Frucht.
Copyright © 2009 by Pearson Education. Published by Prentice Hall. All rights reserved.

Integumentary System at a Glance

Function

The skin provides a protective two-way barrier between our internal environment and the outside world. It also plays an important role in temperature regulation, houses sensory receptors to detect the environment around us and secretes important fluids.

Organs

skin   **hair**   **nails**   **sebaceous glands**   **sweat glands**

Combining Forms

albin/o	white	**melan/o**	black
bi/o	life	**myc/o**	fungus
cry/o	cold	**necr/o**	death
cutane/o	skin	**onych/o**	nail
cyan/o	blue	**pil/o**	hair
derm/o	skin	**phot/o**	light
dermat/o	skin	**py/o**	pus
diaphor/o	profuse sweating	**rhytid/o**	wrinkle
electr/o	electricity	**scler/o**	hard
erythr/o	red	**seb/o**	oil
hidr/o	sweat	**trich/o**	hair
ichthy/o	scaly, dry	**ungu/o**	nail
kerat/o	hard, horny	**vesic/o**	bladder
leuk/o	white	**xer/o**	dry
lip/o	fat		

Suffixes

-derma	skin
-opsy	view of
-tome	instrument used to cut

Prefixes

allo-	other, different from usual
xeno-	strange, foreign

Integumentary System Illustrated

hair

Provides some protection; associated with sensory receptors

skin

Protective barrier, houses sensory receptors, secretes sweat and sebum, temperature regulation

nail

Covers and protects tips of digits

Anatomy and Physiology of the Integumentary System

cutaneous membrane (kew-TAY-nee-us)
hair
integument (in-TEG-you-mint)
integumentary system
  (in-teg-you-MEN-tah-ree)
nails

pathogens (PATH-oh-jenz)
sebaceous glands (see-BAY-shus)
sensory receptors
skin
sweat glands

The **skin** and its accessory organs—**sweat glands**, **sebaceous glands**, **hair**, and **nails**—are known as the **integumentary system**, with **integument** and **cutaneous membrane** being alternate terms for skin. In fact, the skin is the largest organ of the body and can weigh more than 20 pounds in an adult. The skin serves many purposes for the body: protecting, housing nerve receptors, secreting fluids, and regulating temperature.

The primary function of the skin is protection. It forms a two-way barrier capable of keeping **pathogens** (disease-causing organisms) and harmful chemicals from entering the body. It also stops critical body fluids from escaping the body and prevents injury to the internal organs lying underneath the skin.

Sensory receptors that detect temperature, pain, touch, and pressure are located in the skin. The messages for these sensations are conveyed to the spinal cord and brain from the nerve endings in the middle layer of the skin.

Fluids are produced in two types of skin glands: sweat and sebaceous. Sweat glands assist the body in maintaining its internal temperature by creating a cooling effect as sweat evaporates. The sebaceous glands, or oil glands, produce an oily substance that lubricates the skin surface.

The structure of skin aids in the regulation of body temperature through a variety of means. As noted previously, the evaporation of sweat cools the body. The body also lowers its internal temperature by dilating superficial blood vessels in the skin. This brings more blood to the surface of the skin, which allows the release of heat. If the body needs to conserve heat, it constricts superficial blood vessels, keeping warm blood away from the surface of the body. Finally, the continuous layer of fat that makes up the subcutaneous layer of the skin acts as insulation.

The Skin

dermis (DER-mis)
epidermis (ep-ih-DER-mis)

subcutaneous layer (sub-kyoo-TAY-nee-us)

Moving from the outer surface of the skin inward, the three layers are as follows (see Figure 1 ■):

1. **Epidermis** is the thin, outer membrane layer.
2. **Dermis** is the middle, fibrous connective tissue layer.
3. The **subcutaneous layer** (Subcu, Subq) is the innermost layer, containing fatty tissue.

Epidermis

basal layer (BAY-sal)
keratin (KAIR-ah-tin)
melanin (MEL-ah-nin)

melanocytes (mel-AN-oh-sights)
stratified squamous epithelium (STRAT-ih-fyde SKWAY-mus ep-ih-THEE-lee-um)

The epidermis is composed of **stratified squamous epithelium** (see Figure 2 ■). This type of epithelial tissue consists of flat scale-like cells arranged in overlapping layers or strata. The epidermis does not have a blood supply or any connective tissue, so it is dependent for nourishment on the deeper layers of skin.

Epidermis

Dermis

Subcutaneous layer

Sensory receptors

Sebaceous gland

Arrector pili muscle

Hair

Nerve
Vein
Artery

Sweat gland

■ **Figure 1** Skin structure, including the three layers of the skin and the accessory organs: sweat gland, sebaceous gland, and hair.

The deepest layer within the epidermis is called the **basal layer**. Cells in this layer continually grow and multiply. New cells that are forming push the old cells toward the outer layer of the epidermis. During this process the cells shrink, die, and become filled with a hard protein called **keratin**. These dead, overlapping, keratinized cells allow the skin to act as an effective barrier to infection and also make it waterproof.

The basal layer also contains special cells called **melanocytes**, which produce the black pigment **melanin**. Not only is this pigment responsible for the color of the skin, but it also protects against damage from the ultraviolet rays of the sun. This damage may be in the form of leatherlike skin and wrinkles, which are not hazardous, or it may be one of several forms of skin cancer. Dark-skinned people have more melanin and are generally less likely to get wrinkles or skin cancer.

Med Term Tip

We lose 30,000 to 50,000 old dead skin cells per minute and replace them with new younger cells. In fact, because of this process, our skin is replaced entirely about every seven years.

Med Term Tip

A suntan can be thought of as a protective response to the rays of the sun. However, when the melanin in the skin is not able to absorb all the rays of the sun, the skin burns and DNA may be permanently and dangerously damaged.

■ **Figure 2** Photomicrograph of the epidermis layer of the skin.

Dermis

collagen fibers (KOL-ah-jen) **corium** (KOH-ree-um)

The dermis, also referred to as the **corium**, is the middle layer of skin, located between the epidermis and the subcutaneous layer. Its name means "true skin." Unlike the thinner epidermis, the dermis is living tissue with a very good blood supply. The dermis itself is composed of connective tissue and **collagen fibers**. Collagen fibers are made from a strong, fibrous protein present in connective tissue, forming a flexible "glue" that gives connective tissue its strength. The dermis houses hair follicles, sweat glands, sebaceous glands, blood vessels, lymph vessels, sensory receptors, nerve fibers, and muscle fibers.

Subcutaneous Layer

hypodermis (high-poh-DER-mis) **lipocytes** (LIP-oh-sights)

The third and deepest layer of the skin is the subcutaneous layer, also called the **hypodermis**. This layer of tissue, composed of fat cells called **lipocytes**, protects the deeper tissues of the body and acts as insulation for heat and cold.

Accessory Organs

The accessory organs of the skin are the anatomical structures located within the dermis, including the hair, nails, sebaceous glands, and sweat glands.

Hair

arrector pili (ah-REK-tor pee-lie) **hair root**
hair follicle (FALL-ikl) **hair shaft**

The fibers that make up hair are composed of the protein keratin, the same hard protein material that fills the cells of the epidermis. The process of hair formation is much like the process of growth in the epidermal layer of the skin. The deeper cells in the **hair root** force older keratinized cells to move upward, forming the **hair shaft**. The hair shaft grows toward the skin surface within the **hair follicle**. Melanin gives hair its color. Sebaceous glands release oil directly into the hair follicle. Each hair has a small slip of smooth muscle attached to it called the **arrector pili** muscle (see Figure 3 ■). When this muscle contracts the hair shaft stands up and results in "goose bumps."

Nails

cuticle (KEW-tikl) **nail bed**
free edge **nail body**
lunula (LOO-nyoo-lah) **nail root**

Nails are a flat plate of keratin called the **nail body** that covers the ends of fingers and toes. The nail body is connected to the tissue underneath by the **nail bed**. Nails grow longer from the **nail root**, which is found at the base of the nail and is covered and protected by the soft tissue **cuticle**. The **free edge** is the exposed edge that is trimmed when nails become too long. The light-colored half-moon area at the base of the nail is the **lunula** (see Figure 4 ■).

Sebaceous Glands

sebum

Sebaceous glands, found in the dermis, secrete the oil **sebum**, which lubricates the hair and skin, thereby helping to prevent drying and cracking. These glands secrete

■ **Figure 3** Structure of a hair and its associated sebaceous gland.

Epidermis

Sebaceous glands

Arrector pili

Shaft of hair

Hair follicle

Dermis

Hair root

Papilla

Subcutaneous layer

Muscle fibers

sebum directly into hair follicles, rather than a duct (see Figure 1). Secretion from the sebaceous glands increases during adolescence, playing a role in the development of acne. Sebum secretion begins to diminish as age increases. A loss of sebum in old age, along with sun exposure, can account for wrinkles and dry skin.

Sweat Glands

apocrine glands (APP-oh-krin)
perspiration
sudoriferous glands (sue-doh-RIF-er-us)

sweat duct
sweat pore

About two million sweat glands, also called **sudoriferous glands**, are found throughout the body. These highly coiled glands are located in the dermis. Sweat travels to the surface of the skin in a **sweat duct**. The surface opening of a sweat duct is called a **sweat pore** (see Figure 1).

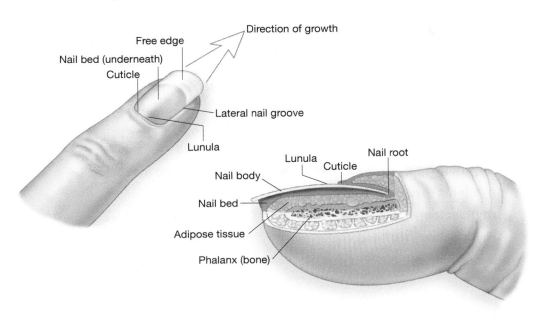

■ **Figure 4** External and internal structures of nails.

Direction of growth

Free edge

Nail bed (underneath)

Cuticle

Lateral nail groove

Lunula

Lunula

Cuticle

Nail root

Nail body

Nail bed

Adipose tissue

Phalanx (bone)

Med Term Tip

Word Watch — be careful when using *hydro-* meaning "water" and *hidr/o* meaning "sweat."

Sweat glands function to cool the body as sweat evaporates. Sweat or **perspiration** contains a small amount of waste product but is normally colorless and odorless. However, there are sweat glands called **apocrine glands** in the pubic and underarm areas that secrete a thicker sweat, which can produce an odor when it comes into contact with bacteria on the skin. This is what we recognize as body odor.

Word Building

The following list contains examples of medical terms built directly from word parts. The definition for these terms can be determined by a straightforward translation of the word parts.

COMBINING FORM	COMBINED WITH	MEDICAL TERM	DEFINITION
cutane/o	sub- -ous	**subcutaneous** (sub-kyoo-TAY-neeus)	pertaining to under the skin
derm/o	epi- -al	**epidermal** (ep-ih-DER-mal)	pertaining to upon the skin
	hypo- -ic	**hypodermic** (high-poh-DER-mik)	pertaining to under the skin
	intra- -al	**intradermal** (in-trah-DER-mal)	pertaining to within the skin
dermat/o	-itis	**dermatitis** (der-mah-TYE-tis)	inflammation of the skin
	-logist	**dermatologist** (der-mah-TALL-oh-jist)	specialist in skin
	-osis	**dermatosis** (der-mah-TOH-sis)	abnormal condition of skin
	-pathy	**dermatopathy** (der-mah-TOP-ah-thee)	skin disease
	-plasty	**dermatoplasty** (DER-mah-toh-plas-tee)	surgical repair of the skin
hidr/o	an- -osis	**anhidrosis** (an-hi-DROH-sis)	abnormal condition of no sweat
	hyper- -osis	**hyperhidrosis** (high-per-hi-DROH-sis)	abnormal condition of excessive sweat
lip/o	-ectomy	**lipectomy** (lih-PECK-toh-mee)	removal of fat
	-oma	**lipoma** (lip-OH-mah)	fatty mass
melan/o	-oma	**melanoma** (mel-ah-NOH-mah)	black tumor
	-cyte	**melanocyte** (meh-LAN-oh-sight)	black cell
necr/o	-osis	**necrosis** (neh-KROH-sis)	abnormal condition of death
onych/o	-ectomy	**onychectomy** (on-ee-KECK-toh-mee)	removal of a nail
	-malacia	**onychomalacia** (on-ih-koh-mah-LAY-she-ah)	softening of nails
	myc/o -osis	**onychomycosis** (on-ih-koh-my-KOH-sis)	abnormal condition of nail fungus
	-phagia	**onychophagia** (on-ih-koh-FAY-jee-ah)	nail eating (nail biting)
py/o	-genic	**pyogenic** (pye-oh-JEN-ik)	pus forming
rhytid/o	-ectomy	**rhytidectomy** (rit-ih-DECK-toh-mee)	removal of wrinkles
	-plasty	**rhytidoplasty** (RIT-ih-doh-plas-tee)	surgical repair of wrinkles
seb/o	-rrhea	**seborrhea** (seb-or-EE-ah)	oily discharge

■ Word Building *(continued)*

COMBINING FORM	COMBINED WITH	MEDICAL TERM	DEFINITION
trich/o	myc/o -osis	**trichomycosis** (trik-oh-my-KOH-sis)	abnormal condition of hair fungus
ungu/o	-al	**ungual** (UNG-gwal)	pertaining to the nails

SUFFIX	COMBINED WITH	MEDICAL TERM	MEANING
-derma	erythr/o	**erythroderma** (eh-rith-roh-DER-mah)	red skin
	ichthy/o	**ichthyoderma** (ick-thee-oh-DER-mah)	scaly and dry skin
	leuk/o	**leukoderma** (loo-koh-DER-mah)	white skin
	py/o	**pyoderma** (pye-oh-DER-mah)	pus skin
	scler/o	**scleroderma** (sklair-ah-DER-mah)	hard skin
	xer/o	**xeroderma** (zee-roh-DER-mah)	dry skin

■ Vocabulary

TERM	DEFINITION
abrasion (ah-BRAY-zhun)	A scraping away of the skin surface by friction.
cicatrix (SICK-ah-trix)	A scar.
comedo (KOM-ee-do)	Collection of hardened sebum in hair follicle. Also called a *blackhead*.
contusion	Injury caused by a blow to the body; causes swelling, pain, and bruising. The skin is not broken.
cyanosis (sigh-ah-NOH-sis)	Bluish tint to the skin caused by deoxygenated blood.

■ **Figure 5** A cyanotic infant. Note the bluish tinge to the skin around the lips, chin, and nose. *(St. Bartholomew's Hospital, London/Photo Researchers, Inc.)*

depigmentation (dee-pig-men-TAY-shun)	Loss of normal skin color or pigment.
dermatology (Derm, derm) (der-mah-TALL-oh-jee)	Branch of medicine involving diagnosis and treatment of conditions and diseases of the integumentary system. Physician is a *dermatologist*.
diaphoresis (dye-ah-for-REE-sis)	Profuse sweating.

Vocabulary *(continued)*

TERM	DEFINITION
ecchymosis (ek-ih-MOH-sis)	Skin discoloration caused by blood collecting under the skin following blunt trauma to the skin. A bruise (see Figure 6A ■).
erythema (er-ih-THEE-mah)	Redness or flushing of the skin.
eschar (ESH-shar)	A thick layer of dead tissue and tissue fluid that develops over a deep burn area.
hirsutism (HER-soot-izm)	Excessive hair growth over the body.
hyperemia (high-per-EE-mee-ah)	Redness of the skin due to increased blood flow.
hyperpigmentation (high-per-pig-men-TAY-shun)	Abnormal amount of pigmentation in the skin.
keloid (KEE-loyd)	Formation of a raised and thickened hypertrophic scar after an injury or surgery.

■ **Figure 7** Keloids, hypertrophic scarring on the back. *(Martin Rotker/ Phototake NYC)*

keratosis (kair-ah-TOH-sis)	Term for any skin condition involving an overgrowth and thickening of the epidermis layer.
lesion (LEE-shun)	A general term for a wound, injury, or abnormality.
nevus (NEV-us)	Pigmented skin blemish, birthmark, or mole. Usually benign but may become cancerous.
pallor (PAL-or)	Abnormal paleness of the skin.
petechiae (peh-TEE-kee-eye)	Pinpoint purple or red spots from minute hemorrhages under the skin (see Figure 6B ■).

A.

B.

C.

■ **Figure 6** A) Male lying supine with large ecchymosis on lateral rib cage and shoulder. B) Petechiae, pinpoint skin hemorrhages. *(Custom Medical Stock Photo, Inc.)* C) Purpura, hemorrhaging into the skin due to fragile blood vessels. *(Caroll H. Weiss/Camera M.D. Studios)*

Vocabulary *(continued)*

TERM	DEFINITION
photosensitivity (foh-toh-sen-sih-TIH-vih-tee)	Condition in which the skin reacts abnormally when exposed to light, such as the ultraviolet (UV) rays of the sun.
plastic surgery	Surgical specialty involved in repair, reconstruction, or improvement of body structures such as the skin that are damaged, missing, or misshapen. Physician is a *plastic surgeon*.
pruritus (proo-RIGH-tus)	Severe itching.
purpura (PER-pew-rah)	Hemorrhages into the skin due to fragile blood vessels. Commonly seen in elderly people (see Figure 6C ■).
	Med Term Tip
	Purpura comes from the Latin word for "purple," which refers to the color of these pinpoint hemorrhages.
purulent (PYUR-yoo-lent)	Containing pus or an infection that is producing pus. Pus consists of dead bacteria, white blood cells, and tissue debris.
strawberry hemangioma (hee-man-jee-OH-ma) ■ **Figure 8** Strawberry hemangioma, a birthmark caused by a collection of blood vessels in the skin. *(H.C. Robinson/Science Photo Library/Photo Researchers, Inc.)*	Congenital collection of dilated blood vessels causing a red birthmark that fades a few months after birth.
suppurative (SUP-pure-a-tiv)	Containing or producing pus.
urticaria (er-tih-KAY-ree-ah)	Also called *hives;* a skin eruption of pale reddish wheals with severe itching. Usually associated with food allergy, stress, or drug reactions.
verruca (ver-ROO-kah)	Commonly called *warts;* a benign growth caused by a virus. Has a rough surface that is removed by chemicals and/or laser therapy.

Pathology

■ Surface Lesions

cyst (SIST)

Fluid-filled sac under the skin (see Figures 9A & 9B ■).

(Bart's Medical Library/Phototake NYC)

fissure (FISH-er)

Crack-like lesion or groove on the skin (see Figures 9C & 9D ■).

(Phototake NYC)

laceration   A torn or jagged wound; incorrectly used to describe a cut.

macule (MACK-yool)

Flat, discolored area that is flush with the skin surface. An example would be a freckle or a birthmark (see Figures 9E & 9F ■).

(Phototake NYC)

nodule (NOD-yool)

Firm, solid mass of cells in the skin larger than 0.5 cm in diameter (see Figures 9G & 9H ■).

(Phototake NYC)

papule (PAP-yool)

Small, solid, circular raised spot on the surface of the skin less than 0.5 cm in diameter (see Figures 9I & 9J ■).

(ISM/Phototake NYC)

pustule (PUS-tyool)

Raised spot on the skin containing pus (see Figures 9E and 9K & 9L ■).

(P. Marazzi/Science Photo Library/Photo Researchers, Inc.)

Pathology *(continued)*

ulcer (ULL-ser)

Open sore or lesion in skin or mucous membrane (see Figures 9M & 9N).

M

N

(Dr. P. Marazzi/Photo Researchers, Inc.)

vesicle (VESS-ikl)

A blister; small, fluid-filled raised spot on the skin (see Figures 9O & 9P).

O

P

(ISM/Phototake NYC)

wheal (WEEL)

Small, round, swollen area on the skin; typically seen in allergic skin reactions such as *hives* and usually accompanied by urticaria (see Figures 9Q & 9R).

Q

R

(Charles Stewart MD FACEP, FAAEM)

TERM	DEFINITION
■ *Skin*	
abscess (AB-sess)	A collection of pus in the skin.
acne (ACK-nee)	Inflammatory disease of the sebaceous glands and hair follicles resulting in papules and pustules.
acne rosacea (ACK-nee roh-ZAY-she-ah)	Chronic form of acne seen in adults involving redness, tiny pimples, and broken blood vessels, primarily on the nose and cheeks.
acne vulgaris (ACK-nee vul-GAY-ris)	Common form of acne seen in teenagers. Characterized by comedo, papules, and pustules.
albinism (al-BIH-nizm)	A genetic condition in which the body is unable to make melanin. Characterized by white hair and skin and red pupils due to the lack of pigment. The person with albinism is called an *albino*.
basal cell carcinoma (BCC) (BAY-sal sell kar-sin-NOH-ma)	Cancerous tumor of the basal cell layer of the epidermis. A frequent type of skin cancer that rarely metastasizes or spreads. These cancers can arise on sun exposed skin.

■ **Figure 10** Basal cell carcinoma. A frequent type of skin cancer that rarely metastasizes. *(ISM/Phototake NYC)*

Pathology *(continued)*

TERM	DEFINITION
burn	Damage to the skin that can result from exposure to open fire, electricity, ultraviolet light from the sun, or caustic chemicals. Seriousness depends on the amount of body surface involved and the depth of the burn. Depth of the burns is determined by the amount of damage to each layer skin and burns are categorized as 1st degree, 2nd degree, or 3rd degree. See Figure 11 ■ for a description of the damage associated with each degree of burn. Extent of a burn is estimated using the Rule of Nines (see Figure 12 ■).

Superficial
First Degree

Skin reddened

(Moynahan Medical Center)

Partial thickness
Second Degree

Blisters

(Charles Stewart MD FACEP, FAAEM)

Full thickness
Third Degree

Charring

■ **Figure 11** Comparison of the level of skin damage as a result of the three different degrees of burns.

Figure 12 Rule of Nines. A method for determining percentage of body burned. Each differently colored section represents a percentage of the body surface. All sections added together will equal 100%.

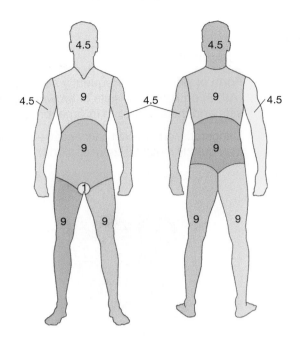

Pathology *(continued)*

TERM	DEFINITION
cellulitis (sell-you-LYE-tis)	A diffuse, acute infection and inflammation of the connective tissue found in the skin.
decubitus ulcer (decub) (dee-KYOO-bih-tus)	Open sore caused by pressure over bony prominences cutting off the blood flow to the overlying skin. These can appear in bedridden patients who lie in one position too long and can be difficult to heal. Also called *bedsore* or *pressure sore.* **Med Term Tip** *Decubitus* comes from the Latin word *decumbo*, meaning "lying down," which leads to the use of the term for a bedsore or pressure sore.
dry gangrene (GANG-green)	Late stages of gangrene characterized by the affected area becoming dried, blackened, and shriveled; referred to as *mummified*.
eczema (EK-zeh-mah)	Superficial dermatitis of unknown cause accompanied by redness, vesicles, itching, and crusting.
gangrene (GANG-green)	Tissue necrosis usually due to deficient blood supply.
ichthyosis (ick-thee-OH-sis)	Condition in which the skin becomes dry, scaly, and keratinized.
impetigo (im-peh-TYE-goh)	A highly infections bacterial infection of the skin with pustules that rupture and become crusted over.

Figure 13 Impetigo, a highly contagious bacterial infection. Note the extensive crusting around the eye.
(Bart's Medical Library/Phototake NYC)

Pathology *(continued)*

TERM	DEFINITION
Kaposi's sarcoma (KAP-oh-seez sar-KOH-mah)	Form of skin cancer frequently seen in acquired immunodeficiency syndrome (AIDS) patients. Consists of brownish-purple papules that spread from the skin and metastasize to internal organs.
malignant melanoma (MM) (mah-LIG-nant mel-a-NOH-ma)	Dangerous form of skin cancer caused by an uncontrolled growth of melanocytes. May quickly metastasize or spread to internal organs.

■ Figure 14 Malignant melanoma. This tumor demonstrates the highly characteristic color of this tumor. *(ISM/Phototake NYC)*

pediculosis (peh-dik-you-LOH-sis)	Infestation with lice. The eggs laid by the lice are called nits and cling tightly to hair.
psoriasis (soh-RYE-ah-sis)	Chronic inflammatory condition consisting of papules forming "silvery scale" patches with circular borders.

■ Figure 15 Psoriasis. This photograph demonstrates the characteristic white skin patches of this condition.

rubella (roo-BELL-ah)	Contagious viral skin infection. Commonly called *German measles*.
scabies (SKAY-bees)	Contagious skin disease caused by an egg-laying mite that burrows through the skin and causes redness and intense itching; often seen in children.
sebaceous cyst (see-BAY-shus SIST)	Sac under the skin filled with sebum or oil from a sebaceous gland. This can grow to a large size and may need to be excised.
squamous cell carcinoma (SCC) (SKWAY-mus sell kar-sih-NOH-mah)	Cancer of the epidermis layer of skin that may invade deeper tissue and metastasize. Often begins as a sore that does not heal.
systemic lupus erythematosus (SLE) (sis-TEM-ik LOO-pus air-ih-them-ah-TOH-sis)	Chronic disease of the connective tissue that injures the skin, joints, kidneys, nervous system, and mucous membranes. May produce a characteristic red, scaly butterfly rash across the cheeks and nose.
tinea (TIN-ee-ah)	Fungal skin disease resulting in itching, scaling lesions.
tinea capitis (TIN-ee-ah CAP-it-is)	Fungal infection of the scalp. Commonly called *ringworm.*
tinea pedis (TIN-ee-ah PED-is)	Fungal infection of the foot. Commonly called *athlete's foot.*

Pathology *(continued)*

TERM	DEFINITION
varicella (VAIR-ih-chell-a)	Contagious viral skin infection. Commonly called *chicken pox*.
■ **Figure 16** Varicella or chicken pox, a viral skin infection. In this photograph, the rash is beginning to form scabs.	
vitiligo (vit-ill-EYE-go)	Disappearance of pigment from the skin in patches, causing a milk-white appearance. Also called *leukoderma*.
wet gangrene (GANG-green)	An area of gangrene that becomes secondarily infected by pus-producing bacteria.
■ *Hair*	
alopecia (al-oh-PEE-she-ah)	Absence or loss of hair, especially of the head. Commonly called *baldness*.
carbuncle (CAR-bung-kl)	Furuncle involving several hair follicles.
furuncle (FOO-rung-kl)	Bacterial infection of a hair follicle. Characterized by redness, pain, and swelling. Also called a *boil*.
■ *Nails*	
onychia (oh-NICK-ee-ah)	Infected nail bed.
paronychia (pair-oh-NICK-ee-ah)	Infection of the skin fold around a nail.

Diagnostic Procedures

TERM	DEFINITION
■ *Clinical Laboratory Tests*	
culture and sensitivity (C&S)	A laboratory test that grows a colony of bacteria removed from an infected area in order to identify the specific infecting bacteria and then determine its sensitivity to a variety of antibiotics.
■ *Biopsy Procedures*	
biopsy (BX, bx) (BYE-op-see)	A piece of tissue is removed by syringe and needle, knife, punch, or brush to examine under a microscope. Used to aid in diagnosis.
	Med Term Tip
	Word Watch — be careful when using *bi-* meaning "two" and *bi/o* meaning "life."
exfoliative cytology (ex-FOH-lee-ah-tiv sigh-TALL-oh-jee)	Scraping cells from tissue and then examining them under a microscope.
frozen section (FS)	A thin piece of tissue is cut from a frozen specimen for rapid examination under a microscope.
fungal scrapings	Scrapings, taken with a curette or scraper, of tissue from lesions are placed on a growth medium and examined under a microscope to identify fungal growth.

TERM	DEFINITION
Skin Grafting	
allograft (AL-oh-graft)	Skin graft from one person to another; donor is usually a cadaver.
autograft (AW-toh-graft) ■ **Figure 17** A freshly applied autograft. Note that the donor skin has been perforated so that it can be stretched to cover a larger burned area. _(Courtesy of Dr. William Dominic, Community Regional Medical Center)_	Skin graft from a person's own body.
dermatome (DER-mah-tohm)	Instrument for cutting the skin or thin transplants of skin.
dermatoplasty (DER-mah-toh-plas-tee)	Skin grafting; transplantation of skin.
heterograft (HET-ur-oh-graft)	Skin graft from an animal of another species (usually a pig) to a human. Also called _xenograft_.
skin graft (SG)	The transfer of skin from a normal area to cover another site. Used to treat burn victims and after some surgical procedures. Also called _dermatoplasty_.
xenograft (ZEN-oh-graft)	Skin graft from an animal of another species (usually a pig) to a human. Also called _heterograft_.
Surgical Procedures	
cauterization (kaw-ter-ih-ZAY-shun)	Destruction of tissue by using caustic chemicals, electric currents, heat, or by freezing.
cryosurgery (cry-oh-SER-jer-ee)	The use of extreme cold to freeze and destroy tissue.
curettage (koo-REH-tahz)	Removal of superficial skin lesions with a curette (surgical instrument shaped like a spoon) or scraper.
debridement (de-BREED-mint)	Removal of foreign material and dead or damaged tissue from a wound.
electrocautery (ee-leck-troh-KAW-teh-ree)	To destroy tissue with an electric current.
incision and drainage (I&D)	Making an incision to create an opening for the drainage of material such as pus.
Plastic Surgery Procedures	
chemabrasion (kee-moh-BRAY-zhun)	Abrasion using chemicals. Also called a _chemical peel_.
dermabrasion (DERM-ah-bray-shun)	Abrasion or rubbing using wire brushes or sandpaper. Performed to remove acne scars, tattoos, and scar tissue.
laser therapy	Removal of skin lesions and birthmarks using a laser beam that emits intense heat and power at a close range. The laser converts frequencies of light into one small, powerful beam.
liposuction (LIP-oh-suck-shun)	Removal of fat beneath the skin by means of suction.
rhytidectomy (rit-ih-DECK-toh-mee)	Surgical removal of excess skin to eliminate wrinkles. Commonly referred to as a _face lift_.

Pharmacology

CLASSIFICATION	ACTION	GENERIC AND BRAND NAMES
anesthetics (an-es-THET-tics)	Applied to the skin to deaden pain.	lidocaine, Xylocaine; procaine, Novocain
antibiotics (an-tye-bye-AW-tics)	Kill bacteria causing skin infections.	bacitracin/neomycin/polymixinB, Neosporin ointment
antifungals (an-tye-FUNG-alls)	Kill fungi infecting the skin.	miconazole, Monistat; clotrimazole, Lotrimin
antiparasitics (an-tye-pair-ah-SIT-tics)	Kill mites or lice.	lindane, Kwell; permethrin, Nix
antipruritics (an-tye-proo-RIGH-tiks)	Reduce severe itching.	diphenhydramine, Benadryl; camphor/pramoxine/zinc, Caladryl
antiseptics (an-tye-SEP-tics)	Used to kill bacteria in skin cuts and wounds or at a surgical site.	isopropyl alcohol; hydrogen peroxide
anti-virals	Treats herpes simplex infection.	valacyclovir, Valtrex; famcyclovir, Famvir; acyclovir, Zovirax
corticosteroid cream	Specific type of powerful anti-inflammatory cream.	hydrocortisone, Cortaid; triamcinolone, Kenalog

Abbreviations

BCC	basal cell carcinoma	**MM**	malignant melanoma
BX, bx	biopsy	**SCC**	squamous cell carcinoma
C&S	culture and sensitivity	**SG**	skin graft
decub	decubitus ulcer	**SLE**	systemic lupus erythematosus
Derm, derm	dermatology	**STSG**	split-thickness skin graft
FS	frozen section	**subcu, SC, sc,**	subcutaneous
HSV	herpes simplex virus	**subq**	
I&D	incision and drainage	**UV**	ultraviolet
ID	intradermal		

Med Term Tip

Word Watch—be careful when using the abbreviation *ID* meaning "intradermal" and *I&D* meaning "incision and drainage."

Chapter Review

Terminology Checklist

 Below are all anatomy and physiology key terms, word building, vocabulary, pathology, diagnostic, therapeutic, and pharmacology terms presented in this chapter. Use this list as a study tool by placing a check in the box in front of each term as you master its meaning.

- ☐ abrasion
- ☐ abscess
- ☐ acne
- ☐ acne rosacea
- ☐ acne vulgaris
- ☐ albinism
- ☐ allograft
- ☐ alopecia
- ☐ anesthetics
- ☐ anhidrosis
- ☐ antibiotics
- ☐ antifungals
- ☐ antiparasitics
- ☐ antipruritics
- ☐ antiseptics
- ☐ anti-virals
- ☐ apocrine glands
- ☐ arrector pili
- ☐ autograft
- ☐ basal cell carcinoma
- ☐ basal layer
- ☐ biopsy
- ☐ burn
- ☐ carbuncle
- ☐ cauterization
- ☐ cellulitis
- ☐ chemabrasion
- ☐ cicatrix
- ☐ collagen fibers
- ☐ comedo
- ☐ contusion
- ☐ corium
- ☐ corticosteroid cream
- ☐ cryosurgery
- ☐ culture and sensitivity
- ☐ curettage
- ☐ cutaneous membrane
- ☐ cuticle

- ☐ cyanosis
- ☐ cyst
- ☐ debridement
- ☐ decubitus ulcer
- ☐ depigmentation
- ☐ dermabrasion
- ☐ dermatitis
- ☐ dermatologist
- ☐ dermatology
- ☐ dermatome
- ☐ dermatopathy
- ☐ dermatoplasty
- ☐ dermatosis
- ☐ dermis
- ☐ diaphoresis
- ☐ dry gangrene
- ☐ ecchymosis
- ☐ eczema
- ☐ electrocautery
- ☐ epidermal
- ☐ epidermis
- ☐ erythema
- ☐ erythroderma
- ☐ eschar
- ☐ exfoliative cytology
- ☐ fissure
- ☐ free edge
- ☐ frozen section
- ☐ fungal scrapings
- ☐ furuncle
- ☐ gangrene
- ☐ hair
- ☐ hair follicle
- ☐ hair root
- ☐ hair shaft
- ☐ heterograft
- ☐ hirsutism
- ☐ hyperemia

- ☐ hyperhidrosis
- ☐ hyperpigmentation
- ☐ hypodermic
- ☐ hypodermis
- ☐ ichthyoderma
- ☐ ichthyosis
- ☐ impetigo
- ☐ incision and drainage
- ☐ integument
- ☐ integumentary system
- ☐ intradermal
- ☐ Kaposi's sarcoma
- ☐ keloid
- ☐ keratin
- ☐ keratosis
- ☐ laceration
- ☐ laser therapy
- ☐ lesion
- ☐ leukoderma
- ☐ lipectomy
- ☐ lipocytes
- ☐ lipoma
- ☐ liposuction
- ☐ lunula
- ☐ macule
- ☐ malignant melanoma
- ☐ melanin
- ☐ melanocytes
- ☐ melanoma
- ☐ nail bed
- ☐ nail body
- ☐ nail root
- ☐ nails
- ☐ necrosis
- ☐ nevus
- ☐ nodule
- ☐ onychectomy
- ☐ onychia

- ☐ onychomalacia
- ☐ onychomycosis
- ☐ onychophagia
- ☐ pallor
- ☐ papule
- ☐ paronychia
- ☐ pathogens
- ☐ pediculosis
- ☐ perspiration
- ☐ petechiae
- ☐ photosensitivity
- ☐ plastic surgery
- ☐ pruritus
- ☐ psoriasis
- ☐ purpura
- ☐ purulent
- ☐ pustule
- ☐ pyoderma
- ☐ pyogenic
- ☐ rhytidectomy
- ☐ rhytidoplasty
- ☐ rubella
- ☐ scabies
- ☐ scleroderma
- ☐ sebaceous cyst
- ☐ sebaceous gland
- ☐ seborrhea
- ☐ sebum
- ☐ sensory receptors
- ☐ skin
- ☐ skin graft
- ☐ squamous cell carcinoma
- ☐ stratified squamous epithelium
- ☐ strawberry hemangioma
- ☐ subcutaneous
- ☐ subcutaneous layer
- ☐ sudoriferous glands
- ☐ suppurative
- ☐ sweat duct
- ☐ sweat glands
- ☐ sweat pore
- ☐ systemic lupus erythematosus
- ☐ tinea
- ☐ tinea capitis
- ☐ tinea pedis
- ☐ trichomycosis
- ☐ ulcer
- ☐ ungual
- ☐ urticaria
- ☐ varicella
- ☐ verruca
- ☐ vesicle
- ☐ vitiligo
- ☐ wet gangrene
- ☐ wheal
- ☐ xenograft
- ☐ xeroderma

Practice Exercises

A. Complete the following statements.

1. The three layers of skin in order starting with the most superficial layer are _epidermis_, _dermis_, and _subcutaneous_

2. The _dermis_ layer is the only living layer of the epidermis.

3. The subcutaneous layer of skin is composed primarily of _lipocytes_.

4. Sensory receptors are located in the _dermis_ layer of skin.

5. Nails and hair are composed of a hard protein called _keratin_.

6. _Melanin_ is the pigment that gives skin its color.

7. Another name for the dermis is _corium_.

8. The nail body is connected to underlying tissue by the _nailbed_.

9. _Sebaceous_ glands release their product directly into hair follicles while _sudoriferous_ glands release their product into a duct.

10. _Apocrine_ glands are sweat glands found in the underarm and pubic areas.

B. State the terms described using the combining forms provided.

The combining form *dermat/o* refers to the skin. Use it to write a term that means:

1. inflammation of the skin _dermatitis_

2. any abnormal skin condition _dermatosis_

Integumentary System

3. an instrument for cutting the skin dermatome

4. specialist in skin dermatologist

5. surgical repair of the skin dermatoplasty

6. study of the skin dermatology

The combining form *melan/o* means black. Use it to write a term that means a:

7. black tumor melanoma

8. black cell melanocyte

The suffix *-derma* means skin. Use it to write a term that means:

9. scaly skin ichthyoderma

10. white skin leukoderma

11. red skin erythroderma

The combining form *onych/o* refers to the nail. Use it to write a term that means:

12. softening of the nails onychomalacia

13. infection around the nail paronychia

14. nail eating (biting) onychophagia

15. removal of the nail onychectomy

C. Define the following combining forms and use them to form integumentary terms.

		Definition	Integumentary term
1.	cry/o	cold	cryosurgery
2.	cutane/o	skin	subcutaneous
3.	diaphor/o	profuse sweating	diaphoresis
4.	py/o	pus	pyoderma
5.	cyan/o	blue	cyanosis
6.	ungu/o	nail	ungual
7.	lip/o	fat	lipoma
8.	hidr/o	sweat	hyperhidrosis
9.	rhytid/o	wrinkle	rhytidectomy
10.	seb/o	oil	sebaceous
11.	trich/o	hair	trichomycosis
12.	necr/o	death	necrosis

Integumentary System

D. Define the following terms.

1. macule _flat, discolored area that is flush w/ the skin surface_
2. papule _small, solid, circular raised spot on the skin less than 0.5cm in diameter_
3. cyst _fluid-filled sac under the skin_
4. fissure _crack-like lesion or groove on the skin_
5. pustule _raised spot on the skin containing pus_
6. wheal _small, round, swollen area on the skin_
7. vesicle _a blister; small, fluid-filled raised spot on the skin_
8. ulcer _open sore or lesion in skin or mucous membrane_
9. nodule _firm, solid mass of cells in the skin larger than 0.5cm in diameter_
10. laceration _a torn or jagged wound_

E. Describe the following types of burns.

1. first degree _superficial, skin reddened_
2. second degree _partial thickness, blisters_
3. third degree _full thickness, charring_

F. Match each term to its definition.

1. _e_ eczema
2. _f_ nevus
3. _i_ lipoma
4. _j_ urticaria
5. _a_ bedsore
6. _c_ acne rosacea
7. _l_ acne vulgaris
8. _g_ hirsutism
9. _k_ alopecia
10. _h_ gangrene
11. _d_ scleroderma
12. _b_ albinism

a. decubitus ulcer

b. lack of skin pigment

c. acne commonly seen in adults

d. hardened skin

e. redness, vesicles, itching, crusts

f. birthmark

g. excessive hair growth

h. caused by deficient blood supply

i. fatty tumor

j. hives

k. baldness

l. acne of adolescence

G. Match each term to its definition.

1. _h_ debridement
2. _i_ cauterization
3. _j_ chemabrasion
4. _e_ dermatoplasty
5. _c_ liposuction
6. _a_ rhytidectomy
7. _f_ curettage
8. _g_ dermabrasion
9. _b_ dermatome
10. _d_ cryosurgery

a. surgical removal of wrinkled skin

b. instrument to cut thin slices of skin

c. removal of fat with suction

d. use extreme cold to destroy tissue

e. skin grafting

f. removal of lesions with scraper

g. removal of skin with brushes

h. removal of damaged skin

i. destruction of tissue with electric current

j. chemical peel

H. Write the abbreviations for the following terms.

1. frozen section ___FS___

2. incision and drainage ___I&D___

3. intradermal ___ID___

4. subcutaneous ___subcu, SC, sc, subq___

5. ultraviolet ___UV___

6. biopsy ___BX, bx___

I. Identify the following abbreviations.

1. C & S ___culture and sensitivity___

2. BCC ___basal cell carcinoma___

3. derm ___dermatology___

4. SG ___skin graft___

5. decub ___decubitus ulcer___

6. MM ___malignant melanoma___

J. Use the following terms in the sentences that follow.

| impetigo | tinea | keloid | exfoliative cytology | xeroderma |
| petechiae | frozen section | paronychia | scabies | Kaposi's sarcoma |

1. The winter climates can cause dry skin. The medical term for this is ___xeroderma___.

2. Kim has experienced small pinpoint purplish spots caused by bleeding under the skin. This is called ___petechiae___.

3. Janet has a fungal skin disease. This is called ___tinea___.

4. A contagious skin disease caused by a mite is ___scabies___.

5. An infection around the entire nail is called __paronychia__.

6. A form of skin cancer affecting AIDS patients is called __Kaposi's sarcoma__.

7. Latrivia has a bacterial skin infection that results in pustules crusting and rupturing. It is called __impetigo__.

8. James's burn scar became a hypertrophic __keloid__.

9. For a(n) __exfoliative cytology__ test, cells scraped off the skin are examined under a microscope.

10. During surgery a __frozen section__ was ordered for a rapid exam of tissue cut from a tumor.

K. Use the following prefixes to write a word that means

epi-   sub-   intra-   hypo-

1. under the skin __hypodermic__ or __subcutaneous__

2. within the skin __intradermal__

3. on the skin __epidermal__

L. Distinguish between the following types of skin graft.

1. allograft __skin graft from one person to another; donor is usually a cadaver__

2. heterograft __skin graft from an animal of another species (usually a pig) to a human__

3. autograft __skin graft from a person's own body__

4. xenograft __same as heterograft__

M. Fill in the classification for each drug description, then match the brand name.

Drug Description	Classification	Brand Name
1. __f__ kills fungi	antifungals	a. Kwell
2. __d__ reduces severe itching	antipruritics	b. Cortaid
3. __a__ kills mites and lice	antiparasitics	c. Valtrex
4. __c__ treats herpes simplex infection	anti-virals	d. Benadryl
5. __b__ powerful anti-inflammatory	corticosteroid cream	e. Neosporin
6. __g__ deadens pain	anesthetics	f. Monistat
7. __e__ kills bacteria	antibiotics	g. Xylocaine

Medical Record Analysis

Below is an item from a patient's medical record. Read it carefully, make sure you understand all the medical terms used, and then answer the questions that follow.

Dermatology Consultation Report

Reason for Consultation:	Evaluate patient for excision of recurrent basal cell carcinoma, left cheek.
History of Present Illness:	Patient is a 74-year-old male first seen by his regular physician five years ago for persistent facial lesions. Biopsies revealed basal cell carcinoma in two lesions, one on the nasal tip and the other on the left cheek. These were excised and healed with a normal cicatrix. The patient noted that the left cheek lesion returned approximately one year ago. Patient admits to not following his physician's advice to use sunscreen and a hat. Patient reports pruritus and states the lesion is growing larger. Patient has been referred for dermatology evaluation regarding deep excision of the lesion and dermatoplasty.
Past Medical History:	Patient's activity level is severely restricted due to congestive heart failure (CHF) with dyspnea, lower extremity edema, and cyanosis. He takes several cardiac medications daily and occasionally requires oxygen by nasal cannula. History is negative for other types of cancer.
Results of Physical Exam:	Examination revealed a 10 × 14 mm lesion on left cheek 20 mm anterior to the ear. The lesion displays marked erythema and poorly defined borders. The area immediately around the lesion shows depigmentation with vesicles. There is a well-healed cicatrix on the nasal tip with no evidence of the neoplasm returning.
Assessment:	Even without a biopsy, this is most likely a recurrence of this patient's basal cell carcinoma.
Recommendations:	Due to the lesion's size, shape, and reoccurrence, recommend deep excision of the neoplasm through the epidermis and dermis layers. The patient will then require dermatoplasty. The most likely donor site will be the proximal-medial thigh. This patient is at high risk for basal cell carcinoma and should never go outside without sunscreen and a hat. I have discussed the surgical procedure with the patient, and he fully understands the procedure, risks, and alternate treatment choices. In light of his cardiac status, if he decides to proceed with the surgery, he will need a thorough workup by his cardiologist.

Critical Thinking Questions

1. Which of the following symptoms was reported by the patient?
   a. easy bruising
   b. excessive scarring
   c. intense itching
   d. yellow skin

2. In your own words, describe the lesion on the patient's face. 10×14mm on left cheek, 20mm in front of the ear, shows marked redness & poorly defined borders, area immediately around lesion shows loss of normal skin color with blisters

Integumentary System

3. What advice did this patient fail to follow? Using sunscreen & hat

What happened, in part, because he did not follow instructions? recurrence of basal cell carcinoma

4. This patient has a serious health condition other than his facial lesion. Name that condition and describe it in your own words. Congestive heart failure (CHF) - reduced outflow of blood from the left side of the heart

What is the abbreviation for this condition? (CHF)

This patient has three symptoms of this condition. List the three symptoms and describe each in your own words. This condition and its symptoms use terminology that has not been introduced yet. You will need to use your text as a reference to answer this question.

dyspnea - difficult breathing

lower extremity edema - swelling

cyanosis - blue skin due to lack of oxygen

5. What procedure was performed on the original lesion that confirmed the diagnosis? Explain, in your own words, what this procedure involves. biopsy - removing a piece of the tissue & examining it under a microscope

6. Briefly describe, in your own words, the two stages of the surgical procedure the physician recommends.

Deep excision - removal of the lesion through the epidermal & dermal layers

Dermatoplasty - surgical repair of the skin

Chart Note Transcription

The chart note below contains ten phrases that can be reworded with a medical term that you learned in this chapter. Each phrase is identified with an underline. Determine the medical term and write your answers in the spaces provided.

Current Complaint:	A 64-year-old female with an <u>open sore</u> ❶ on her right leg is seen by the <u>specialist in treating diseases of the skin</u>. ❷
Past History:	Patient states she first noticed an area of pain, <u>severe itching</u>, ❸ and <u>redness of the skin</u> ❹ just below her right knee about six weeks ago. One week later <u>raised spots containing pus</u> ❺ appeared. Patient states the raised spots containing pus ruptured and the open sore appeared.
Signs and Symptoms:	Patient has a deep open sore 5 × 3 cm: It is 4 cm distal to the knee on the lateral aspect of the right leg. It appears to extend into the <u>middle skin layer</u>, ❻ and the edges show signs of <u>tissue death</u>. ❼ The open sore has a small amount of drainage but there is no odor. A <u>sample of the drainage that was grown in the lab to identify the microorganism and determine the best antibiotic</u> ❽ of the drainage revealed *Staphylococcus* bacteria in the open sore.
Diagnosis:	<u>Inflammation of connective tissue in the skin.</u> ❾
Treatment:	<u>Removal of damaged tissue</u> ❿ of the open sore followed by application of an antibiotic cream. Patient was instructed to return to the specialist in treating diseases of the skin's office in two weeks, or sooner if the open sore does not heal, or if it begins draining pus.

❶ ulcer

❷ dermatologist

❸ pruritis

❹ erythema

❺ pustules

❻ dermis

❼ necrosis

❽ culture & sensitivity (C&S)

❾ dermatitis

❿ debridement

Labeling Exercise

A. System Review

Write the labels for this figure on the numbered lines provided.

5. sweat duct

6. hair

7. sebaceous gland

8. arrector pili muscle

1. epidermis

2. dermis

9. sensory receptors

3. subcutaneous layer

4. sweat gland

B. Anatomy Challenge

1. Write the labels for this figure on the numbered lines provided.

4. Sebaceous gland

5. arrector pili muscle

6. Shaft of hair

7. hair follicle

8. hair root

9. papilla

1. epidermas

2. dermis

3. subcutaneous layer

2. Write the labels for this figure on the numbered lines provided.

1. free edge

2. lateral nail groove

5. nail body

6. cuticle

7. nail root

3. lunula

4. nail bed

Multimedia Preview

Additional interactive resources and activities for this chapter can be found on the Companion Website.

Website Highlights—www.prenhall.com/fremgen

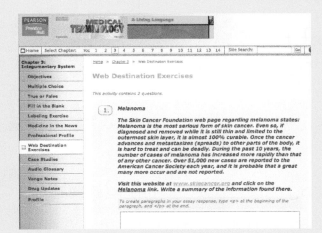

WEB DESTINATION EXERCISES

Surf the net to investigate key topics and then report your findings. This online activity challenges you to visit selected web links where you can explore important issues to reinforce your understanding.

Musculoskeletal System

Learning Objectives

Upon completion of this chapter, you will be able to:

- Identify and define the combining forms, prefixes, and suffixes introduced in this chapter.

- Correctly spell and pronounce medical terms and major anatomical structures relating to the musculoskeletal system.

- Locate and describe the major organs of the musculoskeletal system and their functions.

- Correctly place bones in either the axial or the appendicular skeleton.

- List and describe the components of a long bone.

- Identify bony projections and depressions.

- Identify the parts of a synovial joint.

- Describe the characteristics of the three types of muscle tissue.

- Use movement terminology correctly.

- Build and define musculoskeletal system medical terms from word parts.

- Identify and define musculoskeletal system vocabulary terms.

- Identify and define selected musculoskeletal system pathology terms.

- Identify and define selected musculoskeletal system diagnostic procedures.

- Identify and define selected musculoskeletal system therapeutic procedures.

- Identify and define selected medications relating to the musculoskeletal system.

- Define selected abbreviations associated with the musculoskeletal system.

From Chapter 4 of *Medical Terminology: A Living Language*, 4/e. Bonnie F. Fremgen. Suzanne S. Frucht. Copyright © 2009 by Pearson Education. Published by Prentice Hall. All rights reserved.

Section I: Skeletal System at a Glance

Function

The skeletal system consists of 206 bones that make up the internal framework of the body, called the skeleton. The skeleton supports the body, protects internal organs, serves as a point of attachment for skeletal muscles for body movement, produces blood cells, and stores minerals.

Organs

bones   **joints**

Combining Forms

ankyl/o	stiff joint	**metacarp/o**	metacarpals
arthr/o	joint	**metatars/o**	metatarsals
articul/o	joint	**myel/o**	bone marrow, spinal cord
burs/o	sac	**orth/o**	straight
carp/o	wrist	**oste/o**	bone
cervic/o	neck	**patell/o**	patella
chondr/o	cartilage	**ped/o**	child, foot
clavicul/o	clavicle	**pelv/o**	pelvis
coccyg/o	coccyx	**phalang/o**	phalanges
cortic/o	outer portion	**pod/o**	foot
cost/o	rib	**pub/o**	pubis
crani/o	skull	**radi/o**	radius
femor/o	femur	**sacr/o**	sacrum
fibul/o	fibula	**scapul/o**	scapula
humer/o	humerus	**scoli/o**	crooked, bent
ili/o	ilium	**spondyl/o**	vertebrae
ischi/o	ischium	**stern/o**	sternum
kyph/o	hump	**synovi/o**	synovial membrane
lamin/o	lamina, part of vertebra	**synov/o**	synovial membrane
lord/o	bent backwards	**tars/o**	ankle
lumb/o	loin	**thorac/o**	chest
mandibul/o	mandible	**tibi/o**	tibia
maxill/o	maxilla	**uln/o**	ulna
medull/o	inner portion	**vertebr/o**	vertebra

Suffixes

-blast	immature, embryonic
-clasia	to surgically break
-desis	stabilize, fuse
-listhesis	slipping
-porosis	porous

Skeletal System Illustrated

Skull

Maxilla

Mandible

Cervical vertebrae

Scapula

Sternum

Humerus

Ribs

Thoracic
vertebrae (T11)

Ulna

Radius

Lumbar
vertebrae (L4)

Ilium

Sacrum

Coccyx

Pubis

Carpals

Metacarpals

Phalanges

Ischium

Femur

Patella

Tibia

Fibula

Tarsals

Metatarsals

Phalanges

Anatomy and Physiology of the Skeletal System

bone marrow	ligaments (LIG-ah-ments)
bones	skeleton
joints	

Each bone in the human body is a unique organ that carries its own blood supply, nerves, and lymphatic vessels. However, when the **bones** are connected to each other, forming the framework of the body, it is called a **skeleton**. In addition, the skeleton protects vital organs and stores minerals. **Bone marrow** is the site of blood cell production. A **joint** is the place where two bones meet and are held together by **ligaments**. This gives flexibility to the skeleton. The skeleton, joints, and muscles work together to produce movement.

Bones

cartilage (CAR-tih-lij)	osteoblasts (OSS-tee-oh-blasts)
osseous tissue (OSS-ee-us)	osteocytes (OSS-tee-oh-sights)
ossification (oss-sih-fih-KAY-shun)	

Bones, also called **osseous tissue**, are one of the hardest materials in the body. Bones are formed from a gradual process beginning before birth called **ossification**. The fetal skeleton is formed from a **cartilage** model. This flexible tissue is gradually replaced by **osteoblasts**, immature bone cells. In adult bones, the osteoblasts have matured into **osteocytes**. The formation of strong bones is greatly dependent on an adequate supply of minerals such as calcium and phosphorus.

Bone Structure

articular cartilage (ar-TIK-yoo-lar)	long bones
cancellous bone (CAN-sell-us)	medullary cavity (MED-you-lair-ee)
compact bone	periosteum (pair-ee-AH-stee-um)
cortical bone (KOR-ti-kal)	red bone marrow
diaphysis (dye-AFF-ih-sis)	short bones
epiphysis (eh-PIFF-ih-sis)	spongy bone
flat bones	yellow bone marrow
irregular bones	

Several different types of bones are found throughout the body. They fall into four categories based on their shape: **long bones**, **short bones**, **flat bones**, and **irregular bones** (see Figure 1 ■). Long bones are longer than they are wide. Examples are the femur and humerus. Short bones are roughly as long as they are wide; examples being the carpals and tarsals. Irregular bones received their name because the shapes of the bones are very irregular; for example, the vertebrae are irregular bones. Flat bones are usually plate-shaped bones such as the sternum, scapulae, and pelvis.

The majority of bones in the human body are long bones. These bones have similar structure with a central shaft or **diaphysis** that widens at each end, which is called an **epiphysis**. Each epiphysis is covered by a layer of cartilage called **articular cartilage** to prevent bone from rubbing directly on bone. The remaining surface of each bone is covered with a thin connective tissue membrane called the **periosteum**, which contains numerous blood vessels, nerves, and lymphatic vessels. The dense and hard exterior surface bone is called **cortical** or **compact bone**.

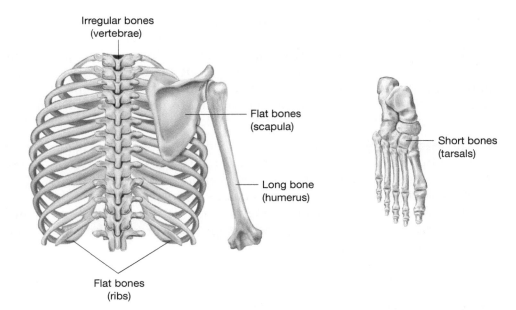

Irregular bones
(vertebrae)

Flat bones
(scapula)

Long bone
(humerus)

Flat bones
(ribs)

Short bones
(tarsals)

Cancellous or **spongy bone** is found inside the bone. As its name indicates, spongy bone has spaces in it, giving it a spongelike appearance. These spaces contain **red bone marrow**. Red bone marrow manufactures most of the blood cells and is found in some parts of all bones.

The center of the diaphysis contains an open canal called the **medullary cavity**. This cavity contains **yellow bone marrow**, which is mainly fat cells. Figure 2 ■ contains an illustration of the structure of long bones.

Bone Projections and Depressions

condyle (KON-dile)
epicondyle (ep-ih-KON-dile)
fissure (FISH-er)
foramen (for-AY-men)
fossa (FOSS-ah)
head

neck
process
sinus (SIGH-nus)
trochanter (tro-KAN-ter)
tubercle (TOO-ber-kl)
tuberosity (too-ber-OSS-ih-tee)

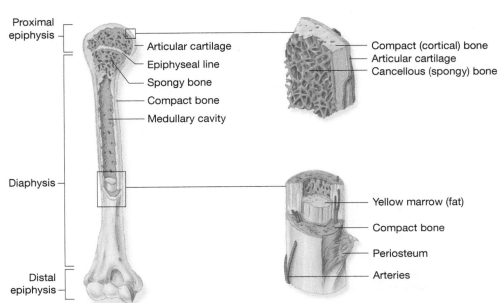

Proximal epiphysis

Articular cartilage
Epiphyseal line
Spongy bone
Compact bone
Medullary cavity

Compact (cortical) bone
Articular cartilage
Cancellous (spongy) bone

Diaphysis

Yellow marrow (fat)

Compact bone

Periosteum

Arteries

Distal epiphysis

■ **Figure 2** Components of a long bone. The entire long bone is on the left side accompanied by a blow-up of the proximal epiphysis and a section of the diaphysis.

Med Term Tip

The elbow, commonly referred to as the *funny bone*, is actually a projection of the ulna called the olecranon process.

Bones have many projections and depressions. Some are rounded and smooth in order to articulate with another bone in a joint. Others are rough to provide muscles with attachment points. The general term for any bony projection is a **process**. Then there are specific terms to describe the different shapes and locations of various processes. These terms are commonly used on operative reports and in physicians' records for clear identification of areas on the individual bones. Some of the common bony processes include the following:

1. The **head** is a large smooth ball-shaped end on a long bone. It may be separated from the body or shaft of the bone by a narrow area called the **neck**.
2. A **condyle** refers to a smooth rounded portion at the end of a bone.
3. The **epicondyle** is a projection located above or on a condyle.
4. The trochanter refers to a large rough process for the attachment of a muscle.
5. A **tubercle** is a small, rough process that provides the attachment for tendons and muscles.
6. The **tuberosity** is a large, rough process that provides the attachment of tendons and muscles.

See Figure 3 ■ for an illustration of the processes found on the femur.

In addition, bones have hollow regions or depressions. The most common depressions are as follows:

1. A **sinus**, which is a hollow cavity within a bone.
2. A **foramen**, which is a smooth round opening for nerves and blood vessels.
3. A **fossa**, which consists of a shallow cavity or depression on the surface of a bone.
4. A **fissure**, which is a slit-type opening.

■ **Figure 3** Bony processes found on the femur.

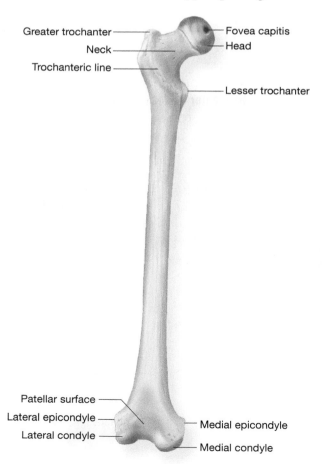

Greater trochanter

Fovea capitis

Neck

Head

Trochanteric line

Lesser trochanter

Patellar surface

Lateral epicondyle

Medial epicondyle

Lateral condyle

Medial condyle

Skeleton

appendicular skeleton (app-en-DIK-yoo-lar)   **axial skeleton** (AK-see-al)

The human skeleton has two divisions: the **axial skeleton** and the **appendicular skeleton**. Figures 4 and 8 illustrate the axial and appendicular skeletons.

Axial Skeleton

cervical vertebrae
coccyx (COCK-six)
cranium (KRAY-nee-um)
ethmoid bone (ETH-moyd)
facial bones
frontal bone
hyoid bone (HIGH-oyd)
intervertebral disc (in-ter-VER-teh-bral)
lacrimal bone (LACK-rim-al)
lumbar vertebrae
mandible (MAN-dih-bl)
maxilla (mack-SIH-lah)
nasal bone

occipital bone (ock-SIP-eh-tal)
palatine bone (PAL-ah-tine)
parietal bone (pah-RYE-eh-tal)
rib cage
sacrum (SAY-crum)
sphenoid bone (SFEE-noyd)
sternum (STER-num)
temporal bone (TEM-por-al)
thoracic vertebrae
vertebral column (VER-teh-bral)
vomer bone (VOH-mer)
zygomatic bone (zeye-go-MAT-ik)

The axial skeleton includes the bones in the head, neck, spine, chest, and trunk of the body (see Figure 4 ▪). These bones form the central axis for the whole body and protect many of the internal organs such as the brain, lungs, and heart.

The head or skull is divided into two parts consisting of the **cranium** and **facial bones**. These bones surround and protect the brain, eyes, ears, nasal cavity, and oral cavity from injury. The muscles for chewing and moving the head are attached to the cranial bones. The cranium encases the brain and consists of the **frontal, parietal, temporal, ethmoid, sphenoid,** and **occipital bones**. The facial bones surround the mouth, nose, and eyes and include the **mandible, maxilla, zygomatic, vomer, palatine, nasal,** and **lacrimal bones**. The cranial and facial bones are illustrated in Figure 5 ▪ and described in Table 1 ▪.

The **hyoid bone** is a single U-shaped bone suspended in the neck between the mandible and larynx. It is a point of attachment for swallowing and speech muscles.

The trunk of the body consists of the **vertebral column, sternum,** and **rib cage**. The vertebral or spinal column is divided into five sections: **cervical vertebrae, thoracic vertebrae, lumbar vertebrae, sacrum,** and **coccyx** (see Figure 6 ▪ and Table 2 ▪). Located between each pair of vertebrae, from the cervical through the lumbar regions, is an **intervertebral disc**. Each disc is composed of fibrocartilage to provide a cushion between the vertebrae. The rib cage has twelve pairs of ribs attached at the back to the vertebral column. Ten of the pairs are also attached to the sternum in the front (see Figure 7 ▪). The lowest two pairs are called *floating ribs* and are attached only to the vertebral column. The rib cage serves to provide support for organs, such as the heart and lungs.

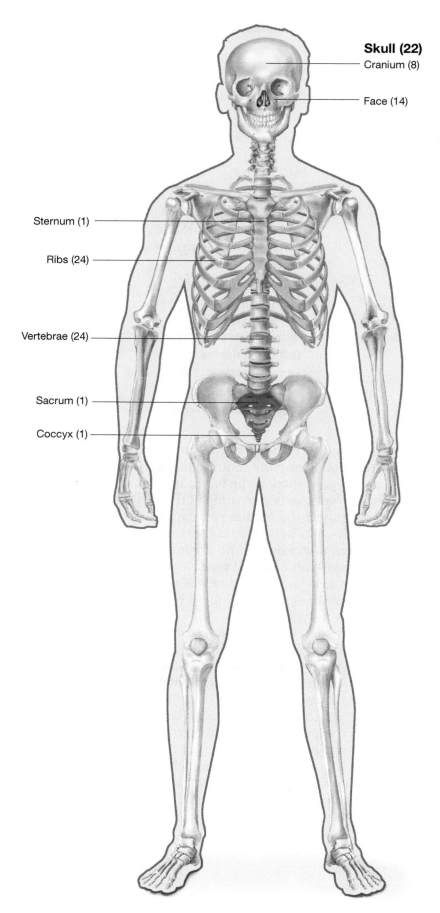

Skull (22)
Cranium (8)
Face (14)
Sternum (1)
Ribs (24)
Vertebrae (24)
Sacrum (1)
Coccyx (1)

■ Figure 4 Bones of the axial skeleton.

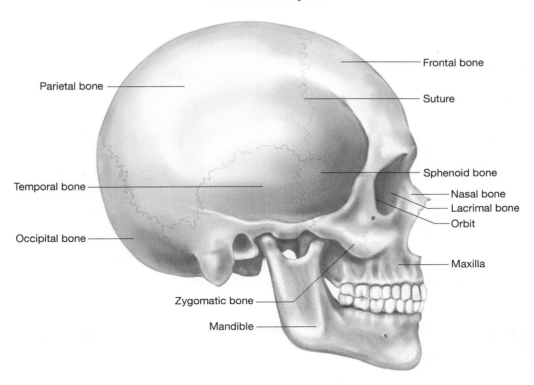

Figure 5 Bones of the skull.

Table 1	Bones of the Skull	
NAME	**NUMBER**	**DESCRIPTION**
Cranial Bones		
Frontal bone	1	Forehead
Parietal bone	2	Upper sides of cranium and roof of skull
Occipital bone	1	Back and base of skull
Temporal bone	2	Sides and base of cranium
Sphenoid bone	1	Bat-shaped bone that forms part of the base of the skull, floor, and sides of eye orbit
Ethmoid bone	1	Forms part of eye orbit, nose, and floor of cranium
Facial Bones		
Lacrimal bone	2	Inner corner of each eye
Nasal bone	2	Form part of nasal septum and support bridge of nose
Maxilla	1	Upper jaw
Mandible	1	Lower jawbone; only movable bone of the skull
Zygomatic bone	2	Cheekbones
Vomer bone	1	Base of nasal septum
Palatine bone	1	Hard palate (PAH lat) of mouth and floor of the nose

Figure 6 Divisions of the vertebral column.

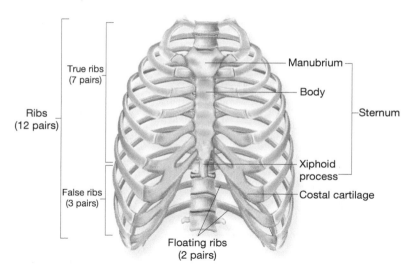

Figure 7 The structure of the rib cage.

Table 2	Bones of the Vertebral/Spinal Column	
NAME	**NUMBER**	**DESCRIPTION**
Cervical vertebra	7	Vertebrae in the neck region
Thoracic vertebra	12	Vertebrae in the chest region with ribs attached
Lumbar vertebra	5	Vertebrae in the small of the back, about waist level
Sacrum	1	Five vertebrae that become fused into one triangular-shaped flat bone at the base of the vertebral column
Coccyx	1	Three to five very small vertebrae attached to the sacrum, often become fused

Appendicular Skeleton

carpals (CAR-pals)
clavicle (CLAV-ih-kl)
femur (FEE-mer)
fibula (FIB-yoo-lah)
humerus (HYOO-mer-us)
ilium (ILL-ee-um)
innominate bone (ih-NOM-ih-nayt)
ischium (ISS-kee-um)
lower extremities
metacarpals (met-ah-CAR-pals)
metatarsals (met-ah-TAHR-sals)
os coxae (OSS KOK-sigh)

patella (pah-TELL-ah)
pectoral girdle
pelvic girdle
phalanges (fah-LAN-jeez)
pubis (PYOO-bis)
radius (RAY-dee-us)
scapula (SKAP-yoo-lah)
tarsals (TAHR-sals)
tibia (TIB-ee-ah)
ulna (UHL-nah)
upper extremities

Med Term Tip

The term *girdle*, meaning something that encircles or confines, refers to the entire bony structure of the shoulder and the pelvis. If just one bone from these areas is being discussed, like the ilium of the pelvis, it would be named as such. If, however, the entire pelvis is being discussed, it would be called the pelvic girdle.

The appendicular skeleton consists of the **pectoral girdle, upper extremities, pelvic girdle,** and **lower extremities** (see Figure 8 ■). These are the bones for our appendages or limbs and along with the muscles attached to them, they are responsible for body movement.

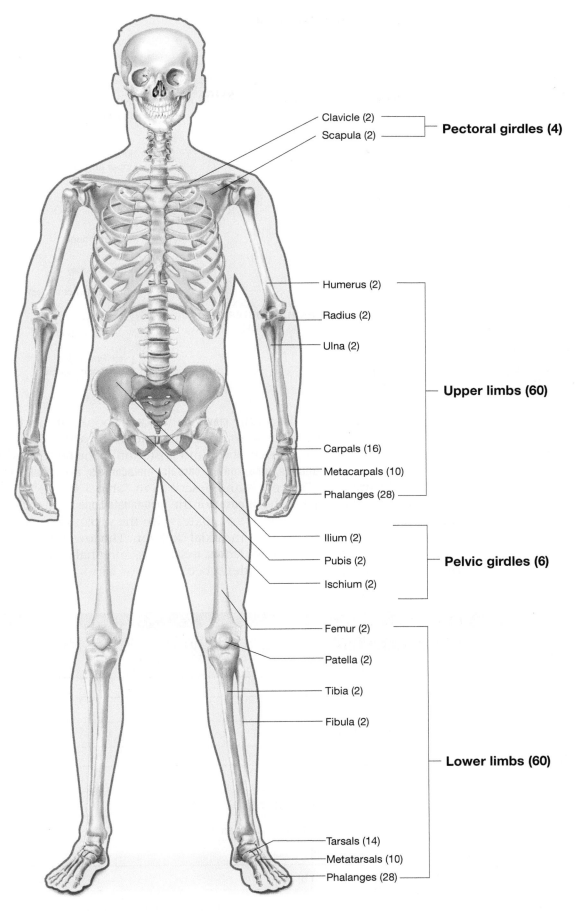

Pectoral girdles (4)
- Clavicle (2)
- Scapula (2)

Upper limbs (60)
- Humerus (2)
- Radius (2)
- Ulna (2)
- Carpals (16)
- Metacarpals (10)
- Phalanges (28)

Pelvic girdles (6)
- Ilium (2)
- Pubis (2)
- Ischium (2)

Lower limbs (60)
- Femur (2)
- Patella (2)
- Tibia (2)
- Fibula (2)
- Tarsals (14)
- Metatarsals (10)
- Phalanges (28)

■ **Figure 8** Bones of the appendicular skeleton.

Figure 9
Anatomical and
common names for the
pectoral girdle and
upper extremity.

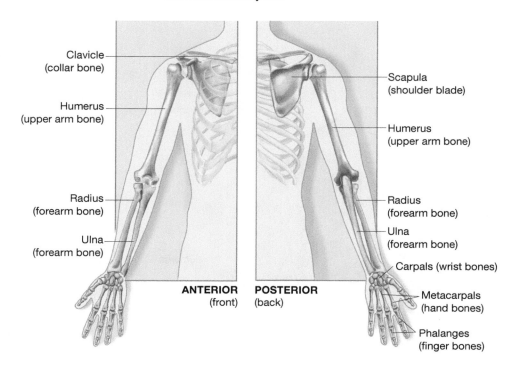

The pectoral girdle consists of the **clavicle** and **scapula** bones. It functions to attach the upper extremity, or arm, to the axial skeleton by articulating with the sternum anteriorly and the vertebral column posteriorly. The bones of the upper extremity include the **humerus, ulna, radius, carpals, metacarpals**, and **phalanges**. These bones are illustrated in Figure 9 ■ and described in Table 3 ■.

The pelvic girdle is called the **os coxae** or the **innominate bone** or hipbone. It contains the **ilium, ischium**, and **pubis**. It articulates with the sacrum posteriorly to attach the lower extremity, or leg, to the axial skeleton. The lower extremity bones include the **femur, patella, tibia, fibula, tarsals, metatarsals**, and phalanges. These bones are illustrated in Figure 10 ■ and described in Table 4 ■.

Table 3	Bones of the Pectoral Girdle and Upper Extremity	
NAME	**NUMBER**	**DESCRIPTION**
Pectoral Girdle		
Clavicle	2	Collar bone
Scapula	2	Shoulder blade
Upper Extremity		
Humerus	2	Upper arm bone
Radius	2	Forearm bone on thumb side of lower arm
Ulna	2	Forearm bone on little finger side of lower arm
Carpal	16	Bones of wrist
Metacarpals	10	Bones in palm of hand
Phalanges	28	Finger bones; three in each finger and two in each thumb

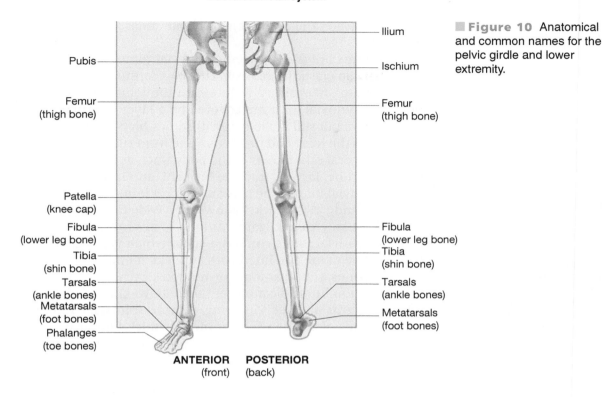

Pubis

Femur
(thigh bone)

Patella
(knee cap)

Fibula
(lower leg bone)

Tibia
(shin bone)

Tarsals
(ankle bones)

Metatarsals
(foot bones)

Phalanges
(toe bones)

Ilium

Ischium

Femur
(thigh bone)

Fibula
(lower leg bone)

Tibia
(shin bone)

Tarsals
(ankle bones)

Metatarsals
(foot bones)

ANTERIOR   **POSTERIOR**
(front)   (back)

■ Figure 10 Anatomical and common names for the pelvic girdle and lower extremity.

Joints

articulation (ar-tik-yoo-LAY-shun)   **joint capsule**
bursa (BER-sah)   **synovial fluid**
cartilaginous joints (car-tih-LAJ-ih-nus)   **synovial joint** (sin-OH-vee-al)
fibrous joints (FYE-bruss)   **synovial membrane**

Joints are formed when two or more bones meet. This is also referred to as an **articulation**. There are three types of joints based on the amount of movement

Table 4	Bones of the Pelvic Girdle and Lower Extremity	
NAME	**NUMBER**	**DESCRIPTION**
Pelvic Girdle/Os Coxae		
Ilium	2	Part of the hipbone
Ischium	2	Part of the hipbone
Pubis	2	Part of the hipbone
Lower Extremity		
Femur	2	Upper leg bone; thigh bone
Patella	2	Knee cap
Tibia	2	Shin bone; thicker lower leg bone
Fibula	2	Thinner, long bone in lateral side of lower leg
Tarsals	14	Ankle and heel bones
Metatarsals	10	Forefoot bones
Phalanges	28	Toe bones; three in each toe and two in each great toe

allowed between the bones: **synovial joints**, **cartilaginous joints**, and **fibrous joints** (see Figure 11 ■).

Most joints are freely moving synovial joints (see Figure 12 ■), which are enclosed by an elastic **joint capsule**. The joint capsule is lined with **synovial membrane**, which secretes **synovial fluid** to lubricate the joint. As noted earlier, the ends of bones in a synovial joint are covered by a layer of articular cartilage. Cartilage is very tough, but still flexible. It withstands high levels of stress to act as a shock absorber for the joint and prevents bone from rubbing against bone. Cartilage is found in several other areas of the body, such as the nasal septum, external ear, eustachian tube, larynx, trachea, bronchi, and intervertebral disks. One example of a synovial joint is the ball-and-socket joint found at the shoulder and hip. The ball rotating in the socket allows for a wide range of motion. Bands of strong connective tissue called ligaments bind bones together at the joint.

Some synovial joints contain a **bursa**, which is a saclike structure composed of connective tissue and lined with synovial membrane. Most commonly found between bones and ligaments or tendons, bursas function to reduce friction. Some common bursa locations are the elbow, knee, and shoulder joints.

Not all joints are freely moving. Fibrous joints allow almost no movement since the ends of the bones are joined by thick fibrous tissue, which may even fuse into solid bone. The sutures of the skull are an example of a fibrous joint. Cartilaginous joints allow for slight movement but hold bones firmly in place by a solid piece of cartilage. An example of this type of joint is the pubic symphysis, the point at which the left and right pubic bones meet in the front of the lower abdomen.

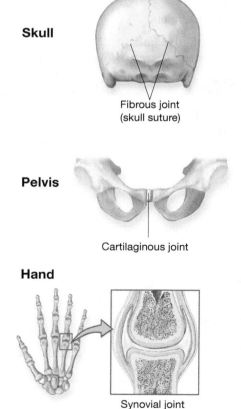

Figure 11 Examples of three types of joints found in the body.

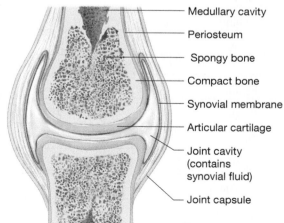

Figure 12 Structure of a generalized synovial joint.

Word Building

The following list contains examples of medical terms built directly from word parts. The definition for these terms can be determined by a straightforward translation of the word parts.

COMBINING FORM	COMBINED WITH	MEDICAL TERM	DEFINITION
arthr/o	-algia	**arthralgia** (ar-THRAL-jee-ah)	joint pain
	-centesis	**arthrocentesis** (ar-thro-sen-TEE-sis)	puncture to withdraw fluid from a joint
	-clasia	**arthroclasia** (ar-throh-KLAY-see-ah)	surgically breaking a joint
	-desis	**arthrodesis** (ar-throh-DEE-sis)	fusion of a joint
	-gram	**arthrogram** (AR-throh-gram)	record of a joint
	-itis	**arthritis** (ar-THRY-tis)	joint inflammation
	-otomy	**arthrotomy** (ar-THROT-oh-mee)	incision into a joint
	-scope	**arthroscope** (AR-throw-skop)	instrument to view inside a joint
burs/o	-ectomy	**bursectomy** (ber-SEK-toh-mee)	removal of a bursa
	-itis	**bursitis** (ber-SIGH-tis)	inflammation of a bursa
chondr/o	-ectomy	**chondrectomy** (kon-DREK-toh-mee)	removal of cartilage
	-malacia	**chondromalacia** (kon-droh-mah-LAY-she-ah)	cartilage softening
	-oma	**chondroma** (kon-DROH-mah)	cartilage tumor
	-plasty	**chondroplasty** (KON-droh-plas-tee)	surgical repair of cartilage
cortic/o	-al	**cortical** (KOR-ti-kal)	pertaining to the outer portion
crani/o	intra- -al	**intracranial** (in-trah-KRAY-nee-al)	pertaining to inside the skull
	-otomy	**craniotomy** (kray-nee-OTT-oh-mee)	incision into the skull
medull/o	-ary	**medullary** (MED-you-lair-ee)	pertaining to the inner portion
myel/o	-oma	**myeloma** (my-ah-LOH-mah)	bone marrow tumor
oste/o	-algia	**ostealgia** (oss-tee-AL-jee-ah)	bone pain
	chondr/o -oma	**osteochondroma** (oss-tee-oh-kon-DROH-mah)	bone and cartilage tumor
	-clasia	**osteoclasia** (oss-tee-oh-KLAY-see-ah)	to surgically break a bone
	myel/o -itis	**osteomyelitis** (oss-tee-oh-mi-ell-EYE-tis)	inflammation of bone and bone marrow
	-otomy	**osteotomy** (oss-tee-OTT-ah-me)	incision into a bone
	-pathy	**osteopathy** (oss-tee-OPP-ah-thee)	bone disease
	-tome	**osteotome** (OSS-tee-oh-tohm)	instrument to cut bone
synov/o	-itis	**synovitis** (sih-no-VI-tis)	inflammation of synovial membrane
	-ectomy	**synovectomy** (sih-no-VEK-toh-mee)	removal of the synovial membrane
vertebr/o	inter- -al	**intervertebral** (in-ter-VER-teh-bral)	pertaining to between vertebrae

Building Adjective Forms of Bone Names

It is important to learn the names and combining forms of all the bones in medical terminology because they are so frequently used as adjectives to indicate location.

ADJECTIVE SUFFIX	COMBINED WITH	ADJECTIVE FORM	NOUN FORM
-ac	ili/o	**iliac** (ILL-ee-ack)	ilium
-al	carp/o	**carpal** (CAR-pal)	carpus
	cervic/o	**cervical** (CER-vih-kal)	neck
	cost/o	**costal** (COAST-all)	rib
	crani/o	**cranial** (KRAY-nee-all)	cranium
	femor/o	**femoral** (FEM-or-all)	femur
	humer/o	**humeral** (HYOO-mer-all)	humerus
	ischi/o	**ischial** (ISH-ee-all)	ischium
	metacarp/o	**metacarpal** (met-ah-CAR-pal)	metacarpus
	metatars/o	**metatarsal** (met-ah-TAHR-sal)	metatarsus
	radi/o	**radial** (RAY-dee-all)	radius
	sacr/o	**sacral** (SAY-kral)	sacrum
	stern/o	**sternal** (STER-nal)	sternum
	tars/o	**tarsal** (TAHR-sal)	tarsus
	tibi/o	**tibial** (TIB-ee-all)	tibia
-ar	clavicul/o	**clavicular** (cla-VIK-yoo-lar)	clavicle
	fibul/o	**fibular** (FIB-yoo-lar)	fibula
	lumb/o	**lumbar** (LUM-bar)	low back
	mandibul/o	**mandibular** (man-DIB-yoo-lar)	mandible
	patell/o	**patellar** (pa-TELL-ar)	patella
	scapul/o	**scapular** (SKAP-yoo-lar)	scapula
	uln/o	**ulnar** (UHL-nar)	ulna
-ary	maxill/o	**maxillary** (mack-sih-LAIR-ree)	maxilla
-eal	coccyg/o	**coccygeal** (cock-eh-JEE-all)	coccyx
	phalang/o	**phalangeal** (fay-lan-JEE-all)	phalanges
-ic	pelv/o	**pelvic** (PEL-vik)	pelvis
	pub/o	**pubic** (PYOO-bik)	pubis
	thorac/o	**thoracic** (tho-RASS-ik)	thorax

Vocabulary

TERM	DEFINITION
callus (KAL-us)	The mass of bone tissue that forms at a fracture site during its healing.
cast	Application of a solid material to immobilize an extremity or portion of the body as a result of a fracture, dislocation, or severe injury. It may be made of plaster of Paris or fiberglass.
chiropractic (ki-roh-PRAK-tik)	Healthcare profession concerned with diagnosis and treatment of malalignment conditions of the spine and musculoskeletal system with the intention of affecting the nervous system and improving health. Healthcare professional is a *chiropractor.*
crepitation (krep-ih-TAY-shun)	The noise produced by bones or cartilage rubbing together in conditions such as arthritis. Also called *crepitus.*
exostosis (eck-sos-TOH-sis)	A bone spur.
kyphosis (ki-FOH-sis)	Abnormal increase in the outward curvature of the thoracic spine. Also known as *hunchback* or *humpback*. See Figure 13 ■ for an illustration of abnormal spine curvatures.

Kyphosis
(excessive posterior thoracic
curvature - hunchback)

Lordosis
(excessive anterior lumbar
curvature - swayback)

Scoliosis
(lateral curvature)

■ **Figure 13** Abnormal spinal curvatures: kyphosis, lordosis, and scoliosis.

Vocabulary *(continued)*

TERM	DEFINITION
lordosis (lor-DOH-sis)	Abnormal increase in the forward curvature of the lumbar spine. Also known as *swayback*. See Figure 13 for an illustration of abnormal spine curvatures.
orthopedics (or-thoh-PEE-diks)	Branch of medicine specializing in the diagnosis and treatment of conditions of the musculoskeletal system. Also called *orthopedic surgery*. Physician is an *orthopedist* or *orthopedic surgeon*. Name derived from straightening (*orth/o*) deformities in children (*ped/o*).
orthotic (or-THOT-ik)	A brace or splint used to prevent or correct deformities. Person skilled in making and adjusting orthotics is an *orthotist*.
podiatry (po-DYE-ah-tree)	Healthcare profession specializing in diagnosis and treatment of disorders of the feet and lower legs. Healthcare professional is a *podiatrist*.
prosthesis (pross-THEE-sis)	Artificial device that is used as a substitute for a body part that is either congenitally missing or absent as a result of accident or disease. An example would be an artificial leg.
prosthetics (pross-THET-iks)	Healthcare profession specializing in making artificial body parts. Person skilled in making and adjusting prostheses is a *prosthetist*.

Pathology

TERM	DEFINITION
■ *Fractures*	
closed fracture ■ **Figure 14** A) Closed (or simple) fracture and B) open (or compound) fracture.	Fracture in which there is no open skin wound. Also called a *simple fracture*.

A

B

Pathology *(continued)*

TERM	DEFINITION
Colles' (COL-eez) **fracture** ■ **Figure 15** Colles' fracture. *(Charles Stewart MD FACEP, FAAEM)*	A common type of wrist fracture.
comminuted fracture (kom-ih-NYOOT-ed)	Fracture in which the bone is shattered, splintered, or crushed into many small pieces or fragments.
compound fracture	Fracture in which the skin has been broken through to the fracture. Also called an *open fracture* (see also Figure 14B).
compression fracture	Fracture involving loss of height of a vertebral body. It may be the result of trauma, but in older persons, especially women, it may be caused by conditions like osteoporosis.
fracture (FX, Fx)	A broken bone.
greenstick fracture	Fracture in which there is an incomplete break; one side of bone is broken and the other side is bent. This type of fracture is commonly found in children due to their softer and more pliable bone structure.
impacted fracture	Fracture in which bone fragments are pushed into each other.
oblique (oh-BLEEK) **fracture** ■ **Figure 16** X-ray showing oblique fracture of the humerus. *(Charles Stewart MD FACEP, FAAEM)*	Fracture at an angle to the bone.
pathologic (path-a-LOJ-ik) **fracture**	Fracture caused by diseased or weakened bone.
spiral fracture	Fracture in which the fracture line spirals around the shaft of the bone. Can be caused by a twisting injury and is often slower to heal than other types of fractures.
stress fracture	A slight fracture caused by repetitive low-impact forces, like running, rather than a single forceful impact.

Pathology (continued)

TERM	DEFINITION
transverse fracture	Complete fracture that is straight across the bone at right angles to the long axis of the bone (see Figure 17 ■).

■ Bones

TERM	DEFINITION
Ewing's sarcoma (YOO-wings sar-KOH-mah)	Malignant growth found in the shaft of long bones that spreads through the periosteum. Removal is treatment of choice, because this tumor will metastasize or spread to other organs.
osteogenic sarcoma (oss-tee-oh-GIN-ik sark-OH-mah)	The most common type of bone cancer. Usually begins in osteocytes found at the ends of long bones.
osteomalacia (oss-tee-oh-mah-LAY-she-ah)	Softening of the bones caused by a deficiency of calcium. It is thought that in children the cause is insufficient sunlight and vitamin D.
osteoporosis (oss-tee-oh-por-ROH-sis)	Decrease in bone mass that results in a thinning and weakening of the bone with resulting fractures. The bone becomes more porous, especially in the spine and pelvis.
Paget's (PAH-jets) **disease**	A fairly common metabolic disease of the bone from unknown causes. It usually attacks middle-aged and elderly people and is characterized by bone destruction and deformity. Named for Sir James Paget, a British surgeon.
rickets (RIK-ets)	Deficiency in calcium and vitamin D found in early childhood that results in bone deformities, especially bowed legs.

■ Spinal Column

TERM	DEFINITION
ankylosing spondylitis (ang-kih-LOH-sing spon-dih-LYE-tis)	Inflammatory spinal condition that resembles rheumatoid arthritis. Results in gradual stiffening and fusion of the vertebrae. More common in men than women.
herniated nucleus pulposus (HNP) (HER-nee-ated NOO-klee-us pull-POH-sus)	Herniation or protrusion of an intervertebral disk; also called *herniated disk* or *ruptured disk*. May require surgery (see Figure 18 ■).
scoliosis (skoh-lee-OH-sis)	Abnormal lateral curvature of the spine. See Figure 13 for an illustration of abnormal spine curvatures.
spina bifida (SPY-nah BIF-ih-dah)	Congenital anomaly that occurs when a vertebra fails to fully form around the spinal cord.
spinal stenosis (ste-NOH-sis)	Narrowing of the spinal canal causing pressure on the cord and nerves.
spondylolisthesis (spon-dih-loh-liss-THEE-sis)	The forward sliding of a lumbar vertebra over the vertebra below it.
spondylosis (spon-dih-LOH-sis)	Specifically refers to ankylosing of the spine, but commonly used in reference to any degenerative condition of the vertebral column.
whiplash	Injury to the bones in the cervical spine as a result of a sudden movement forward and backward of the head and neck. Can occur as a result of a rear-end auto collision.

■ Joints

TERM	DEFINITION
bunion (BUN-yun)	Inflammation of the bursa of the first metatarsophalangeal joint (base of the big toe).

Figure 17 X-ray showing transverse fracture of radius. *(James Stevenson/Science Photo Library/ Photo Researchers, Inc.)*

Figure 18 Color enhanced magnetic resonance imaging (MRI) image demonstrating a herniated nucleus pulposus putting pressure on the spinal cord (see arrows). *(ISM/Phototake NYC)*

Pathology *(continued)*

TERM	DEFINITION
dislocation	Occurs when the bones in a joint are displaced from their normal alignment and the ends of the bones are no longer in contact.
osteoarthritis (OA) (oss-tee-oh-ar-THRY-tis)	Arthritis resulting in degeneration of the bones and joints, especially those bearing weight. Results in bone rubbing against bone.
rheumatoid arthritis (RA) (ROO-mah-toyd ar-THRY-tis) **Figure 19** Patient with typical rheumatoid arthritis contractures.	Chronic form of arthritis with inflammation of the joints, swelling, stiffness, pain, and changes in the cartilage that can result in crippling deformities; considered to be an autoimmune disease. *(Michal Heran/Pearson Education/PH College)*
sprain	Damage to the ligaments surrounding a joint due to overstretching, but no dislocation of the joint or fracture of the bone.
subluxation (sub-LUCKS-a-shun)	An incomplete dislocation, the joint alignment is disrupted, but the ends of the bones remain in contact.
systemic lupus erythematosus (SLE) (sis-TEM-ik LOOP-us air-ih-them-ah-TOH-sis)	Chronic inflammatory autoimmune disease of connective tissue affects many systems that may include joint pain and arthritis. May be mistaken for rheumatoid arthritis.
talipes (TAL-ih-peez)	Congenital deformity causing misalignment of the ankle joint and foot. Also referred to as a *clubfoot*.

Diagnostic Procedures

TERM	DEFINITION
■ Diagnostic Imaging	
arthrography (ar-THROG-rah-fee)	Visualization of a joint by radiographic study after injection of a contrast medium into the joint space.
bone scan	A nuclear medicine procedure in which the patient is given a radioactive dye and then scanning equipment is used to visualize bones. It is especially useful in identifying stress fractures, observing progress of treatment for osteomyelitis and locating cancer metastases to the bone.
dual-energy absorptiometry (DXA) (ab-sorp-she-AHM-eh-tree)	Measurement of bone density using low dose x-ray for the purpose of detecting osteoporosis.
myelography (my-eh-LOG-rah-fee)	Study of the spinal column after injecting opaque contrast material; particularly useful in identifying herniated nucleus pulposus pinching a spinal nerve.
radiography	A diagnostic imaging procedure using x-rays to study the internal structure of the body; especially useful for visualizing bones and joints.
■ Endoscopic Procedures	
arthroscopy (ar-THROS-koh-pee)	Examination of the interior of a joint by entering the joint with an *arthroscope*. The arthroscope contains a small television camera that allows the physician to view the interior of the joint on a monitor during the procedure. Some joint conditions can be repaired during arthroscopy.

Therapeutic Procedures

TERM	DEFINITION
■ Surgical Procedures	
amputation (am-pew-TAY-shun)	Partial or complete removal of a limb for a variety of reasons, including tumors, gangrene, intractable pain, crushing injury, or uncontrollable infection.
arthroscopic surgery (ar-throh-SKOP-ic)	Performing a surgical procedure while using an arthroscope to view the internal structure, such as a joint.
bone graft	Piece of bone taken from the patient used to take the place of a removed bone or a bony defect at another site.
bunionectomy (bun-yun-ECK-toh-mee)	Removal of the bursa at the joint of the great toe.
laminectomy (lam-ih-NEK-toh-mee)	Removal of the vertebral posterior arch to correct severe back problems and pain caused by compression of a spinal nerve.
percutaneous diskectomy (per-kyou-TAY-nee-us disk-EK-toh-mee)	A thin catheter tube is inserted into the intervertebral disk through the skin and the herniated or ruptured disk material is sucked out or a laser is used to vaporize it.
spinal fusion	Surgical immobilization of adjacent vertebrae. This may be done for several reasons, including correction for a herniated disk.
total hip arthroplasty (THA) (ar-thro-PLAS-tee)	Surgical reconstruction of a hip by implanting a prosthetic or artificial hip joint. Also called *total hip replacement (THR)* (see Figure 20).

■ Figure 20 Prosthetic hip joint. *(Lawrence Livermore National Library/Science Photo Library/Photo Researchers, Inc.)*

Therapeutic Procedures *(continued)*

TERM	DEFINITION
total knee arthroplasty (TKA) (ar-thro-PLAS-tee)	Surgical reconstruction of a knee joint by implanting a prosthetic knee joint. Also called *total knee replacement (TKR)*.
■ Fracture Care	
fixation	A procedure to stabilize a fractured bone while it heals. *External fixation* includes casts, splints, and pins inserted through the skin. *Internal fixation* includes pins, plates, rods, screws, and wires that are applied during an *open reduction*.
reduction	Correcting a fracture by realigning the bone fragments. *Closed reduction* is doing this manipulation without entering the body. *Open reduction* is the process of making a surgical incision at the site of the fracture to do the reduction. This is necessary when bony fragments need to be removed or *internal fixation* such as plates or pins are required.
traction	Applying a pulling force on a fractured or dislocated limb or the vertebral column in order to restore normal alignment.

Pharmacology

CLASSIFICATION	ACTION	GENERIC AND BRAND NAMES
bone reabsorption inhibitors	Conditions that result in weak and fragile bones, such as osteoporosis and Paget's disease, are improved by medications that reduce the reabsorption of bones.	alendronate, Fosamax; ibandronate, Boniva
calcium supplements and Vitamin D therapy	Maintaining high blood levels of calcium in association with vitamin D helps maintain bone density; used to treat osteomalacia, osteoporosis, and rickets.	calcium carbonate, Oystercal, Tums; calcium citrate, Cal-Citrate, Citracal
corticosteroids	A hormone produced by the adrenal cortex that has very strong anti-inflammatory properties. It is particularly useful in treating rheumatoid arthritis.	prednisone; methylprednisolone, Medrol; dexamethasone, Decadron
nonsteroidal anti-inflammatory drugs (NSAIDs)	A large group of drugs that provide mild pain relief and anti-inflammatory benefits for conditions such as arthritis.	ibuprofen, Advil, Motrin; naproxen, Aleve, Naprosyn; salicylates, Aspirin

Abbreviations

AE	above elbow
AK	above knee
BDT	bone density testing
BE	below elbow
BK	below knee
BMD	bone mineral density
C1, C2, etc.	first cervical vertebra, second cervical vertebra, etc.
Ca	calcium
DJD	degenerative joint disease
DXA	dual-energy absorptiometry
FX, Fx	fracture
HNP	herniated nucleus pulposus
JRA	juvenile rheumatoid arthritis
L1, L2, etc.	first lumbar vertebra, second lumbar vertebra, etc.
LE	lower extremity
LLE	left lower extremity
LUE	left upper extremity
NSAID	nonsteroidal anti-inflammatory drug
OA	osteoarthritis
ORIF	open reduction–internal fixation
Orth, ortho	orthopedics
RA	rheumatoid arthritis
RLE	right lower extremity
RUE	right upper extremity
SLE	systemic lupus erythematosus
T1, T2, etc.	first thoracic vertebra, second thoracic vertebra, etc.
THA	total hip arthroplasty
THR	total hip replacement
TKA	total knee arthroplasty
TKR	total knee replacement
UE	upper extremity

Section II: Muscular System at a Glance

Function

Muscles are bundles, sheets, or rings of tissue that produce movement by contracting and pulling on the structures to which they are attached.

Organs

muscles

Combining Forms

fasci/o	fibrous band
fibr/o	fibers
kinesi/o	movement
muscul/o	muscle
my/o	muscle
myocardi/o	heart muscle
myos/o	muscle
plant/o	sole of foot
ten/o	tendon
tend/o	tendon
tendin/o	tendon

Suffixes

-asthenia	weakness
-kinesia	movement
-tonia	tone

Prefixes

ab-	away from
ad-	toward
circum-	around

Muscular System Illustrated

Masseter

Sternocleidomastoid

Deltoid

Pectoralis Major

Triceps

Biceps

Rectus abdominis

External oblique

Adductor femoris

Sartorius

Quadriceps femoris

Vastus medialis

Gastrocnemius

Tibialis anterior

Anatomy and Physiology of the Muscular System

muscle tissue fibers   **muscles**

Muscles are bundles of parallel **muscle tissue fibers**. As these fibers contract (shorten in length) they produce movement of or within the body. The movement may take the form of bringing two bones closer together, pushing food through the digestive system, or pumping blood through blood vessels. In addition to producing movement, muscles also hold the body erect and generate heat.

Types of Muscles

cardiac muscle   **smooth muscle**
involuntary muscles   **voluntary muscles**
skeletal muscle

The three types of muscle tissue are **skeletal muscle**, **smooth muscle**, and **cardiac muscle** (see Figure 21 ■). Muscle tissue may be either voluntary or involuntary. **Voluntary muscles** mean that a person consciously chooses which muscles to contract and how long and how hard to contract them. The skeletal muscles of the arm and leg are examples of this type of muscle. **Involuntary muscles** are under the control of the subconscious regions of the brain. The smooth muscles found in internal organs and cardiac muscles are examples of involuntary muscle tissue.

Med Term Tip

The term *muscle* is the diminutive form of the Latin word *mus* or "little mouse." This is thought to describe how the skin ripples when a muscle contracts, like a little mouse running.

■ **Figure 21** The three types of muscles: skeletal, smooth, and cardiac.

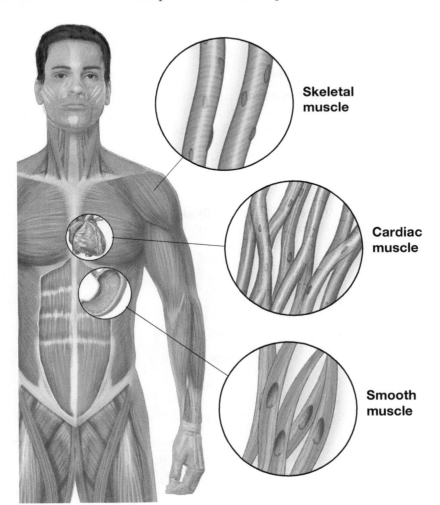

Skeletal muscle

Cardiac muscle

Smooth muscle

Skeletal Muscle

fascia (FASH-ee-ah)
motor neurons
myoneural junction (MY-oh-NOO-rall)

striated muscle (stry-a-ted)
tendon (TEN-dun)

Skeletal muscles are directly or indirectly attached to bones and produce voluntary movement of the skeleton. It is also referred to as **striated muscle** because of its striped appearance under the microscope (see Figure 22 ■). Each muscle is wrapped in layers of fibrous connective tissue called **fascia**. The fascia tapers at each end of a skeletal muscle to form a very strong **tendon**. The tendon then inserts into the periosteum covering a bone to anchor the muscle to the bone. Skeletal muscles are stimulated by **motor neurons** of the nervous system. The point at which the motor nerve contacts a muscle fiber is called the **myoneural junction**.

Smooth Muscle

visceral muscle (vis-she-ral)

Smooth muscle tissue is found in association with internal organs. For this reason, it is also referred to as **visceral muscle**. The name smooth muscle refers to the muscle's microscopic appearance—it lacks the striations of skeletal muscle (see Figure 22). Smooth muscle is found in the walls of the hollow organs, such as the stomach, tube-shaped organs, such as the respiratory airways, and blood vessels. It is responsible for the involuntary muscle action associated with movement of the internal organs, such as churning food, constricting a blood vessel, and uterine contractions.

Cardiac Muscle

myocardium (my-oh-CAR-dee-um)

Cardiac muscle, or **myocardium**, makes up the wall of the heart (see Figure 22). With each involuntary contraction the heart squeezes to pump blood out of its chambers and through the blood vessels.

■ **Figure 22** Characteristics of the three types of muscles.

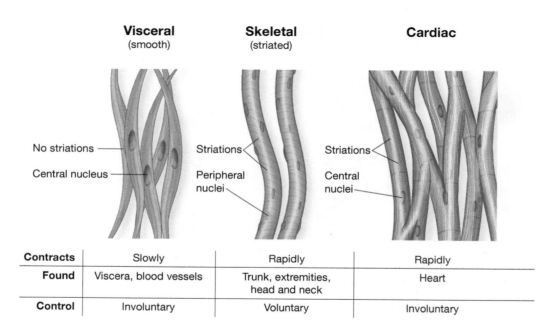

	Visceral (smooth)	Skeletal (striated)	Cardiac
Contracts	Slowly	Rapidly	Rapidly
Found	Viscera, blood vessels	Trunk, extremities, head and neck	Heart
Control	Involuntary	Voluntary	Involuntary

Naming Skeletal Muscles

biceps (BYE-seps)

extensor carpi

external oblique

flexor carpi

gluteus maximus (GLOO-tee-us
MACKS-ih-mus)

rectus abdominis (REK-tus ab-DOM-ih-nis)

sternocleidomastoid (STER-noh-KLY-doh-
MASS-toid)

The name of a muscle often reflects its location, origin and insertion, size, action, fiber direction, or number of attachment points, as the following examples illustrate.

- **Location:** The term **rectus abdominis** means straight (rectus) abdominal muscle.
- **Origin and insertion:** The **sternocleidomastoid** is named for its two origins (stern/o for sternum and cleid/o for clavicle) and single insertion (mastoid process).
- **Size:** When gluteus, meaning rump area, is combined with maximus, meaning large, we have the term **gluteus maximus**.
- **Action:** The **flexor carpi** and **extensor carpi** muscles are named because they produce flexion and extension at the wrist.
- **Fiber direction:** The **external oblique** muscle is an abdominal muscle whose fibers run at an oblique angle.
- **Number of attachment points:** The term *bi*, meaning two, can form the medical term **biceps**, which refers to the muscle in the upper arm that has two heads or connecting points.

Skeletal Muscle Actions

action

antagonistic pairs

insertion

origin

Skeletal muscles are attached to two different bones and overlap a joint. When a muscle contracts, the two bones move, but not usually equally. The less movable of the two bones is considered to be the starting point of the muscle and is called the **origin**. The more movable bone is considered to be where the muscle ends and is called the **insertion**. The type of movement a muscle produces is called its **action**. Muscles are often arranged around joints in **antagonistic pairs**, meaning they produce opposite actions. For example, one muscle will bend a joint while its antagonist is responsible for straightening the joint. Some common terminology for muscle actions are described in Table 5 ■.

Table 5	Muscle Actions
ACTION	**DESCRIPTION**
Grouped by antagonistic pairs	
abduction (ab-DUCK-shun)	Movement away from midline of the body (see Figure 23 ■)
adduction (ah-DUCK-shun)	Movement toward midline of the body (see Figure 23)
flexion (FLEK-shun)	Act of bending or being bent (see Figure 24 ■)
extension (eks-TEN-shun)	Movement that brings limb into or toward a straight condition (see Figure 24)
dorsiflexion (dor-see-FLEK-shun)	Backward bending, as of hand or foot (see Figure 25A ■)
plantar flexion (PLAN-tar-FLEK-shun)	Bending sole of foot; pointing toes downward (see Figure 25B ■)

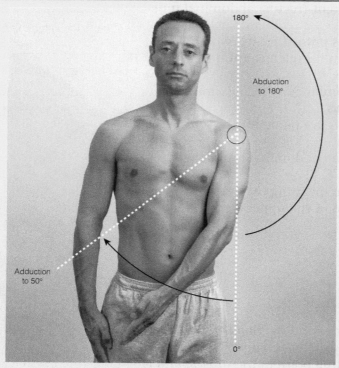

■ **Figure 23** Abduction and adduction of the shoulder joint.

■ **Figure 24** Flexion and extension of the elbow joint.

■ **Figure 25** Dorsiflexion (a) and plantar flexion (b) of the ankle joint.

Table 5	Muscle Actions (continued)
ACTION	**DESCRIPTION**
eversion (ee-VER-zhun)	Turning outward (see Figure 26 ▪)
inversion (in-VER-zhun)	Turning inward (see Figure 26)
pronation (proh-NAY-shun)	To turn downward or backward as with the hand or foot (see Figure 27 ▪)
supination (soo-pin-NAY-shun)	Turning the palm or foot upward (see Figure 27)
elevation	To raise a body part, as in shrugging the shoulders
depression	A downward movement, as in dropping the shoulders
	The circular actions described below are an exception to the antagonistic pair arrangement
circumduction (sir-kum-DUCK-shun)	Movement in a circular direction from a central point. Imagine drawing a large circle in the air
opposition	Moving thumb away from palm; the ability to move the thumb into contact with the other fingers **Med Term Tip** Primates are the only animals with opposable thumbs.
rotation	Moving around a central axis

■ **Figure 26** Eversion and inversion of the foot.

■ **Figure 27** Pronation and supination of the forearm.

Word Building

The following list contains examples of medical terms built directly from word parts. The definition for these terms can be determined by a straightforward translation of the word parts.

COMBINING FORM	COMBINED WITH PREFIX	MEDICAL TERM	DEFINITION
fasci/o	-al	**fascial** (FAS-ee-all)	pertaining to fascia
	-itis	**fasciitis** (fas-ee-EYE-tis)	inflammation of fascia
	-otomy	**fasciotomy** (fas-ee-OT-oh-mee)	incision into fascia
kinesi/o	-logy	**kinesiology** (kih-NEE-see-oh-loh-jee)	study of movement
muscul/o	-ar	**muscular** (MUSS-kew-lar)	pertaining to muscles
my/o	-algia	**myalgia** (my-AL-jee-ah)	muscle pain
	-asthenia	**myasthenia** (my-ass-THEE-nee-ah)	muscle weakness
	electr/o -gram	**electromyogram** (EMG) (ee-lek-troh-MY-oh-gram)	record of muscle electricity
	cardi/o -al	**myocardial** (my-oh-CAR-dee-al)	pertaining to heart muscle
	-pathy	**myopathy** (my-OPP-ah-thee)	muscle disease
	-plasty	**myoplasty** (MY-oh-plas-tee)	surgical repair of muscle
	-rrhaphy	**myorrhaphy** (MY-or-ah-fee)	suture a muscle
	-rrhexis	**myorrhexis** (my-oh-REK-sis)	muscle rupture
myos/o	poly- -itis	**polymyositis** (pol-ee-my-oh-SIGH-tis)	inflammation of many muscles
ten/o	-dynia	**tenodynia** (ten-oh-DIN-ee-ah)	tendon pain
	-plasty	**tenoplasty** (TEN-oh-plas-tee)	surgical repair of a tendon
	-rrhaphy	**tenorrhaphy** (tah-NOR-ah-fee)	suture a tendon
tend/o	-plasty	**tendoplasty** (TEN-doh-plas-tee)	surgical repair of tendon
	-otomy	**tendotomy** (tend-OT-oh-mee)	incision into tendon
tendin/o	-itis	**tendinitis** (ten-dih-NIGH-tis)	inflammation of tendon
	-ous	**tendinous** (TEN-din-us)	pertaining to tendons

SUFFIX	COMBINED WITH PREFIX	MEDICAL TERM	DEFINITION
-kinesia	brady-	**bradykinesia** (brad-ee-kih-NEE-see-ah)	slow movement
	dys-	**dyskinesia** (dis-kih-NEE-see-ah)	difficult or painful movement
	hyper-	**hyperkinesia** (high-per-kih-NEE-see-ah)	excessive movement
	hypo-	**hypokinesia** (HI-poh-kih-NEE-see-ah)	insufficient movement
-tonia	a-	**atonia**	lack of tone
	dys-	**dystonia**	abnormal tone
	hyper-	**hypertonia**	excessive tone
	hypo-	**hypotonia**	insufficient tone
	my/o	**myotonia**	muscle tone

Vocabulary

TERM	DEFINITION
adhesion	Scar tissue forming in the fascia surrounding a muscle, making it difficult to stretch the muscle.
atrophy (AT-rah-fee)	Poor muscle development as a result of muscle disease, nervous system disease, or lack of use; commonly referred to as *muscle wasting*.
contracture (kon-TRACK-chur)	Abnormal shortening of muscle fibers, tendons, or fascia making it difficult to stretch the muscle.
hypertrophy (high-PER-troh-fee)	Increase in muscle bulk as a result of using it, as in lifting weights
intermittent claudication (klaw-dih-KAY-shun)	Attacks of severe pain and lameness caused by ischemia of the muscles, typically the calf muscles; brought on by walking even very short distances.
spasm	Sudden, involuntary, strong muscle contraction.
torticollis (tore-tih-KOLL-iss)	Severe neck spasms pulling the head to one side. Commonly called *wryneck* or a *crick in the neck*.

Pathology

TERM	DEFINITION
■ *Muscles*	
fibromyalgia (figh-broh-my-AL-jee-ah)	Condition with widespread aching and pain in the muscles and soft tissue.
lateral epicondylitis (ep-ih-kon-dih-LYE-tis)	Inflammation of the muscle attachment to the lateral epicondyle of the elbow. Often caused by strongly gripping. Commonly called *tennis elbow*.
muscular dystrophy (MD) (MUSS-kew-ler DIS-troh-fee)	Inherited disease causing a progressive muscle degeneration, weakness, and atrophy.
pseudohypertrophic muscular dystrophy (soo-doh-HIGH-per-troh-fic)	One type of inherited muscular dystrophy in which the muscle tissue is gradually replaced by fatty tissue, making the muscle look strong. Also called *Duchenne's muscular dystrophy*.
■ *Tendons, Muscles, and/or Ligaments*	
carpal tunnel syndrome (CTS)	Repetitive motion disorder with pain caused by compression of the finger flexor tendons and median nerve as they pass through the carpal tunnel of the wrist.
ganglion cyst (GANG-lee-on)	Cyst that forms on tendon sheath, usually on hand, wrist, or ankle.
repetitive motion disorder	Group of chronic disorders involving the tendon, muscle, joint, and nerve damage, resulting from the tissue being subjected to pressure, vibration, or repetitive movements for prolonged periods.
rotator cuff injury	The rotator cuff consists of the joint capsule of the shoulder joint reinforced by the tendons from several shoulder muscles. The high degree of flexibility at the shoulder joint puts the rotator cuff at risk for strain and tearing.
strain	Damage to the muscle, tendons, or ligaments due to overuse or overstretching.

Diagnostic Procedures

TERM	DEFINITION
■ Clinical Laboratory Test	
creatine phosphokinase (CPK) (KREE-ah-teen foss-foe-KYE-nase)	Muscle enzyme found in skeletal muscle and cardiac muscle. Blood levels become elevated in disorders such as heart attack, muscular dystrophy, and other skeletal muscle pathologies.
■ Additional Diagnostic Procedures	
deep tendon reflexes (DTR)	Muscle contraction in response to a stretch caused by striking the muscle tendon with a reflex hammer. Test used to determine if muscles are responding properly.
electromyography (EMG) (ee-lek-troh-my-OG-rah-fee)	Study and record of the strength and quality of muscle contractions as a result of electrical stimulation.
muscle biopsy (BYE-op-see)	Removal of muscle tissue for pathological examination.

Treatment Procedures

TERM	DEFINITION
■ Surgical Procedures	
carpal tunnel release	Surgical cutting of the ligament in the wrist to relieve nerve pressure caused by carpal tunnel syndrome, which can result from repetitive motion such as typing.
tenodesis (ten-oh-DEE-sis)	Surgical procedure to stabilize a joint by anchoring down the tendons of the muscles that move the joint.

Pharmacology

CLASSIFICATION	ACTION	GENERIC AND BRAND NAMES
skeletal muscle relaxants	Medication to relax skeletal muscles in order to reduce muscle spasms. Also called *antispasmodics*.	cyclobenzaprine, Flexeril; carisoprodol, Soma

Abbreviations

CTS	carpal tunnel syndrome	**EMG**	electromyogram
CPK	creatine phosphokinase	**IM**	intramuscular
DTR	deep tendon reflex	**MD**	muscular dystrophy

Chapter Review

Terminology Checklist

Below are all Anatomy and Physiology key terms, Word Building, Vocabulary, Pathology, Diagnostic, Therapeutic, and Pharmacology terms presented in this chapter. Use this list as a study tool by placing a check in the box in front of each term as you master its meaning.

- ☐ abduction
- ☐ action
- ☐ adduction
- ☐ adhesion
- ☐ amputation
- ☐ ankylosing spondylitis
- ☐ antagonistic pairs
- ☐ appendicular skeleton
- ☐ arthralgia
- ☐ arthritis
- ☐ arthrocentesis
- ☐ arthroclasia
- ☐ arthrodesis
- ☐ arthrogram
- ☐ arthrography
- ☐ arthroscope
- ☐ arthroscopic surgery
- ☐ arthroscopy
- ☐ arthrotomy
- ☐ articular cartilage
- ☐ articulation
- ☐ atonia
- ☐ atrophy
- ☐ axial skeleton
- ☐ biceps
- ☐ bone graft
- ☐ bone marrow
- ☐ bone reabsorption inhibitors
- ☐ bones
- ☐ bone scan
- ☐ bradykinesia
- ☐ bunion
- ☐ bunionectomy
- ☐ bursa
- ☐ bursectomy
- ☐ bursitis
- ☐ calcium supplements
- ☐ callus
- ☐ cancellous bone
- ☐ cardiac muscle
- ☐ carpal
- ☐ carpal tunnel release
- ☐ carpal tunnel syndrome
- ☐ cartilage
- ☐ cartilaginous joints
- ☐ cast
- ☐ cervical
- ☐ cervical vertebrae
- ☐ chiropractic
- ☐ chondrectomy
- ☐ chondroma
- ☐ chondromalacia
- ☐ chondroplasty
- ☐ circumduction
- ☐ clavicle
- ☐ clavicular
- ☐ closed fracture
- ☐ coccygeal
- ☐ coccyx
- ☐ Colles' fracture
- ☐ comminuted fracture
- ☐ compact bone
- ☐ compound fracture
- ☐ compression fracture
- ☐ condyle
- ☐ contracture
- ☐ cortical
- ☐ cortical bone
- ☐ corticosteroids
- ☐ costal
- ☐ cranial
- ☐ craniotomy
- ☐ cranium
- ☐ creatine phosphokinase
- ☐ crepitation
- ☐ deep tendon reflex
- ☐ diaphysis
- ☐ dislocation
- ☐ dorsiflexion
- ☐ dual-energy absorptiometry
- ☐ dyskinesia
- ☐ dystonia
- ☐ electromyogram
- ☐ electromyography
- ☐ elevation
- ☐ epicondyle
- ☐ epiphysis
- ☐ ethmoid bone
- ☐ eversion
- ☐ Ewing's sarcoma
- ☐ exostosis
- ☐ extension
- ☐ extensor carpi
- ☐ external oblique
- ☐ facial bones
- ☐ fascia
- ☐ fascial
- ☐ fasciitis
- ☐ fasciotomy
- ☐ femoral
- ☐ femur
- ☐ fibromyalgia
- ☐ fibrous joints
- ☐ fibula
- ☐ fibular
- ☐ fissure
- ☐ fixation
- ☐ flat bones
- ☐ flexion
- ☐ flexor carpi
- ☐ foramen
- ☐ fossa
- ☐ fracture
- ☐ frontal bone
- ☐ ganglion cyst
- ☐ gluteus maximus
- ☐ greenstick fracture

- head
- herniated nucleus pulposus
- humeral
- humerus
- hyoid bone
- hyperkinesia
- hypertonia
- hypertrophy
- hypokinesia
- hypotonia
- iliac
- ilium
- impacted fracture
- innominate bone
- insertion
- intermittent claudication
- intervertebral
- intervertebral disc
- intracranial
- inversion
- involuntary muscle
- irregular bones
- ischial
- ischium
- joint capsule
- joints
- kinesiology
- kyphosis
- lacrimal bone
- laminectomy
- lateral epicondylitis
- ligaments
- long bones
- lordosis
- lower extremities
- lumbar
- lumbar vertebrae
- mandible
- mandibular
- maxilla
- maxillary
- medullary
- medullary cavity
- metacarpal
- metatarsal
- motor neurons
- muscle biopsy
- muscles
- muscle tissue fibers
- muscular
- muscular dystrophy
- myalgia
- myasthenia
- myelography
- myeloma
- myocardial
- myocardium
- myoneural junction
- myopathy
- myoplasty
- myorrhaphy
- myorrhexis
- myotonia
- nasal bone
- neck
- nonsteroidal anti-inflammatory drugs
- oblique fracture
- occipital bone
- opposition
- origin
- orthopedics
- orthotic
- os coxae
- osseous tissue
- ossification
- ostealgia
- osteoarthritis
- osteoblasts
- osteochondroma
- osteoclasia
- osteocytes
- osteogenic sarcoma
- osteomalacia
- osteomyelitis
- osteopathy
- osteoporosis
- osteotome
- osteotomy
- Paget's disease
- palatine bone
- parietal bone
- patella
- patellar
- pathologic fracture
- pectoral girdle
- pelvic
- pelvic girdle
- percutaneous diskectomy
- periosteum
- phalangeal
- phalanges
- plantar flexion
- podiatry
- polymyositis
- process
- pronation
- prosthesis
- prosthetics
- pseudohypertrophic muscular dystrophy
- pubic
- pubis
- radial
- radiography
- radius
- rectus abdominis
- red bone marrow
- reduction
- repetitive motion disorder
- rheumatoid arthritis
- rib cage
- rickets
- rotation
- rotator cuff injury
- sacral
- sacrum
- scapula
- scapular
- scoliosis
- short bones
- sinus
- skeletal muscle
- skeletal muscle relaxants
- skeleton

- ☐ smooth muscle
- ☐ spasm
- ☐ sphenoid bone
- ☐ spina bifida
- ☐ spinal fusion
- ☐ spinal stenosis
- ☐ spiral fracture
- ☐ spondylolisthesis
- ☐ spondylosis
- ☐ spongy bone
- ☐ sprain
- ☐ sternal
- ☐ sternocleidomastoid
- ☐ sternum
- ☐ strain
- ☐ stress fracture
- ☐ striated muscle
- ☐ subluxation
- ☐ supination
- ☐ synovectomy

- ☐ synovial fluid
- ☐ synovial joint
- ☐ synovial membrane
- ☐ synovitis
- ☐ systemic lupus erythematosus
- ☐ talipes
- ☐ tarsal
- ☐ temporal bone
- ☐ tendinitis
- ☐ tendinous
- ☐ tendon
- ☐ tendoplasty
- ☐ tendotomy
- ☐ tenodesis
- ☐ tenodynia
- ☐ tenoplasty
- ☐ tenorrhaphy
- ☐ thoracic
- ☐ thoracic vertebrae
- ☐ tibia

- ☐ tibial
- ☐ torticollis
- ☐ total hip arthroplasty
- ☐ total knee arthroplasty
- ☐ traction
- ☐ transverse fracture
- ☐ trochanter
- ☐ tubercle
- ☐ tuberosity
- ☐ ulna
- ☐ ulnar
- ☐ upper extremities
- ☐ vertebral column
- ☐ visceral muscle
- ☐ Vitamin D therapy
- ☐ voluntary muscle
- ☐ vomer bone
- ☐ whiplash
- ☐ yellow bone marrow
- ☐ zygomatic bone

Practice Exercises

A. Complete the following statements.

1. The two divisions of the human skeleton are the __axial__ and __appendicular__.

2. Another name for visceral muscle is __smooth__ muscle.

3. The five functions of the skeletal system are to __support the body__, __protect internal organs__, __produce blood cells__, __store minerals__, and __point of attachment for skeletal muscles for body movement.__

4. Nerves contact skeletal muscle fibers at the __myoneural__ junction.

5. __Short__ bones are roughly as long as they are wide.

6. The membrane covering bones is called the __periosteum__.

7. A Colles' fracture occurs in the __wrist__.

8. Another name for spongy bone is __cancellous__ bone.

9. __Synovial__ joints are the most common joints in the body.

10. The three types of muscle are __skeletal__, __smooth__, and __cardiac__.

11. A __foramen__ is a smooth round opening in bones.

12. The __diaphysis__ is the shaft of a long bone.

Musculoskeletal System

B. State the terms described using the combining forms provided.

The combining form *oste/o* refers to bone. Use it to write a term that means:

1. bone cell _____ osteocyte

2. embryonic bone cell _____ osteoblast

3. porous bone _____ osteoporosis

4. disease of the bone _____ osteopathy

5. incision of the bone _____ osteotomy

6. instrument to cut bone _____ osteotome

7. inflammation of the bone and bone marrow _____ osteomyelitis

8. softening of the bones _____ osteomalacia

9. tumor composed of both bone and cartilage _____ osteochondroma

The combining form *my/o* refers to muscle. Use it to write a term that means:

10. muscle disease _____ myopathy

11. surgical repair of muscle _____ myoplasty

12. suture of muscle _____ myorrhaphy

13. record of muscle electricity _____ electromyogram

14. muscle weakness _____ myasthenia

The combining form *ten/o* refers to tendons. Use it to write a term that means:

15. tendon pain _____ tenodynia

16. tendon suture _____ tenorrhaphy

The combining form *arthr/o* refers to the joints. Use it to write a term that means:

17. surgical fusion of a joint _____ arthrodesis

18. surgical repair of a joint _____ arthroplasty

19. incision into a joint _____ arthrotomy

20. inflammation of a joint _____ arthritis

21. puncture to withdraw fluid from a joint _____ arthrocentesis

22. pain in the joints _____ arthralgia

The combining form *chondr/o* refers to cartilage. Use it to write a term that means:

23. cartilage removal _____ chondrectomy

24. cartilage tumor _____ chondroma

25. cartilage softening _____ chondromalacia

C. Write the suffix for each expression and provide an example of its use from the chapter.

	Suffix	Musculoskeletal Term
1. fuse	-desis	tenodesis
2. weakness	-asthenia	myasthenia
3. slipping	-listhesis	spondylolisthesis
4. to surgically break	-clasia	arthroclasia
5. movement	-kinesia	kinesiology
6. porous	-porosis	osteoporosis

D. Give the adjective form for the following bones.

1. femur	femoral	6. tibia	tibial
2. sternum	sternal	7. patella	patellar
3. clavicle	clavicular	8. phalanges	phalangeal
4. coccyx	coccygeal	9. humerus	humeral
5. maxilla	maxillary	10. pubis	pubic

E. Define the following combining forms and use them to form musculoskeletal terms.

	Definition	Musculoskeletal Term
1. lamin/o	lamina, part of vertebra	laminectomy
2. ankyl/o	stiff joint	ankylosing spondylitis
3. chondr/o	cartilage	chondroma
4. spondyl/o	vertebrae	spondylosis
5. my/o	muscle	myopathy
6. orth/o	straight	orthotic
7. kyph/o	hump	kyphosis
8. tend/o	tendon	tendinitis
9. myel/o	bone marrow, spinal cord	myeloma
10. articul/o	joint	articulation

F. Define the following terms.

1. chondroplasty — surgical repair of cartilage

2. bradykinesia — slow movement

3. osteoporosis _porous bone - decrease in bone mass_

4. lordosis _(bent backwards) abnormal increase in forward curvature of lumbar spine_

5. atrophy _poor muscle development as a result of muscle disease, nervous sys disease, or lack of use_

6. myeloma _bone marrow tumor_

7. prosthesis _artificial device used as a substitute for a missing body part_

8. craniotomy _incision into the skull_

9. arthrocentesis _puncture to withdraw fluid from a joint_

10. bursitis _inflammation of a bursa_

G. Name the five regions of the spinal column and indicate the number of bones in each area.

Name	Number of Bones
1. cervical vertebrae	7
2. thoracic vertebrae	12
3. lumbar vertebrae	5
4. sacrum	1
5. coccyx	1

H. Circle the prefix and/or suffix and place a *P* for prefix or an *S* for suffix over these word parts. In the space provided, define the term.

1. arthro(scopy)[S] _process of visually examining a joint_

2. (inter)[P]verteb(ral)[S] _pertaining to between vertebrae_

3. chondro(malacia)[S] _cartilage softening_

4. disk(ectomy)[S] _surgical removal of a disk_

5. (intra)[P]crani(al)[S] _pertaining to inside the skull_

6. (sub)[P]scapul(ar)[S] _pertaining to under the scapula_

I. Match each term to its definition.

1. _e_ abduction   a. backward bending of the foot

2. _d_ rotation   b. bending the foot to point toes toward the ground

3. _b_ plantar flexion   c. straightening motion

4. _c_ extension   d. motion around a central axis

5. _a_ dorsiflexion   e. motion away from the body

6. _h_ flexion   f. moving the thumb away from the palm

Musculoskeletal System

7. __g__ adduction   g. motion toward the body

8. __f__ opposition   h. bending motion

J. Match each fracture type to its definition.

1. __c__ comminuted   a. fracture line is at an angle

2. __h__ greenstick   b. fracture line curves around the bone

3. __f__ compound   c. bone is splintered or crushed

4. __g__ simple   d. bone is pressed into itself

5. __d__ impacted   e. fracture line is straight across bone

6. __e__ transverse   f. skin has been broken

7. __a__ oblique   g. no open wound

8. __b__ spiral   h. bone only partially broken

K. Define the following medical specialties and specialists.

1. orthopedics __bone specialists (musculoskeletal)__

2. chiropractic __pertaining to specialist in the spine (musculoskeletal)__

3. podiatry __specializing in the feet__

4. orthotics __use of equipment to support a muscle, promote a motion or correct musculoskeletal deformities__

5. prosthetics __artificial devices that replace a missing body part__

L. Write the anatomical name for each of the following common bone names.

1. knee cap __patella__

2. ankle bones __tarsals__

3. collar bone __clavicle__

4. thigh bone __femur__

5. toe bones __phalanges__

6. wrist bones __carpals__

7. shin bone __tibia__

8. shoulder blade __scapula__

9. finger bones __phalanges__

M. Identify the following abbreviations.

1. DJD __degenerative joint disease__

2. EMG __electromyogram__

3. C1 __first cervical vertebra__

4. T6 __sixth thoracic vertebra__

5. IM __intramuscular__

Musculoskeletal System

6. DTR _deep tendon reflex_

7. JRA _juvenile rheumatoid arthritis_

8. LLE _left lower extremity_

9. ortho _orthopedics_

10. CTS _carpal tunnel syndrome_

N. Write the abbreviations for the following terms.

1. intramuscular _IM_

2. total knee replacement _TKR_

3. herniated nucleus pulposus _HNP_

4. deep tendon reflex _DTR_

5. upper extremity _UE_

6. fifth lumbar vertebra _L5_

7. bone density testing _BDT_

8. above the knee _AK_

9. fracture _FX, Fx_

10. nonsteroidal anti-inflammatory drug _NSAID_

O. Use the following terms in the sentences that follow.

carpal tunnel syndrome	rickets	lateral epicondylitis	systemic lupus
scoliosis	osteogenic sarcoma	pseudohypertrophic	erythematosus
herniated nucleus	osteoporosis	muscular dystrophy	
pulposus	spondylolisthesis		

1. Mrs. Lewis, age 84, broke her hip. Her physician will be running tests for what potential ailment? _osteoporosis_

2. Jamie, age 6 months, is being given orange juice and vitamin supplements to avoid what condition? _rickets_

3. George has severe elbow pain after playing tennis four days in a row. He may have _lateral epicondylitis_

4. Marshall's doctor told him that he had a ruptured disk. The medical term for this is? _herniated nucleus pulposis_

5. Mr. Jefferson's physician has discovered a tumor at the end of his femur. He has been admitted to the hospital for a biopsy to rule out what type of bone cancer? _osteogenic sarcoma_

6. The school nurse has asked Janelle to bend over so that she may examine her back to see if she is developing a lateral curve. What is the nurse looking for? _scoliosis_

7. Gerald has experienced a gradual loss of muscle strength over the past five years even though his muscles look large and healthy. The doctors believe he has an inherited muscle disease. What is that disease? _pseudohypertrophic muscular dystrophy_

8. Roberta has suddenly developed arthritis in her hands and knees. Rheumatoid arthritis had been ruled out, but what other auto-immune disease might Roberta have? _systemic lupus erythematosus_

9. Mark's x-ray demonstrated forward sliding of a lumbar vertebra; the radiologist diagnosed _spondylolisthesis_

10. The orthopedist determined that Marcia's repetitive wrist movements at work caused her to develop _carpal tunnel syndrome_

P. Fill in the classification for each drug description, then match the brand name.

	Drug Description	Classification	Brand Name
1. _____	Treats mild pain and anti-inflammatory	_____	a. Flexeril
2. _____	Hormone with anti-inflammatory properties	_____	b. Aleve
3. _____	Reduces muscle spasms	_____	c. Fosamax
4. _____	Treats conditions of weakened bones	_____	d. Oystercal
5. _____	Maintains blood calcium levels	_____	e. Medrol

Medical Record Analysis

Below is an item from a patient's medical record. Read it carefully, make sure you understand all the medical terms used, and then answer the questions that follow.

Discharge Summary

Admitting Diagnosis:	Osteoarthritis bilateral knees.
Final Diagnosis:	Osteoarthritis bilateral knees with prosthetic right knee replacement.
History of Present Illness:	Patient is a 68-year-old male. He reports he has experienced occasional knee pain and swelling since he injured his knees playing football in high school. These symptoms became worse while he was in his 50s and working on a concrete surface. The right knee has always been more painful than the left. Arthroscopy twelve years ago revealed a torn lateral meniscus and chondromalacia of the patella on the right. He had an arthroscopic meniscectomy with a 50% improvement in symptoms at that time. He returned to his orthopedic surgeon six months ago because of constant knee pain and swelling severe enough to interfere with sleep and all activities. He required a cane to walk. CT scan indicated severe bilateral osteoarthritis, with complete loss of the joint space on the right. He was referred to a physiatrist who prescribed Motrin; physical therapy for ROM; strengthening exercises; and a low-fat, low-calorie weight loss diet for moderate obesity that greatly added to the strain on his knees. Over the course of the next two months, the left knee improved, but the right knee did not. Due to the failure of conservative treatment, he is admitted to the hospital at this time for prosthetic replacement of the right knee. Patient's other medical history is significant for hypertension and coronary artery disease that is controlled with medication. He has lost weight through diet, which has improved his hypertension, if not his knee pain.
Summary of Hospital Course:	Patient tolerated the surgical procedure well. He began intensive physical therapy for lower extremity ROM and strengthening exercises and gait training with a walker. He received occupational therapy instruction in ADLs, especially dressing and personal care. He was able to transfer himself out of bed by the third post-op day and was able to ambulate 150 ft with a walker and dress himself on the fifth post-op day. His right knee flexion was 90° and he lacked 5° of full extension.
Discharge Plans:	Patient was discharged home with his wife one week post-op. He will continue rehabilitation as an outpatient. Return to office for post-op checkup in one week.

Critical Thinking Questions

1. What is the specialty of a physiatrist? Describe in your own words what the physiatrist ordered for this patient.

   A physiatrist is a rehabilitation specialist / physical therapist.
   He ordered Motrin for pain + inflammation, physical therapy to increase range of motion, strengthening exercises + weight loss.

Musculoskeletal System

2. What surgical procedure did the patient have twelve years ago? What two pathologies were revealed by that procedure? What surgical procedure was performed to correct his problems at that time?

They visually examined his joints 12yrs ago & found a torn side meniscus on the left knee & softening of the knee cap cartilage on the rt. knee. He had surgical repair of the meniscus.

3. The following medical terms are not defined in your text. Based on your reading of this discharge summary, what do you think each term means in general—not the specifics of this patient?
   a. conservative treatment _non-surgical, non-invasive treatment_
   b. outpatient _outside of the hospital_

4. What two types of post-op therapy did this patient receive? Describe the treatment each type of therapy provided for this patient.

Physical therapy to increase strength & range of motion & training to use a walker. Occupational therapy to help him with daily activities post-op.

5. Describe how much the patient could move his right knee when he was discharged from the hospital.

He could bend his knee 90° & lacked 5° of fully straightening it.

6. The following medical terms were not defined to you in this chapter. Use your text as a dictionary to describe, in your own words, what each term means.
   a. coronary artery disease _disease of the arteries of the heart_
   b. hypertension _high blood pressure_

Musculoskeletal System

Chart Note Transcription

The chart note below contains eleven phrases that can be reworded with a medical term that you learned in this chapter. Each phrase is identified with an underline. Determine the medical term and write your answers in the space provided.

Current Complaint:	An 82-year-old female was transported to the Emergency Room via ambulance with severe left hip pain following a fall on the ice.
Past History:	Patient suffered a <u>wrist broken bone</u> ❶ two years earlier that required <u>immobilization by solid material</u>. ❷ Following this <u>broken bone</u>, ❸ her <u>physician who specializes in treatment of bone conditions</u> ❹ diagnosed her with moderate <u>porous bones</u> ❺ on the basis of a <u>computer-assisted X-ray</u>. ❻
Signs and Symptoms:	Patient reported severe left hip pain, rating it as 8 on a scale of 1 to 10. She held her hip <u>in a bent position</u> ❼ and could not tolerate <u>movement toward a straight position</u>. ❽ X-rays of the left hip and leg were taken.
Diagnosis:	<u>Shattered broken bone</u> ❾ in the neck of the left <u>thigh bone</u>. ❿
Treatment:	<u>Implantation of an artificial hip joint</u> ⑪ on the left.

❶ Colles' fracture

❷ fixation - cast

❸ fracture

❹ orthopedist - orthopedic doctor

❺ osteoporosis

❻ dual-anergy absorptiometry (DXA)

❼ ~~adduction~~ ~~& flexion~~ extension

❽ & adduction

❾ comminuted fracture

❿ femur

⑪ total hip arthroplasty (THA)

Labeling Exercise

A. System Review

Write the labels for this figure on the numbered lines provided.

1. cranium _skull_
2. caryical vertebrae
3. sternum
4. ribs
5. thoracic vertebrae
6. lumbar vertebrae
7. Ilium
8. Pubis
9. Ischium
10. Femur
11. Patella
12. Tibia
13. Fibula
14. Tarsals
15. Metatarsals
16. Phalanges
17. maxilla
18. mandible
19. scapula
20. Humerus
21. Ulna
22. radius
23. sacrum
24. coccyx
25. carpals
26. metacarpals
27. phalanges

B. Anatomy Challenge

1. Write the labels for this figure on the numbered lines provided.

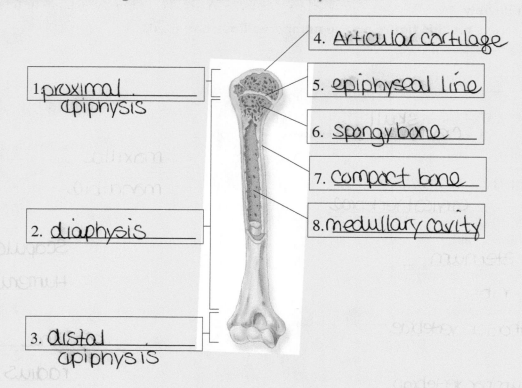

1. proximal epiphysis

2. diaphysis

3. distal epiphysis

4. Articular cartilage

5. epiphyseal line

6. spongy bone

7. compact bone

8. medullary cavity

2. Write the labels for this figure on the numbered lines provided.

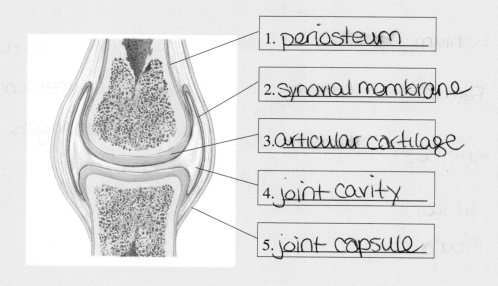

1. periosteum

2. synovial membrane

3. articular cartilage

4. joint cavity

5. joint capsule

Multimedia Preview

Additional interactive resources and activities for this chapter can be found on the Companion Website.

Website Highlights—www.prenhall.com/fremgen

AUDIO GLOSSARY

Click here and take advantage of the free-access on-line study guide that accompanies your textbook. You'll find an audio glossary with definitions and audio pronunciations for every term in the book. By clicking on this URL you'll also access a variety of quizzes with instant feedback, links to download mp3 audio reviews, and current news articles.

Cardiovascular System

Learning Objectives

Upon completion of this chapter, you will be able to:

- Identify and define the combining forms and suffixes introduced in this chapter.
- Correctly spell and pronounce medical terms and major anatomical structures relating to the cardiovascular system.
- Describe the major organs of the cardiovascular system and their functions.
- Describe the anatomy of the heart.
- Describe the flow of blood through the heart.
- Explain how the electrical conduction system controls the heartbeat.
- List and describe the characteristics of the three types of blood vessels.
- Define pulse and blood pressure.
- Build and define cardiovascular system medical terms from word parts.
- Identify and define cardiovascular system vocabulary terms.
- Identify and define selected cardiovascular system pathology terms.
- Identify and define selected cardiovascular system diagnostic procedures.
- Identify and define selected cardiovascular system therapeutic procedures.
- Identify and define selected medications relating to the cardiovascular system.
- Define selected abbreviations associated with the cardiovascular system.

From Chapter 5 of *Medical Terminology: A Living Language*, 4/e. Bonnie F. Fremgen. Suzanne S. Frucht. Copyright © 2009 by Pearson Education. Published by Prentice Hall. All rights reserved.

Cardiovascular System at a Glance

Function

The cardiovascular system consists of the pump and vessels that distribute blood to all areas of the body. This system allows for the delivery of needed substances to the cells of the body as well as for the removal of wastes.

Organs

blood vessels
- arteries
- capillaries
- veins

heart

Combining Forms

angi/o	vessel	**sphygm/o**	pulse
aort/o	aorta	**steth/o**	chest
arteri/o	artery	**thromb/o**	clot
ather/o	fatty substance	**valv/o**	valve
atri/o	atrium	**valvul/o**	valve
cardi/o	heart	**vascul/o**	blood vessel
coron/o	heart	**vas/o**	vessel, duct
hemangi/o	blood vessel	**ven/o**	vein
phleb/o	vein	**ventricul/o**	ventricle

Suffixes

-manometer	instrument to measure pressure
-ole	small
-tension	pressure
-ule	small

Cardiovascular System Illustrated

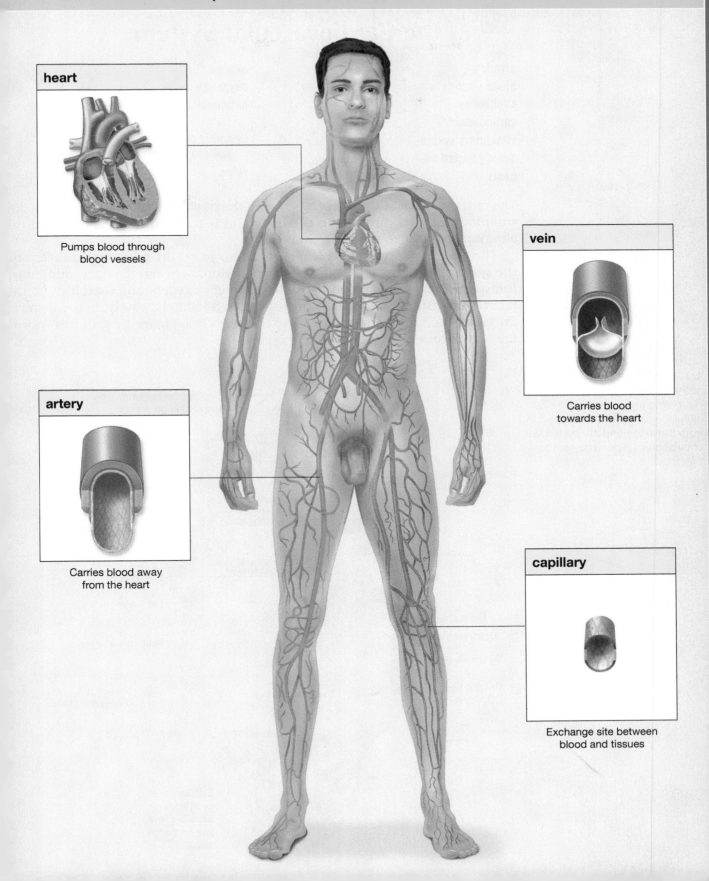

heart

Pumps blood through blood vessels

artery

Carries blood away from the heart

vein

Carries blood towards the heart

capillary

Exchange site between blood and tissues

Anatomy and Physiology of the Cardiovascular System

arteries
blood vessels
capillaries
carbon dioxide
circulatory system
deoxygenated (dee-OK-sih-jen-ay-ted)
heart

oxygen
oxygenated (OK-sih-jen-ay-ted)
pulmonary circulation
   (PULL-mon-air-ee ser-kew-LAY-shun)
systemic circulation
   (sis-TEM-ik ser-kew-LAY-shun)
veins

The cardiovascular (CV) system, also called the **circulatory system,** maintains the distribution of blood throughout the body and is composed of the **heart** and the **blood vessels—arteries, capillaries**, and **veins.**

The circulatory system is composed of two parts: the **pulmonary circulation** and the **systemic circulation**. The pulmonary circulation, between the heart and lungs, transports **deoxygenated** blood to the lungs to get oxygen, and then back to the heart. The systemic circulation carries **oxygenated** blood away from the heart to the tissues and cells, and then back to the heart (see Figure 1 ■). In this way all the body's cells receive blood and oxygen.

■ Figure 1 A schematic of the circulatory system illustrating the pulmonary circulation picking up oxygen from the lungs and the systemic circulation delivering oxygen to the body.

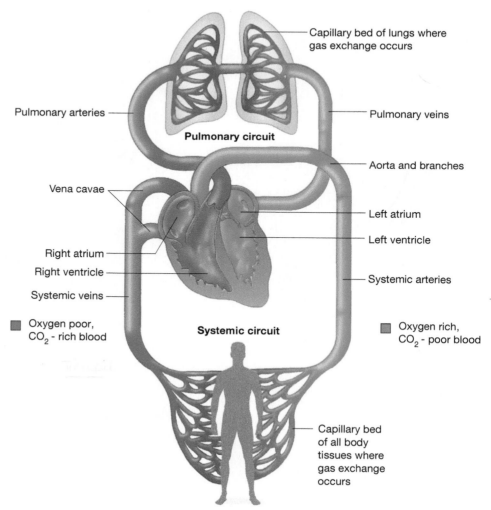

Capillary bed of lungs where gas exchange occurs

Pulmonary arteries

Pulmonary circuit

Pulmonary veins

Aorta and branches

Vena cavae

Left atrium

Left ventricle

Right atrium

Right ventricle

Systemic arteries

Systemic veins

Oxygen poor, CO_2 - rich blood

Systemic circuit

Oxygen rich, CO_2 - poor blood

Capillary bed of all body tissues where gas exchange occurs

In addition to distributing **oxygen** and other nutrients, such as glucose and amino acids, the cardiovascular system also collects the waste products from the body's cells. **Carbon dioxide** and other waste products produced by metabolic reaction are transported by the cardiovascular system to the lungs, liver, and kidneys where they are eliminated from the body.

Heart

apex (AY-peks)   **cardiac muscle** (CAR-dee-ak)

The heart is a muscular pump made up of **cardiac muscle** fibers that could be considered a muscle rather than an organ. It has four chambers, or cavities, and beats an average of 60 to 100 beats per minute (bpm) or about 100,000 times in one day. Each time the cardiac muscle contracts, blood is ejected from the heart and pushed throughout the body within the blood vessels.

The heart is located in the mediastinum in the center of the chest cavity, however, it is not exactly centered; more of the heart is on the left side of the mediastinum than the right. At about the size of a fist and shaped like an upside-down pear the heart lies directly behind the sternum. The tip of the heart at the lower edge is called the **apex** (see Figure 2 ■).

Heart Layers

endocardium (en-doh-CAR-dee-um)
epicardium (ep-ih-CAR-dee-um)
myocardium (my-oh-CAR-dee-um)
parietal pericardium
  (pah-RYE-eh-tal pair-ih-CAR-dee-um)

pericardium (pair-ih-CAR-dee-um)
visceral pericardium
  (VISS-er-al pair-ih-CAR-dee-um)

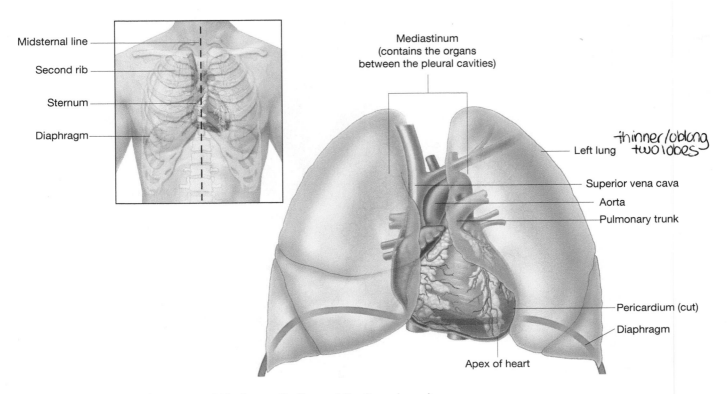

■ Figure 2 Location of the heart within the mediastinum of the thoracic cavity.

Cardiovascular System

The wall of the heart is quite thick and composed of three layers (see Figures 3 ■ and 4 ■):

Med Term Tip

These layers become important when studying the disease conditions affecting the heart. For instance, when the prefix *endo-* is added to *carditis*, forming *endocarditis*, we know that the inflammation is within the "inner layer of the heart." In discussing the muscular action of the heart the prefix *myo-*, meaning "muscle," is added to *cardium* to form the word *myocardium*. The diagnosis *myocardial infarction* (MI), or heart attack, means that the patient has an infarct or "dead tissue in the muscle of the heart." The prefix *peri-*, meaning "around," when added to the word *cardium* refers to the sac "surrounding the heart." Therefore, *pericarditis* is an "inflammation of the outer sac of the heart."

1. The **endocardium** is the inner layer of the heart lining the heart chambers. It is a very smooth, thin layer that serves to reduce friction as the blood passes through the heart chambers.
2. The **myocardium** is the thick muscular middle layer of the heart. Contraction of this muscle layer develops the pressure required to pump blood through the blood vessels.
3. The **epicardium** is the outer layer of the heart. The heart is enclosed within a double-layered pleural sac, called the **pericardium**. The epicardium is the **visceral pericardium**, or inner layer of the sac. The outer layer of the sac is the **parietal pericardium**. Fluid between the two layers of the sac reduces friction as the heart beats.

Heart Chambers

atria (AY-tree-ah)
interatrial septum
  (in-ter-AY-tree-al SEP-tum)

interventricular septum
  (in-ter-ven-TRIK-yoo-lar SEP-tum)
ventricles (VEN-trik-lz)

Med Term Tip

The term *ventricle* comes from the Latin term *venter*, which means "little belly." Although it originally referred to the abdomen and then the stomach, it came to stand for any hollow region inside an organ.

The heart is divided into four chambers or cavities (see Figures 3 and 4). There are two **atria**, or upper chambers, and two **ventricles**, or lower chambers. These chambers are divided into right and left sides by walls called the **interatrial septum** and the **interventricular septum**. The atria are the receiving chambers of the heart. Blood returning to the heart via veins first collects in the atria. The ventricles are the pumping chambers. They have a much thicker myocardium and their contraction ejects blood out of the heart and into the great arteries.

■ **Figure 3** Internal view of the heart illustrating the heart chambers, heart layers, heart valves, and major blood vessels associated with the heart.

134

Right atrium

Pulmonary
semilunar
valve

Right ventricle

Interventricular
septum

Aorta

Aortic
semilunar
valve

Left atrium

Bicuspid valve

Chordae tendineae

Papillary muscle

Left ventricle

■ Figure 4 Internal view of heart specimen illustrating heart chambers, septum, and heart valves.

Heart Valves

aortic valve (ay-OR-tik)

atrioventricular valve
  (ay-tree-oh-ven-TRIK-yoo-lar)

bicuspid valve (bye-CUSS-pid)

cusps

mitral valve (MY-tral)

pulmonary valve (PULL-mon-air-ee)

semilunar valve (sem-ih-LOO-nar)

tricuspid valve (try-CUSS-pid)

Four valves act as restraining gates to control the direction of blood flow. They are situated at the entrances and exits to the ventricles (see Figures 4 ■ and 5 ■). Properly functioning valves allow blood to flow only in the forward direction by blocking it from returning to the previous chamber.

The four valves are as follows:

1. **Tricuspid valve:** an **atrioventricular valve** (AV), meaning that it controls the opening between the right atrium and the right ventricle. Once the blood enters the right ventricle, it cannot go back up into the atrium again. The prefix *tri-*, meaning three, indicates that this valve has three leaflets or **cusps**.
2. **Pulmonary valve:** a **semilunar valve**. The prefix *semi-*, meaning half, and the term **lunar**, meaning moon, indicate that this valve looks like a half moon. Located between the right ventricle and the pulmonary artery, this valve prevents blood that has been ejected into the pulmonary artery from returning to the right ventricle as it relaxes.
3. **Mitral valve:** also called the **bicuspid valve**, indicating that it has two cusps. Blood flows through this atrioventricular valve to the left ventricle and cannot go back up into the left atrium.
4. **Aortic valve:** a semilunar valve located between the left ventricle and the aorta. Blood leaves the left ventricle through this valve and cannot return to the left ventricle.

Med Term Tip

The heart makes two distinct sounds referred to as "lub-dupp." These sounds are produced by the forceful snapping shut of the heart valves. *Lub* is the closing of the atrioventricular valves. *Dupp* is the closing of the semilunar valves.

Blood Flow Through the Heart

aorta (ay-OR-tah)

diastole (dye-ASS-toe-lee)

inferior vena cava (VEE-nah KAY-vah)

pulmonary artery (PULL-mon-air-ee)

pulmonary veins

superior vena cava

systole (SIS-toe-lee)

Figure 5 Superior view of heart valves illustrating position, size, and shape of each valve.

Pulmonary valve
(right semilunar valve)

Aortic valve
(left semilunar valve)

Mitral valve
(left atrioventricular valve)

Tricuspid valve
(right atrioventricular valve)

The flow of blood through the heart is very orderly (see Figure 6 ■). It progresses through the heart to the lungs, where it receives oxygen; then goes back to the heart; and then out to the body tissues and parts. The normal process of blood flow is as follows:

1. Deoxygenated blood from all the tissues in the body enters a relaxed right atrium via two large veins called the **superior vena cava** and **inferior vena cava**.
2. The right atrium contracts and blood flows through the tricuspid valve into the relaxed right ventricle.
3. The right ventricle then contracts and blood is pumped through the pulmonary valve into the **pulmonary artery**, which carries it to the lungs for oxygenation.
4. The left atrium receives blood returning to the heart after being oxygenated by the lungs. This blood enters the relaxed left atrium from the four **pulmonary veins**.
5. The left atrium contracts and blood flows through the mitral valve into the relaxed left ventricle.
6. When the left ventricle contracts, the blood is pumped through the aortic valve and into the **aorta**, the largest artery in the body. The aorta carries blood to all parts of the body.

It can be seen that the heart chambers alternate between relaxing in order to fill and contracting to push blood forward. The period of time a chamber is relaxed is **diastole**. The contraction phase is **systole**.

Conduction System of the Heart

atrioventricular bundle

atrioventricular node

autonomic nervous system (aw-toh-NOM-ik NER-vus SIS-tem)

bundle branches

bundle of His

pacemaker

Purkinje fibers (per-KIN-gee)

sinoatrial node (sigh-noh-AY-tree-al)

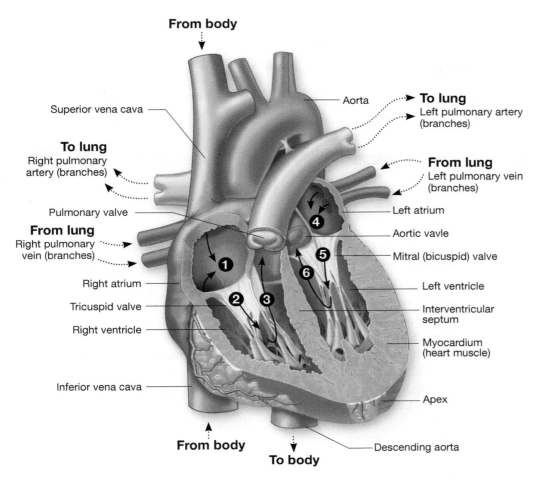

Figure 6 The path of blood flow through the chambers of the left and right side of the heart, including the veins delivering blood to the heart and arteries receiving blood ejected from the heart.

The heart rate is regulated by the **autonomic nervous system**; therefore, we have no voluntary control over the beating of our heart. Special tissue within the heart is responsible for conducting an electrical impulse stimulating the different chambers to contract in the correct order.

The path that the impulses travel is as follows (see Figure 7 ■):

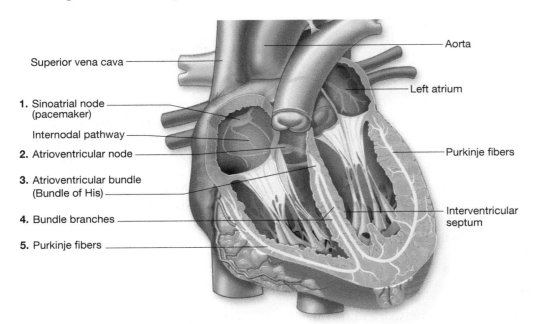

Figure 7 The conduction system of the heart; traces the path of the electrical impulse that stimulates the heart chambers to contract in the correct sequence.

■ **Figure 8** An electrocardiogram (EKG) wave, record of the electrical signal as it moves through the conduction system of the heart. This signal stimulates the chambers of the heart to contract and relax in the proper sequence.

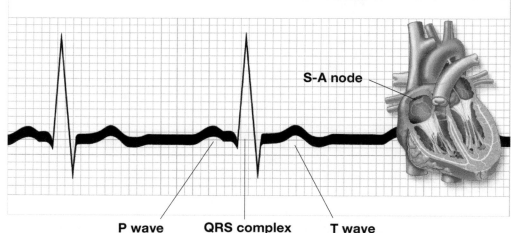

S-A node

P wave
precedes atrial systole

QRS complex
precedes ventricular systole

T wave
precedes ventricular diastole

1. The **sinoatrial (SA) node**, or **pacemaker**, is where the electrical impulses begin. From the sinoatrial node a wave of electricity travels through the atria, causing them to contract, or go into systole.
2. The **atrioventricular node** is stimulated.
3. This node transfers the stimulation wave to the **atrioventricular bundle** (formerly called **bundle of His**).
4. The electrical signal next travels down the **bundle branches** within the interventricular septum.
5. The **Purkinje fibers** out in the ventricular myocardium are stimulated, resulting in ventricular systole.

Blood Vessels

lumen (LOO-men)

There are three types of blood vessels: arteries, capillaries, and veins (see Figure 9 ■). These are the pipes that circulate blood through out the body. The **lumen** is the channel within these vessels through which blood flows.

Arteries

arterioles (ar-TEE-ree-ohlz)   **coronary arteries** (KOR-ah-nair-ee
                                                      AR-te-reez)

The arteries are the large, thick-walled vessels that carry the blood away from the heart. The walls of arteries contain a thick layer of smooth muscle that can contract or relax to change the size of the arterial lumen. The pulmonary artery carries deoxygenated blood from the right ventricle to the lungs. The largest artery, the aorta, begins from the left ventricle of the heart and carries oxygenated blood to all the body systems. The **coronary arteries** then branch from the aorta and provide blood to the myocardium (see Figure 10 ■). As they travel through the body, the arteries branch into progressively smaller sized arteries. The smallest of the arteries, called **arterioles**, deliver blood to the capillaries. Figure 11 ■ illustrates the major systemic arteries.

Capillaries

capillary bed

Capillaries are a network of tiny blood vessels referred to as a **capillary bed**. Arterial blood flows into a capillary bed, and venous blood flows back out (see Figure

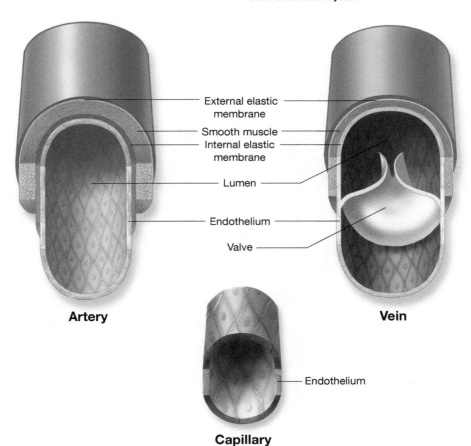

■ **Figure 9** Comparative structure of arteries, capillaries, and veins.

External elastic membrane
Smooth muscle
Internal elastic membrane
Lumen
Endothelium
Valve

Artery

Vein

Endothelium

Capillary

9). Capillaries are very thin walled, allowing for the diffusion of the oxygen and nutrients from the blood into the body tissues. Likewise, carbon dioxide and waste products are able to diffuse out of the body tissues and into the bloodstream to be carried away. Since the capillaries are so small in diameter, the blood will not flow as quickly through them as it does through the arteries and veins. This means that the blood has time for an exchange of nutrients, oxygen, and waste material to take place. As blood exits a capillary bed, it returns to the heart through a vein.

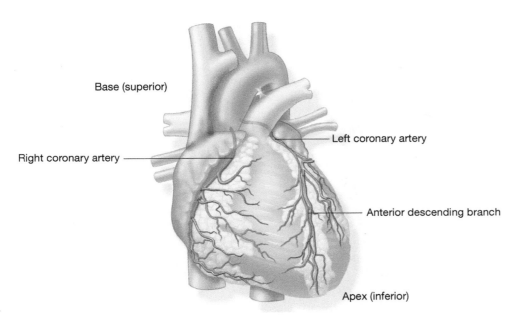

■ **Figure 10** The coronary arteries.

Base (superior)
Left coronary artery
Right coronary artery
Anterior descending branch
Apex (inferior)

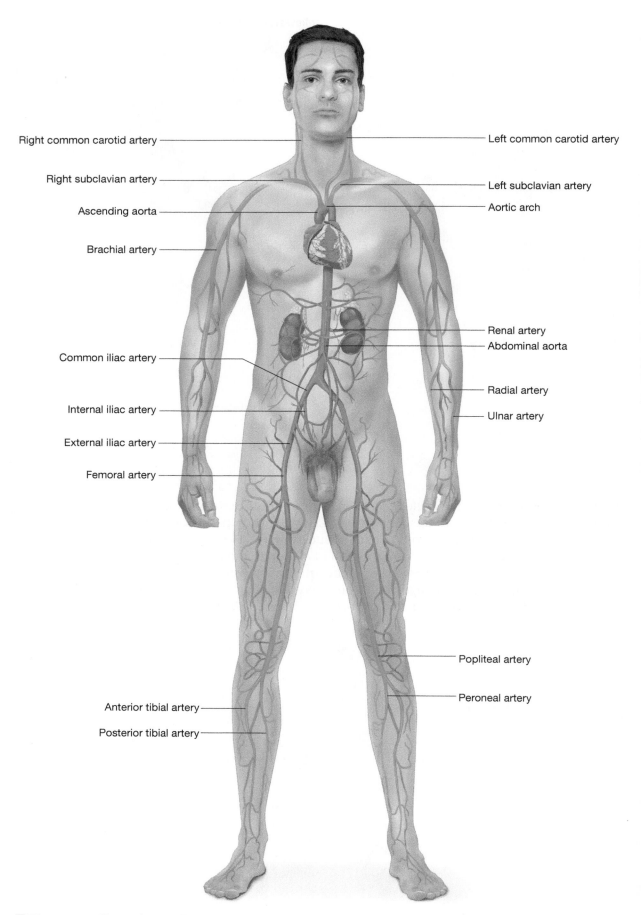

Right common carotid artery

Right subclavian artery

Ascending aorta

Brachial artery

Common iliac artery

Internal iliac artery

External iliac artery

Femoral artery

Anterior tibial artery

Posterior tibial artery

Left common carotid artery

Left subclavian artery

Aortic arch

Renal artery

Abdominal aorta

Radial artery

Ulnar artery

Popliteal artery

Peroneal artery

■ **Figure 11** The major arteries of the body.

Veins

venules (VEN-yools)

The veins carry blood back to the heart. Blood leaving capillaries first enters small **venules**, which then merge into larger veins. Veins have much thinner walls than arteries, causing them to collapse easily. The veins also have valves that allow the blood to move only toward the heart. These valves prevent blood from backflowing; ensuring that blood always flows toward the heart (see Figure 9). The two large veins that enter the heart are the superior vena cava, which carries blood from the upper body, and the inferior vena cava, which carries blood from the lower body. Blood pressure in the veins is much lower than in the arteries. Muscular action against the veins and skeletal muscle contractions help in the movement of blood. Figure 12 ■ illustrates the major systemic veins.

Pulse and Blood Pressure

blood pressure (BP)   **pulse**
diastolic pressure (dye-ah-STOL-ik)   **systolic pressure** (sis-TOL-ik)

Blood pressure (BP) is a measurement of the force exerted by blood against the wall of a blood vessel. During ventricular systole, blood is under a lot of pressure from the ventricular contraction, giving the highest blood pressure reading—the **systolic pressure**. The **pulse** felt at the wrist or throat is the surge of blood caused by the heart contraction. This is why pulse rate is normally equal to heart rate. During ventricular diastole, blood is not being pushed by the heart at all and the blood pressure reading drops to its lowest point—the **diastolic pressure**. Therefore, to see the full range of what is occurring with blood pressure, both numbers are required. Blood pressure is also affected by several other characteristics of the blood and the blood vessels. These include the elasticity of the arteries, the diameter of the blood vessels, the viscosity of the blood, the volume of blood flowing through the vessels, and the amount of resistance to blood flow.

Med Term Tip

The instrument used to measure blood pressure is called a *sphygmomanometer*. The combining form *sphygm/o* means "pulse" and the suffix *-manometer* means "instrument to measure pressure." A blood pressure reading is reported as two numbers, for example, 120/80. The 120 is the systolic pressure and the 80 is the diastolic pressure. There is not one "normal" blood pressure number. The normal range for blood pressure in an adult is 90/60 to 140/90.

Word Building

The following list contains examples of medical terms built directly from word parts. The definition for these terms can be determined by a straightforward translation of the word parts.

COMBINING FORM	COMBINED WITH	MEDICAL TERM	DEFINITION
angi/o	-gram	**angiogram** (AN-jee-oh-gram)	record of a vessel
	-itis	**angiitis** (an-jee-EYE-tis)	inflammation of a vessel
	-plasty	**angioplasty** (AN-jee-oh-plas-tee)	surgical repair of a vessel
	-spasm	**angiospasm** (AN-jee-oh-spazm)	involuntary muscle contraction of a vessel
	-stenosis	**angiostenosis** (an-jee-oh-sten-OH-sis)	narrowing of a vessel
aort/o	-ic	**aortic** (ay-OR-tik)	pertaining to the aorta
arteri/o	-al	**arterial** (ar-TEE-ree-al)	pertaining to the artery
	-ole	**arteriole** (ar-TEE-ree-ohl)	small artery
	-rrhexis	**arteriorrhexis** (ar-tee-ree-oh-REK-sis)	ruptured artery
ather/o	-ectomy	**atherectomy** (ath-er-EK-toh-mee)	removal of fatty substance

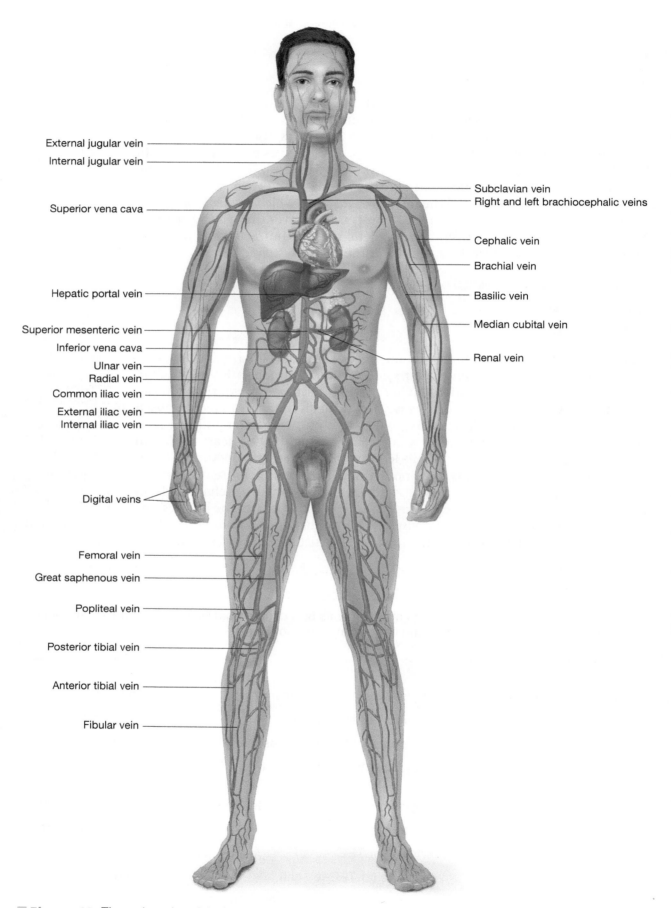

External jugular vein

Internal jugular vein

Superior vena cava

Hepatic portal vein

Superior mesenteric vein

Inferior vena cava

Ulnar vein

Radial vein

Common iliac vein

External iliac vein

Internal iliac vein

Digital veins

Femoral vein

Great saphenous vein

Popliteal vein

Posterior tibial vein

Anterior tibial vein

Fibular vein

Subclavian vein

Right and left brachiocephalic veins

Cephalic vein

Brachial vein

Basilic vein

Median cubital vein

Renal vein

■ **Figure 12** The major veins of the body.

Word Building (continued)

COMBINING FORM	COMBINED WITH	MEDICAL TERM	DEFINITION
	-oma	**atheroma** (ath-er-OH-mah)	fatty substance tumor/growth
atri/o	-al	**atrial** (AY-tree-al)	pertaining to the atrium
	inter- -al	**interatrial** (in-ter-AY-tree-al)	pertaining to between the atria
cardi/o	-ac	**cardiac** (CAR-dee-ak)	pertaining to the heart
	brady- -ia	**bradycardia** (brad-ee-CAR-dee-ah)	state of slow heart
	electr/o -gram	**electrocardiogram** (ee-lek-tro-CAR-dee-oh-gram)	record of heart electricity
	-megaly	**cardiomegaly** (car-dee-oh-MEG-ah-lee)	enlarged heart
	my/o -al	**myocardial** (my-oh-CAR-dee-al)	pertaining to heart muscle
	-ologist	**cardiologist** (car-dee-ALL-oh-jist)	specialist in the heart
	-rrhexis	**cardiorrhexis** (card-dee-oh-REK-sis)	ruptured heart
	tachy- -ia	**tachycardia** (tak-ee-CAR-dee-ah)	state of fast heart
coron/o	-ary	**coronary** (KOR-ah-nair-ee)	pertaining to the heart
phleb/o	-itis	**phlebitis** (fleh-BYE-tis)	inflammation of a vein
valv/o	-plasty	**valvoplasty** (VAL-voh-plas-tee)	surgical repair of a valve
valvul/o	-itis	**valvulitis** (val-view-LYE-tis)	inflammation of a valve
	-ar	**valvular** (VAL-view-lar)	pertaining to a valve
vascul/o	-ar	**vascular** (VAS-kwee-lar)	pertaining to a blood vessel
ven/o	-ous	**venous** (VEE-nus)	pertaining to a vein
	-ule	**venule** (VEN-yool)	small vein
	-gram	**venogram** (VEN-oh-gram)	record of a vein
ventricul/o	-ar	**ventricular** (ven-TRIK-yoo-lar)	pertaining to a ventricle
	inter- -ar	**interventricular** (in-ter-ven-TRIK-yoo-lar)	pertaining to between the ventricles

Vocabulary

TERM	DEFINITION
auscultation (oss-kul-TAY-shun)	The process of listening to the sounds within the body by using a stethoscope.
cardiology (car-dee-ALL-oh-jee)	The branch of medicine involving diagnosis and treatment of conditions and diseases of the cardiovascular system. Physician is a *cardiologist*.
catheter (KATH-eh-ter)	A flexible tube inserted into the body for the purpose of moving fluids into or out of the body. In the cardiovascular system a catheter is used to place dye into blood vessels so they may be visualized on x-rays.
infarct (IN-farkt)	An area of tissue within an organ or part that undergoes necrosis (death) following the loss of its blood supply.
ischemia (is-KEYH-mee-ah)	The localized and temporary deficiency of blood supply due to an obstruction to the circulation.

Vocabulary (continued)

TERM	DEFINITION
murmur (MUR-mur)	An abnormal heart sound such as a soft blowing sound or harsh click. It may be quiet and heard only with a stethoscope, or so loud it can be heard several feet away. Also referred to as a *bruit*.
orthostatic hypotension (or-thoh-STAT-ik)	The sudden drop in blood pressure a person experiences when standing up suddenly.
palpitations (pal-pih-TAY-shunz)	Pounding, racing heartbeats.
plaque (plak)	A yellow, fatty deposit of lipids in an artery that are the hallmark of atherosclerosis.
regurgitation (re-ger-gih-TAY-shun)	To flow backwards. In the cardiovascular system this refers to the backflow of blood through a valve.
sphygmomanometer (sfig-moh-mah-NOM-eh-ter)	Instrument for measuring blood pressure. Also referred to as a *blood pressure cuff* (see Figure 13 ■).
stent	A stainless steel tube placed within a blood vessel or a duct to widen the lumen (see Figure 14 ■).
stethoscope (STETH-oh-scope)	Instrument for listening to body sounds (auscultation), such as the chest, heart, or intestines.

Pathology

TERM	DEFINITION
■ *Heart*	
angina pectoris (an-JYE-nah PECK-tor-is)	Condition in which there is severe pain with a sensation of constriction around the heart. Caused by a deficiency of oxygen to the heart muscle.

■ **Figure 13** Using a sphygmomanometer to measure blood pressure.

■ **Figure 14** The process of placing a stent in a blood vessel. A) A catheter is used to place a collapsed stent next to an atherosclerotic plaque; B) stent is expanded; C) catheter is removed, leaving the expanded stent behind.

Pathology *(continued)*

TERM	DEFINITION
arrhythmia (ah-RITH-mee-ah)	Irregularity in the heartbeat or action. Comes in many different forms; some are not serious, while others are life threatening.
bundle branch block (BBB)	Occurs when the electrical impulse is blocked from traveling down the bundle of His or bundle branches. Results in the ventricles beating at a different rate than the atria. Also called a *heart block*.
cardiac arrest	Complete stopping of heart activity.
cardiomyopathy (car-dee-oh-my-OP-ah-thee)	General term for a disease of the myocardium. Can be caused by alcohol abuse, parasites, viral infection, and congestive heart failure. One of the most common reasons a patient may require a heart transplant.
congenital septal defect (CSD)	A hole, present at birth, in the septum between two heart chambers; results in a mixture of oxygenated and deoxygenated blood. There can be an *atrial septal defect* (ASD) and a *ventricular septal defect* (VSD).
congestive heart failure (CHF) (kon-JESS-tiv)	Pathological condition of the heart in which there is a reduced outflow of blood from the left side of the heart because the left ventricle myocardium has become too weak to efficiently pump blood. Results in weakness, breathlessness, and edema.
coronary artery disease (CAD) (KOR-ah-nair-ee AR-ter-ee dis-EEZ)	Insufficient blood supply to the heart muscle due to an obstruction of one or more coronary arteries. May be caused by atherosclerosis and may cause angina pectoris and myocardial infarction.

Med Term Tip

All types of cardiovascular disease have been the number one killer of Americans since the 19th century. This disease kills more people annually than the next six causes of death combined.

■ **Figure 15** Formation of an atherosclerotic plaque within a coronary artery; may lead to coronary artery disease, angina pectoris, and myocardial infarction.

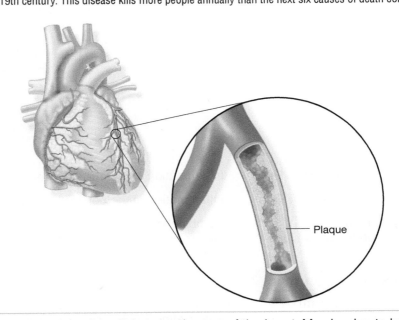

Plaque

endocarditis (en-doh-car-DYE-tis)	Inflammation of the lining membranes of the heart. May be due to bacteria or to an abnormal immunological response. In bacterial endocarditis, the mass of bacteria that forms is referred to as *vegetation*.
fibrillation (fih-brill-AY-shun)	An extremely serious arrhythmia characterized by an abnormal quivering or contraction of heart fibers. When this occurs in the ventricles, cardiac arrest and death can occur. Emergency equipment to defibrillate, or convert the heart to a normal beat, is necessary.

Pathology *(continued)*

TERM	DEFINITION
flutter	An arrhythmia in which the atria beat too rapidly, but in a regular pattern.
heart valve prolapse (PROH-laps)	Condition in which the cusps or flaps of the heart valve are too loose and fail to shut tightly, allowing blood to flow backward through the valve when the heart chamber contracts. Most commonly occurs in the mitral valve, but may affect any of the heart valves.
heart valve stenosis (steh-NOH-sis)	The cusps or flaps of the heart valve are too stiff. Therefore, they are unable to open fully, making it difficult for blood to flow through, or shut tightly, allowing blood to flow backward. This condition may affect any of the heart valves.
myocardial infarction (MI) (my-oh-CAR-dee-al in-FARC-shun)	Condition caused by the partial or complete occlusion or closing of one or more of the coronary arteries. Symptoms include a squeezing pain or heavy pressure in the middle of the chest (angina pectoris). A delay in treatment could result in death. Also referred to as a *heart attack*.

■ **Figure 16** External and cross-sectional view of an infarct caused by a myocardial infarction.

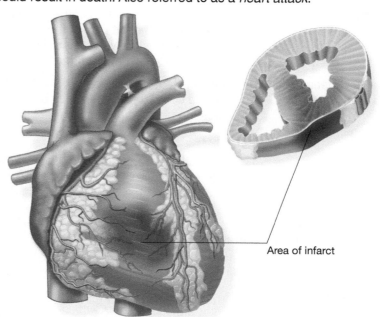

Area of infarct

myocarditis (my-oh-car-DYE-tis)	Inflammation of the muscle layer of the heart wall.
pericarditis (pair-ih-car-DYE-tis)	Inflammation of the pericardial sac around the heart.
tetralogy of Fallot (teh-TRALL-oh-jee of fal-LOH)	Combination of four congenital anomalies: pulmonary stenosis, an interventricular septal defect, improper placement of the aorta, and hypertrophy of the right ventricle. Needs immediate surgery to correct.

■ *Blood Vessels*

aneurysm (AN-yoo-rizm)	Weakness in the wall of an artery resulting in localized widening of the artery. Although an aneurysm may develop in any artery, common sites include the aorta in the abdomen and the cerebral arteries in the brain (see Figure 17 ■).
arteriosclerosis (ar-tee-ree-oh-skleh-ROH-sis)	Thickening, hardening, and loss of elasticity of the walls of the arteries. Most often due to atherosclerosis.

Pathology *(continued)*

TERM	DEFINITION
atherosclerosis (ath-er-oh-skleh-ROH-sis)	The most common form of arteriosclerosis. Caused by the formation of yellowish plaques of cholesterol on the inner walls of arteries (see Figure 18 ■).
coarctation of the aorta (CoA) (koh-ark-TAY-shun)	Severe congenital narrowing of the aorta.
embolus (EM-boh-lus)	The obstruction of a blood vessel by a blood clot that has broken off from a thrombus somewhere else in the body and traveled to the point of obstruction. If it occurs in a coronary artery, it may result in a myocardial infarction (see Figure 19 ■).
hemorrhoid (HIM-oh-royd)	Varicose veins in the anal region.

■ **Figure 17** Illustration of a large aneurysm in the abdominal aorta which has ruptured.

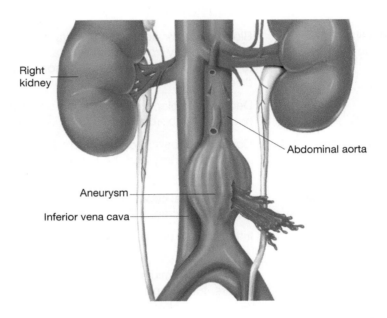

Right kidney

Abdominal aorta

Aneurysm

Inferior vena cava

■ **Figure 18** Development of an atherosclerotic plaque that progressively narrows the lumen of an artery to the point that a thrombus fully occludes the lumen.

A

Lumen
Smooth muscle
Plaque
Endothelium lining of vessel

Plaque formed in artery wall

Damage to epithelium

Platelets and fibrin deposit on plaque forming a clot

B

Moderate narrowing of lumen

Thrombus partially occluding lumen

Thrombus completely occluding lumen

Figure 19 Illustration of an embolus floating in an artery. The embolus will eventually lodge in an artery that is smaller than it is, resulting in occlusion of that artery.

Pathology *(continued)*

TERM	DEFINITION
hypertension (HTN) (high-per-TEN-shun)	Blood pressure above the normal range. *Essential* or *primary hypertension* occurs directly from cardiovascular disease. *Secondary hypertension* refers to high blood pressure resulting from another disease such as kidney disease.
hypotension (high-poh-TEN-shun)	Decrease in blood pressure. Can occur in shock, infection, cancer, anemia, or as death approaches.
patent ductus arteriosus (PDA) (PAY-tent DUCK-tus ar-tee-ree-OH-sis)	Congenital heart anomaly in which the fetal connection between the pulmonary artery and the aorta fails to close at birth. This condition requires surgery.
peripheral vascular disease (PVD)	Any abnormal condition affecting blood vessels outside the heart. Symptoms may include pain, pallor, numbness, and loss of circulation and pulses.
polyarteritis (pol-ee-ar-ter-EYE-tis)	Inflammation of several arteries.
Raynaud's phenomenon (ray-NOZ)	Periodic ischemic attacks affecting the extremities of the body, especially the fingers, toes, ears, and nose. The affected extremities become cyanotic and very painful. These attacks are brought on by arterial constriction due to extreme cold or emotional stress.
thrombophlebitis (throm-boh-fleh-BYE-tis)	Inflammation of a vein resulting in the formation of blood clots within the vein.
thrombus (THROM-bus)	A blood clot forming within a blood vessel (see Figure 18). May partially or completely occlude the blood vessel.
varicose veins (VAIR-ih-kohs)	Swollen and distended veins, usually in the legs.

Diagnostic Procedures

TERM	DEFINITION
■ *Clinical Laboratory Tests*	
cardiac enzymes (CAR-dee-ak EN-zyms)	Blood test to determine the level of enzymes specific to heart muscles in the blood. An increase in the enzymes may indicate heart muscle damage such as a myocardial infarction. These enzymes include creatine phosphokinase (CPK), lactate dehydrogenase (LDH), and glutamic oxaloacetic transaminase (GOT).
serum lipoprotein level (SEE-rum lip-oh-PROH-teen)	Blood test to measure the amount of cholesterol and triglycerides in the blood. An indicator of atherosclerosis risk.

Diagnostic Procedures *(continued)*

TERM	DEFINITION
■ *Diagnostic Imaging*	
angiography (an-jee-OG-rah-fee)	X-rays taken after the injection of an opaque material into a blood vessel. Can be performed on the aorta as an aortic angiogram, on the heart as an angiocardiogram, and on the brain as a cerebral angiogram.
cardiac scan	Patient is given radioactive thallium intravenously and then scanning equipment is used to visualize the heart. It is especially useful in determining myocardial damage.
Doppler ultrasonography (DOP-ler ul-trah-son-OG-rah-fee)	Measurement of sound-wave echoes as they bounce off tissues and organs to produce an image. In this system, used to measure velocity of blood moving through blood vessels to look for blood clots or deep vein thromboses.
echocardiography (ek-oh-car-dee-OG-rah-fee)	Noninvasive diagnostic method using ultrasound to visualize internal cardiac structures. Cardiac valve activity can be evaluated using this method.
venography (vee-NOG-rah-fee)	X-ray of the veins by tracing the venous pulse. May be used to identify a thrombus. Also called *phlebography*.
■ *Cardiac Function Tests*	
cardiac catheterization (CAR-dee-ak cath-eh-ter-ih-ZAY-shun)	Passage of a thin tube catheter through a blood vessel leading to the heart. Done to detect abnormalities, to collect cardiac blood samples, and to determine the blood pressure within the heart.
electrocardiography (ECG, EKG) (ee-lek-troh-car-dee-OG-rah-fee)	Process of recording the electrical activity of the heart. Useful in the diagnosis of abnormal cardiac rhythm and heart muscle (myocardium) damage.
Holter monitor	Portable ECG monitor worn by a patient for a period of a few hours to a few days to assess the heart and pulse activity as the person goes through the activities of daily living. Used to assess a patient who experiences chest pain and unusual heart activity during exercise and normal activities.
stress testing	Method for evaluating cardiovascular fitness. The patient is placed on a treadmill or a bicycle and then subjected to steadily increasing levels of work. An EKG and oxygen levels are taken while the patient exercises. The test is stopped if abnormalities occur on the EKG. Also called an *exercise test* or a *treadmill test*

■ **Figure 20** Man undergoing a stress test on a treadmill while physician monitors his condition. *(Jonathan Nourok/PhotoEdit Inc.)*

Therapeutic Procedures

TERM	DEFINITION

■ Medical Procedures

TERM	DEFINITION
cardiopulmonary resuscitation (CPR) (car-dee-oh-PULL-mon-air-ee ree-suss-ih-TAY-shun)	Procedure to restore cardiac output and oxygenated air to the lungs for a person in cardiac arrest. A combination of chest compressions (to push blood out of the heart) and artificial respiration (to blow air into the lungs) performed by one or two CPR-trained rescuers.
defibrillation (dee-fib-rih-LAY-shun)	A procedure that converts serious irregular heartbeats, such as fibrillation, by giving electric shocks to the heart using an instrument called a defibrillator. Also called *cardioversion*.

■ Figure 21 An emergency medical technician positions defibrillator paddles on the chest of a supine male patient.

TERM	DEFINITION
extracorporeal circulation (ECC) (EX-tra-core-poor-EE-al)	During open-heart surgery, the routing of blood to a heart-lung machine so it can be oxygenated and pumped to the rest of the body.
implantable cardioverter-defibrillator (CAR-dee-oh-ver-ter de-FIB-rih-lay-tor)	A device implanted in the heart that delivers an electrical shock to restore a normal heart rhythm. Particularly useful for persons who experience ventricular fibrillation.
pacemaker implantation	Electrical device that substitutes for the natural pacemaker of the heart. It controls the beating of the heart by a series of rhythmic electrical impulses. An external pacemaker has the electrodes on the outside of the body. An internal pacemaker has the electrodes surgically implanted within the chest wall (see Figure 22 ■).
thrombolytic therapy (throm-boh-LIT-ik THAIR-ah-pee)	Process in which drugs, such as streptokinase (SK) or tissue-type plasminogen activator (tPA), are injected into a blood vessel to dissolve clots and restore blood flow.

■ Surgical Procedures

TERM	DEFINITION
aneurysmectomy (an-yoo-riz-MEK-toh-mee)	The surgical removal of the sac of an aneurysm.
arterial anastomosis (ar-TEE-ree-all ah-nas-toe-MOE-sis)	The surgical joining together of two arteries. Performed if an artery is severed or if a damaged section of an artery is removed.
coronary artery bypass graft (CABG) (KOR-ah-nair-ee)	Open-heart surgery in which a blood vessel from another location in the body (often a leg vein) is grafted to route blood around a blocked coronary artery.
embolectomy (em-boh-LEK-toh-mee)	The removal of an embolus or clot from a blood vessel.
endarterectomy (end-ar-teh-REK-toh-mee)	Removal of the diseased or damaged inner lining of an artery. Usually performed to remove atherosclerotic plaques.

Therapeutic Procedures *(continued)*

TERM	DEFINITION
heart transplantation	Replacement of a diseased or malfunctioning heart with a donor's heart.
intracoronary artery stent (in-trah-KOR-ah-nair-ee AR-ter-ee)	Placing of a stent within a coronary artery to treat coronary ischemia due to atherosclerosis (see Figure 14).
ligation and stripping (lye-GAY-shun)	Surgical treatment for varicose veins. The damaged vein is tied off (ligation) and removed (stripping).
percutaneous transluminal coronary angioplasty (PTCA) (per-kyoo-TAY-nee-us trans-LOO-mih-nal KOR-ah-nair-ee AN-jee-oh-plas-tee)	The method for treating localized coronary artery narrowing. A balloon catheter is inserted through the skin into the coronary artery and inflated to dilate the narrow blood vessel (see Figure 23 ▦).
valve replacement	Removal of a diseased heart valve and replacement with an artificial valve.

▦ **Figure 22** Color enhanced X-ray showing a pacemaker implanted in the left side of the chest and the electrode wires running to the heart muscle. *(UHB Trust/Getty Images Inc.—Stone Allstock)*

▦ **Figure 23** Balloon angioplasty: A) deflated balloon catheter is approaching an atherosclerotic plaque; B) plaque is compressed by inflated balloon; C) plaque remains compressed after balloon catheter is removed.

Pharmacology

CLASSIFICATION	ACTION	GENERIC AND BRAND NAMES
ACE inhibitor drugs	Produce vasodilation and decrease blood pressure.	benazepril, Lotensin; catopril, Capoten
antiarrhythmic (an-tye-a-RHYTH-mik)	Reduces or prevents cardiac arrhythmias.	flecainide, Tambocor; ibutilide, Corvert
anticoagulant (an-tye-koh-AG-you-lant)	Prevent blood clot formation.	warfarin sodium, Coumadin, Warfarin
antilipidemic (an-tye-lip-ih-DEM-ik)	Reduces amount of cholesterol and lipids in the bloodstream; treats hyperlipidemia.	atorvastatin, Lipitor; simvastatin, Zocor

Pharmacology *(continued)*

CLASSIFICATION	ACTION	GENERIC AND BRAND NAMES
beta-blocker drugs	Treats hypertension and angina pectoris by lowering the heart rate.	metoprolol, Lopressor; propranolol, Inderal
calcium channel blocker drugs	Treats hypertension, angina pectoris, and congestive heart failure by causing the heart to beat less forcefully and less often.	diltiazem, Cardizem; nifedipine, Procardia
cardiotonic (card-ee-oh-TAHN-ik)	Increases the force of cardiac muscle contraction; treats congestive heart failure.	digoxin, Lanoxin
diuretic (dye-you-RET-ik)	Increases urine production by the kidneys, which works to reduce plasma and therefore blood volume, resulting in lower blood pressure.	furosemide, Lasix
thrombolytic (throm-boh-LIT-ik)	Dissolves existing blood clots.	clopidogrel, Plavix; alteplase, Activase
vasoconstrictor (vaz-oh-kon-STRICK-tor)	Contracts smooth muscle in walls of blood vessels; raises blood pressure.	metaraminol, Aramine
vasodilator (vaz-oh-DYE-late-or)	Relaxes the smooth muscle in the walls of arteries, thereby increasing diameter of the blood vessel. Used for two main purposes: increasing circulation to an ischemic area; reducing blood pressure.	nitroglycerine, Nitro-Dur; isoxsuprine, Vasodilan

 # Abbreviations

AF	atrial fibrillation		**IV**	intravenous
AMI	acute myocardial infarction		**LDH**	lactate dehydrogenase
AS	arteriosclerosis		**LVAD**	left ventricular assist device
ASD	atrial septal defect		**LVH**	left ventricular hypertrophy
ASHD	arteriosclerotic heart disease		**MI**	myocardial infarction, mitral insufficiency
AV, A-V	atrioventricular		**mm Hg**	millimeters of mercury
BBB	bundle branch block (L for left; R for right)		**MR**	mitral regurgitation
BP	blood pressure		**MS**	mitral stenosis
bpm	beats per minute			
CABG	coronary artery bypass graft			
CAD	coronary artery disease			
cath	catheterization			

Med Term Tip

Word alert – be careful using the abbreviation *MS* which can mean either "mitral stenosis" or "multiple sclerosis."

CC	cardiac catheterization, chief complaint		**MVP**	mitral valve prolapse
CCU	coronary care unit		**P**	pulse
CHF	congestive heart failure		**PAC**	premature atrial contraction
CoA	coarctation of the aorta		**PDA**	patent ductus arteriosus
CP	chest pain		**PTCA**	percutaneous transluminal coronary angioplasty
CPK	creatine phosphokinase			
CPR	cardiopulmonary resuscitation		**PVC**	premature ventricular contraction
CSD	congenital septal defect		**S1**	first heart sound
CV	cardiovascular		**S2**	second heart sound
DVT	deep vein thrombosis		**SA, S-A**	sinoatrial
ECC	extracorporeal circulation		**SGOT**	serum glutamic oxaloacetic transaminase
ECG, EKG	electrocardiogram		**SK**	streptokinase
ECHO	echocardiogram		**tPA**	tissue-type plasminogen activator
GOT	glutamic oxaloacetic transaminase		**Vfib**	ventricular fibrillation
HTN	hypertension		**VSD**	ventricular septal defect
ICU	intensive care unit		**VT**	ventricular tachycardia

Chapter Review

Terminology Checklist

 Below are all Anatomy and Physiology key terms, Word Building, Vocabulary, Pathology, Diagnostic, Therapeutic, and Pharmacology terms presented in this chapter. Use this list as a study tool by placing a check in the box in front of each term as you master its meaning.

- ☐ ACE inhibitor drugs
- ☐ aneurysm
- ☐ aneurysmectomy
- ☐ angiitis
- ☐ angina pectoris
- ☐ angiogram
- ☐ angiography
- ☐ angioplasty
- ☐ angiospasm
- ☐ angiostenosis
- ☐ antiarrhythmic
- ☐ anticoagulant
- ☐ antilipidemic
- ☐ aorta
- ☐ aortic
- ☐ aortic valve
- ☐ apex
- ☐ arrhythmia
- ☐ arterial
- ☐ arterial anastomosis
- ☐ arteries
- ☐ arterioles
- ☐ arteriorrhexis
- ☐ arteriosclerosis
- ☐ atherectomy
- ☐ atheroma
- ☐ atherosclerosis
- ☐ atria
- ☐ atrial
- ☐ atrioventricular bundle
- ☐ atrioventricular node
- ☐ atrioventricular valve
- ☐ auscultation
- ☐ autonomic nervous system
- ☐ beta blocker drugs
- ☐ bicuspid valve
- ☐ blood pressure
- ☐ blood vessels

- ☐ bradycardia
- ☐ bundle branch block
- ☐ bundle branches
- ☐ bundle of His
- ☐ calcium channel blocker drugs
- ☐ capillaries
- ☐ capillary bed
- ☐ carbon dioxide
- ☐ cardiac
- ☐ cardiac arrest
- ☐ cardiac catheterization
- ☐ cardiac enzymes
- ☐ cardiac muscle
- ☐ cardiac scan
- ☐ cardiologist
- ☐ cardiology
- ☐ cardiomegaly
- ☐ cardiomyopathy
- ☐ cardiopulmonary resuscitation
- ☐ cardiorrhexis
- ☐ cardiotonic
- ☐ catheter
- ☐ circulatory system
- ☐ coarctation of the aorta
- ☐ congenital septal defect
- ☐ congestive heart failure
- ☐ coronary
- ☐ coronary arteries
- ☐ coronary artery bypass graft
- ☐ coronary artery disease
- ☐ cusps
- ☐ defibrillation
- ☐ deoxygenated
- ☐ diastole
- ☐ diastolic pressure
- ☐ diuretic
- ☐ Doppler ultrasonography
- ☐ echocardiography

- ☐ electrocardiogram
- ☐ electrocardiography
- ☐ embolectomy
- ☐ embolus
- ☐ endarterectomy
- ☐ endocarditis
- ☐ endocardium
- ☐ epicardium
- ☐ extracorporeal circulation
- ☐ fibrillation
- ☐ flutter
- ☐ heart
- ☐ heart transplantation
- ☐ heart valve prolapse
- ☐ heart valve stenosis
- ☐ hemorrhoid
- ☐ Holter monitor
- ☐ hypertension
- ☐ hypotension
- ☐ implantable cardioverter-defibrillator
- ☐ infarct
- ☐ inferior vena cava
- ☐ interatrial
- ☐ interatrial septum
- ☐ interventricular
- ☐ interventricular septum
- ☐ intracoronary artery stent
- ☐ ischemia
- ☐ ligation and stripping
- ☐ lumen
- ☐ mitral valve
- ☐ murmur
- ☐ myocardial
- ☐ myocardial infarction
- ☐ myocarditis
- ☐ myocardium
- ☐ orthostatic hypotension

- ☐ oxygen
- ☐ oxygenated
- ☐ pacemaker
- ☐ pacemaker implantation
- ☐ palpitations
- ☐ parietal pericardium
- ☐ patent ductus arteriosus
- ☐ percutaneous transluminal coronary angioplasty
- ☐ pericarditis
- ☐ pericardium
- ☐ peripheral vascular disease
- ☐ phlebitis
- ☐ phlebogram
- ☐ plaque
- ☐ polyarteritis
- ☐ pulmonary artery
- ☐ pulmonary circulation
- ☐ pulmonary valve
- ☐ pulmonary vein

- ☐ pulse
- ☐ Purkinje fibers
- ☐ Raynaud's phenomenon
- ☐ regurgitation
- ☐ semilunar valves
- ☐ serum lipoprotein
- ☐ sinoatrial node
- ☐ sphygmomanometer
- ☐ stent
- ☐ stethoscope
- ☐ stress testing
- ☐ superior vena cava
- ☐ systemic circulation
- ☐ systole
- ☐ systolic pressure
- ☐ tachycardia
- ☐ tetralogy of Fallot
- ☐ thrombolytic
- ☐ thrombolytic therapy

- ☐ thrombophlebitis
- ☐ thrombus
- ☐ tricuspid valve
- ☐ valve replacement
- ☐ valvoplasty
- ☐ valvular
- ☐ valvulitis
- ☐ varicose veins
- ☐ vascular
- ☐ vasoconstrictor
- ☐ vasodilator
- ☐ veins
- ☐ venography
- ☐ venous
- ☐ ventricles
- ☐ ventricular
- ☐ venules
- ☐ visceral pericardium

Practice Exercises

A. Complete the following statements.

1. The study of the heart is called _Cardiology_.

2. The three layers of the heart are _endocardium_, _myocardium_, and _epicardium_.

3. The impulse for the heartbeat (the pacemaker) originates in the _Sinoatrial (SA) node_.

4. Arteries carry blood _away_ the heart.

5. The four heart valves are _tricuspid valve_, _pulmonary valve_, _mitral valve_, and _aortic valve_.

6. The _atria_ are the receiving chambers of the heart and the _ventricles_ are the pumping chambers.

7. The _pulmonary_ circulation carries blood to and from the lungs.

8. The pointed tip of the heart is called the _apex_.

9. The _interatrial septum & interventricular septum?_ divides the heart into left and right halves.

10. _Systole_ is the contraction phase of the heart beat and _diastole_ is the relaxation phase.

B. State the terms described using the combining forms provided.

The combining form *cardi/o* refers to the heart. Use it to write a term that means:

1. pertaining to the heart ___cardiac___

2. disease of the heart muscle ___cardiomyopathy___

3. enlargement of the heart ___cardiomegaly___

4. abnormally fast heart rate ___tachycardia___

5. abnormally slow heart rate ___bradycardia___

6. rupture of the heart ___~~cardiorrhexxis~~ cardiorrhexis___

The combining form *angi/o* refers to the vessel. Use it to write a term that means:

7. vessel narrowing ___angiostenosis___

8. vessel inflammation ___angitis___

9. involuntary muscle contraction of a vessel ___angiospasm___

The combining form *arteri/o* refers to the artery. Use it to write a term that means:

10. pertaining to an artery ___arterial___

11. hardening of an artery ___arteriosclerosis___

12. small artery ___arteriole___

C. Add a prefix to *-carditis* to form the term for:

1. inflammation of the inner lining of the heart ___endocarditis___

2. inflammation of the outer layer of the heart ___epicarditis___

3. inflammation of the muscle of the heart ___myocarditis___

D. Define the following combining forms and use them to form cardiovascular terms.

	Definition	Cardiovascular Term
1. cardi/o	heart	myocardial
2. valvul/o	valve	valvular
3. steth/o	chest	stethoscope
4. arteri/o	artery	arteriole
5. phleb/o	vein	phlebitis
6. angi/o	vessel	angiogram
7. ventricul/o	ventricle	ventricular

8. thromb/o ___Clot___ ___thrombus___

9. atri/o ___atrium___ ___atrial___

10. ather/o ___fatty substance___ ___artherectomy___

E. Write medical terms for the following definitions.

1. pertaining to a vein ___venous___

2. study of the heart ___cardiology___

3. record of a vein ___venogram___

4. process of recording electrical activity of heart ___electrocardiography___

5. high blood pressure ___hypertension___

6. low blood pressure ___hypotension___

7. surgical repair of valve ___valvoplasty___

8. pertaining to between ventricles ___intervantricular___

9. removal of fatty substance ___artherectomy___

10. narrowing of the arteries ___arteriostenosis___

F. Write the suffix for each expression and provide an example of its use.

	Suffix	Example
1. pressure	-tension	hypertension
2. abnormal narrowing	-stenosis	arteriostenosis
3. instrument to measure pressure	-manometer	sphygmomanometer
4. small	-ole, -ule	arteriole, vanule
5. hardening	-sclerosis	arteriosclerosis

G. Identify the following abbreviations.

1. BP ___blood pressure___

2. CHF ___congestive heart failure___

3. MI ___myocardial infarction, mitral insufficiency___

4. CCU ___coronary care unit___

5. PVC ___premature ventricular contraction___

6. CPR ___cardiopulmonary resuscitation___

7. CAD ___coronary artery disease___

8. CP _____ chest pain _____

9. EKG _____ electrocardiogram _____

10. S1 _____ first heart sound _____

H. Write the abbreviations for the following terms.

1. mitral valve prolapse ___ MVP _____

6. lactate dehydrogenase ___ LDH _____

2. ventricular septal defect ___ VSD _____

7. coarctation of the aorta ___ CoA _____

3. percutaneous transluminal coronary angioplasty _____
___ PTCA _____

8. tissue-type plasminogen activator _____
___ tPA _____

4. ventricular fibrillation ___ Vfib _____

9. cardiovascular ___ CV _____

5. deep vein thrombosis ___ DVT _____

10. extracorporeal circulation ___ ECC _____

I. Match each term to its definition.

1. ___ f ___ arrhythmia

a. swollen, distended veins

2. ___ h ___ thrombus

b. inflammation of vein

3. ___ d ___ bradycardia

c. serious congenital anomaly

4. ___ g ___ murmur

d. slow heart rate

5. ___ b ___ phlebitis

e. insertion of thin tubing

6. ___ i ___ hypotension

f. irregular heartbeat

7. ___ a ___ varicose vein

g. an abnormal heart sound

8. ___ c ___ tetralogy of Fallot

h. clot in blood vessel

9. ___ e ___ catheterization

i. low blood pressure

10. ___ j ___ sphygmomanometer

j. blood pressure cuff

J. Define the following terms.

1. catheter ___ a flexible tube inserted in the body to move fluids in or out

2. infarct ___ an area of tissue within an organ or part that undergoes necrosis following a loss of it's blood supply.

3. thrombus ___ blood clot

4. palpitation ___ pounding, racing heart beats

5. regurgitation ___ to flow backwards, back flow of blood through a valve

6. aneurysm ___ weakness in the wall of an artery resulting in localized widening of the artery

7. cardiac arrest ___ complete stopping of heart activity

Cardiovascular System

8. fibrillation _an extremely serious arrhythmia characterized by an abnormal_ quivering or contraction of heart fibers

9. myocardial infarction _condition caused by partial or complete occlusion or closing of_ one or more coronary arteries - heart attack

10. hemorrhoid _varicose veins in the anal region_

K. Match each procedure to its definition.

1. __C__ cardiac enzymes
2. __g__ Doppler ultrasound
3. __j__ Holter monitor
4. __a__ cardiac scan
5. __d__ stress testing
6. __b__ echocardiography
7. __i__ extracorporeal circulation
8. __e__ ligation and stripping
9. __f__ thrombolytic therapy
10. __h__ PTAC

a. visualizes heart after patient is given radioactive thallium

b. uses ultrasound to visualize heart beating

c. blood test that indicates heart muscle damage

d. uses treadmill to evaluate cardiac fitness

e. removes varicose veins

f. clot dissolving drugs

g. measures velocity of blood moving through blood vessels

h. balloon angioplasty

i. use of a heart-lung machine

j. portable EKG monitor

L. Fill in the classification for each drug description, then match the brand name.

	Drug Description	Classification		Brand Name
1. __e__	prevents arrhythmia	antiarrhythmic	a.	Plavix
2. __g__	reduces cholesterol	antilipidemic	b.	Coumadin
3. __f__	increases force of heart contraction	cardiotonic	c.	Cardizem
4. __h__	increases urine production	diuretic	d.	Nitro-Dur
5. __b__	prevents blood clots	anticoagulant	e.	Tambocor
6. __a__	dissolves blood clots	thrombolytic	f.	Lanoxin
7. __d__	relaxes smooth muscle in artery wall	vasodilator	g.	Lipitor
8. __c__	cause heart to beat less forcefully	calcium channel blocker drugs	h.	Lasix

M. Use the following terms in the sentences that follow.

angiography   murmur   varicose veins   echocardiogram   pacemaker   CHF
defibrillation   angina pectoris   Holter monitor   hypertension   MI   CCU

1. Tiffany was born with a congenital condition resulting in an abnormal heart sound called a(n) _murmur_.

2. Joseph suffered an arrhythmia resulting in a cardiac arrest. The emergency team used an instrument to give electric shocks to the heart to create a normal heart rhythm. This procedure is called _defibrillation_.

3. Marguerite has been placed on a low-sodium diet and medication to bring her blood pressure down to a normal range. She suffers from _hypertension_.

4. Tony has had an artificial device called a(n) _pacemaker_ inserted to control the beating of his heart by producing rhythmic electrical impulses.

5. Derrick's physician determined that he had _varicose veins_ after examining his legs and finding swollen, tortuous veins.

6. Laura has persistent chest pains that require medication. The term for the pain is _angina pectoris_.

7. La Tonya will be admitted to what hospital unit after surgery to correct her heart condition? _CCU_

8. Stephen is going to have a coronary artery bypass graft to correct the blockage in his coronary arteries. He recently suffered a heart attack as a result of this occlusion. His attack is called a(n) _MI_.

9. Stephen's physician scheduled a(n) _angiography_, an X-ray to determine the extent of his blood vessel damage.

10. A patient scheduled to have a diagnostic procedure that uses ultrasound to produce an image of the heart valves is going to have a(n) _echocardiogram_

11. Eric must wear a device for 24 hours that will keep track of his heart activity as he performs his normal daily routine. This device is called a(n) _Holter monitor_

12. Lydia is 82 years old and is suffering from a heart condition that causes weakness, edema, and breathlessness. Her heart failure is the cause of her lung congestion. This condition is called _CHF_.

Medical Record Analysis

Below is an item from a patient's medical record. Read it carefully, make sure you understand all the medical terms used, and then answer the questions that follow.

Discharge Summary

Admitting Diagnosis:
Difficulty breathing, hypertension, tachycardia

Final Diagnosis:
CHF secondary to mitral valve prolapse

History of Present Illness:
Patient was brought to the Emergency Room by her family because of SOB, tachycardia, and anxiety. Patient reports that she has experienced these symptoms for the past six months, brought on by exertion. The current episode began while she was cleaning house and is more severe than any previous episode. Upon admission in the ER, HR was 120 beats per minute and blood pressure was 180/110. The patient was cyanotic around the lips and nail beds and had severe edema in feet and lower legs. The results of an EKG and cardiac enzyme blood tests were normal. Medication improved the symptoms, but she was admitted for observation and a complete cardiac workup for tachycardia, hypertension.

Summary of Hospital Course:
Patient underwent a full battery of cardiac diagnostic tests. A prolapsed mitral valve was observed on an echocardiogram. A treadmill test had to be stopped early due to onset of severe difficulty in breathing and cyanosis of the lips. Arterial blood gases showed low oxygen, and supplemental oxygen per nasal canula was required to resolve cyanosis. Angiocardiography failed to demonstrate significant coronary artery thrombosis. Blood pressure, tachycardia, anxiety, and pitting edema were controlled with medications. Patient took Lopressor to control blood pressure, Norpace to slow heart rate, Valium for the anxiety, and Lasix to reduce edema. At discharge, HR was 88 beats per minute, blood pressure was 165/98, and there was no evidence of edema unless she was on her feet too long.

Discharge Plans:
There was no evidence of a myocardial infarction and with lack of significant coronary thrombosis, angioplasty is not indicated for this patient. Patient was placed on a low-salt and low-cholesterol diet. She received instructions on beginning a carefully graded exercise program. She is to continue Lasix, Norpace, Valium, and Lopressor. If symptoms are not controlled by these measures, a mitral valve replacement will be considered.

Critical Thinking Questions

1. List the four medications this patient was given in the hospital and describe in your own words what condition each medication treats.
   a. Lopressor - high blood pressure
   b. Norpace - rapid heart rate
   c. Valium - anxiety
   d. Lasix - swelling

2. Two diagnostic tests conducted in the Emergency Room were normal. List them and describe each test in your own words. Because the results from these two tests were normal, a very serious heart condition could be ruled out. This is noted in the discharge plans. Identify the serious heart condition and describe it in your own words.

EKG - electrocardiogram - record of electrical activity in the heart
Cardiac Enzyme blood test - looks for increased enzymes indicating heart muscle damage
Myocardial Infarction - heart attack

3. Explain in your own words why the treadmill test had to be stopped. The patient had difficulty breathing and lips were turning blue.

4. Which of the following is NOT one of the admitting diagnoses?
   a. high blood pressure
   b. dizziness
   c. difficulty breathing
   d. fast heartbeat

5. The physician has two treatment options for this patient: medication and surgery. If the medication fails to control her condition, then describe what surgery will be considered. Mitral Valve Replacement - replacement of the valve

6. Compare and contrast valve stenosis and valve prolapse. Valve stenosis is a narrowing of the valve - they are stiff & unable to open fully. Valve prolapse cusps are too loose & fail to shut tightly. Both defects allow blood to flow backward.

Chart Note Transcription

The chart note below contains eleven phrases that can be reworded with a medical term that you learned in this chapter. Each phrase is identified with an underline. Determine the medical term and write your answers in the space provided.

Current Complaint:	A 56-year-old male was admitted to the Cardiac Care Unit from the Emergency Room with left arm pain, severe pain around the heart, ❶ an abnormally slow heartbeat, ❷ nausea, and vomiting.
Past History:	Patient reports no heart problems prior to this episode. He has taken medication for high blood pressure ❸ for the past five years. His family history is significant for a father and brother who both died in their 50s from death of heart muscle. ❹
Signs and Symptoms:	Patient reports severe pain around the heart that radiates into his left jaw and arm. A record of the heart's electrical activity ❺ and a blood test to determine the amount of heart damage ❻ were abnormal.
Diagnosis:	An acute death of heart muscle ❹ resulting from insufficient blood flow to heart muscle due to obstruction of coronary artery. ❼
Treatment:	First, provide supportive care during the acute phase. Second, evaluate heart damage by passing a thin tube through a blood vessel into the heart to detect abnormalities ❽ and evaluate heart fitness by having patient exercise on a treadmill. ❾ Finally, perform surgical intervention by either inflating a balloon catheter to dilate a narrow vessel ❿ or by open heart surgery to create a shunt around a blocked vessel. ⓫

1. angina pectoris
2. bradycardia
3. hypertension
4. myocardial infarction
5. EKG
6. Cardiac Enzyme Test
7. ~~myocardial infarction~~ ⑦ coronary artery disease
8. ⑧ cardiac catheterization ⑨ stress test
9.
10. PTCA
11. intracoronary artery stent

Labeling Exercise

A. System Review

Write the labels for this figure on the numbered lines provided.

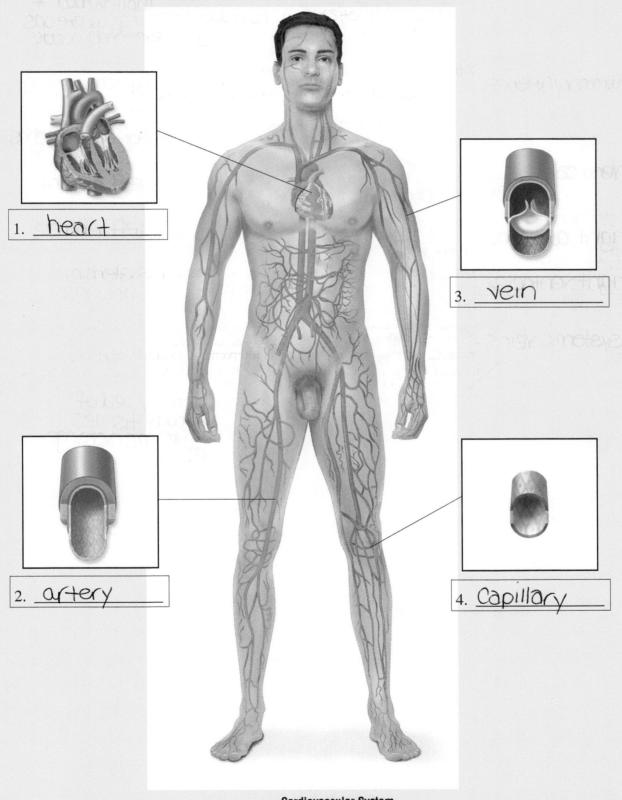

1. heart

2. artery

3. vein

4. Capillary

Cardiovascular System

B. Anatomy Challenge

1. Write the labels for this figure on the numbered lines provided.

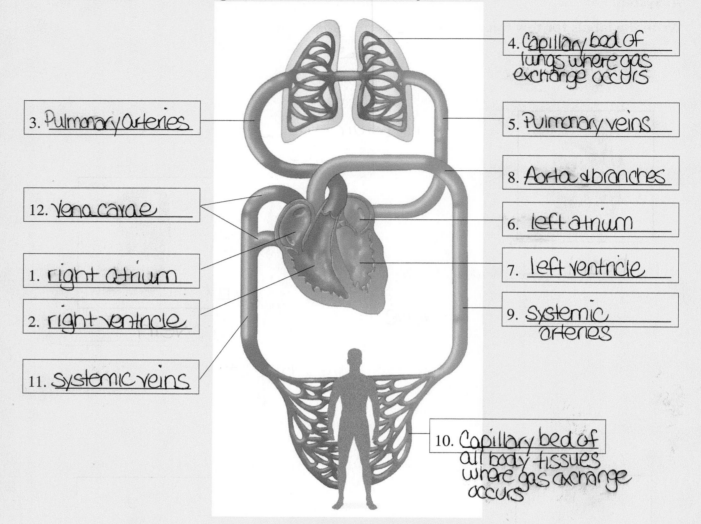

3. Pulmonary Arteries

12. Vena cavae

1. right atrium

2. right ventricle

11. systemic veins

4. Capillary bed of lungs where gas exchange occurs

5. Pulmonary veins

8. Aorta & branches

6. left atrium

7. left ventricle

9. systemic arteries

10. Capillary bed of all body tissues where gas exchange occurs

2. Write the labels for this figure on the numbered lines provided.

13. superior vena cava

12. Aorta

5. Pulmonary trunk

4. Pulmonary valve

1. right atrium

2. tricuspid valve

3. right ventricle

14. inferior vena cava

6. left pulmonary artery branches

7. left pulmonary vein branches

8. left atrium

11. aortic valve

9. mitral valve

10. left ventricle

15. endocardium

16. myocardium

17. pericardium

Multimedia Preview

Additional interactive resources and activities for this chapter can be found on the Companion Website.

Website Highlights — www.prenhall.com/fremgen

LABELING EXERCISE

Click here and take advantage of the free-access on-line study guide that accompanies your textbook. You'll find a figure labeling quiz that corresponds to this chapter. By clicking on this URL you'll also access links to download mp3 audio reviews, current news articles, and an audio glossary.

Blood and the Lymphatic and Immune Systems

Learning Objectives

Upon completion of this chapter, you will be able to:

- Recognize the combining forms and suffixes introduced in this chapter.
- Gain the ability to pronounce medical terms and major anatomical structures.
- List the major components, structures, and organs of the blood and lymphatic and immune systems and their functions.
- Describe the blood typing systems.
- Discuss immunity, the immune response, and standard precautions.
- Build blood and lymphatic and immune system medical terms from word parts.
- Define vocabulary, pathology, diagnostic, and therapeutic medical terms relating to the blood and lymphatic and immune system.
- Recognize types of medication associated with blood and the lymphatic and immune systems.
- Interpret abbreviations associated with blood and the lymphatic and immune systems.

From Chapter 6 of *Medical Terminology: A Living Language*, 4/e. Bonnie F. Fremgen. Suzanne S. Frucht. Copyright © 2009 by Pearson Education. Published by Prentice Hall. All rights reserved.

Section I: Blood at a Glance

Function

Blood transports to all areas of the body gases, nutrients, and wastes either attached to red blood cells or dissolved in the plasma. White blood cells fight infection and disease, and platelets initiate the blood clotting process.

Components

formed elements
- **erythrocytes**
- **platelets** -- thrombocytes
- **leukocytes**

plasma

Combining Forms

agglutin/o	clumping, clotting, coagulate	**hem/o**	blood
bas/o	base	**hemat/o**	blood
chrom/o	color	**leuk/o**	white
coagul/o	clotting	**morph/o**	shape
eosin/o	rosy red	**neutr/o**	neutral
erythr/o	red	**phag/o**	eat, swallow
fibrin/o	fibers, fibrous	**sanguin/o**	blood
granul/o	granules	**thromb/o**	clot

Suffixes

-apheresis	removal, carry away
-cytosis	more than the normal number of cells
-emia	blood condition
-globin	protein
-penia	abnormal decrease, too few thrombocytopenia
-phil	attracted to
-poiesis	formation
-stasis	standing still

Blood Illustrated

Whole blood

Blood specimen collected

Centrifuge

Blood separated

Plasma

Red blood cells

Platelets

Neutrophil

Monocyte

Basophil

Eosinophil

Lymphocyte

Anatomy and Physiology of Blood

erythrocytes (eh-RITH-roh-sights)
formed elements
hematopoiesis (hee-mah-toh-poy-EE-sis)
leukocytes (LOO-koh-sights)

plasma (PLAZ-mah)
platelets (PLAYT lets)
red blood cells
white blood cells

The average adult has about five liters of blood that circulates throughout the body within the blood vessels of the cardiovascular system. Blood is a mixture of cells floating in watery **plasma**. As a group, these cells are referred to as **formed elements**, but there are three different kinds: **erythrocytes** or **red blood cells**, **leukocytes** or **white blood cells**, and **platelets**. Blood cells are produced in the red bone marrow by a process called **hematopoiesis**. Plasma and erythrocytes are responsible for transporting substances, leukocytes protect the body from invading microorganisms, and platelets play a role in controlling bleeding.

Plasma

albumin (al-BEW-min)
amino acids (ah-MEE-noh)
calcium (KAL-see-um)
creatinine (kree-AT-in-in)
fats
fibrinogen (fye-BRIN-oh-jen)
gamma globulin (GAM-ah GLOB-yoo-lin)

globulins (GLOB-yew-lenz)
glucose (GLOO-kohs)
plasma proteins
potassium (poh-TASS-ee-um)
sodium
urea (yoo-REE-ah)

> **Med Term Tip**
>
> Word watch—plasma and *serum* are not interchangeable words. Serum is plasma, but with fibrinogen removed or inactivated. This way it can be handled and tested without it clotting. The term *serum* is also sometimes used to mean antiserum or antitoxin.

Liquid plasma composes about 55% of whole blood in the average adult and is 90 to 92% water. The remaining 8 to 10% portion of plasma is dissolved substances, especially **plasma proteins** such as **albumin**, **globulins**, and **fibrinogen**. Albumin helps transport fatty substances that cannot dissolve in the watery plasma. There are three main types of globulins. The most commonly known one of these, **gamma globulin**, acts as antibodies. Fibrinogen is a blood-clotting protein. In addition to the plasma proteins, smaller amounts of other important substances are also dissolved in the plasma for transport: **calcium**, **potassium**, **sodium**, **glucose**, **amino acids**, **fats**, and waste products such as **urea** and **creatinine**.

Erythrocytes

bilirubin (bil-ly-ROO-bin)
enucleated (ee-NEW-klee-ate-ed)

hemoglobin (hee-moh-GLOH-bin)

Erythrocytes, or red blood cells (RBCs), are biconcave disks that are **enucleated**, meaning they no longer contain a nucleus (see Figure 1 ■). Red blood cells appear red in color because they contain **hemoglobin**, which is an iron-containing pigment. Hemoglobin is the part of the red blood cell that picks up oxygen from the lungs and delivers it to the tissues of the body.

> **Med Term Tip**
>
> Your body makes about 2 million erythrocytes every second. Of course, it must then destroy 2 million every second to maintain a relatively constant 30 trillion red blood cells.

There are about five million erythrocytes per cubic millimeter of blood. The total number in an average-sized adult is 35 trillion, with males having more red blood cells than females. Erythrocytes have an average life span of 120 days, and then the spleen removes the worn-out and damaged ones from circulation. Much of the red blood cell, such as the iron, can be reused, but one portion, **bilirubin**, is a waste product disposed of by the liver.

Basophil

Monocyte

Eosinophil

Neutrophil

Lymphocyte

■ **Figure 1** The biconcave disk shape of erythrocytes (red blood cells).

■ **Figure 2** The five different types of leukocytes (white blood cells).

Leukocytes

agranulocytes (ah-GRAN-yew-loh-sights)

granulocytes (GRAN-yew-loh-sights)

pathogens (PATH-oh-ginz)

Leukocytes, also referred to as white blood cells (WBCs), provide protection against the invasion of **pathogens** such as bacteria, viruses, and other foreign material. In general, white blood cells have a spherical shape with a large nucleus, and there are about 8,000 per cubic millimeter of blood (see Figure 2 ■). There are five different types of white blood cells, each with its own strategy for protecting the body. The five can be subdivided into two categories: **granulocytes** (with granules in the cytoplasm) and **agranulocytes** (without granules in the cytoplasm). The name and function of each type is presented in Table 1 ■.

Med Term Tip

A *phagocyte* is a cell that has the ability to ingest (eat) and digest bacteria and other foreign particles. This process, *phagocytosis*, is critical for the control of bacteria within the body.

Table 1	Leukocyte Classification
LEUKOCYTE	**FUNCTION**
Granulocytes	
Basophils (basos) (BAY-soh-fillz)	Release histamine and heparin to damaged tissues
Eosinophils (eosins) (ee-oh-SIN-oh-fillz)	Destroy parasites and increase during allergic reactions
Neutrophils (NOO-troh-fillz)	Important for phagocytosis; most numerous of the leukocytes
Agranulocytes	
Monocytes (monos) (MON-oh-sights)	Important for phagocytosis
Lymphocytes (lymphs) (LIM-foh-sights)	Plays several different roles in immune response

Platelets

agglutinate (ah-GLOO-tih-nayt) **thrombin** (THROM-bin)
fibrin (FYE-brin) **thrombocyte** (THROM-boh-sight)
hemostasis (hee-moh-STAY-sis) **thromboplastin** (throm-boh-PLAS-tin)
prothrombin (proh-THROM-bin)

■ **Figure 3** Platelet structure.

Platelet, the modern term for **thrombocyte,** refers to the smallest of all the formed blood elements. Platelets are not whole cells, but rather are formed when the cytoplasm of a large precursor cell shatters into small plate-like fragments (see Figure 3 ■). There are between 200,000 and 300,000 per cubic millimeter in the body.

Platelets play a critical part in the blood-clotting process or **hemostasis**. They **agglutinate** or clump together into small clusters when a blood vessel is cut or damaged. Platelets also release a substance called **thromboplastin**, which, in the presence of calcium, reacts with **prothrombin**, a clotting protein in the blood, to form **thrombin**. Then thrombin, in turn, works to convert fibrinogen to **fibrin**, which eventually becomes the meshlike blood clot.

Blood Typing

ABO system **Rh factor**
blood typing

Each person's blood is different due to the presence of antigens or markers on the surface of erythrocytes. Before a person receives a blood transfusion, it is important to do **blood typing.** This laboratory test determines if the donated blood is compatible with the recipient's blood. There are many different subgroups of blood markers, but the two most important ones are the **ABO system** and **Rh factor.**

ABO System

type A **type O**
type AB **universal donor**
type B **universal recipient**

In the ABO blood system there are two possible red blood cell markers, A and B. A marker is one method by which cells identify themselves. A person with an A marker is said to have **type A** blood. Type A blood produces anti-B antibodies that will attack type B blood. The presence of a B marker gives **type B** blood and anti-A antibodies (that will attack type A blood). If both markers are present, the blood is **type AB** and does not contain any antibodies. Therefore, type AB blood will not attack any other blood type. The absence of either an A or a B marker results in **type O** blood, which contains both anti-A and anti-B antibodies. Type O blood will attack all other blood types, A, B, and AB. For further information on antibodies, refer to the lymphatic section later in this chapter.

Because type O blood does not have either marker A or B, it will not react with anti-A or anti-B antibodies. For this reason, a person with type O blood is referred to as a **universal donor.** In extreme cases, type O blood may be given to a person with any of the other blood types. Similarly, type AB blood is the **universal recipient**. A person with type AB blood has no antibodies against the other blood types and, therefore, in extreme cases, can receive any type of blood.

Rh Factor

Rh-negative **Rh-positive**

Rh factor is not as difficult to understand as the ABO system. A person with the Rh factor on his or her red blood cells is said to be **Rh-positive** (Rh+). Since this person has the factor, he or she will not make anti-Rh antibodies. A person without the Rh factor is **Rh-negative** (Rh−) and will produce anti-Rh antibodies. Therefore, an Rh+ person may receive both an Rh+ and an Rh− transfusion, but an Rh− person can receive only Rh− blood.

Word Building

The following list contains examples of medical terms built directly from word parts. Their definitions can be determined by a straightforward translation of the word parts.

COMBINING FORM	COMBINED WITH	MEDICAL TERM	DEFINITION
fibrin/o	-gen	**fibrinogen** (fye-BRIN-oh-jen)	fiber producing
	-lysis	**fibrinolysis** (fye-brin-oh-LYE-sis)	destruction of fibers
	-ous	**fibrinous** (fye-brin-us)	pertaining to fibers
hem/o	-globin	**hemoglobin** (hee-moh-GLOH-bin)	blood protein
	-lysis	**hemolysis** (hee-MALL-ih-sis)	blood destruction
	-lytic	**hemolytic** (hee-moh-LIH-tik)	blood destruction
	-rrhage	**hemorrhage** (HEM-er-rij)	rapid flow of blood
hemat/o	-ologist	**hematologist** (hee-mah-TALL-oh-jist)	blood specialist
	-ic	**hematic** (hee-MAT-ik)	pertaining to blood
sanguin/o	-ous	**sanguinous** (SANG-gwih-nus)	pertaining to blood
SUFFIX	COMBINED WITH	MEDICAL TERM	DEFINITION
-cyte	erythr/o	**erythrocyte** (eh-RITH-roh-sight)	red cell
	leuk/o	**leukocyte** (LOO-koh-sight)	white cell
	thromb/o	**thrombocyte** (THROM-boh-sight)	clotting cell
	granul/o	**granulocyte** (GRAN-yew-loh-sight)	granular cell
	a- granul/o	**agranulocyte** (ah-GRAN-yew-loh-sight)	nongranular cell
-cytosis	erythr/o	**erythrocytosis** (ee-RITH-row-sigh-toe-sis)	too many red cells
	leuk/o	**leukocytosis** (LOO-koh-sigh-toh-sis)	too many white cells
	thromb/o	**thrombocytosis** (throm-boh-sigh-TOH-sis)	too many clotting cells
-penia	erythr/o	**erythropenia** (ee-RITH-row-pen-ee-ah)	too few red (cells)
	leuk/o	**leukopenia** (LOO-koh-pen-ee-ah)	too few white (cells)
	thromb/o	**thrombopenia** (THROM-boh-pen-ee-ah)	too few clotting (cells)
	pan- cyt/o	**pancytopenia** (pan-sigh-toe-PEN-ee-ah)	too few of all cells
-poiesis	erythr/o	**erythropoiesis** (eh-rith-roh-poy-EE-sis)	red (cell) producing
	hemat/o	**hematopoiesis** (hee-mah-toh-poy-EE-sis)	blood producing
	leuk/o	**leukopoiesis** (loo-koh-poy-EE-sis)	white (cell) producing
	thromb/o	**thrombopoiesis** (throm-boh-poy-EE-sis)	clotting (cell) producing

Vocabulary

TERM	DEFINITION
blood clot	The hard collection of fibrin, blood cells, and tissue debris that is the end result of hemostasis or the blood-clotting process.

■ **Figure 4** Electronmicrograph showing a blood clot. It is composed of fibrin, red blood cells, and tissue debris.

(CNRI/Photo Researchers, Inc.)

TERM	DEFINITION
coagulate (koh-ag-YOO-late)	To convert from a liquid to a gel or solid, as in blood coagulation.
dyscrasia (dis-CRAZ-ee-ah)	A general term indicating the presence of a disease affecting blood.
hematology (hee-mah-TALL-oh-jee)	The branch of medicine that specializes in treating diseases and conditions of the blood. Physician is a *hematologist*.
hematoma (hee-mah-TOH-mah)	The collection of blood under the skin as the result of blood escaping into the tissue from damaged blood vessels. Commonly referred to as a *bruise*. **Med Term Tip** Word watch—the term *hematoma* is confusing. Its simple translation is "blood tumor." However, it is used to refer to blood that has leaked out of a blood vessel and pooled in the tissues.
hemostasis (hee-moh-STAY-sis)	To stop bleeding or the stagnation of blood flow through the tissues.
packed cells	A transfusion of only the formed elements and without plasma.
whole blood	Refers to the mixture of both plasma and formed elements.

Pathology

TERM	DEFINITION
■ *Blood*	
hemophilia (hee-moh-FILL-ee-ah)	Hereditary blood disease in which blood-clotting time is prolonged due to a lack of one vital clotting factor. It is transmitted by a sex-linked trait from females to males, appearing almost exclusively in males.
hyperlipidemia (HYE-per-lip-id-ee-mee-ah)	Condition of having too high a level of lipids such as cholesterol in the bloodstream. A risk factor for developing atherosclerosis and coronary artery disease.

Pathology *(continued)*

TERM	DEFINITION
septicemia (sep-tih-SEE-mee-ah)	Having bacteria or their toxins in the bloodstream. *Sepsis* is a term that means putrefaction. Commonly referred to as *blood poisoning*.
■ *Erythrocytes*	
anemia (an-NEE-mee-ah)	A large group of conditions characterized by a reduction in the number of red blood cells or the amount of hemoglobin in the blood; results in less oxygen reaching the tissues.
aplastic anemia (a-PLAS-tik an-NEE-mee-ah)	Severe form of anemia that develops as a consequence of loss of functioning red bone marrow. Results in a decrease in the number of all the formed elements. Treatment may eventually require a bone marrow transplant.
hemolytic anemia (hee-moh-LIT-ik an-NEE-mee-ah)	An anemia that develops as the result of the excessive loss of erythrocytes.
hemolytic reaction (hee-moh-LIT-ik)	The destruction of a patient's erythrocytes that occurs when receiving a transfusion of an incompatible blood type. Also called a *transfusion reaction*.
hypochromic anemia (hi-poe-CHROME-ik an-NEE-mee-ah)	Anemia resulting from having insufficient hemoglobin in the erythrocytes. Named because the hemoglobin molecule is responsible for the dark red color of the erythrocytes.
iron-deficiency anemia	Anemia that results from having insufficient iron to manufacture hemoglobin.
pernicious anemia (PA) (per-NISH-us an-NEE-mee-ah)	Anemia associated with insufficient absorption of vitamin B_{12} by the digestive system. Vitamin B_{12} is necessary for erythrocyte production.
polycythemia vera (pol-ee-sigh-THEE-mee-ah VAIR-rah)	Production of too many red blood cells by the bone marrow. Blood becomes too thick to easily flow through the blood vessels.
sickle cell anemia	A genetic disorder in which erythrocytes take on an abnormal curved or "sickle" shape. These cells are fragile and are easily damaged, leading to a hemolytic anemia.

■ **Figure 5** Comparison of normal-shaped erythrocytes and the abnormal sickle shape noted in patients with sickle cell anemia.

Normal red blood cells　　　**Sickled cells**

thalassemia (thal-ah-SEE-mee-ah)	A genetic disorder in which the body is unable to make functioning hemoglobin, resulting in anemia.
■ *Leukocytes*	
leukemia (loo-KEE-mee-ah)	Cancer of the white blood cell-forming red bone marrow resulting in a large number of abnormal and immature white blood cells circulating in the blood.

Diagnostic Procedures

TERM	DEFINITION
■ Clinical Laboratory Tests	
blood culture and sensitivity (C&S)	Sample of blood is incubated in the laboratory to check for bacterial growth. If bacteria are present, they are identified and tested to determine which antibiotics they are sensitive to.
complete blood count (CBC)	Combination of blood tests including: red blood cell count (RBC), white blood cell count (WBC), hemoglobin (Hgb), hematocrit (Hct), white blood cell differential, and platelet count.
erythrocyte sedimentation rate (ESR, sed rate) (eh-RITH-roh-sight sed-ih-men-TAY-shun)	Blood test to determine the rate at which mature red blood cells settle out of the blood after the addition of an anticoagulant. This is an indicator of the presence of an inflammatory disease.
hematocrit (HCT, Hct, crit) (hee-MAT-oh-krit)	Blood test to measure the volume of red blood cells (erythrocytes) within the total volume of blood.
hemoglobin (Hgb, hb) (hee-moh-GLOH-bin)	A blood test to measure the amount of hemoglobin present in a given volume of blood.
platelet count (PLAYT-let)	Blood test to determine the number of platelets in a given volume of blood.
prothrombin time (Pro time, PT) (proh-THROM-bin)	A measure of the blood's coagulation abilities by measuring how long it takes for a clot to form after prothrombin has been activated.
red blood cell count (RBC)	Blood test to determine the number of erythrocytes in a volume of blood. A decrease in red blood cells may indicate anemia; an increase may indicate polycythemia.
red blood cell morphology	Examination of a specimen of blood for abnormalities in the shape (morphology) of the erythrocytes. Used to determine diseases like sickle cell anemia.
sequential multiple analyzer computer (SMAC)	Machine for doing multiple blood chemistry tests automatically.
white blood cell count (WBC)	Blood test to measure the number of leukocytes in a volume of blood. An increase may indicate the presence of infection or a disease such as leukemia. A decrease in white blood cells may be caused by radiation therapy or chemotherapy.
white blood cell differential (diff) (diff-er-EN-shal)	Blood test to determine the number of each variety of leukocytes.
■ Medical Procedures	
bone marrow aspiration (as-pih-RAY-shun)	Sample of bone marrow is removed by aspiration with a needle and examined for diseases such as leukemia or aplastic anemia.

Diagnostic Procedures *(continued)*

TERM	DEFINITION
phlebotomy (fleh-BOT-oh-me)	Incision into a vein in order to remove blood for a diagnostic test. Also called *venipuncture.*

■ **Figure 6** Phlebotomist using a needle to withdraw blood.

Therapeutic Procedures

TERM	DEFINITION
■ *Medical Procedures*	
autologous transfusion (aw-TALL-oh-gus trans-FYOO-zhun)	Procedure for collecting and storing a patient's own blood several weeks prior to the actual need. It can then be used to replace blood lost during a surgical procedure.
blood transfusion (trans-FYOO-zhun)	Artificial transfer of blood into the bloodstream. **Med Term Tip** Before a patient receives a blood transfusion, the laboratory performs a *type and crossmatch*. This test first double checks the blood type of both the donor's and recipient's blood. Then a crossmatch is performed. This process mixes together small samples of both bloods and observes the mixture for adverse reactions.
bone marrow transplant (BMT)	Patient receives red bone marrow from a donor after the patient's own bone marrow has been destroyed by radiation or chemotherapy.
homologous transfusion (hoh-MALL-oh-gus trans-FYOO-zhun)	Replacement of blood by transfusion of blood received from another person.
plasmapheresis (plaz-mah-fah-REE-sis)	Method of removing plasma from the body without depleting the formed elements. Whole blood is removed and the cells and plasma are separated. The cells are returned to the patient along with a donor plasma transfusion.

Pharmacology

CLASSIFICATION	ACTION	GENERIC AND BRAND NAMES
anticoagulant (an-tih-koh-AG-yoo-lant)	Substance that prevents blood clot formation. Commonly referred to as *blood thinners*.	heparin, HepLock; warfarin, coumadin
antihemorrhagic (an-tih-hem-er-RAJ-ik)	Substance that prevents or stops hemorrhaging; a *hemostatic agent*.	aminocaproic acid, Amicar; vitamin K
antiplatelet agents (an-tih-PLATE-let)	Substance that interferes with the action of platelets. Prolongs bleeding time. Used to prevent heart attacks and strokes.	clopidogrel, Plavix; ticlopidine, Ticlid
hematinic (hee-mah-TIN-ik)	Substance that increases the number of erythrocytes or the amount of hemoglobin in the blood.	epoetin alfa, Procrit; darbepoetin alfa, Aranesp
thrombolytic (throm-boh-LIT-ik)	Term meaning able to dissolve existing blood clots.	alteplase, Activase; streptokinase, Streptase

Abbreviations

ALL	acute lymphocytic leukemia	**lymphs**	lymphocytes
AML	acute myelogenous leukemia	**monos**	monocytes
basos	basophils	**PA**	pernicious anemia
BMT	bone marrow transplant	**PCV**	packed cell volume
CBC	complete blood count	**PMN, polys**	polymorphonuclear neutrophil
CLL	chronic lymphocytic leukemia	**PT, pro-time**	prothrombin time
CML	chronic myelogenous leukemia	**RBC**	red blood cell
diff	differential	**Rh+**	Rh-positive
eosins, eos	eosinophils	**Rh−**	Rh-negative
ESR, SR, sed rate	erythrocyte sedimentation rate	**segs**	segmented neutrophils
HCT, Hct, crit	hematocrit	**SMAC**	sequential multiple analyzer computer
Hgb, Hb, HGB	hemoglobin	**WBC**	white blood cell

Section II: The Lymphatic and Immune Systems at a Glance

Function

The lymphatic system consists of a network of lymph vessels that pick up excess tissue fluid, cleanse it, and return it to the circulatory system. It also picks up fats that have been absorbed by the digestive system. The immune system fights disease and infections.

Organs

lymph nodes
lymphatic vessels
spleen
thymus gland
tonsils

Combining Forms

adenoid/o	adenoids
immun/o	protection
lymph/o	lymph
lymphaden/o	lymph node
lymphangi/o	lymph vessel
path/o	disease
splen/o	spleen
thym/o	thymus
tonsill/o	tonsils
tox/o	poison

Suffixes Relating

-globulin	protein

The Lymphatic and Immune Systems Illustrated

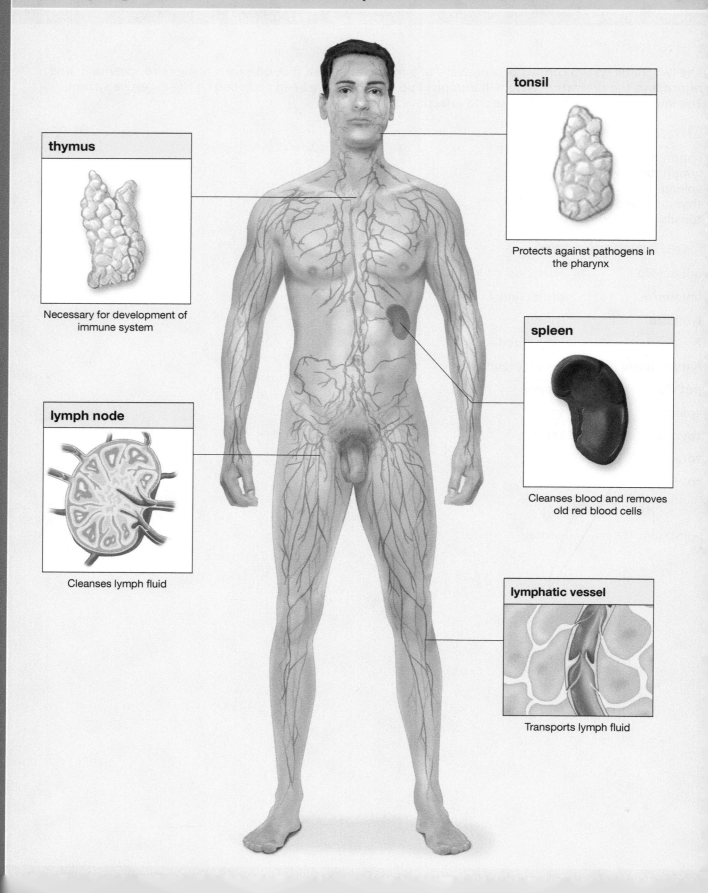

thymus

Necessary for development of immune system

lymph node

Cleanses lymph fluid

tonsil

Protects against pathogens in the pharynx

spleen

Cleanses blood and removes old red blood cells

lymphatic vessel

Transports lymph fluid

Anatomy and Physiology of the Lymphatic and Immune Systems

lacteals (lack-TEE-als)
lymph (LIMF)
lymph nodes
lymphatic vessels (lim-FAT-ik)

spleen
thymus gland (THIGH-mus)
tonsils (TON-sulls)

The lymphatic system consists of a network of **lymphatic vessels**, **lymph nodes**, the **spleen**, the **thymus gland**, and the **tonsils**. These organs perform several quite diverse functions for the body. First, they collect excess tissue fluid throughout the body and return it to the circulatory system. The fluid, once it is inside a lymphatic vessel, is referred to as **lymph**. Lymph vessels around the small intestines, called **lacteals**, are able to pick up absorbed fats for transport. Additionally, the lymphatic system works with the immune system to form the groups of cells, tissues, organs, and molecules that serve as the body's primary defense against the invasion of pathogens. These systems work together defending the body against foreign invaders and substances, as well as removing our own cells that have become diseased.

Lymphatic Vessels

lymphatic capillaries (CAP-ih-lair-eez)
lymphatic ducts
right lymphatic duct

thoracic duct
valves

The lymphatic vessels form an extensive network of vessels throughout the entire body. However, unlike the circulatory system, these vessels are not in a closed loop. Instead, they serve as one-way pipes conducting lymph from the tissues toward the thoracic cavity (see Figure 7 ■). These vessels begin as very

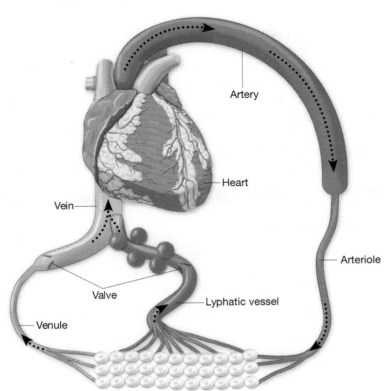

■ **Figure 7** Lymphatic vessels (green) pick up excess tissue fluid, purify it in lymph nodes, and return it to the circulatory system.

A   B

■ **Figure 8** A) Lymphatic vessel with valves within tissue cells; B) Photomicrograph of lymphatic vessel with valve clearly visible. *(Michael Abbey/Photo Researchers, Inc.)*

Med Term Tip

The term *capillary* is also used to describe the minute blood vessels within the circulatory system. This is one of several general medical terms, such as valves, cilia, and hair that are used in several systems.

small **lymphatic capillaries** in the tissues. Excessive tissue fluid enters these capillaries to begin the trip back to the circulatory system. The capillaries merge into larger lymphatic vessels. This is a very low pressure system, so these vessels have **valves** along their length to ensure that lymph can only move forward toward the thoracic cavity (see Figure 8 ■). These vessels finally drain into one of two large **lymphatic ducts**, the **right lymphatic duct** or the **thoracic duct**. The smaller right lymphatic duct drains the right arm and the right side of the neck and chest. This duct empties lymph into the right subclavian vein. The larger thoracic duct drains lymph from the rest of the body and empties into the left subclavian vein (see Figure 9 ■).

Lymph Nodes

lymph glands

Med Term Tip

In surgical procedures to remove a malignancy from an organ, such as a breast, the adjacent lymph nodes are also tested for cancer. If cancerous cells are found in the tested lymph nodes, the disease is said to have spread or *metastasized*. Tumor cells may then spread to other parts of the body by means of the lymphatic system.

Lymph nodes are small organs composed of lymphatic tissue located along the route of the lymphatic vessels. These nodes, also referred to as **lymph glands**, house lymphocytes and antibodies and therefore work to remove pathogens and cell debris as lymph passes through them on its way back to the thoracic cavity (see Figure 10 ■). Lymph nodes also serve to trap and destroy cells from cancerous tumors. Although found throughout the body, lymph nodes are particularly concentrated in several regions. For example, lymph nodes concentrated in the neck region drain lymph from the head. See Table 2 ■ and Figure 9 for a description of some of the most important sites for lymph nodes.

Table 2	Sites for Lymph Nodes	
NAME	**LOCATION**	**FUNCTION**
Axillary (AK-sih-lair-ee)	Armpits	Drain arms and shoulder region; cancer cells from breasts may be present
Cervical (SER-vih-kal)	Neck	Drain head and neck; may be enlarged during upper respiratory infections
Inguinal (ING-gwih-nal)	Groin	Drain legs and lower pelvis
Mediastinal (mee-dee-ass-TYE-nal)	Chest	Drain chest cavity

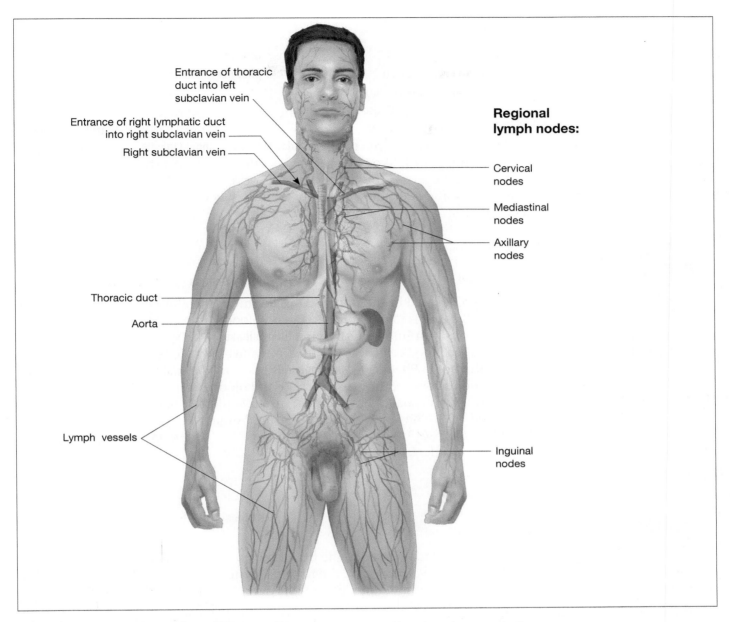

Entrance of thoracic
duct into left
subclavian vein

Entrance of right lymphatic duct
into right subclavian vein

Right subclavian vein

Thoracic duct

Aorta

Lymph vessels

**Regional
lymph nodes:**

Cervical
nodes

Mediastinal
nodes

Axillary
nodes

Inguinal
nodes

■ **Figure 9** Location of lymph vessels, lymphatic ducts, and areas of lymph node concentrations.

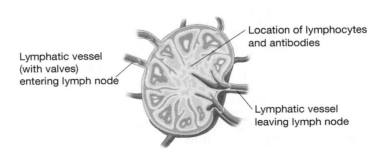

Lymphatic vessel
(with valves)
entering lymph node

Location of lymphocytes
and antibodies

Lymphatic vessel
leaving lymph node

■ **Figure 10** Structure of a lymph node.

Tonsils

adenoids (ADD-eh-noydz)

pharyngeal tonsils (fair-IN-jee-al)

lingual tonsils (LING-gwal)

pharynx (FAIR-inks)

palatine tonsils (PAL-ah-tyne)

■ **Figure 11** The shape of a tonsil.

The tonsils are collections of lymphatic tissue located on each side of the throat or **pharynx** (see Figure 11 ■). There are three sets of tonsils: **palatine tonsils**; **pharyngeal tonsils**, commonly referred to as the **adenoids**; and **lingual tonsils**. All tonsils contain a large number of leukocytes and act as filters to protect the body from the invasion of pathogens through the digestive or respiratory systems. Tonsils are not vital organs and can safely be removed if they become a continuous site of infection.

Spleen

blood sinuses

macrophages (MACK-roh-fayj-ez)

■ **Figure 12** The shape of the spleen.

The spleen, located in the upper left quadrant of the abdomen, consists of lymphatic tissue that is highly infiltrated with blood vessels (see Figure 12 ■). These vessels spread out into slow-moving **blood sinuses.** The spleen filters out and destroys old red blood cells, recycles the iron, and also stores some of the blood supply for the body. Phagocytic **macrophages** line the blood sinuses in the spleen to engulf and remove pathogens. Because the blood is moving through the organ slowly, the macrophages have time to carefully identify pathogens and worn-out red blood cells. The spleen is also not a vital organ and can be removed due to injury or disease. However, without the spleen, a person's susceptibility to a bloodstream infection may be increased.

Thymus Gland

T cells

thymosin (thigh-MOH-sin)

T lymphocytes

■ **Figure 13** The shape of the thymus gland.

The thymus gland, located in the upper portion of the mediastinum, is essential for the proper development of the immune system (see Figure 13 ■). It assists the body with the immune function and the development of antibodies. This organ's hormone, **thymosin**, changes lymphocytes to **T lymphocytes** (simply called **T cells**), which play an important role in the immune response. The thymus is active in the unborn child and throughout childhood until adolescence, when it begins to shrink in size.

Immunity

acquired immunity

immunizations (im-yoo-nih-ZAY-shuns)

active acquired immunity

natural immunity

bacteria (bak-TEE-ree-ah)

passive acquired immunity

cancerous tumors

protozoans (proh-toh-ZOH-anz)

fungi (FUN-jee)

toxins

immune response

vaccinations (vak-sih-NAY-shuns)

immunity (im-YOO-nih-tee)

viruses

Immunity is the body's ability to defend itself against pathogens, such as **bacteria**, **viruses**, **fungi**, **protozoans**, **toxins**, and **cancerous tumors**. Immunity comes in two forms: **natural immunity** and **acquired immunity**. Natural immunity, also called *innate immunity*, is not specific to a particular disease and does not require prior exposure to the pathogenic agent. A good example of natural immunity is the macrophage. These leukocytes are present throughout all the tissues of the body, but are concentrated in areas of high exposure to invading bacteria, like the lungs and digestive system. They are very active phagocytic cells, ingesting and digesting any pathogen they encounter (see Figure 14 ■).

Acquired immunity is the body's response to a specific pathogen and may be established either passively or actively. **Passive acquired immunity** results when a person receives protective substances produced by another human or animal. This may take the form of maternal antibodies crossing the placenta to a baby or an antitoxin or gamma globulin injection. **Active acquired immunity** develops following direct exposure to the pathogenic agent. The agent stimulates the body's **immune response**, a series of different mechanisms all geared to neutralize the agent. For example, a person typically can catch chickenpox only once because once the body has successfully fought the virus, it will be able to more quickly recognize and kill it in the future. **Immunizations** or **vaccinations** are special types of active acquired immunity. Instead of actually being exposed to the infectious agent and having the disease, a person is exposed to a modified or weakened pathogen that is still capable of stimulating the immune response but not actually causing the disease.

Immune Response

antibody (AN-tih-bod-ee)	**cell-mediated immunity**
antibody-mediated immunity	**cellular immunity**
antigen–antibody complex	**cytotoxic** (sigh-toh-TOK-sik)
antigens (AN-tih-jens)	**humoral immunity** (HYOO-mor-al)
B cells	**natural killer** (NK) **cells**
B lymphocytes	

Disease-causing agents are recognized as being foreign because they display proteins that are different from a person's own natural proteins. Those foreign proteins, called **antigens**, stimulate the immune response. The immune response consists of two distinct and different processes: **humoral immunity** (also called **antibody-mediated immunity**) and **cellular immunity** (also called **cell-mediated immunity**).

■ **Figure 14** Color enhanced photomicrograph showing a macrophage (purple) attacking *Escherichia coli* (yellow), a type of bacteria. *(Dennis Kunkel/Phototake NYC)*

Humoral immunity refers to the production of **B lymphocytes**, also called **B cells**, which respond to antigens by producing a protective protein, an **antibody**. Antibodies combine with the antigen to form an **antigen–antibody complex**. This complex either targets the foreign substance for phagocytosis or prevents the infectious agent from damaging healthy cells.

Cellular immunity involves the production of T cells and **natural killer** (NK) **cells**. These defense cells are **cytotoxic**, meaning that they physically attack and destroy pathogenic cells.

Standard Precautions

cross infection	reinfection
nosocomial infection (no-so-KOH-mee-all)	self-inoculation
Occupational Safety and Health Administration (OSHA)	

Hospital and other healthcare settings contain a large number of infective pathogens. Patients and healthcare workers are exposed to each other's pathogens and sometimes become infected. An infection acquired in this manner, as a result of hospital exposure, is referred to as a **nosocomial infection**. Nosocomial infections can spread in several ways. **Cross infection** occurs when a person, either a patient or healthcare worker, acquires a pathogen from another patient or healthcare worker. **Reinfection** takes place when a patient becomes infected again with the same pathogen that originally brought him or her to the hospital. **Self-inoculation** occurs when a person becomes infected in a different part of the body by a pathogen from another part of his or her own body—such as intestinal bacteria spreading to the urethra.

With the appearance of the human immunodeficiency virus (HIV) and the hepatitis B virus (HBV) in the mid-1980s, the fight against spreading infections took on even greater significance. In 1987 the **Occupational Safety and Health Administration** (OSHA) issued mandatory guidelines to ensure that all employees at risk of exposure to body fluids are provided with personal protective equipment. These guidelines state that all human blood, tissue, and body fluids must be treated as if they were infected with HIV, HBV, or other bloodborne pathogens. These guidelines were expanded in 1992 and 1996 to encourage the fight against not just bloodborne pathogens, but all nosocomial infections spread by contact with blood, mucous membranes, nonintact skin, and all body fluids (including amniotic fluid, vaginal secretions, pleural fluid, cerebrospinal fluid, peritoneal fluid, pericardial fluid, and semen). These guidelines are commonly referred to as the Standard Precautions:

1. Wash hands before putting on and after removing gloves and before and after working with each patient or patient equipment.
2. Wear gloves when in contact with any body fluid, mucous membrane, or nonintact skin or if you have chapped hands, a rash, or open sores.
3. Wear a nonpermeable gown or apron during procedures that are likely to expose you to any body fluid, mucous membrane, or nonintact skin.
4. Wear a mask and protective equipment or a face shield when patients are coughing often or if body fluid droplets or splashes are likely.
5. Wear a facemask and eyewear that seal close to the face during procedures that cause body tissues to be vaporized.
6. Remove for proper cleaning any shared equipment—such as a thermometer, stethoscope, or blood pressure cuff—that has come into contact with body fluids, mucous membrane, or nonintact skin.

Word Building

The following list contains examples of medical terms built directly from word parts. The definition for these terms can be determined by a straightforward translation of the word parts.

COMBINING FORM	COMBINED WITH	MEDICAL TERM	DEFINITION
adenoid/o	-ectomy	adenoidectomy (add-eh-noyd-EK-toh-mee)	removal of the adenoids
	-itis	adenoiditis (add-eh-noyd-EYE-tis)	inflammation of the adenoids
immun/o	-logist	immunologist (im-yoo-NALL-oh-jist)	immunity specialist
lymph/o	aden/o –ectomy	lymphadenectomy (lim-fad-eh-NEK-toh-mee)	removal of lymph gland
	aden/o –pathy	lymphadenopathy (lim-fad-eh-NOP-ah-thee)	lymph gland disease
	angi/o –gram	lymphangiogram (lim-FAN-jee-oh-gram)	record of lymph vessels
	angi/o -oma	lymphangioma (lim-fan-jee-OH-mah)	lymph vessel tumor
	-oma	lymphoma (lim-FOH-mah)	lymph tumor
	-tic	lymphatic (lim-FAT-ik)	pertaining to lymph
path/o	-genic	pathogenic (path-oh-JEN-ik)	disease producing
	-logy	pathology (path-OL-oh-gee)	study of disease
splen/o	-ectomy	splenectomy (splee-NEK-toh-mee)	removal of spleen
	-megaly	splenomegaly (splee-noh-MEG-ah-lee)	enlarged spleen
thym/o	-ectomy	thymectomy (thigh-MEK-toh-mee)	removal of the thymus
	-oma	thymoma (thigh-MOH-mah)	thymus tumor
tonsill/o	-ar	tonsillar (ton-sih-lar)	pertaining to tonsils
	-ectomy	tonsillectomy (ton-sih-LEK-toh-mee)	removal of the tonsils
	-itis	tonsillitis (ton-sil-EYE-tis)	inflammation of the tonsils

Vocabulary

TERM	DEFINITION
allergen (AL-er-jin)	An antigen that causes an allergic reaction.
allergist (AL-er-jist)	A physician who specializes in testing for and treating allergies.
allergy (AL-er-jee)	Hypersensitivity to a common substance in the environment or to a medication.
autoimmune disease	A disease resulting from the body's immune system attacking its own cells as if they were pathogens. Examples include systemic lupus erythematosus, rheumatoid arthritis, and multiple sclerosis.
hives	Appearance of wheals as part of an allergic reaction.

Vocabulary (continued)

TERM	DEFINITION
human immunodeficiency virus (HIV) (im-yoo-noh-dee-FIH-shen-see)	Virus that causes AIDS; also known as a **retrovirus.**

■ **Figure 15** Color enhanced scanning electron micrograph of HIV virus (red) infecting T-helper cells (green). *(NIBSC/Science Photo Library/Photo Researchers, Inc.)*

TERM	DEFINITION
immunocompromised (im-you-noh-KOM-pro-mized)	Having an immune system that is unable to respond properly to pathogens. Also called *immunodeficiency disorder.*
immunoglobulins (im-yoo-noh-GLOB-yoo-linz)	Antibodies secreted by the B cells. All antibodies are immunoglobulins and assist in protecting the body and its surfaces from the invasion of bacteria. For example, the immunoglobulin IgA in colostrum, the first milk from the mother, helps to protect the newborn from infection.
immunology (im-yoo-NALL-oh-jee)	A branch of medicine concerned with diagnosis and treatment of infectious diseases and other disorders of the immune system. Physician is an *immunologist.*
inflammation (in-flah-MA-shun)	The tissues' response to injury from pathogens or physical agents. Characterized by redness, pain, swelling, and feeling hot to touch.

> **Med Term Tip**
>
> Word watch—the terms *inflammation* and *inflammatory* are spelled with two "m"s, while *inflame* and *inflamed* each have only one "m." These may be the most commonly misspelled terms by medical terminology students.

■ **Figure 16** Inflammation as illustrated by cellulitis of the arm. Note that the area is red and swollen. It is also painful and hot to touch.

TERM	DEFINITION
lymphedema (limf-eh-DEE-mah)	Edema appearing in the extremities due to an obstruction of the lymph flow through the lymphatic vessels.
opportunistic infections	Infectious diseases associated with patients who have compromised immune systems and therefore a lowered resistance to infections and parasites. May be the result of HIV infection.
urticaria (er-tih-KAY-ree-ah)	Severe itching associated with hives, usually linked to food allergy, stress, or drug reactions.

Pathology

TERM	DEFINITION
■ Allergic Reactions	
anaphylactic shock (an-ah-fih-LAK-tik)	Life-threatening condition resulting from a severe allergic reaction. Examples of instances that may trigger this reaction include bee stings, medications, or the ingestion of foods. Circulatory and respiratory problems occur, including respiratory distress, hypotension, edema, tachycardia, and convulsions. Also called **anaphylaxis**.
■ Lymphatic System	
elephantiasis (el-eh-fan-TYE-ah-sis)	Inflammation, obstruction, and destruction of the lymph vessels resulting in enlarged tissues due to edema.
Hodgkin's disease (HD) (HOJ-kins dih-ZEEZ) ■ Figure 17 Late-stage Hodgkin's disease with tumor eroding skin above cancerous lymph node.	Also called *Hodgkin's lymphoma*. Cancer of the lymphatic cells found in concentration in the lymph nodes. Named after Thomas Hodgkin, a British physician, who first described it.
lymphadenitis (lim-fad-en-EYE-tis)	Inflammation of the lymph nodes. Referred to as *swollen glands*.
mononucleosis (mono) (mon-oh-nook-lee-OH-sis)	Acute infectious disease with a large number of abnormal lymphocytes. Caused by the Epstein–Barr virus. Abnormal liver function may occur.
non-Hodgkin's lymphoma (NHL)	Cancer of the lymphatic tissues other than Hodgkin's lymphoma.
■ Immune System	
acquired immunodeficiency syndrome (AIDS) (ac-quired im-you-noh-dee-FIH-shen-see SIN-drohm)	Disease involving a defect in the cell-mediated immunity system. A syndrome of opportunistic infections occurring in the final stages of infection with the human immunodeficiency virus (HIV). This virus attacks T4 lymphocytes and destroys them, reducing the person's ability to fight infection.
AIDS-related complex (ARC)	Early stage of AIDS. There is a positive test for the virus, but only mild symptoms of weight loss, fatigue, skin rash, and anorexia.
graft vs. host disease (GVHD)	Serious complication of bone marrow transplant (graft). Immune cells from the donor bone marrow attack the recipient's (host's) tissues.
Kaposi's sarcoma (KS) (KAP-oh-seez sar-KOH-mah)	Form of skin cancer frequently seen in patients with AIDS. It consists of brownish-purple papules that spread from the skin and metastasize to internal organs. Named for Moritz Kaposi, an Austrian dermatologist.
Pneumocystis carinii **pneumonia** (PCD) (noo-moh-SIS-tis kah-RYE-nee-eye new-MOH-nee-ah)	Pneumonia common in patients with AIDS that is caused by infection with an opportunistic parasite.
sarcoidosis (sar-koyd-OH-sis)	Disease of unknown cause that forms fibrous lesions commonly appearing in the lymph nodes, liver, skin, lungs, spleen, eyes, and small bones of the hands and feet.
severe combined immunodeficiency syndrome (SCIDS)	Disease seen in children born with a nonfunctioning immune system. Often these children are forced to live in sealed sterile rooms.

Diagnostic Procedures

TERM	DEFINITION
■ *Clinical Laboratory Tests*	
enzyme-linked immunosorbent assay (ELISA) (EN-zym LINK'T im-yoo-noh-sor-bent ASS-say)	A blood test for an antibody to the AIDS virus. A positive test means that the person has been exposed to the virus. There may be a false-positive reading, and then the Western blot test would be used to verify the results.
Western blot	Test used as a backup to the ELISA blood test to detect the presence of the antibody to HIV (AIDS virus) in the blood.
■ *Diagnostic Imaging*	
lymphangiography (lim-FAN-jee-oh-graf-ee)	X-ray taken of the lymph vessels after the injection of dye into the foot. The lymph flow through the chest is traced.
■ *Additional Diagnostic Procedures*	
Monospot	Test for infectious mononucleosis.
scratch test	Form of allergy testing in which the body is exposed to an allergen through a light scratch in the skin.

A.

B.

■ Figure 18 A) Scratch test; patient is exposed to allergens through light scratch in the skin. B) Positive scratch test results. Inflammation indicates person is allergic to that substance. *(James King-Holmes/Science Photo Library/Photo Researchers, Inc.)*

Therapeutic Procedures

TERM	DEFINITION
Medical Procedures	
immunotherapy (IM-yoo-noh-thair-ah-pee)	Giving a patient an injection of immunoglobulins or antibodies in order to treat a disease. The antibodies may be produced by another person or animal, for example, antivenom for snake bites. More recent developments include treatments to boost the activity of the immune system, especially to treat cancer and AIDS.
vaccination (vak-sih-NAY-shun)	Exposure to a weakened pathogen that stimulates the immune response and antibody production in order to confer protection against the full-blown disease. Also called *immunization*.
Surgical Procedures	
lymphadenectomy (lim-fad-eh-NEK-toh-mee)	Removal of a lymph node. This is usually done to test for malignancy.

Pharmacology

CLASSIFICATION	ACTION	GENERIC AND BRAND NAMES
antihistamine (an-tih-HIST-ah-meen)	Blocks the effects of histamine released by the body during an allergic reaction.	cetirizine, Zyrtec; diphenhydramine, Benadryl
corticosteroids (core-tih-koh-STARE-royds)	A hormone produced by the adrenal cortex that has very strong anti-inflammatory properties. Particularly useful in treating autoimmune diseases.	prednisone; methylprednisolone, Solu-Medrol
immunosuppressants (im-yoo-noh-sue-PRESS-antz)	Blocks certain actions of the immune system. Required to prevent rejection of a transplanted organ.	mycophenolate mofetil, CellCept; cyclosporine, Neoral
protease inhibitor drugs (PROH-tee-ace)	Inhibits protease, an enzyme viruses need to reproduce.	indinavir, Crixivan; saquinavir, Fortovase
reverse transcriptase inhibitor drugs (trans-KRIP-tays)	Inhibits reverse transcriptase, an enzyme needed by viruses to reproduce.	lamivudine, Epivir; zidovudine, Retrovir

Abbreviations

AIDS	acquired immunodeficiency syndrome	**KS**	Kaposi's sarcoma
ARC	AIDS-related complex	**mono**	mononucleosis
ELISA	enzyme-linked immunosorbent assay	**NHL**	non-Hodgkin's lymphoma
GVHD	graft vs. host disease	**NK**	natural killer cells
HD	Hodgkin's disease	**PCP**	*Pneumocystis carinii* pneumonia
HIV	human immunodeficiency virus	**SCIDS**	severe combined immunodeficiency
Ig	immunoglobulins (IgA, IgD, IgE, IgG, IgM)		syndrome

Chapter Review

Terminology Checklist

Below are all Anatomy and Physiology key terms, Word Building, Vocabulary, Pathology, Diagnostic, Therapeutic, and Pharmacology terms presented in this chapter. Use this list as a study tool by placing a check in the box in front of each term as you master its meaning.

- ☐ ABO system
- ☐ acquired immunity
- ☐ acquired immunodeficiency syndrome
- ☐ active acquired immunity
- ☐ adenoidectomy
- ☐ adenoiditis
- ☐ adenoids
- ☐ agglutinate
- ☐ agranulocytes
- ☐ AIDS-related complex
- ☐ albumin
- ☐ allergen
- ☐ allergist
- ☐ allergy
- ☐ amino acids
- ☐ anaphylactic shock
- ☐ anaphylaxis
- ☐ anemia
- ☐ antibody
- ☐ antibody-mediated immunity
- ☐ anticoagulant
- ☐ antigen
- ☐ antigen–antibody complex
- ☐ antihemorrhagic
- ☐ antihistamine
- ☐ antiplatelet agent
- ☐ aplastic anemia
- ☐ autoimmune disease
- ☐ autologous transfusion
- ☐ axillary
- ☐ bacteria
- ☐ basophils
- ☐ B cells
- ☐ bilirubin
- ☐ blood clot
- ☐ blood culture and sensitivity
- ☐ blood sinuses

- ☐ blood transfusion
- ☐ blood typing
- ☐ B lymphocytes
- ☐ bone marrow aspiration
- ☐ bone marrow transplant
- ☐ calcium
- ☐ cancerous tumors
- ☐ cell-mediated immunity
- ☐ cellular immunity
- ☐ cervical
- ☐ coagulate
- ☐ complete blood count
- ☐ corticosteroids
- ☐ creatinine
- ☐ cross infection
- ☐ cytotoxic
- ☐ dyscrasia
- ☐ elephantiasis
- ☐ enucleated
- ☐ enzyme-linked immunosorbent assay (ELISA)
- ☐ eosinophils
- ☐ erythrocytes
- ☐ erythrocyte sedimentation rate
- ☐ erythrocytosis
- ☐ erythropenia
- ☐ erythropoiesis
- ☐ fats
- ☐ fibrin
- ☐ fibrinogen
- ☐ fibrinolysis
- ☐ fibrinous
- ☐ formed elements
- ☐ fungi
- ☐ gamma globulin
- ☐ globulins
- ☐ glucose
- ☐ graft vs. host disease

- ☐ granulocyte
- ☐ hematic
- ☐ hematinic
- ☐ hematocrit
- ☐ hematologist
- ☐ hematology
- ☐ hematoma
- ☐ hematopoiesis
- ☐ hemoglobin
- ☐ hemolysis
- ☐ hemolytic
- ☐ hemolytic anemia
- ☐ hemolytic reaction
- ☐ hemophilia
- ☐ hemorrhage
- ☐ hemostasis
- ☐ hives
- ☐ Hodgkin's disease
- ☐ homologous transfusion
- ☐ human immunodeficiency virus
- ☐ humoral immunity
- ☐ hyperlipidemia
- ☐ hypochromic anemia
- ☐ immune response
- ☐ immunity
- ☐ immunization
- ☐ immunocompromised
- ☐ immunoglobulins
- ☐ immunologist
- ☐ immunology
- ☐ immunosuppressants
- ☐ immunotherapy
- ☐ inflammation
- ☐ inguinal
- ☐ iron-deficiency anemia
- ☐ Kaposi's sarcoma
- ☐ lacteals
- ☐ leukemia

- leukocytes
- leukocytosis
- leukopenia
- leukopoiesis
- lingual tonsils
- lymph
- lymphadenectomy
- lymphadenitis
- lymphadenopathy
- lymphangiogram
- lymphangiography
- lymphangioma
- lymphatic
- lymphatic capillaries
- lymphatic ducts
- lymphatic vessels
- lymphedema
- lymph glands
- lymph nodes
- lymphocytes
- lymphoma
- macrophage
- mediastinal
- metastasize
- monocytes
- mononucleosis
- Monospot
- natural immunity
- natural killer cells
- neutrophils
- non-Hodgkin's lymphoma
- nosocomial infection
- Occupational Safety and Health Administration
- opportunistic infections
- packed cells
- palatine tonsils
- pancytopenia
- passive acquired immunity
- pathogenic
- pathogens

- pathology
- pernicious anemia
- phagocyte
- phagocytosis
- pharyngeal tonsils
- pharynx
- phlebotomy
- plasma
- plasmapheresis
- plasma proteins
- platelet count
- platelets
- *Pneumocystis carinii* pneumonia
- polycythemia vera
- potassium
- protease inhibitor drugs
- prothrombin
- prothrombin time
- protozoans
- red blood cell count
- red blood cell morphology
- red blood cells
- reinfection
- reverse transcriptase inhibitor drugs
- Rh factor
- Rh-negative
- Rh-positive
- right lymphatic duct
- sanguinous
- sarcoidosis
- scratch test
- self-inoculation
- septicemia
- sequential multiple analyzer computer
- serum
- severe combined immunodeficiency syndrome
- sickle cell anemia
- sodium

- spleen
- splenectomy
- splenomegaly
- T cells
- thalassemia
- thoracic duct
- thrombin
- thrombocyte
- thrombocytosis
- thrombolytic
- thrombopenia
- thromboplastin
- thrombopoiesis
- thymectomy
- thymoma
- thymosin
- thymus gland
- T lymphocytes
- tonsillar
- tonsillectomy
- tonsillitis
- tonsils
- toxins
- type A
- type AB
- type and crossmatch
- type B
- type O
- universal donor
- universal recipient
- urea
- urticaria
- vaccination
- valves
- viruses
- Western blot
- white blood cell count
- white blood cell differential
- white blood cells
- whole blood

Practice Exercises

A. Complete the following statements.

1. The study of the blood is called _hematology_.

2. The organs of the lymphatic system other than lymphatic vessels and lymph nodes are the _spleen_, _thymus gland_, and _tonsils_.

3. The two lymph ducts are the _rt. lymphatic duct_ and _thoracic duct_.

4. The primary concentrations of lymph nodes are the _axillary_, _cervical_, _inguinal_, and _mediastinal_ regions.

5. The process whereby cells ingest and destroy bacteria within the body is _phagocytosis_.

6. The formed elements of blood are the, _erythrocytes_, _leukocytes_, and _platelets_.

7. The fluid portion of blood is called _plasma_.

8. _Active aquired_ immunity develops following direct exposure to a pathogen.

9. Humoral immunity is also referred to as _antibody-mediated_ immunity.

10. The medical term for blood clotting is _hemostasis_.

B. State the terms described using the combining forms provided.

The combining form *splen/o* refers to the spleen. Use it to write a term that means:

1. enlargement of the spleen _splenomegaly_

2. surgical removal of the spleen _splenectomy_

3. incision into the spleen _splenotomy_

The combining form *lymph/o* refers to the lymph. Use it to write a term that means:

4. lymph cells _lymphocytes_

5. tumor of the lymph system _lymphoma_

The combining form *lymphaden/o* refers to the lymph glands. Use it to write a term that means:

6. disease of a lymph gland _lymphadenopathy_

7. tumor of a lymph gland _lymphadenoma_

8. inflammation of a lymph gland _lymphadenitis_

The combining form *immun/o* refers to the immune system. Use it to write a term that means:

9. specialist in the study of the immune system _immunologist_

10. immune protein _immunoglobulin_

Blood and the Lymphatic and Immune Systems

11. study of the immune system __immunology__

The combining form *hemat/o* refers to blood. Use it to write a term that means:

12. relating to the blood __hematic__

13. blood tumor or mass __hematoma__

14. blood formation __hematopoiesis__

The combining form *hem/o* refers to blood. Use it to write a term that means:

15. blood destruction __hemolysis__

16. blood protein __hemoglobin__

C. Use the following suffixes to create medical terms for the following definitions.

-penia   -globin   -cytosis   -cyte   -globulin

1. too few white (cells) __leukopenia__

2. too few red (cells) __erythropenia__

3. too few clotting (cells) __thrombopenia__

4. too few of all cells __pancytopenia__

5. increase in white cells __leukocytosis__

6. increase in red cells __erythrocytosis__

7. increase in clotting cells __thrombocytosis__

8. blood protein __hemoglobin__

9. immunity protein __immunoglobulin__

10. red cell __erythrocyte__

11. white cell __leukocyte__

12. lymph cell __lymphocyte__

D. Write the combining form for each definition and then use it to form a medical term.

	Combining Form	Medical Term
1. lymph node	lymphaden/o	lymphadenectomy
2. clot	thromb/o	thrombosis
3. blood	hemat/o	hematic
4. tonsil	tonsill/o	tonsillectomy
5. poison	tox/o	toxic
6. eat/swallow	phag/o	phagocytosis

Blood and the Lymphatic and Immune Systems

7. lymph vessel **lymphangi/o**   lymphangiotomy

8. disease **path/o**   pathogen

9. spleen **splen/o**   splenectomy

10. lymph **lymph/o**   lymphocyte

E. Identify the following abbreviations.

1. basos **basophils**

2. CBC **complete blood count**

3. Hgb **hemoglobin**

4. PT **prothrombin time**

5. GVHD **graft vs. host disease**

6. RBC **red blood cell**

7. PCV **packed cell volume**

8. ESR **erythrocyte sedimentation rate**

9. diff **differential**

10. lymphs **lymphocytes**

F. Write the abbreviations for the following terms.

1. acquired immunodeficiency
   syndrome **AIDS**

2. AIDS-related complex **ARC**

3. human immunodeficiency
   virus **HIV**

4. acute lymphocytic leukemia **ALL**

5. bone marrow transplant **BMT**

6. mononucleosis **mono**

7. Kaposi's sarcoma **KS**

8. eosinophils **eosins) eos**

9. immunoglobulin **Ig**

10. severe combined immunodeficiency
    syndrome **SCIDS**

G. Match each blood term to its definition.

1. **g** thalassemia

2. **i** lacteals

3. **e** A, B, AB, O

4. **a** plasma

5. **h** dyscrasia

a. fluid portion of blood

b. disease in which blood does not clot

c. conditions with reduced number of RBCs

d. mass of blood

e. blood type

6. __d__ hematoma
7. __c__ anemia
8. __j__ serum
9. __b__ hemophilia
10. __f__ fibrinogen

f. blood clotting protein
g. type of anemia
h. general term for blood disorders
i. lymph vessels around intestine
j. plasma with inactivated fibrinogen

H. Match each lymphatic and immune system term to its definition.

1. __c__ allergy
2. __h__ nosocomial
3. __d__ phagocytosis
4. __a__ hives
5. __e__ antibody
6. __b__ antigen
7. __f__ Hodgkin's disease
8. __g__ sarcoidosis
9. __j__ vaccination
10. __i__ ELISA

a. seen in an allergic reaction
b. substance that stimulates antibody formation
c. a hypersensitivity reaction
d. engulfing
e. protective blood protein
f. a type of cancer
g. autoimmune disease
h. infection acquired in the hospital
i. blood test for AIDS
j. immunization

I. Match each blood test to its definition.

1. __d__ culture and sensitivity
2. __f__ hematocrit
3. __b__ complete blood count
4. __g__ erythrocyte sedimentation rate
5. __a__ prothrombin time
6. __e__ white cell differential
7. __c__ red cell morphology

a. measure of blood's clotting ability
b. counts number of each type of blood cell
c. examines cells for abnormal shape
d. checks blood for bacterial growth and best antibiotic to use
e. determines number of each type of white blood cell
f. measures percent of whole blood that is red blood cells
g. an indicator of the presence of an inflammatory condition

J. Fill in the classification for each drug description, then match the brand name.

Drug Description	Classification	Brand Name
1. _____ inhibits enzyme needed for viral reproduction	_____	a. HepLock
2. _____ prevents blood clot formation	_____	b. Activase
3. _____ stops bleeding	_____	c. Solu-Medrol
4. _____ blocks effects of histamine	_____	d. Amicar
5. _____ prevents rejection of a transplanted organ	_____	e. Epivir
6. _____ dissolves existing blood clots	_____	f. CellCept
7. _____ increases number of erythrocytes	_____	g. Procrit
8. _____ strong anti-inflammatory properties	_____	h. Zyrtec
9. _____ interferes with action of platelets	_____	i. Plavix

K. Use the following terms in the sentences below.

Kaposi's sarcoma	mononucleosis	Hodgkin's disease	aplastic
polycythemia vera	anaphylactic shock	AIDS	pernicious
Pneumocystis carinii	HIV		

1. The condition characterized by the production of too many red blood cells is called Polycythemia vera.

2. The Epstein–Barr virus is thought to be responsible for what infectious disease? mononucleosis.

3. A life-threatening allergic reaction is anaphylactic shock.

4. The virus responsible for causing AIDS is HIV.

5. A cancer that is seen frequently in AIDS patients is Kaposi's sarcoma.

6. An ELISA is used to test for AIDS.

7. Malignant tumors concentrate in lymph nodes with this disease: Hodgkin's disease

8. A type of pneumonia seen in AIDS patients is Pneumocystis carinii pneumonia.

9. Aplastic anemia is a severe form of anemia caused by nonfunctioning red bone marrow.

10. Pernicious anemia is the result of a vitamin B_{12} deficiency

Medical Record Analysis

Below is an item from a patient's medical record. Read it carefully, make sure you understand all the medical terms used, and then answer the questions that follow.

Discharge Summary

Admitting Diagnosis:	Splenomegaly, weight loss, diarrhea, fatigue, chronic cough
Final Diagnosis:	Non-Hodgkin's lymphoma, primary site spleen; splenectomy
History of Present Illness:	Patient is a 36-year-old businessman who was first seen in the office with complaints of feeling generally "run down," intermittent diarrhea, weight loss, and, more recently, a dry cough. He states he has been aware of these symptoms for approximately six months, but admits it may have been "coming on" for closer to one year. A screening test for mononucleosis was negative. A chest x-ray was negative for pneumonia or bronchitis, but did reveal suspicious nodules in the left thoracic cavity. In spite of a 35-pound weight loss, he has abdominal swelling and splenomegaly detected with abdominal palpation. He was admitted to the hospital for further evaluation and treatment.
Summary of Hospital Course:	Blood tests were negative for the Epstein–Barr virus and hepatitis B. Abdominal ultrasound confirmed generalized splenomegaly and located a 3-cm encapsulated tumor. A lymphangiogram identified the thoracic nodules to be enlarged lymph glands. Biopsies taken from the spleen tumor and thoracic lymph glands confirmed the diagnosis of non-Hodgkin's lymphoma. A full body MRI failed to demonstrate any additional metastases in the liver or brain. The patient underwent splenectomy for removal of the primary tumor.
Discharge Plans:	Patient was discharged home following recovery from the splenectomy. The abdominal swelling and diarrhea were resolved, but the dry cough persisted. He was referred to an oncologist for evaluation and establishment of a chemotherapy and radiation therapy protocol to treat the metastatic thoracic lymphadenomas and ongoing surveillance for additional metastases.

Critical Thinking Questions

1. What complaints caused the patient to go to the doctor? He felt run down, had intermittent diarrhea, weight loss & a dry cough.

2. Explain in your own words what negative, as in "chest x-ray was negative for pneumonia," means. The chest x-ray did not support a diagnosis of pneumonia or bronchitis.

3. This discharge summary contains four medical terms that have not been introduced yet. Describe each of these terms in your own words. Use your text as a dictionary.

a. primary site _main/originating site - where malignant tumor 1st appeared_

b. encapsulated _growth enclosed in a sheath of tissue that prevents tumor cells from invading surrounding tissue_

c. ascites _collection or accumulation of fluid in the peritoneal cavity_

d. metastases _the spreading of a cancerous tumor from its original site to different locations in the body_

4. What is the name of a diagnostic procedure that produces an image from high-frequency sound waves? The

procedure is _Ultrasound_.

5. Which of the following pathological conditions was discovered using this procedure?
   a. inflammatory liver disease
   b. an acute infection with a large number of lymphocytes
   c. a malignant tumor of the thymus gland
   d. an enlarged spleen

6. What diagnostic test failed to find any cancer in other organs of the body? Which organs are free of cancer?
   A full body MRI

7. When the patient was discharged from the hospital, which symptoms were resolved and which persisted?
   Resolved: _abdominal swelling & diarrhea_
   Persisted: _dry cough_

Chart Note Transcription

The chart note below contains ten phrases that can be reworded with a medical term that you learned in this chapter. Each phrase is identified with an underline. Determine the medical term and write your answers in the space provided.

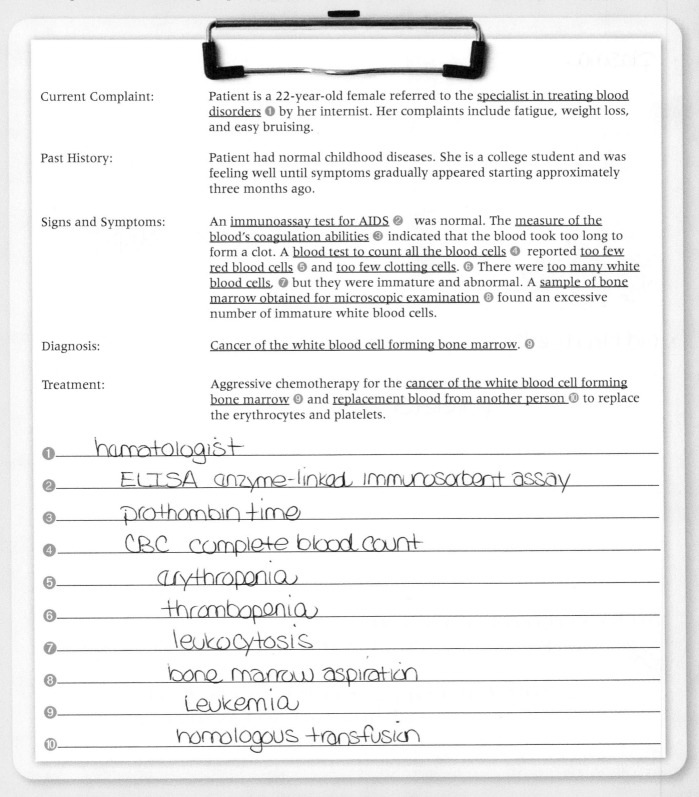

Current Complaint:	Patient is a 22-year-old female referred to the <u>specialist in treating blood disorders</u> ❶ by her internist. Her complaints include fatigue, weight loss, and easy bruising.
Past History:	Patient had normal childhood diseases. She is a college student and was feeling well until symptoms gradually appeared starting approximately three months ago.
Signs and Symptoms:	An <u>immunoassay test for AIDS</u> ❷ was normal. The <u>measure of the blood's coagulation abilities</u> ❸ indicated that the blood took too long to form a clot. A <u>blood test to count all the blood cells</u> ❹ reported <u>too few red blood cells</u> ❺ and <u>too few clotting cells.</u> ❻ There were <u>too many white blood cells,</u> ❼ but they were immature and abnormal. A <u>sample of bone marrow obtained for microscopic examination</u> ❽ found an excessive number of immature white blood cells.
Diagnosis:	<u>Cancer of the white blood cell forming bone marrow.</u> ❾
Treatment:	Aggressive chemotherapy for the <u>cancer of the white blood cell forming bone marrow</u> ❾ and <u>replacement blood from another person</u> ❿ to replace the erythrocytes and platelets.

❶ _hematologist_

❷ _ELISA enzyme-linked immunosorbent assay_

❸ _prothombin time_

❹ _CBC complete blood count_

❺ _erythropenia_

❻ _thrombopenia_

❼ _leukocytosis_

❽ _bone marrow aspiration_

❾ _leukemia_

❿ _homologous transfusion_

Labeling Exercise

A. System Review

Write the labels for this figure on the numbered lines provided.

1. plasma

2. red blood cells

3. platelets

4. white blood cells

B. Anatomy Challenge

1. Write the labels for this figure on the numbered lines provided.

1. _thymus_

2. _lymph node_

3. _tonsil_

4. _spleen_

5. _lymphatic vessel_

2. Write the labels for this figure on the numbered lines provided.

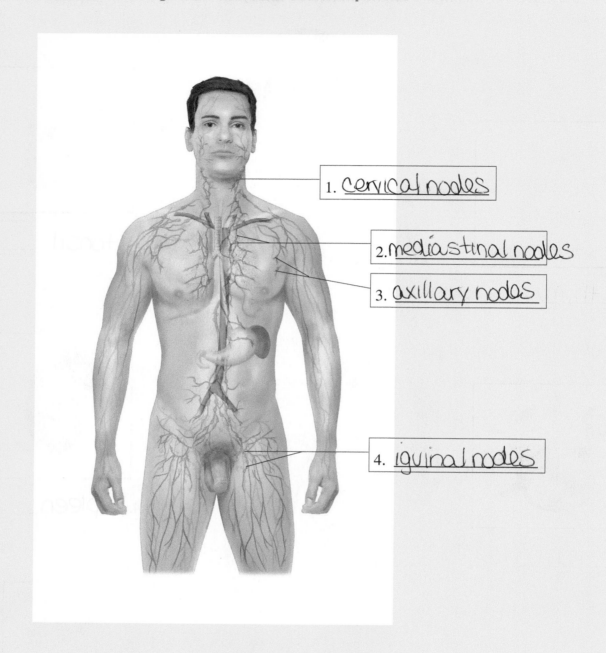

1. cervical nodes

2. mediastinal nodes

3. axillary nodes

4. iguinal nodes

Multimedia Preview

Additional interactive resources and activities for this chapter can be found on the Companion Website.

Website Highlights—www.prenhall.com/fremgen

MEDICINE IN THE NEWS

Click here and take advantage of the free-access on-line study guide that accompanies your textbook. You'll be able to stay current with a link to medical news articles updated daily by *The New York Times*. By clicking on this URL you'll also access a variety of quizzes with instant feedback, links to download mp3 audio reviews, and an audio glossary.

206

Respiratory System

Learning Objectives

Upon completion of this chapter, you will be able to:

- Identify and define the combining forms and suffixes introduced in this chapter.
- Correctly spell and pronounce medical terms and major anatomical structures relating to the respiratory system.
- Locate and describe the major organs of the respiratory system and their functions.
- List and describe the lung volumes and capacities.
- Describe the process of respiration.
- Build and define respiratory system medical terms from word parts.
- Identify and define respiratory system vocabulary terms.
- Identify and define selected respiratory system pathology terms.
- Identify and define selected respiratory system diagnostic procedures.
- Identify and define selected respiratory system therapeutic procedures.
- Identify and define selected medications relating to the respiratory system.
- Define selected abbreviations associated with the respiratory system.

From Chapter 7 of *Medical Terminology: A Living Language*, 4/e. Bonnie F. Fremgen. Suzanne S. Frucht. Copyright © 2009 by Pearson Education. Published by Prentice Hall. All rights reserved.

Respiratory System at a Glance

Function

The organs of the respiratory system are responsible for bringing fresh air into the lungs, exchanging oxygen for carbon dioxide between the air sacs of the lungs and the blood stream, and exhaling the stale air.

Organs

nasal cavity
pharynx
larynx
trachea
bronchial tubes
lungs

Combining Forms

alveol/o	alveolus; air sac	**orth/o**	straight, upright
anthrac/o	coal	**ox/o, ox/i**	oxygen
atel/o	incomplete	**pharyng/o**	pharynx
bronch/o	bronchus	**pleur/o**	pleura
bronchi/o	bronchus	**pneum/o**	lung, air
bronchiol/o	bronchiole	**pneumon/o**	lung, air
coni/o	dust	**pulmon/o**	lung
diaphragmat/o	diaphragm	**rhin/o**	nose
epiglott/o	epiglottis	**sinus/o**	sinus, cavity
laryng/o	larynx	**spir/o**	breathing
lob/o	lobe	**trache/o**	trachea, windpipe
nas/o	nose		

Suffixes

-capnia	carbon dioxide
-ectasis	dilated, expansion
-osmia	smell
-phonia	voice
-pnea	breathing
-ptysis	spitting
-thorax	chest

Respiratory System Illustrated

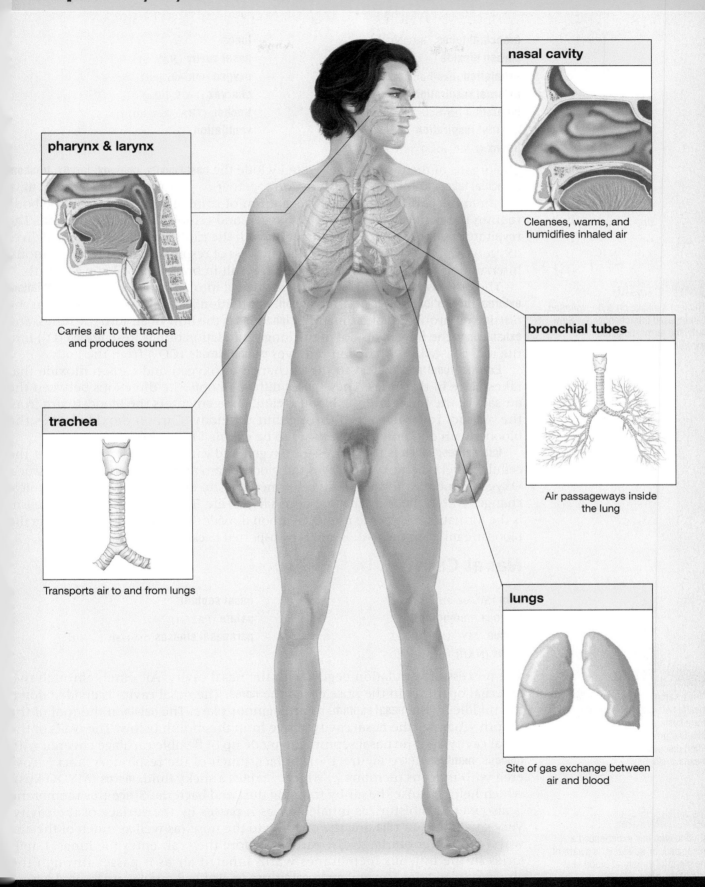

nasal cavity

Cleanses, warms, and humidifies inhaled air

pharynx & larynx

Carries air to the trachea and produces sound

bronchial tubes

Air passageways inside the lung

trachea

Transports air to and from lungs

lungs

Site of gas exchange between air and blood

Anatomy and Physiology of the Respiratory System

bronchial tubes (BRONG-key-all)

carbon dioxide

exhalation (eks-hah-LAY-shun)

external respiration

inhalation (in-hah-LAY-shun)

internal respiration

larynx (LAIR-inks)

lungs

nasal cavity (NAY-zl)

oxygen (OK-sih-jen)

pharynx (FAIR-inks)

trachea (TRAY-kee-ah)

ventilation

The organs of the respiratory system include the **nasal cavity, pharynx, larynx, trachea, bronchial tubes**, and **lungs**—that function together to perform the mechanical and, for the most part, unconscious mechanism of respiration. The cells of the body require the continuous delivery of oxygen and removal of carbon dioxide. The respiratory system works in conjunction with the cardiovascular system to deliver oxygen to all the cells of the body. The process of respiration must be continuous; interruption for even a few minutes can result in brain damage and/or death.

The process of respiration can be subdivided into three distinct parts: **ventilation, external respiration**, and **internal respiration**. Ventilation is the flow of air between the outside environment and the lungs. **Inhalation** is the flow of air into the lungs, and **exhalation** is the flow of air out of the lungs. Inhalation brings fresh **oxygen** (O_2) into the air sacs, while exhalation removes **carbon dioxide** (CO_2) from the body.

External respiration refers to the exchange of oxygen and carbon dioxide that takes place in the lungs. These gases diffuse in opposite directions between the air sacs of the lungs and the bloodstream. Oxygen enters the bloodstream from the air sacs to be delivered throughout the body. Carbon dioxide leaves the bloodstream and enters the air sacs to be exhaled from the body.

Internal respiration is the process of oxygen and carbon dioxide exchange at the cellular level when oxygen leaves the bloodstream and is delivered to the tissues. Oxygen is needed for the body cells' metabolism, all the physical and chemical changes within the body that are necessary for life. The by-product of metabolism is the formation of a waste product, carbon dioxide. The carbon dioxide enters the bloodstream from the tissues and is transported back to the lungs for disposal.

Nasal Cavity

cilia (SIL-ee-ah)

mucous membrane

mucus (MYOO-kus)

nares (NAIR-eez)

nasal septum

palate (PAL-at)

paranasal sinuses (pair-ah-NAY-zl)

The process of ventilation begins with the nasal cavity. Air enters through two external openings in the nose called the **nares**. The nasal cavity is divided down the middle by the **nasal septum**, a cartilaginous plate. The **palate** in the roof of the mouth separates the nasal cavity above from the mouth below. The walls of the nasal cavity and the nasal septum are made up of flexible cartilage covered with **mucous membrane** (see Figure 1 ■). In fact, much of the respiratory tract is covered with mucous membrane, which secretes a sticky fluid, **mucus** (MYOO kus), which helps cleanse the air by trapping dust and bacteria. Since this membrane is also wet, it moisturizes inhaled air as it passes by the surface of the cavity. Very small hairs or **cilia** line the opening to the nose (as well as much of the airways), and filter out large dirt particles before they can enter the lungs. Capillaries in the mucous membranes warm inhaled air as it passes through the airways. In addition, several **paranasal sinuses** or air-filled cavities are located within

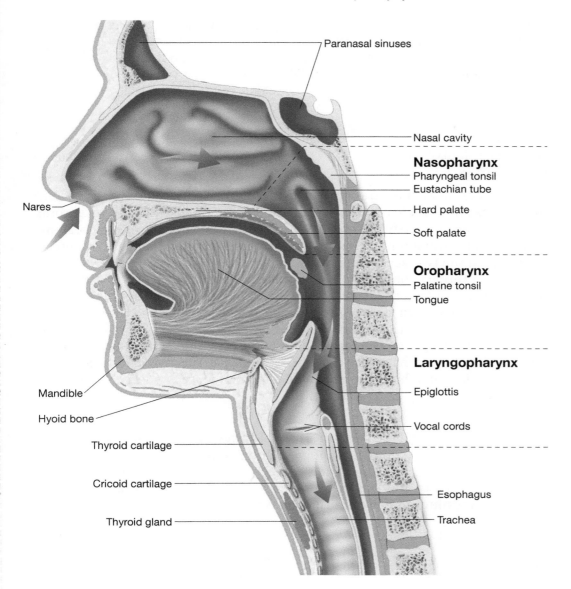

Figure 1 Sagittal section of upper respiratory system illustrating the internal anatomy of the nasal cavity, pharynx, larynx, and trachea.

Paranasal sinuses

Nasal cavity

Nasopharynx
Pharyngeal tonsil
Eustachian tube

Hard palate

Soft palate

Oropharynx
Palatine tonsil
Tongue

Laryngopharynx

Epiglottis

Vocal cords

Esophagus

Trachea

Nares

Mandible

Hyoid bone

Thyroid cartilage

Cricoid cartilage

Thyroid gland

the facial bones. The sinuses act as an echo chamber during sound production and give resonance to the voice.

Pharynx

adenoids (ADD-eh-noydz)
auditory tube
eustachian tube (yoo-STAY-she-en)
laryngopharynx (lair-ring-goh-FAIR-inks)
lingual tonsils (LING-gwal)

nasopharynx (nay-zoh-FAIR-inks)
oropharynx (or-oh-FAIR-inks)
palatine tonsils (PAL-ah-tine)
pharyngeal tonsils (fair-IN-jee-al)

Air next enters the pharynx, also called the *throat*, which is used by both the respiratory and digestive systems. At the end of the pharynx, air enters the trachea while food and liquids are shunted into the esophagus.

The pharynx is roughly a 5-inch-long tube consisting of three parts: the upper **nasopharynx**, middle **oropharynx**, and lower **laryngopharynx** (see Figure 1). Three pairs of tonsils, collections of lymphatic tissue, are located in the pharynx. Tonsils are strategically placed to help keep pathogens from entering the body through either the air breathed or food and liquid swallowed. The nasopharynx, behind the nose, contains the **adenoids** or **pharyngeal tonsils**. The oropharynx, behind the mouth, contains the **palatine tonsils** and the **lingual tonsils**.

The opening of the **eustachian** or **auditory tube** is also found in the nasopharynx. The other end of this tube is in the middle ear. Each time you swallow, this tube opens to equalize air pressure between the middle ear and the outside atmosphere.

Larynx

epiglottis (ep-ih-GLOT-iss)
glottis (GLOT-iss)

thyroid cartilage (THIGH-royd CAR-tih-lij)
vocal cords

The larynx or *voice box* is a muscular structure located between the pharynx and the trachea and contains the **vocal cords** (see Figures 1 and 2 ■). The vocal cords are not actually cordlike in structure, but rather they are folds of membranous tissue that produce sound by vibrating as air passes through the **glottis**, the opening between the two vocal cords.

A flap of cartilaginous tissue, the **epiglottis**, sits above the glottis and provides protection against food and liquid being inhaled into the lungs. The epiglottis covers the larynx and trachea during swallowing and shunts food and liquid from the pharynx into the esophagus. The walls of the larynx are composed of several cartilage plates held together with ligaments and muscles. One of these cartilages, the **thyroid cartilage**, forms what is known as the *Adam's apple*. The thyroid cartilage is generally larger in males than in females and helps to produce the deeper male voice.

Trachea

The trachea, also called the *windpipe*, is the passageway for air that extends from the pharynx and larynx down to the main bronchi (see Figure 3 ■). Measuring approximately 4 inches in length, it is composed of smooth muscle and cartilage rings and is lined by mucous membrane and cilia. Therefore, it also assists in cleansing, warming, and moisturizing air as it travels to the lungs.

Bronchial Tubes

alveoli (al-VEE-oh-lye)
bronchioles (BRONG-key-ohlz)
bronchus (BRONG-kus)

pulmonary capillaries
respiratory membrane

■ **Figure 2** The vocal cords within the larynx, superior view from the pharynx. *(CNRI/Phototake NYC)*

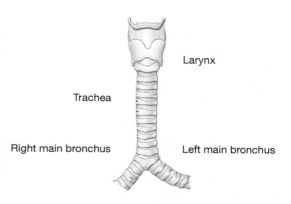

Larynx

Trachea

Right main bronchus

Left main bronchus

■ **Figure 3** Structure of the trachea which extends from the larynx above to the primary bronchi below.

Respiratory System

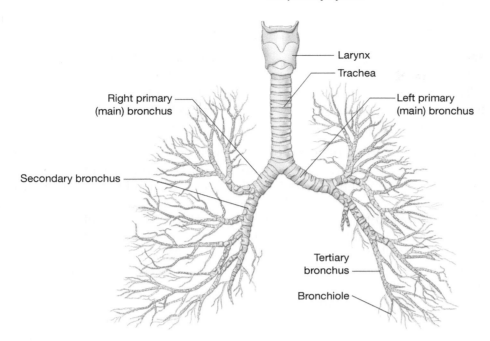

Larynx

Trachea

Right primary (main) bronchus

Left primary (main) bronchus

Secondary bronchus

Tertiary bronchus

Bronchiole

■ **Figure 4** The bronchial tree, each primary (main) bronchus enters a lung and then branches into smaller and smaller secondary bronchi, tertiary bronchi, and bronchioles.

The distal end of the trachea divides to form the left and right primary (main) bronchi. Each **bronchus** enters one of the lungs and branches repeatedly to form secondary and tertiary bronchi. Each branch becomes narrower until the narrowest branches, the **bronchioles**, are formed (see Figure 4 ■). Each bronchiole terminates in a small group of air sacs, called **alveoli**. Each lung has approximately 150 million alveoli. The walls of alveoli are elastic, giving them the ability to expand to hold air and then recoil to their original size. A network of **pulmonary capillaries** from the pulmonary blood vessels tightly encases each alveolus (see Figure 5 ■). In fact, the walls of the alveoli and capillaries are so tightly associated with each other they are referred to as a single unit, the **respiratory membrane**. The exchange of oxygen and carbon dioxide between the air within the alveolus and the blood inside the capillaries takes place across the respiratory membrane.

Med Term Tip

The respiratory system can be thought of as an upside-down tree and its branches. The trunk of the tree consists of the pharynx, larynx, and trachea. The trachea then divides into two branches, the bronchi. Each bronchus divides into smaller and smaller branches. In fact, this branching system of tubes is referred to as the *bronchial tree*.

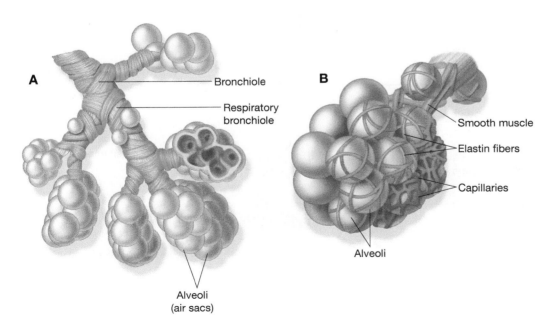

A

Bronchiole

Respiratory bronchiole

B

Smooth muscle

Elastin fibers

Capillaries

Alveoli

Alveoli (air sacs)

■ **Figure 5** A) Each bronchiole terminates in an alveolar sac, a group of alveoli. B) Alveoli encased by network capillaries, forming the respiratory membrane.

Lungs

apex	**parietal pleura** (pah-RYE-eh-tal)
base	**pleura** (PLOO-rah)
hilum (HYE-lum)	**pleural cavity**
lobes	**serous fluid** (SEER-us)
mediastinum (mee-dee-ass-TYE-num)	**visceral pleura** (VISS-er-al)

Each lung is the total collection of the bronchi, bronchioles, and alveoli. They are spongy to the touch because they contain air. The lungs are protected by a double membrane called the **pleura**. The pleura's outer membrane is the **parietal pleura**, which also lines the wall of the chest cavity. The inner membrane or **visceral pleura** adheres to the surface of the lungs. The pleural membrane is folded in such a way that it forms a sac around each lung referred to as the **pleural cavity.** There is normally slippery, watery **serous fluid** between the two layers of the pleura that reduces friction when the two layers rub together as the lungs repeatedly expand and contract.

The lungs contain divisions or **lobes**. There are three lobes in the larger right lung and two in the left lung. The pointed superior portion of each lung is the **apex**, while the broader lower area is the **base**. Entry of structures like the bronchi, pulmonary blood vessels, and nerves into each lung occurs along its medial border in an area called the **hilum**. The lungs within the thoracic cavity are protected from puncture and damage by the ribs. The area between the right and left lung is called the **mediastinum** and contains the heart, aorta, esophagus, thymus gland, and trachea. See Figure 6 ■ for an illustration of the lungs within the chest cavity.

Lung Volumes and Capacities

pulmonary function test   **respiratory therapist**

For some types of medical conditions, like emphysema, it is important to measure the volume of air flowing in and out of the lungs to determine lung capac-

■ Figure 6 Position of the lungs within the thoracic cavity, anterior view illustrating regions of the lungs and their relationship to other thoracic organs.

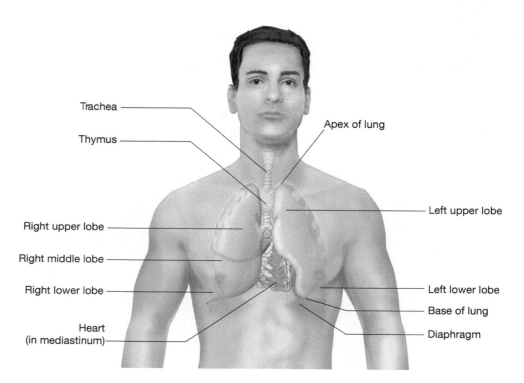

ity. Lung volumes are measured by **respiratory therapists** to aid in determining the functioning level of the respiratory system. Collectively, these measurements are called **pulmonary function tests**. Table 1 ■ lists and defines the four lung volumes and four lung capacities.

Respiratory Muscles

diaphragm   **intercostal muscles** (in-ter-COS-tal)

Air moves in and out of the lungs due to the difference between the atmospheric pressure and the pressure within the chest cavity. This difference in pressure is produced by the **diaphragm**, which is the muscle separating the abdomen from the thoracic cavity. To do this, the diaphragm contracts and moves downward. This increase in thoracic cavity volume causes a decrease in pressure, or negative thoracic pressure, within the chest cavity. Air then flows into the lungs, inhalation, to equalize the pressure. The **intercostal muscles** between the ribs assist in inhalation by raising the rib cage to further enlarge the thoracic cavity. See Figure 7 ■ for an illustration of the role of the diaphragm in inhalation. Similarly, when the diaphragm and intercostal muscles relax, the thoracic cavity becomes smaller. This produces an increase in pressure within the cavity, or positive thoracic pressure, and air flows out of the lungs, resulting in exhalation. Therefore, a quiet, unforced exhalation is a passive process since it does not require any muscle contraction. When a forceful inhalation or exhalation is required, additional chest and neck muscles become active to create larger changes in thoracic pressure.

Med Term Tip

Diaphragmatic breathing is taught to singers and public speakers. You can practice this type of breathing by allowing your abdomen to expand during inhalation and contract during exhalation while your shoulders remain motionless.

Respiratory Rate

vital signs

Respiratory rate (measured in breaths per minute) is one of our **vital signs** (VS), along with heart rate, temperature, and blood pressure. Normally, respiratory rate

Table 1	Lung Volumes and Capacities
TERM	**DEFINITION**
Tidal volume (TV)	The amount of air that enters the lungs in a single inhalation or leaves the lungs in a single exhalation of quiet breathing. In an adult this is normally 500 mL.*
Inspiratory reserve volume (IRV)	The air that can be forcibly inhaled after a normal respiration has taken place. Also called *complemental air*, generally measures around 3,000 mL.*
Expiratory reserve volume (ERV)	The amount of air that can be forcibly exhaled after a normal quiet respiration. This is also called *supplemental air*, approximately 1,000 mL.*
Residual volume (RV)	The air remaining in the lungs after a forced exhalation; about 1,500 mL* in the adult.
Inspiratory capacity (IC)	The volume of air inhaled after a normal exhale.
Functional residual capacity (FRC)	The air that remains in the lungs after a normal exhalation has taken place.
Vital capacity (VC)	The total volume of air that can be exhaled after a maximum inhalation. This amount will be equal to the sum of TV, IRV, and ERV.
Total lung capacity (TLC)	The volume of air in the lungs after a maximal inhalation.

*There is a normal range for measurements of the volume of air exchanged. The numbers given are for the average measurement.

Figure 7 A) Bell jar apparatus demonstrating how downward movement of the diaphragm results in air flowing into the lungs. B) Action of the intercostal muscles lift the ribs to assist the diaphragm in enlarging the volume of the thoracic cavity.

A

- Tube (trachea)
- Bell jar (thoracic cavity)
- Toy balloon (lung)
- Rubber sheet (diaphragm)

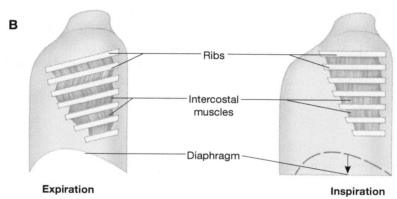

B

- Ribs
- Intercostal muscles
- Diaphragm

Expiration   Inspiration

Med Term Tip

When divers wish to hold their breath longer, they first hyperventilate (breath faster and deeper) in order to get rid of as much CO_2 as possible. This will hold off the urge to breathe longer, allowing a diver to stay submerged longer.

is regulated by the level of CO_2 in the blood. When the CO_2 level is high, we breathe more rapidly to expel the excess. Then, when CO_2 levels drop, our respiratory rate will also drop.

When the respiratory rate falls outside the range of normal, it may indicate an illness or medical condition. For example, when a patient is running an elevated temperature and has shortness of breath (SOB) due to pneumonia, the respiratory rate may increase dramatically. Or a brain injury or some medications, such as those for pain, can cause a decrease in the respiratory rate. See Table 2 ■ for normal respiratory rate ranges for different age groups.

Table 2	Respiratory Rates for Different Age Groups
AGE	RESPIRATIONS PER MINUTE
Newborn	30–60
1-year-old	18–30
16-year-old	16–20
Adult	12–20

Word Building

The following list contains examples of medical terms built directly from word parts. The definition for these terms can be determined by a straightforward translation of the word parts.

COMBINING FORM	COMBINED WITH	MEDICAL TERM	DEFINITION
bronch/o	-gram	**bronchogram** (BRONG-koh-gram)	record of the bronchus
	-itis	**bronchitis** (brong-KIGH-tis)	inflammation of a bronchus
	-plasty	**bronchoplasty** (BRONG-koh-plas-tee)	surgical repair of a bronchus
	-genic	**bronchogenic** (brong-koh-JEN-ik)	produced by the bronchus
	-scope	**bronchoscope** (BRONG-koh-scope)	instrument to view inside of bronchus
	-spasm	**bronchospasm** (BRONG-koh-spazm)	involuntary muscle spasm of bronchus
	-ial	**bronchial** (BRONG-ee-all)	pertaining to a bronchus
bronchi/o	-ectasis	**bronchiectasis** (brong-key-EK-tah-sis)	dilated bronchus
diaphragmat/o	-ic	**diaphragmatic** (dye-ah-frag-MAT-ik)	pertaining to the diaphragm
laryng/o	-ectomy	**laryngectomy** (lair-in-JEK-toh-mee)	removal of the voice box
	-itis	**laryngitis** (lair-in-JYE-tis)	inflammation of the voice box
	-plasty	**laryngoplasty** (lair-RING-goh-plas-tee)	surgical repair of the voice box
	-scope	**laryngoscope** (lair-RING-go-scope)	instrument to view voice box
	-eal	**laryngeal** (lair-in-GEE-all)	pertaining to the voice box
	-plegia	**laryngoplegia** (lair-RING-goh-plee-gee-ah)	paralysis of the voice box
lob/o	-ectomy	**lobectomy** (loh-BEK-toh-mee)	removal of a (lung) lobe
ox/i	-meter	**oximeter** (ox-IM-eh-ter)	instrument to measure oxygen
ox/o	an- -ia	**anoxia** (ah-NOK-see-ah)	condition of no oxygen
	hypo- -emia	**hypoxemia** (high-pox-EE-mee-ah)	insufficient oxygen in the blood
	hypo- -ia	**hypoxia** (high-POX-ee-ah)	insufficient oxygen condition
pleur/o	-centesis	**pleurocentesis** (ploor-oh-sen-TEE-sis)	puncture of the pleura to withdraw fluid
	-ectomy	**pleurectomy** (ploor-EK-toh-mee)	removal of the pleura
	-dynia	**pleurodynia** (ploor-oh-DIN-ee-ah)	pleural pain
pharyng/o	-itis	**pharyngitis** (fair-in-JYE-tis)	throat inflammation (*i.e., sore throat*)
	-eal	**pharyngeal** (fair-in-GEE-all)	pertaining to the throat
	nas/o -itis	**nasopharyngitis** (nay-zoh-fair-in-JYE-tis)	nose and throat inflammation (*i.e., common cold*)
pulmon/o	-logist	**pulmonologist** (pul-mon-ALL-oh-jist)	lung specialist
	-ary	**pulmonary** (PULL-mon-air-ee)	pertaining to the lung
rhin/o	-itis	**rhinitis** (rye-NYE-tis)	inflammation of the nose
	myc/o -osis	**rhinomycosis** (rye-noh-my-KOH-sis)	abnormal condition of nose fungus
	-plasty	**rhinoplasty** (RYE-noh-plas-tee)	surgical repair of the nose

Word Building (continued)

COMBINING FORM	COMBINED WITH	MEDICAL TERM	DEFINITION
	-rrhagia	**rhinorrhagia** (rye-noh-RAH-jee-ah)	rapid flow (of blood) from the nose
	-rrhea	**rhinorrhea** (rye-noh-REE-ah)	nose discharge (*i.e., runny nose*)
sinus/o	pan- -itis	**pansinusitis** (pan-sigh-nus-EYE-tis)	inflammation of all the sinuses
thorac/o	-algia	**thoracalgia** (thor-ah-KAL-jee-ah)	chest pain
	-ic	**thoracic** (tho-RASS-ik)	pertaining to the chest
	-otomy	**thoracotomy** (thor-ah-KOT-oh-mee)	incision into the chest
trache/o	endo- -al	**endotracheal** (en-doh-TRAY-kee-al)	pertaining to inside the trachea
	-otomy	**tracheotomy** (tray-kee-OTT-oh-mee)	incision into the trachea
	-stenosis	**tracheostenosis** (tray-kee-oh-steh-NOH-sis)	narrowing of the trachea

SUFFIX	COMBINED WITH	MEDICAL TERM	DEFINITION
-phonia	a-	**aphonia** (a-FOH-nee-ah)	no voice
	dys-	**dysphonia** (dis-FOH-nee-ah)	abnormal voice
-capnia	a-	**acapnia** (a-CAP-nee-ah)	lack of carbon dioxide
	hyper-	**hypercapnia** (high-per-CAP-nee-ah)	excessive carbon dioxide
-osmia	an-	**anosmia** (ah-NOZ-mee-ah)	lack of (sense of) smell
-pnea	a-	**apnea** (AP-nee-ah)	not breathing
	brady-	**bradypnea** (bray-DIP-nee-ah)	slow breathing
	dys-	**dyspnea** (DISP-nee-ah)	difficult, labored breathing
	eu-	**eupnea** (yoop-NEE-ah)	normal breathing
	hyper-	**hyperpnea** (high-per-NEE-ah)	excessive (deep) breathing
	hypo-	**hypopnea** (high-POP-nee-ah)	insufficient (shallow) breathing
	ortho-	**orthopnea** (or-THOP-nee-ah)	(sitting) straight breathing
	tachy-	**tachypnea** (tak-ip-NEE-ah)	rapid breathing
-thorax	hem/o	**hemothorax** (hee-moh-THOH-raks)	blood in the chest
	py/o	**pyothorax** (pye-oh-THOH-raks)	pus in the chest
	pneum/o	**pneumothorax** (new-moh-THOH-raks)	air in the chest

Vocabulary

TERM	DEFINITION
asphyxia (as-FIK-see-ah)	Lack of oxygen that can lead to unconsciousness and death if not corrected immediately; also called *asphyxiation* or *suffocation*. Some common causes include drowning, foreign body in the respiratory tract, poisoning, and electric shock.

Vocabulary (continued)

TERM	DEFINITION
aspiration (as-peer-RAY-shun)	Refers to withdrawing fluid from a body cavity using suction. For example, using a long needle and syringe to withdraw fluid from the pleural cavity or using a vacuum pump to remove phlegm from a patient's airways. In addition, it also refers to inhaling food, liquid, or a foreign object into the airways. Often leads to the development of pneumonia.
Cheyne–Stokes respiration (CHAIN STOHKS res-pir-AY-shun)	Abnormal breathing pattern in which there are long periods (10 to 60 seconds) of apnea followed by deeper, more rapid breathing. Named for John Cheyne, a Scottish physician, and Sir William Stokes, an Irish surgeon.
clubbing	The abnormal widening and thickening of the ends of the fingers and toes associated with chronic oxygen deficiency. Seen in patients with chronic respiratory conditions or circulatory problems.
cyanosis (sigh-ah-NO-sis)	Refers to the bluish tint of skin that is receiving an insufficient amount of oxygen or circulation.
epistaxis (ep-ih-STAKS-is)	Nosebleed.
hemoptysis (hee-MOP-tih-sis)	To cough up blood or blood-stained sputum.
hyperventilation (HYE-per-vent-ill-a-shun)	To breathe both too fast (tachypnea) and too deep (hyperpnea).
hypoventilation (HYE-poh-vent-ill-a-shun)	To breathe both too slow (bradypnea) and too shallow (hypopnea).
internal medicine	Branch of medicine involving the diagnosis and treatment of diseases and conditions of internal organs such as the respiratory system. The physician is an *internist*.
nasal cannula (CAN-you-lah)	Two-pronged plastic device for delivering oxygen into the nose; one prong is inserted into each naris.
orthopnea (or-THOP-nee-ah)	A term to describe dyspnea that is worsened by lying flat. In other words, the patient is able to breath easier when sitting straight up.
otorhinolaryngology (ENT) (oh-toh-rye-noh-lair-in-GOL-oh-jee)	Branch of medicine involving the diagnosis and treatment of conditions and diseases of the ear, nose, and throat region. The physician is an *otorhinolaryngologist*. This medical specialty may also be referred to as *otolaryngology*.
patent (PAY-tent)	Open or unblocked, such as a patent airway.
percussion (per-KUH-shun)	Use of the fingertips to tap on a surface to determine the condition beneath the surface. Determined in part by the feel of the surface as it is tapped and the sound generated.
phlegm (FLEM)	Thick mucus secreted by the membranes that line the respiratory tract. When phlegm is coughed through the mouth, it is called *sputum*. Phlegm is examined for color, odor, and consistency.
pleural rub (PLOO-ral)	Grating sound made when the two layers of the pleura rub together during respiration. It is caused when one of the surfaces becomes thicker as a result of inflammation or other disease conditions. This rub can be felt through the fingertips when they are placed on the chest wall or heard through the stethoscope.

Vocabulary (continued)

TERM	DEFINITION
pulmonology (pull-mon-ALL-oh-jee)	Branch of medicine involved in diagnosis and treatment of diseases and disorders of the respiratory system. Physician is a *pulmonologist*.
rales (RALZ)	Abnormal crackling sound made during inspiration. Usually indicates the presence of fluid or mucus in the airways.
respiratory therapy	Allied health specialty that assists patients with respiratory and cardiopulmonary disorders. Duties of a *respiratory therapist* include conducting pulmonary function tests, monitoring oxygen and carbon dioxide levels in the blood, administering breathing treatments, and ventilator management.
rhonchi (RONG-kigh)	Somewhat musical sound during expiration, often found in asthma or infection. Caused by spasms of the bronchial tubes. Also called *wheezing*.
shortness of breath (SOB)	Term used to indicate that a patient is having some difficulty breathing; also called *dyspnea*. The causes can range from mild SOB after exercise to SOB associated with heart disease.
sputum (SPEW-tum)	Mucus or phlegm that is coughed up from the lining of the respiratory tract.
	Med Term Tip
	The term *sputum,* from the Latin word meaning "to spit," now refers to the material coughed up and spit out from the respiratory system.
stridor (STRIGH-dor)	Harsh, high-pitched, noisy breathing sound made when there is an obstruction of the bronchus or larynx. Found in conditions such as croup in children.
thoracic surgery (tho-RASS-ik)	Branch of medicine involving diagnosis and treatment of conditions and diseases of the respiratory system by surgical means. Physician is a *thoracic surgeon*.

Pathology

TERM	DEFINITION
■ *Upper Respiratory System*	
croup (KROOP)	Acute respiratory condition found in infants and children that is characterized by a barking type of cough or stridor.
diphtheria (dif-THEAR-ee-ah)	Bacterial upper respiratory infection characterized by the formation of a thick membranous film across the throat and a high mortality rate. Rare now due to the DPT (diphtheria, pertussis, tetanus) vaccine.
pertussis (per-TUH-is)	Commonly called *whooping cough*, due to the whoop sound made when coughing. An infectious bacterial disease of the upper respiratory system that children receive immunization against as part of their DPT shots.
■ *Bronchial Tubes*	
asthma (AZ-mah)	Disease caused by various conditions, like allergens, and resulting in constriction of the bronchial airways, dyspnea, coughing, and wheezing. Can cause violent spasms of the bronchi (bronchospasms) but is generally not a life-threatening condition. Medication can be very effective.
	Med Term Tip
	The term *asthma,* from the Greek word meaning "panting," describes the breathing pattern of a person having an asthma attack.

Pathology *(continued)*

TERM	DEFINITION
bronchiectasis (brong-key-EK-tah-sis)	The abnormal enlargement of bronchi; may be the result of a lung infection. This condition can be irreversible and result in destruction of the bronchial walls. Major symptoms include coughing up a large amount of purulent sputum, rales, and hemoptysis.
bronchogenic carcinoma (brong-koh-JEN-ik car-sin-OH-mah) ■ **Figure 8** Color enchanced X-ray of large malignant tumor in right lower lung. *(ISM/Phototake NYC)*	Malignant tumor originating in the bronchi. Usually associated with a history of cigarette smoking.

■ *Lungs*

TERM	DEFINITION
adult respiratory distress syndrome (ARDS)	Acute respiratory failure in adults characterized by tachypnea, dyspnea, cyanosis, tachycardia, and hypoxemia. May follow trauma, pneumonia, or septic infections. Also called *acute respiratory distress syndrome*.
anthracosis (an-thra-KOH-sis)	A type of pneumoconiosis that develops from the collection of coal dust in the lung. Also called *black lung* or *miner's lung*.
asbestosis (az-bes-TOH-sis)	A type of pneumoconiosis that develops from collection of asbestos fibers in the lungs. May lead to the development of lung cancer.
atelectasis (at-eh-LEK-tah-sis)	Condition in which the alveoli in a portion of the lung collapse, preventing the respiratory exchange of oxygen and carbon dioxide. Can be caused by a variety of conditions, including pressure on the lung from a tumor or other object. Term also used to describe the failure of a newborn's lungs to expand.
chronic obstructive pulmonary disease (COPD) (PULL-mon-air-ee)	Progressive, chronic, and usually irreversible group of conditions, like emphysema, in which the lungs have a diminished capacity for inspiration (inhalation) and expiration (exhalation). The person may have dypsnea upon exertion and a cough.
cystic fibrosis (CF) (SIS-tik fye-BROH-sis)	Hereditary condition causing the exocrine glands to malfunction. The patient produces very thick mucus that causes severe congestion within the lungs and digestive system. Through more advanced treatment, many children are now living into adulthood with this disease.
emphysema (em-fih-SEE-mah)	Pulmonary condition characterized by the destruction of the walls of the alveoli, resulting in fewer overexpanded air sacs. Can occur as a result of long-term heavy smoking. Air pollution also worsens this disease. The patient may not be able to breathe except in a sitting or standing position.

Pathology (continued)

TERM	DEFINITION
histoplasmosis (his-toh-plaz-MOH-sis)	Pulmonary infection caused by the fungus *Histoplasma capsulatum*, found in dust and in the droppings of pigeons and chickens.
infant respiratory distress syndrome (IRDS)	A lung condition most commonly found in premature infants that is characterized by tachypnea and respiratory grunting. The condition is caused by a lack of surfactant necessary to keep the lungs inflated. Also called *hyaline membrane disease* (HMD) and *respiratory distress syndrome of the newborn*.
influenza (in-floo-EN-za)	Viral infection of the respiratory system characterized by chills, fever, body aches, and fatigue. Commonly called the *flu*.
Legionnaire's disease (lee-jen-AYRZ)	Severe, often fatal bacterial infection characterized by pneumonia and liver and kidney damage. Named after people who came down with it at an American Legion convention in 1976.
***Mycoplasma* pneumonia** (MY-koh-plaz-em)	A less severe but longer lasting form of pneumonia caused by the *Mycoplasma pneumoniae* bacteria. Also called *walking pneumonia*.
pneumoconiosis (noo-moh-koh-nee-OH-sis)	Condition that is the result of inhaling environmental particles that become toxic. Can be the result of inhaling coal dust (anthracosis) or asbestos (asbestosis).
***Pneumocystis carinii* pneumonia** (PCP) (noo-moh-SIS-tis kah-RYE-nee-eye new-MOH-nee-ah)	Pneumonia with a nonproductive cough, very little fever, and dyspnea caused by the fungus *Pneumocystis carinii*. An opportunistic infection often seen in those with weakened immune systems, such as AIDS patients.
pneumonia (new-MOH-nee-ah)	Inflammatory condition of the lung that can be caused by bacterial and viral infections, diseases, and chemicals. Results in the filling of the alveoli and air spaces with fluid.
pulmonary edema (PULL-mon-air-ee eh-DEE-mah)	Condition in which lung tissue retains an excessive amount of fluid, especially in the alveoli. Results in dyspnea.
pulmonary embolism (PULL-mon-air-ee EM-boh-lizm)	Blood clot or air bubble in the pulmonary artery or one of its branches. May cause an infarct in the lung tissue.
pulmonary fibrosis (fi-BROH-sis)	Formation of fibrous scar tissue in the lungs that leads to decreased ability to expand the lungs. May be caused by infections, pneumoconiosis, autoimmune diseases, and toxin exposure.
severe acute respiratory syndrome (SARS)	Acute viral respiratory infection that begins like the flu but quickly progresses to severe dyspnea; high fatality rate. First appeared in China in 2003.
silicosis (sil-ih-KOH-sis)	A type of pneumoconiosis that develops from the inhalation of silica (quartz) dust found in quarrying, glass works, sandblasting, and ceramics.
sleep apnea (AP-nee-ah)	Condition in which breathing stops repeatedly during sleep long enough to cause a drop in oxygen levels in the blood.
sudden infant death syndrome (SIDS)	Unexpected and unexplained death of an apparently well infant under one year of age. The child suddenly stops breathing for unknown reasons.
tuberculosis (TB) (too-ber-kyoo-LOH-sis)	Infectious disease caused by the bacteria *Mycobacterium tuberculosis*. Most commonly affects the respiratory system and causes inflammation and calcification in the lungs. Tuberculosis incidence is on the increase and is seen in many patients with weakened immune systems. Multidrug resistant tuberculosis is a particularly dangerous form of the disease because some bacteria have developed a resistance to the standard drug therapy.

Pathology (continued)

TERM	DEFINITION
■ Pleural Cavity	
empyema (em-pye-EE-mah)	Pus within the pleural space usually associated with a bacterial infection. Also called *pyothorax*.
pleural effusion (PLOO-ral eh-FYOO-zhun)	Abnormal accumulation of fluid in the pleural cavity preventing the lungs from fully expanding. Physicians can detect the presence of fluid by tapping the chest (percussion) or listening with a stethoscope (auscultation).
pleurisy (PLOOR-ih-see)	Inflammation of the pleura characterized by sharp chest pain with each breath. Also called *pleuritis*.
pneumothorax (new-moh-THOH-raks)	Collection of air or gas in the pleural cavity, which may result in collapse of the lung.

■ **Figure 9** Pneumothorax. Figure illustrates how puncture of thoracic wall and tearing of pleural membrane allows air into lung and results in a collapsed lung.

Torn pleura

Outside air entering pleural cavity

Left lung

Inspiration

Diaphragm

Diagnostic Procedures

TERM	DEFINITION
■ Clinical Laboratory Tests	
arterial blood gases (ABGs) (ar-TEE-ree-al)	Testing for the gases present in the blood. Generally used to assist in determining the levels of oxygen (O_2) and carbon dioxide (CO_2) in the blood.
sputum culture and sensitivity (C&S) (SPEW-tum)	Testing sputum by placing it on a culture medium and observing any bacterial growth. The specimen is then tested to determine antibiotic effectiveness.
sputum cytology (SPEW-tum sigh-TALL-oh-jee)	Examining sputum for malignant cells.
■ Diagnostic Imaging	
bronchography (brong-KOG-rah-fee)	X-ray of the lung after a radiopaque substance has been inserted into the trachea or bronchial tube. Resulting x-ray is called a *bronchogram*.
chest x-ray (CXR)	Taking a radiographic picture of the lungs and heart from the back and sides.

Diagnostic Procedures *(continued)*

TERM	DEFINITION
pulmonary angiography (PULL-mon-air-ee an-jee-OG-rah-fee)	Injecting dye into a blood vessel for the purpose of taking an x-ray of the arteries and veins of the lungs.
ventilation-perfusion scan (per-FUSE-shun)	A nuclear medicine diagnostic test that is especially useful in identifying pulmonary emboli. Radioactive air is inhaled for the ventilation portion to determine if air is filling the entire lung. Radioactive intravenous injection shows whether blood is flowing to all parts of the lung.

■ *Endoscopic Procedures*

bronchoscopy (Bronch) (brong-KOSS-koh-pee)	Visual examination of the inside of the bronchi; uses an instrument called a *bronchoscope*.

■ **Figure 10** Bronchoscopy. Figure illustrates physician using a bronchoscope to inspect the patient's bronchial tubes. Advances in technology include using a videoscope which projects the internal view of the bronchus onto a video screen.

Cross Section of Scope

Eye piece

Viewing channel
Light source
Biopsy forceps and instrument channel

Flexible bronchoscopic tube

laryngoscopy (lair-in-GOSS-koh-pee)	Examination of the interior of the larynx with a lighted instrument called a *laryngoscope*.

■ *Pulmonary Function Tests*

oximetry (ox-IM-eh-tree)	Measures the oxygen level in the blood using a device, an *oximeter*, placed on the patient's fingertip or ear lobe.
pulmonary function test (PFT) (PULL-mon-air-ee)	A group of diagnostic tests that give information regarding air flow in and out of the lungs, lung volumes, and gas exchange between the lungs and bloodstream.
spirometry (spy-ROM-eh-tree)	Procedure to measure lung capacity using a **spirometer**.

■ *Additional Diagnostic Procedures*

polysomnography (polly-som-NOG-rah-fee)	Monitoring a patient while sleeping to identify sleep apnea. Also called *sleep apnea study*.
sweat test	A test for cystic fibrosis. Patients with this disease have an abnormally large amount of salt in their sweat.
tuberculin skin tests (TB test) (too-BER-kyoo-lin)	Applying the tuberculin purified protein derivative (PPD) under the surface of the skin to determine if the patient has been exposed to tuberculosis. Also called a *Tine* or *Mantoux test*.

Therapeutic Procedures

TERM	DEFINITION
■ *Respiratory Therapy*	
aerosol therapy (AIR-oh-sol)	Medication suspended in a mist that is intended to be inhaled. Delivered by a *nebulizer*, which delivers the mist for a period of time while the patient breathes, or a *metered dose inhaler* (MDI), which delivers a single puff of mist.
endotracheal intubation (en-doh-TRAY-kee-al in-too-BAY-shun)	Placing a tube through the mouth, through the glottis, and into the trachea to create a patent airway.

Epiglottis   Trachea

Esophagus

■ **Figure 11** Endotracheal intubation. First, a lighted scope is used to identify the trachea from the esophagus. Next, the tube is placed through the pharynx and into the trachea. Finally, the scope is removed, leaving the tube in place.

TERM	DEFINITION
intermittent positive pressure breathing (IPPB)	Method for assisting patients in breathing using a mask that is connected to a machine that produces an increased positive thoracic pressure.
postural drainage	Drainage of secretions from the bronchi by placing the patient in a position that uses gravity to promote drainage. Used for the treatment of cystic fibrosis and bronchiectasis.
supplemental oxygen therapy	Providing a patient with additional concentration of oxygen to improve oxygen levels in the bloodstream. Oxygen may be provided by a mask or nasal cannula.
ventilator (VENT-ih-later)	A machine that provides artificial ventilation for a patient unable to breathe on his or her own. Also called a *respirator*.

■ **Figure 12** Patient with tracheostomy tube in place receiving oxygen through mask placed over the tracheostomy opening and attached to a ventilator. *(Ansell Horn/Phototake NYC)*

Therapeutic Procedures *(continued)*

TERM	DEFINITION

■ *Surgical Procedures*

thoracentesis
(thor-ah-sen-TEE-sis)

■ **Figure 13** Thoracentesis. The needle is inserted between the ribs to withdraw fluid from the pleural sac at the base of the left lung.

Surgical puncture of the chest wall for the removal of fluids. Also called *thoracocentesis*.

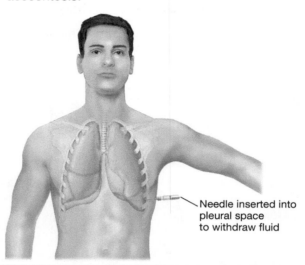

Needle inserted into pleural space to withdraw fluid

---

thoracostomy
(thor-ah-KOS-toh-mee)

Insertion of a tube into the chest for the purpose of draining off fluid or air. Also called *chest tube*.

---

tracheostomy
(tray-kee-OSS-toh-mee)

■ **Figure 14** A tracheostomy tube in place, inserted through an opening in the front of the neck and anchored within the trachea.

A surgical procedure often performed in an emergency that creates an opening directly into the trachea to allow the patient to breathe easier; also called *tracheotomy*.

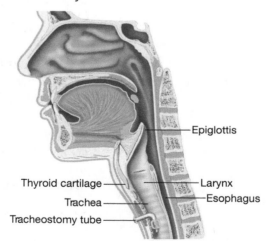

Epiglottis

Thyroid cartilage

Trachea

Tracheostomy tube

Larynx

Esophagus

■ *Additional Procedures*

cardiopulmonary resuscitation
(CPR)
(car-dee-oh-PULL-mon-air-ee ree-suss-ih-TAY-shun)

Emergency treatment provided by persons trained in CPR and given to patients when their respirations and heart stop. CPR provides oxygen to the brain, heart, and other vital organs until medical treatment can restore a normal heart and pulmonary function.

Heimlich maneuver (HYME-lik)

Technique for removing a foreign body from the trachea or pharynx by exerting diaphragmatic pressure. Named for Harry Heimlich, a U.S. thoracic surgeon.

Pharmacology

CLASSIFICATION	ACTION	GENERIC AND BRAND NAMES
antibiotic (an-tih-bye-AW-tic)	Kills bacteria causing respiratory infections.	ampicillin; amoxicillin, Amoxil; ciprofloxacin, Cipro
antihistamine (an-tih-HIST-ah-meen)	Blocks the effects of histamine that has been released by the body during an allergy attack.	fexofenadine, Allegra; loratadine, Claritan; diphenhydramine, Benadryl
antitussive (an-tih-TUSS-ive)	Relieves urge to cough.	hydrocodon, Hycodan; dextromethorphan, Vicks Formula 44
bronchodilator (BRONG-koh-dye-late-or)	Relaxes muscle spasms in bronchial tubes. Used to treat asthma.	albuterol, Proventil, Ventolin; salmetrol, Serevent; theophyllin, Theo-Dur
corticosteroids (core-tih-koh-STAIR-ryods)	Reduces inflammation and swelling in the respiratory tract.	fluticasone, Flonase; mometasone, Nasonex; triamcinolone, Azmacort
decongestant (dee-kon-JES-tant)	Reduces stuffiness and congestion throughout the respiratory system.	oxymetazoline, Afrin, Dristan, Sinex; pseudoephedrine, Drixoral, Sudafed
expectorant (ek-SPEK-toh-rant)	Improves the ability to cough up mucus from the respiratory tract.	guaifenesin, Robitussin, Mucinex
mucolytic (myoo-koh-LIT-ik)	Liquefies mucus so it is easier to cough and clear it from the respiratory tract.	N-acetyl-cysteine, Mucomyst

Abbreviations

ABGs	arterial blood gases	**O$_2$**	oxygen
ARDS	adult (or acute) respiratory distress syndrome	**PCP**	*Pneumocystis carinii* pneumonia
Bronch	bronchoscopy	**PFT**	pulmonary function test
CO$_2$	carbon dioxide	**PPD**	purified protein derivative
COPD	chronic obstructive pulmonary disease	**R**	respiration
CPR	cardiopulmonary resuscitation	**RA**	room air
C&S	culture and sensitivity	**RDS**	respiratory distress syndrome
CTA	clear to auscultation	**RLL**	right lower lobe
CXR	chest x-ray	**RML**	right middle lobe
DOE	dyspnea on exertion	**RRT**	registered respiratory therapist
DPT	diphtheria, pertussis, tetanus injection	**RV**	reserve volume
ENT	ear, nose, and throat	**RUL**	right upper lobe
ERV	expiratory reserve volume	**SARS**	severe acute respiratory syndrome
FRC	functional residual capacity	**SIDS**	sudden infant death syndrome
HMD	hyaline membrane disease	**SOB**	shortness of breath
IC	inspiratory capacity	**TB**	tuberculosis
IPPB	intermittent positive pressure breathing	**TLC**	total lung capacity
IRDS	infant respiratory distress syndrome	**TPR**	temperature, pulse, and respiration
IRV	inspiratory reserve volume	**TV**	tidal volume
LLL	left lower lobe	**URI**	upper respiratory infection
LUL	left upper lobe	**VC**	vital capacity
MDI	metered dose inhaler		

Chapter Review

Terminology Checklist

Below are all Anatomy and Physiology key terms, Word Building, Vocabulary, Pathology, Diagnostic, Therapeutic, and Pharmacology terms presented in this chapter. Use this list as a study tool by placing a check in the box in front of each term as you master its meaning.

☐ acapnia
☐ adenoids
☐ adult respiratory distress syndrome
☐ aerosol therapy
☐ alveoli
☐ anosmia
☐ anoxia
☐ anthracosis
☐ antibiotic
☐ antihistamine
☐ antitussive
☐ apex
☐ aphonia
☐ apnea
☐ arterial blood gases
☐ asbestosis
☐ asphyxia
☐ aspiration
☐ asthma
☐ atelectasis
☐ auditory tube
☐ base
☐ bradypnea
☐ bronchial
☐ bronchial tube
☐ bronchiectasis
☐ bronchioles
☐ bronchitis
☐ bronchodilator
☐ bronchogenic
☐ bronchogenic carcinoma
☐ bronchogram
☐ bronchography
☐ bronchoplasty
☐ bronchoscope
☐ bronchoscopy
☐ bronchospasm

☐ bronchus
☐ carbon dioxide
☐ cardiopulmonary resuscitation
☐ chest x-ray
☐ Cheyne–Stokes respiration
☐ chronic obstructive pulmonary disease
☐ cilia
☐ clubbing
☐ corticosteroids
☐ croup
☐ cyanosis
☐ cystic fibrosis
☐ decongestant
☐ diaphragm
☐ diaphragmatic
☐ diphtheria
☐ dysphonia
☐ dyspnea
☐ emphysema
☐ empyema
☐ endotracheal
☐ endotracheal intubation
☐ epiglottis
☐ epistaxis
☐ eupnea
☐ eustachian tube
☐ exhalation
☐ expectorant
☐ expiratory reserve volume
☐ external respiration
☐ functional residual capacity
☐ glottis
☐ Heimlich maneuver
☐ hemoptysis
☐ hemothorax
☐ hilum
☐ histoplasmosis
☐ hypercapnia

☐ hyperpnea
☐ hyperventilation
☐ hypopnea
☐ hypoventilation
☐ hypoxemia
☐ hypoxia
☐ infant respiratory distress syndrome
☐ influenza
☐ inhalation
☐ inspiratory capacity
☐ inspiratory reserve volume
☐ intercostal muscles
☐ intermittent positive pressure breathing
☐ internal medicine
☐ internal respiration
☐ laryngeal
☐ laryngectomy
☐ laryngitis
☐ laryngopharynx
☐ laryngoplasty
☐ laryngoplegia
☐ laryngoscope
☐ laryngoscopy
☐ larynx
☐ Legionnaire's disease
☐ lingual tonsils
☐ lobectomy
☐ lobes
☐ lungs
☐ mediastinum
☐ mucolytic
☐ mucous membrane
☐ mucus
☐ *Mycoplasma* pneumonia
☐ nares
☐ nasal cannula
☐ nasal cavity

Respiratory System

- [ ] nasal septum
- [ ] nasopharyngitis
- [ ] nasopharynx
- [ ] oropharynx
- [ ] orthopnea
- [ ] otorhinolaryngology
- [ ] oximeter
- [ ] oximetry
- [ ] oxygen
- [ ] palate
- [ ] palatine tonsils
- [ ] pansinusitis
- [ ] paranasal sinuses
- [ ] parietal pleura
- [ ] patent
- [ ] percussion
- [ ] pertussis
- [ ] pharyngeal
- [ ] pharyngeal tonsils
- [ ] pharyngitis
- [ ] pharynx
- [ ] phlegm
- [ ] pleura
- [ ] pleural cavity
- [ ] pleural effusion
- [ ] pleural rub
- [ ] pleurectomy
- [ ] pleurisy
- [ ] pleurocentesis
- [ ] pleurodynia
- [ ] pneumoconiosis
- [ ] *Pneumocystis carinii* pneumonia

- [ ] pneumonia
- [ ] pneumothorax
- [ ] polysomnography
- [ ] postural drainage
- [ ] pulmonary
- [ ] pulmonary angiography
- [ ] pulmonary capillaries
- [ ] pulmonary edema
- [ ] pulmonary embolism
- [ ] pulmonary fibrosis
- [ ] pulmonary function test
- [ ] pulmonologist
- [ ] pulmonology
- [ ] pyothorax
- [ ] rales
- [ ] residual volume
- [ ] respiratory membrane
- [ ] respiratory therapist
- [ ] respiratory therapy
- [ ] rhinitis
- [ ] rhinomycosis
- [ ] rhinoplasty
- [ ] rhinorrhagia
- [ ] rhinorrhea
- [ ] rhonchi
- [ ] serous fluid
- [ ] severe acute respiratory syndrome
- [ ] shortness of breath
- [ ] silicosis
- [ ] sleep apnea
- [ ] spirometer

- [ ] spirometry
- [ ] sputum
- [ ] sputum culture and sensitivity
- [ ] sputum cytology
- [ ] stridor
- [ ] sudden infant death syndrome
- [ ] supplemental oxygen therapy
- [ ] sweat test
- [ ] tachypnea
- [ ] thoracalgia
- [ ] thoracentesis
- [ ] thoracic
- [ ] thoracic surgery
- [ ] thoracostomy
- [ ] thoracotomy
- [ ] thyroid cartilage
- [ ] tidal volume
- [ ] total lung capacity
- [ ] trachea
- [ ] tracheostenosis
- [ ] tracheostomy
- [ ] tracheotomy
- [ ] tuberculin skin tests
- [ ] tuberculosis
- [ ] ventilation
- [ ] ventilation-perfusion scan
- [ ] ventilator
- [ ] visceral pleura
- [ ] vital capacity
- [ ] vital signs
- [ ] vocal cords

Practice Exercises

A. Complete the following statements.

1. The primary function of the respiratory system is <u>respiration</u>.

2. The movement of air in and out of the lungs is called <u>ventilation</u>.

3. Define external respiration: <u>exchange of O2 & CO2 that takes place in the lungs</u>

4. Define internal respiration: <u>process of O2 & CO2 exchange at the cellular level when O2 leaves the bloodstream & is delivered to the tissues.</u>

5. The organs of the respiratory system are <u>nasal cavity</u>, <u>pharynx</u>, <u>larynx</u>, <u>trachea</u>, <u>lungs</u>, and <u>bronchial tubes</u>

Respiratory System

6. The passageway for food, liquids, and air is the _____.

7. The _opiglottis_ helps to keep food out of the respiratory tract.

8. The function of the cilia in the nose is to _filter out large dirt particles before they can enter the lungs._

9. The muscle that divides the thoracic cavity from the abdominal cavity is the _diaphragm_.

10. The respiratory rate for an adult is _12_ to _20_ respirations per minute.

11. The respiratory rate for a newborn is _30_ to _40_ respirations per minute.

12. The right lung has _3_ lobes; the left lung has _2_ lobes.

13. The air sacs at the ends of the bronchial tree are called _alveoli_.

14. The term for the double membrane around the lungs is _pleura_.

15. The nasal cavity is separated from the mouth by the _palate_.

16. The small branches of the bronchi are the _bronchioles_.

B. State the terms described using the combining forms provided.

The combining form *rhin/o* refers to the nose. Use it to write a term that means:

1. inflammation of the nose _rhinitis_

2. rapid flow from the nose _~~rhinorrhea~~ rhinorrhagia_

3. discharge from the nose _rhinorrhea_

4. surgical repair of the nose _rhinoplasty_

The combining form *laryng/o* refers to the larynx or voice box. Use it to write a term that means:

5. inflammation of the larynx _laryngitis_

6. spasm of the larynx _laryngospasm_

7. visual examination of the larynx _laryngoscopy_

8. pertaining to the larynx _laryngeal_

9. incision of the larynx _laryngotomy_

10. removal of the larynx _laryngectomy_

11. surgical repair of the larynx _laryngoplasty_

12. paralysis of the larynx _laryngoplegia_

The combining form *bronch/o* refers to the bronchus. Use it to write a term that means:

13. pertaining to bronchus _bronchial_

14. inflammation of the bronchus _bronchitis_

15. visually examine the interior of the bronchus ___bronchoscopy___

16. produced by bronchus ___bronchogenic___

17. spasm of the bronchus ___bronchospasm___

The combining form *thorac/o* refers to the chest. Use it to write a term that means:

18. surgical repair of the chest ___thoracoplasty___

19. incision into the chest ___thoracotomy___

20. chest pain ___thoracalgia___

21. pertaining to chest ___thoracic___

The combining form *trache/o* refers to the trachea. Use it to write a term that means:

22. cutting into the trachea ___tracheotomy___

23. surgical repair of the trachea ___tracheoplasty___

24. narrowing of the trachea ___tracheostenosis___

25. pertaining to inside trachea ___endo-tracheal___

26. inflammation of the trachea ___tracheaitis___

27. forming an artificial opening into the trachea ___tracheostomy___

C. Define the following combining forms and use them to form respiratory terms.

	Definition	Respiratory Term
1. trache/o	trachea, windpipe	tracheotomy
2. laryng/o	larynx	laryngectomy
3. bronch/o	bronchus	bronchial
4. spir/o	breathing	respiration
5. pneum/o	lung, air	pneumonia
6. rhin/o	nose	rhinoplasty
7. coni/o	dust	pneumoconiosis
8. pleur/o	pleura	pleurocentesis
9. epiglott/o	epiglottis	
10. alveol/o	alveolus, air sac	alveolitis
11. pulmon/o	lung	pulmonary
12. ox/o	oxygen	hypoxia

13. sinus/o _____sinus, cavity_____ _____sinusitis_____

14. lob/o _____lobe_____ _____lobectomy_____

15. nas/o _____nose_____ _____nasopharyngeal_____

D. Define each suffix and use it to form a term from the respiratory system.

	Meaning	Respiratory Term
1. -ectasis	dilated, expansion	bronchiectasis
2. -capnia	carbon dioxide	acapnia
3. -phonia	voice	dysphonia
4. -thorax	chest	hemothorax
5. -pnea	breathing	eupnea
6. -ptysis	spitting	hemoptysis
7. -osmia	smell	anosmia

E. The suffix -pnea means breathing. Use this suffix to write a medical term that means:

1. normal breathing _____eupnea_____

2. difficult or labored breathing _____dyspnea_____

3. rapid breathing _____tachypnea_____

4. can breathe only in an upright position _____orthopnea_____

5. lack of breathing _____apnea_____

F. Define the following terms.

1. total lung capacity _____The volume of air in the lungs after a maximal inhalation._____

2. tidal volume _____Amount of air that enters or leaves the lungs in a single inhalation or exhalation of quiet breathing._____

3. residual volume _____The air remaining in the lungs after a forced exhalation._____

G. Write the medical term for each definition.

1. the process of breathing in _____inhalation_____

2. spitting up of blood _____hemoptysis_____

3. blood clot in the pulmonary artery _____pulmonary embolism_____

4. inflammation of a sinus _____sinusitis_____

5. sore throat _____pharyngitis_____

6. air in the pleural cavity _____pneumothorax_____

Respiratory System

7. whooping cough ___pertussis___

8. incision into the pleura ___pleurotomy___

9. pain in the pleural region ___pleurodynia___

10. common cold ___nasopharyngitis___

H. Write the abbreviations for the following terms.

1. upper respiratory infection ___URI___

2. pulmonary function test ___PFT___

3. left lower lobe ___LLL___

4. oxygen ___O_2___

5. carbon dioxide ___CO_2___

6. intermittent positive pressure breathing ___IPPB___

7. chronic obstructive pulmonary disease ___COPD___

8. bronchoscopy ___Bronch___

9. total lung capacity ___TLC___

10. tuberculosis ___TB___

11. infant respiratory distress syndrome ___IRDS___

I. Identify the following abbreviations.

1. CXR ___chest x-ray___

2. TV ___tidal volume___

3. TPR ___temperature, pulse & respiration___

4. ABGs ___arterial blood gases___

5. DOE ___dyspnea on exertion___

6. RUL ___right upper lobe___

7. SIDS ___sudden infant death syndrome___

8. TLC ___total lung capacity___

9. ARDS ___adult (or acute) respiratory distress syndrome___

10. MDI ___metered dose inhaler___

11. CTA ___clear to auscultation___

12. SARS ___severe acute respiratory syndrome___

J. Match each term to its definition.

1. __e__ inhaling environmental particles
2. __k__ whooping cough
3. __h__ may result in collapsed lung
4. __a__ test to identify sleep apnea
5. __j__ respiratory tract mucus
6. __l__ sweat test
7. __c__ measures oxygen levels in blood
8. __g__ *Mycoplasma* pneumonia
9. __f__ disease with overexpanded air sacs
10. __b__ tuberculin test
11. __d__ nose bleed
12. __i__ pus in the pleural space

a. polysomnography
b. Tine test
c. oximetry
d. epistaxis
e. pneumoconiosis
f. emphysema
g. walking pneumonia
h. pneumothorax
i. empyema
j. phlegm
k. pertussis
l. test for cystic fibrosis

K. Use the following terms in the sentences below.

anthracosis   thoracentesis   supplemental oxygen   sputum cytology
respirator   hyperventilation   cardiopulmonary resuscitation   ventilation-perfusion scan
patent   rhonchi

1. When the patient's breathing and heart stopped, the paramedics began cardiopulmonary resuscitation

2. The physician performed a thoracentesis to remove fluid from the chest.

3. A respirator is also called a ventilator.

4. The patient received supplemental oxygen through a nasal cannula.

5. An endotracheal intubation was performed to establish a patent airway.

6. A ventilation - perfusion scan is a particularly useful test to identify a pulmonary embolism.

7. The result of the sputum cytology was negative for cancer.

8. Hyperventilation involves tachypnea and hyperpnea.

9. Rhonci are wheezing lung sounds.

10. Miners are at risk of developing anthracosis.

L. Fill in the classification for each drug description, then match the brand name.

	Drug Description	Classification	Brand Name
1.	_____ Reduces stuffiness and congestion	_____	a. Hycodan
2.	_____ Relieves the urge to cough	_____	b. Flonase
3.	_____ Kills bacteria	_____	c. Cipro
4.	_____ Improves ability to cough up mucus	_____	d. Ventolin
5.	_____ Liquefies mucus	_____	e. Allegra
6.	_____ Relaxes bronchial muscle spasms	_____	f. Afrin
7.	_____ Blocks allergy attack	_____	g. Robitussin
8.	_____ Reduces inflammation and swelling	_____	h. Mucomyst

Medical Record Analysis

Below is an item from a patient's medical record. Read it carefully, make sure you understand all the medical terms used, and then answer the questions that follow.

Pulmonology Consultation Report

Reason for Consultation:	Evaluation of increasingly severe asthma.
History of Present Illness:	Patient is a 10-year-old male who first presented to the Emergency Room with dyspnea, coughing, and wheezing at 7 years of age. Paroxysmal attacks are increasing in frequency, and there do not appear to be any precipitating factors such as exercise. No other family members are asthmatics.
Results of Physical Examination:	Patient is currently in the ER with a paroxysmal attack with marked dyspnea, cyanosis around the lips, prolonged expiration, and a hacking cough producing thick, nonpurulent phlegm. Thoracic auscultation with stethoscope revealed rhonchi throughout bilateral lung fields. Chest x-ray shows poor pulmonary expansion, with hypoxemia indicated by ABG. A STAT pulmonary function test reveals moderately severe airway obstruction during expiration. This patient responded to oxygen therapy and IV Alupent and steroids, and he is beginning to cough less and breathe with less effort.
Assessment:	Acute asthma attack with severe airway obstruction. There is no evidence of pulmonary infection. In view of increasing severity and frequency of attacks, all his medications should be reevaluated for effectiveness and all attempts to identify precipitating factors should be made.
Recommendations:	Patient is to continue to use Alupent for relief of bronchospasms and steroids to reduce general inflammation. Instructions for taking medications and controlling severity of asthma attacks were carefully reviewed with the patient and his family. A referral to an allergist was made to evaluate this young man for presence of environmental allergies.

Critical Thinking Questions

1. What does the medical term *paroxysmal* mean? _____
   _____

2. What do the following abbreviations stand for?
   a. IV _____intravenous_____
   b. STAT ____at once; immediately_____
   c. ABG _____arterial blood gas_____

3. The patient was discharged and sent home with two medications. Explain in your own words the purpose of each of these medications. Alupent - relaxes muscle spasms in bronchial tubes. Steroids - to reduce inflammation making breathing more difficult

4. What important information regarding this young man's asthma is unknown to the physician? What does this consulting physician recommend to address this problem? The cause. He refers the patient to an allergist to test for environmental allergies.

5. Describe the characteristics related to this patient's cough in your own words. hacking cough w/thick non-pus filled phlegm

6. Which of the following is not one of the symptoms seen in the emergency room?
   a. crackling lung sounds
   b. bluish skin
   c. difficulty breathing
   d. extended breathing out time

Chart Note Transcription

The chart note below contains eleven phrases that can be reworded with a medical term that you learned in this chapter. Each phrase is identified with an underline. Determine the medical term and write your answers in the space provided.

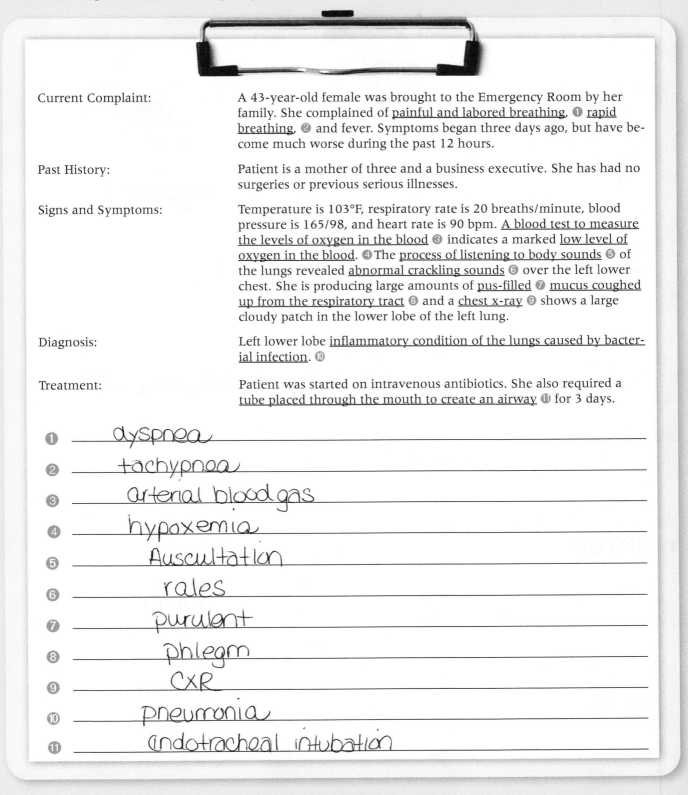

Current Complaint: A 43-year-old female was brought to the Emergency Room by her family. She complained of <u>painful and labored breathing</u>, ❶ <u>rapid breathing</u>, ❷ and fever. Symptoms began three days ago, but have become much worse during the past 12 hours.

Past History: Patient is a mother of three and a business executive. She has had no surgeries or previous serious illnesses.

Signs and Symptoms: Temperature is 103°F, respiratory rate is 20 breaths/minute, blood pressure is 165/98, and heart rate is 90 bpm. <u>A blood test to measure the levels of oxygen in the blood</u> ❸ indicates a marked <u>low level of oxygen in the blood</u>. ❹ The <u>process of listening to body sounds</u> ❺ of the lungs revealed <u>abnormal crackling sounds</u> ❻ over the left lower chest. She is producing large amounts of <u>pus-filled</u> ❼ <u>mucus coughed up from the respiratory tract</u> ❽ and a <u>chest x-ray</u> ❾ shows a large cloudy patch in the lower lobe of the left lung.

Diagnosis: Left lower lobe <u>inflammatory condition of the lungs caused by bacterial infection</u>. ❿

Treatment: Patient was started on intravenous antibiotics. She also required a <u>tube placed through the mouth to create an airway</u> ⓫ for 3 days.

❶ _dyspnea_
❷ _tachypnea_
❸ _arterial blood gas_
❹ _hypoxemia_
❺ _Auscultation_
❻ _rales_
❼ _purulent_
❽ _phlegm_
❾ _CXR_
❿ _pneumonia_
⓫ _endotracheal intubation_

Labeling Exercise

A. System Review

Write the labels for this figure on the numbered lines provided.

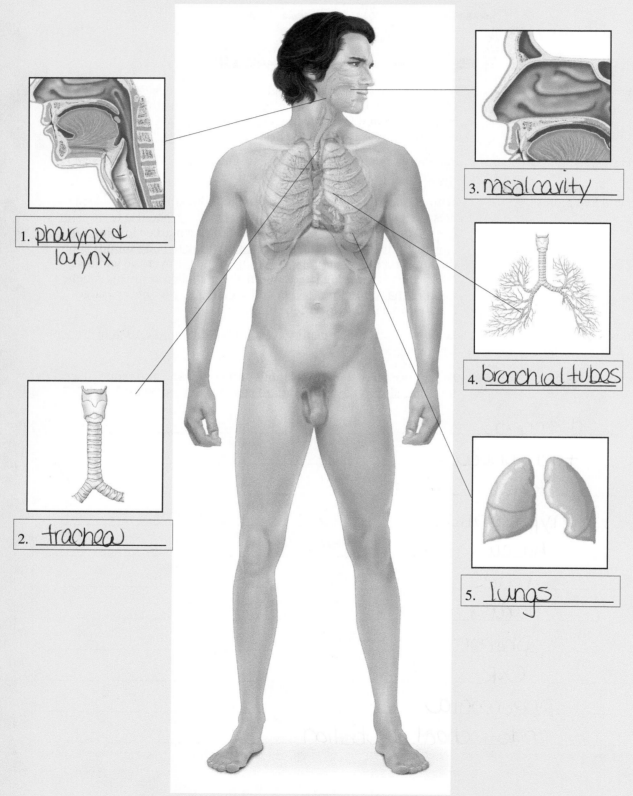

1. pharynx & larynx

2. trachea

3. nasal cavity

4. bronchial tubes

5. lungs

Respiratory System

B. Anatomy Challenge

1. Write the labels for this figure on the numbered lines provided.

2. paranasal sinuses

3. nasal cavity

4. pharyngeal tonsil

5. eustachian tube

6. hard palate

7. soft palate

8. palatine tonsil

9. epiglottis

10. vocal cords

1. nares

11. esophagus

12. trachea

2. Write the labels for this figure on the numbered lines provided.

1. trachea

5. apex of lung

2. right upper lobe

3. right middle lobe

4. right lower lobe

6. left upper lobe

7. left lower lobe

8. diaphragm

Respiratory System

Multimedia Preview

Additional interactive resources and activities for this chapter can be found on the Companion Website.

Website Highlights—www.prenhall.com/fremgen

CASE STUDY

Put your understanding of medical terms to the test within a real-world scenario. Here you'll be presented with a clinical case followed by a series of questions that quiz your grasp of the situation.

Digestive System

Learning Objectives

Upon completion of this chapter, you will be able to:

- Identify and define the combining forms and suffixes introduced in this chapter.
- Correctly spell and pronounce medical terms and major anatomical structures relating to the digestive system.
- Locate and describe the major organs of the digestive system and their functions.
- Describe the function of the accessory organs of the digestive system.
- Identify the shape and function of each type of tooth.
- Build and define digestive system medical terms from word parts.
- Identify and define digestive system vocabulary terms.
- Identify and define selected digestive system pathology terms.
- Identify and define selected digestive system diagnostic procedures.
- Identify and define selected digestive system therapeutic procedures.
- Identify and define selected medications relating to the digestive system.
- Define selected abbreviations associated with the digestive system.

From Chapter 8 of *Medical Terminology: A Living Language*, 4/e. Bonnie F. Fremgen. Suzanne S. Frucht.
Copyright © 2009 by Pearson Education. Published by Prentice Hall. All rights reserved.

Digestive System at a Glance

Function

The digestive system begins breaking down food through mechanical and chemical digestion. After being digested, nutrient molecules are absorbed into the body and enter the blood stream. Any food not digested or absorbed is eliminated as solid waste.

Organs

colon
esophagus
gallbladder (GB)
liver
oral cavity
pancreas
pharynx
salivary glands
small intestine
stomach

Combining Forms

an/o	anus	gloss/o	tongue
append/o	appendix	hepat/o	liver
appendic/o	appendix	ile/o	ileum
bar/o	weight	jejun/o	jejunum
bucc/o	cheek	labi/o	lip
cec/o	cecum	lapar/o	abdomen
chol/e	bile, gall	lingu/o	tongue
cholangi/o	bile duct	lith/o	stone
cholecyst/o	gallbladder	odont/o	tooth
choledoch/o	common bile duct	or/o	mouth
col/o	colon	palat/o	palate
colon/o	colon	pancreat/o	pancreas
dent/o	tooth	pharyng/o	throat, pharynx
duoden/o	duodenum	proct/o	anus and rectum
enter/o	small intestine	pylor/o	pylorus
esophag/o	esophagus	rect/o	rectum
gastr/o	stomach	sialaden/o	salivary gland
gingiv/o	gums	sigmoid/o	sigmoid colon

Suffixes

-emesis	vomit	-phagia	eat, swallow
-lithiasis	condition of stones	-prandial	pertaining to a meal
-orexia	appetite	-tripsy	surgical crushing
-pepsia	digestion		

Digestive System Illustrated

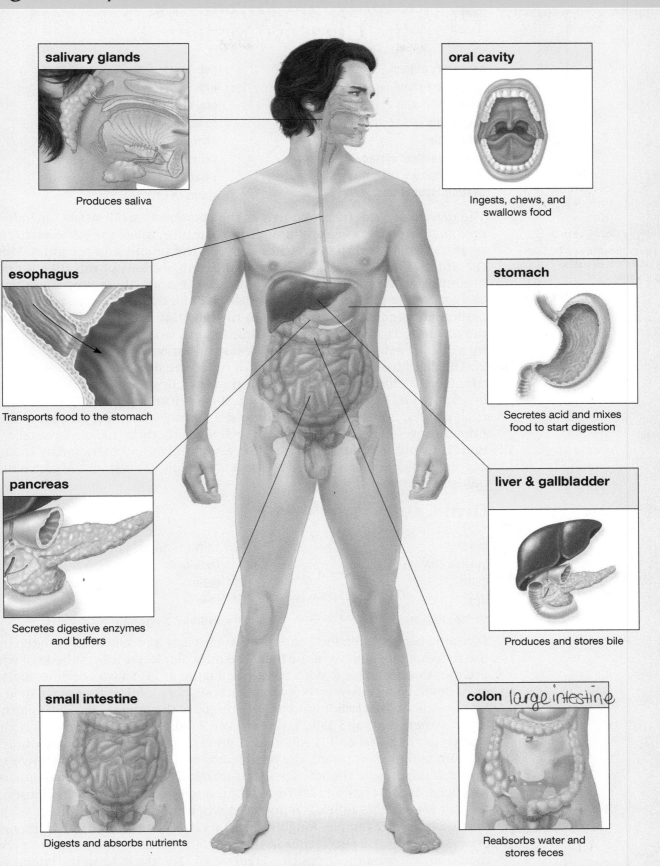

salivary glands

Produces saliva

oral cavity

Ingests, chews, and swallows food

esophagus

Transports food to the stomach

stomach

Secretes acid and mixes food to start digestion

pancreas

Secretes digestive enzymes and buffers

liver & gallbladder

Produces and stores bile

small intestine

Digests and absorbs nutrients

colon large intestine

Reabsorbs water and stores feces

Anatomy and Physiology of the Digestive System

accessory organs	**gut**
alimentary canal (al-ih-MEN-tar-ree)	**liver**
colon (COH-lon)	**oral cavity**
esophagus (eh-SOFF-ah-gus)	**pancreas** (PAN-kree-ass)
gallbladder	**pharynx** (FAIR-inks)
gastrointestinal system	**salivary glands** (SAL-ih-vair-ee)
(gas-troh-in-TESS-tih-nal)	**small intestine**
gastrointestinal tract	**stomach** (STUM-ak)

<table>
<tr><td>

Med Term Tip

The term *alimentary* comes from the Latin term *alimentum* meaning "nourishment."

</td></tr>
</table>

The digestive system, also known as the **gastrointestinal (GI) system,** includes approximately 30 feet of a continuous muscular tube, called the **gut, alimentary canal,** or **gastrointestinal tract** that stretches between the mouth and the anus. Most of the organs in this system are actually different sections of this tube. In order, beginning at the mouth and continuing to the anus, these organs are the **oral cavity, pharynx, esophagus, stomach, small intestine,** and **colon.** The **accessory organs** of digestion are organs that participate in the digestion process, but are not part of the continuous alimentary canal. These organs, which are connected to the gut by a duct, are the **liver, pancreas, gallbladder,** and **salivary glands.**

The digestive system has three main functions: digesting food, absorbing nutrients, and eliminating waste. Digestion includes the physical and chemical breakdown of large food particles into simple nutrient molecules like glucose, triglycerides, and amino acids. These simple nutrient molecules are absorbed from the intestines and circulated throughout the body by the cardiovascular system. They are used for growth and repair of organs and tissues. Any food that cannot be digested or absorbed by the body is eliminated from the gastrointestinal system as a solid waste.

Oral Cavity

cheeks	**saliva** (suh-LYE-vah)
gingiva (JIN-jih-veh)	**taste buds**
gums	**teeth**
lips	**tongue**
palate (PAL-at)	**uvula** (YU-vyu-lah)

Digestion begins when food enters the mouth and is mechanically broken up by the chewing movements of the **teeth**. The muscular **tongue** moves the food within the mouth and mixes it with **saliva** (see Figure 1 ■). Saliva contains digestive enzymes to break down carbohydrates and slippery lubricants to make food easier to swallow. **Taste buds**, found on the surface of the tongue, can distinguish the bitter, sweet, sour, and salty flavors in our food. The roof of the oral cavity is known as the **palate** and is subdivided into the hard palate, the bony anterior portion, and the soft palate, the flexible posterior portion. Hanging down from the posterior edge of the soft palate is the **uvula**. The uvula serves two important functions. First, it has a role in speech production. Second, it is the location of the gag reflex. This reflex is stimulated when food enters the throat without swallowing (for example, laughing with food in your mouth). It is important because swallowing also results in the epiglottis covering the larynx to prevent food from entering the lungs (see Figure 2 ■). The **cheeks** form the lateral walls of this cavity and the **lips** are the anterior opening. The entire oral cavity is lined

Digestive System

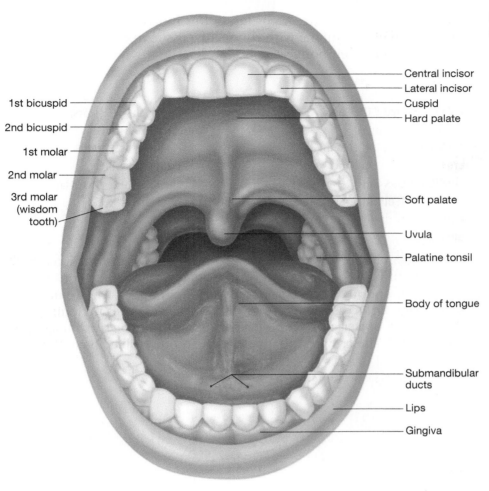

Central incisor
Lateral incisor
Cuspid
Hard palate

1st bicuspid
2nd bicuspid
1st molar
2nd molar
3rd molar (wisdom tooth)

Soft palate

Uvula

Palatine tonsil

Body of tongue

Submandibular ducts

Lips

Gingiva

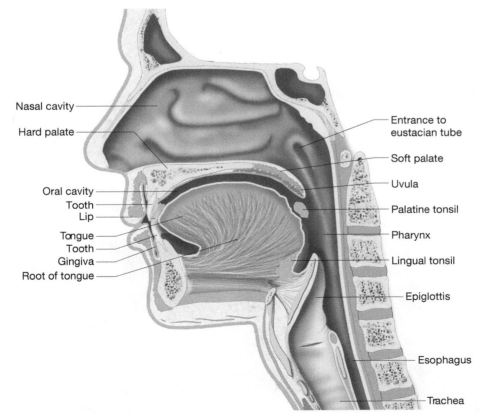

■ **Figure 2** Sagittal view of the head and neck, illustrating structures of the oral cavity, and pharynx, and esophagus.

Nasal cavity

Hard palate

Oral cavity
Tooth
Lip
Tongue
Tooth
Gingiva
Root of tongue

Entrance to eustacian tube

Soft palate

Uvula

Palatine tonsil

Pharynx

Lingual tonsil

Epiglottis

Esophagus

Trachea

with mucous membrane. A portion of this mucous membrane forms the **gums**, or **gingiva**, which combine with connective tissue to cover the jaw bone and seal off the teeth in their bony sockets.

Teeth

bicuspids (bye-CUSS-pids)	**incisors** (in-SIGH-zors)
canines (KAY-nines)	**molars** (MOH-lars)
cementum (see-MEN-tum)	**periodontal ligaments** (pair-ee-on-DON-tal)
crown	**permanent teeth**
cuspids (CUSS-pids)	**premolars** (pree-MOH-lars)
deciduous teeth (dee-SID-yoo-us)	**pulp cavity**
dentin (DEN-tin)	**root**
enamel	**root canal**

Med Term Tip

There are three different molars, simply referred to as the first, second, or third molars. However, the third molar has a more common name, the wisdom tooth. Not every person ever forms all four wisdom teeth. Unfortunately, most people do not have enough room in their jaws for the third molars to properly erupt through the gum, a condition requiring surgical removal of the third molar referred to as an *impacted wisdom tooth*.

Teeth are an important part of the first stage of digestion. The teeth in the front of the mouth bite, tear, or cut food into small pieces. These cutting teeth include the **incisors** and the **cuspids** or **canines** (see Figure 3 ■). The remaining posterior teeth grind and crush food into even finer pieces. These grinding teeth include the **bicuspids**, or **premolars**, and the **molars**. A tooth can be subdivided into the **crown** and the **root**. The crown is that part of the tooth visible above the gum line; the

■ Figure 3 A) The name and shape of the adult teeth. These teeth represent those found in the right side of the mouth. Those of the left side would be a mirror image. The incisors and cuspids are cutting teeth. The bicuspids and molars are grinding teeth. B) Color enhanced x-ray of all teeth. Note the four wisdom teeth (3rd molars) that have not erupted. *(Science Photo Library/Photo Researchers, Inc.)*

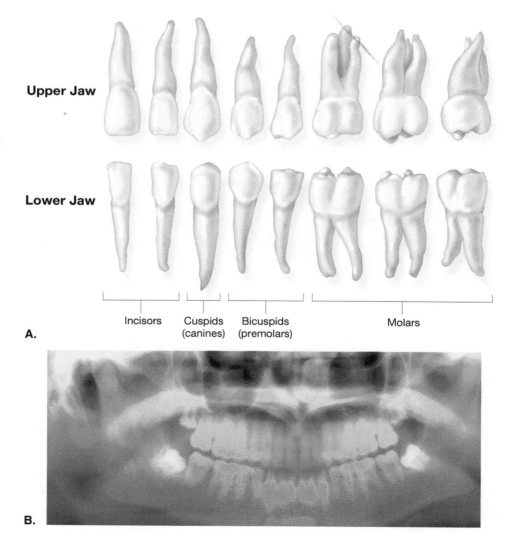

Upper Jaw

Lower Jaw

Incisors Cuspids (canines) Bicuspids (premolars) Molars

A.

B.

root is below the gum line. The root is anchored in the bony socket of the jaw by **cementum** and tiny **periodontal ligaments**. The crown of the tooth is covered by a layer of **enamel**, the hardest substance in the body. Under the enamel layer is **dentin**, the substance that makes up the main bulk of the tooth. The hollow interior of a tooth is called the **pulp cavity** in the crown and the **root canal** in the root. These cavities contain soft tissue made up of blood vessels, nerves, and lymph vessels (see Figure 4 ■).

Humans have two sets of teeth. The first set, often referred to as baby teeth, are **deciduous teeth.** There are 20 teeth in this set that erupt through the gums between the ages of 6 and 28 months. At approximately 6 years of age, these teeth begin to fall out and are replaced by the 32 **permanent teeth**. This replacement process continues until about 18 to 20 years of age.

Med Term Tip

The combining form *dent/o* means teeth. Hence we have terms such as dentist and dentistry. The combining form *odont/o* also means teeth and when combined with *orth/o*, which means straight, we have the speciality of *orthodontics*, or straightening teeth.

Pharynx

epiglottis (ep-ih-GLOT-iss)   **oropharynx**
laryngopharynx

When food is swallowed, it enters the **oropharynx** and then the **laryngopharynx** (see Figure 2). Remember from your study of the respiratory system that air is also traveling through these portions of the pharynx. The **epiglottis** is a cartilaginous flap that folds down to cover the larynx and trachea so that food is prevented from entering the respiratory tract and instead continues into the esophagus.

Esophagus

peristalsis (pair-ih-STALL-sis)

The esophagus is a muscular tube of about 10 inches long in adults. Food entering the esophagus is carried through the thoracic cavity and diaphragm and into the abdominal cavity where it enters the stomach (see Figure 5 ■). Food is

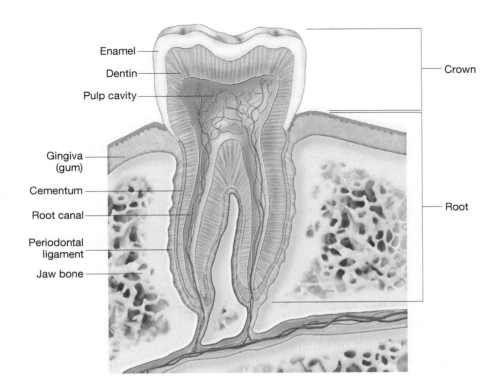

Enamel
Dentin
Pulp cavity
Gingiva (gum)
Cementum
Root canal
Periodontal ligament
Jaw bone
Crown
Root

■ **Figure 4** An adult tooth, longitudinal view showing internal structures of the crown and root.

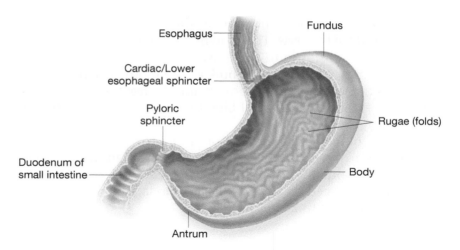

Esophagus

Fundus

Cardiac/Lower esophageal sphincter

Pyloric sphincter

Duodenum of small intestine

Rugae (folds)

Body

Antrum

Med Term Tip

It takes about 10 seconds for swallowed food to reach the stomach.

propelled along the esophagus by wavelike muscular contractions called **peristalsis**. In fact, peristalsis works to push food through the entire gastrointestinal tract.

Stomach

antrum (AN-trum)
body
cardiac sphincter
chyme (KIGHM)
fundus (FUN-dus)
hydrochloric acid

lower esophageal sphincter
(eh-soff-ah-JEE-al SFINGK-ter)
pyloric sphincter (pigh-LOR-ik SFINGK-ter)
rugae (ROO-gay)
sphincters (SFINGK-ters)

The stomach, a J-shaped muscular organ that acts as a bag or sac to collect and churn food with digestive juices, is composed of three parts: the **fundus** or upper region, the **body** or main portion, and the **antrum** or lower region (see Figure 5). The folds in the lining of the stomach are called **rugae**. When the stomach fills with food, the rugae stretch out and disappear. **Hydrochloric acid** (HCl) is secreted by glands in the mucous membrane lining of the stomach. Food mixes with hydrochloric acid and other gastric juices to form a liquid mixture called **chyme**, which then passes through the remaining portion of the digestive system.

Entry into and exit from the stomach is controlled by muscular valves called **sphincters**. These valves open and close to ensure that food can only move forward down the gut tube. The **cardiac sphincter**, named for its proximity to the heart, is located between the esophagus and the fundus. Also called the **lower esophageal sphincter** (LES), it keeps food from flowing backward into the esophagus.

The antrum tapers off into the **pyloric sphincter**, which regulates the passage of food into the small intestine. Only a small amount of the chyme is allowed to enter the small intestine with each opening of the sphincter for two important reasons. First, the small intestine is much narrower than the stomach and cannot hold as much as the stomach can. Second, the chyme is highly acidic and must be thoroughly neutralized as it leaves the stomach.

Med Term Tip

It is easier to remember the function of the pyloric sphincter when you note that *pylor/o* means "gatekeeper." This gatekeeper controls the forward movement of food. Sphincters are rings of muscle that can be opened and closed to control entry and exit from hollow organs like the stomach, colon, and bladder.

Small Intestine

duodenum
(doo-oh-DEE-num / doo-OD-eh-num)
ileocecal valve (ill-ee-oh-SEE-kal)

ileum (ILL-ee-um)
jejunum (jee-JOO-num)

The small intestine, or small bowel, is the major site of digestion and absorption of nutrients from food. It is located between the pyloric sphincter and the colon (see Figure 6 ▪). Because the small intestine is concerned with absorption of food products, an abnormality in this organ can cause malnutrition. The small intestine, with an average length of 20 feet, is the longest portion of the alimentary canal and has three sections: the **duodenum**, the **jejunum**, and the **ileum**.

- The duodenum, which extends from the pyloric sphincter to the jejunum, is about 10 to 12 inches long. Digestion is completed in the duodenum after the liquid chyme from the stomach is mixed with digestive juices from the pancreas and gallbladder.
- The jejunum, or middle portion, extends from the duodenum to the ileum and is about 8 feet long.
- The ileum is the last portion of the small intestine and extends from the jejunum to the colon. At 12 feet in length, it is the longest portion of the small intestine. The ileum connects to the colon with a sphincter called the **ileocecal valve**.

Colon

anal sphincter (AY-nal SFINGK-ter)
anus (AY-nus)
ascending colon
cecum (SEE-kum)
defecation
descending colon

feces (FEE-seez)
rectum (REK-tum)
sigmoid colon (SIG-moyd)
transverse colon
vermiform appendix
(VER-mih-form ah-PEN-diks)

Fluid that remains after the complete digestion and absorption of nutrients in the small intestine enters the colon or large intestine (see Figure 7 ▪). Most of this fluid is water that is reabsorbed into the body. The material that remains after absorption is solid waste called **feces** (or stool). This is the product evacuated in bowel movements (BM).

The colon is approximately 5 feet long and extends from the ileocecal valve of the small intestine to the **anus**. The **cecum** is a pouch or saclike area in the first two to three inches at the beginning of the colon. The **vermiform appendix** is a small worm-shaped outgrowth at the end of the cecum. The remaining colon consists of the **ascending colon**, **transverse colon**, **descending colon**, and **sigmoid colon**. The ascend-

Med Term Tip

Word watch—Be careful not to confuse the word root *ile/o* meaning "ileum," a portion of the small intestines, and *ili/o* meaning "ilium," a pelvic bone.

Med Term Tip

We can survive without a portion of the small intestine. For example, in cases of cancer, much of the small intestine and/or colon may have to be removed. The surgeon then creates an opening between the remaining intestine and the abdominal wall. The combining form for the section of intestine connected to the abdominal wall and the suffix *-ostomy* are used to describe this procedure. For example, if a person has a *jejunostomy*, the jejunum is connected to the abdominal wall and the ileum (and remainder of the gut tube) has been removed.

Med Term Tip

The term *colon* refers to the large intestine. However, you should be aware that many people use it incorrectly as a general term referring to the entire intestinal system, both small and large intestines.

■ **Figure 6** The small intestine. Anterior view of the abdominopelvic cavity illustrating how the three sections of small intestine—duodenum, jejunum, ileum—begin at the pyloric sphincter and end at the colon, but are not arranged in a orderly fashion.

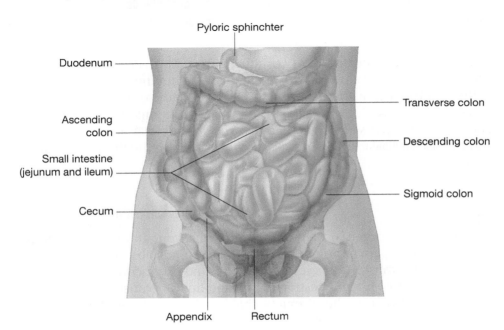

Pyloric sphinchter
Duodenum
Ascending colon
Small intestine (jejunum and ileum)
Cecum
Transverse colon
Descending colon
Sigmoid colon
Appendix
Rectum

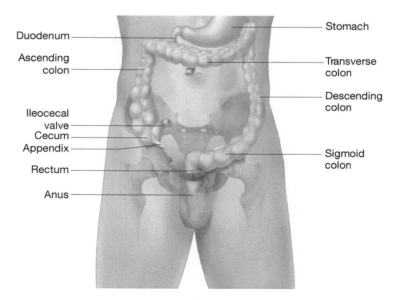

■ **Figure 7** The regions of the colon beginning with the cecum and ending at the anus.

Labels: Duodenum, Ascending colon, Ileocecal valve, Cecum, Appendix, Rectum, Anus, Stomach, Transverse colon, Descending colon, Sigmoid colon

ing colon on the right side extends from the cecum to the lower border of the liver. The transverse colon begins where the ascending colon leaves off and moves horizontally across the upper abdomen toward the spleen. The descending colon then travels down the left side of the body to where the sigmoid colon begins. The sigmoid colon curves in an S-shape back to the midline of the body and ends at the **rectum**. The rectum, where feces is stored, leads into the anus, which contains the **anal sphincter**. This sphincter consists of rings of voluntary and involuntary muscles to control the evacuation of feces or **defecation**.

Accessory Organs of the Digestive System

As described earlier, the accessory organs of the digestive system are the salivary glands, the liver, the pancreas, and the gallbladder. In general, these organs function by producing much of the digestive fluids and enzymes necessary for the chemical breakdown of food. Each is attached to the gut tube by a duct.

Salivary Glands

amylase (AM-ill-ace)
bolus
parotid glands (pah-ROT-id)
sublingual glands (sub-LING-gwal)
submandibular glands (sub-man-DIB-yoo-lar)

Salivary glands in the oral cavity produce saliva. This very watery and slick fluid allows food to be swallowed with less danger of choking. Saliva mixed with food in the mouth forms a **bolus**, chewed food that is ready to swallow. Saliva also contains the digestive enzyme **amylase** that begins the digestion of carbohydrates. There are three pairs of salivary glands. The **parotid glands** are in front of the ears, and the **submandibular glands** and **sublingual glands** are in the floor of the mouth (see Figure 8 ■).

Liver

bile (BYE-al)
emulsification (ee-mull-sih-fih-KAY-shun)

The liver, a large organ located in the right upper quadrant of the abdomen, has several functions, including processing the nutrients absorbed by the intestines, detoxifying harmful substances in the body, and producing **bile** (see Figure 9 ■). Bile is important for the digestion of fats and lipids because it breaks up large fat globules into much smaller droplets, making them easier to digest in the watery environment inside the intestines. The process is called **emulsification**.

Med Term Tip

In anatomy the term *accessory* generally means that the structure is auxiliary to a more important structure. This is not true for these organs. Digestion would not be possible without the digestive juices produced by these organs.

Med Term Tip

The liver weighs about 4 pounds and has so many important functions that people cannot live without it. It has become a major transplant organ. The liver is also able to regenerate itself. You can lose more than half of your liver, and it will regrow.

Digestive System

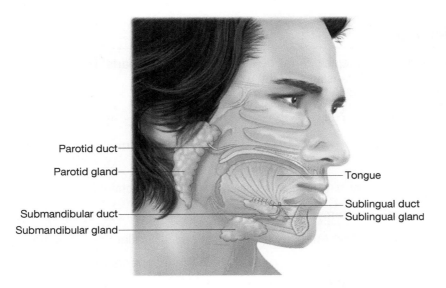

■ **Figure 8** The salivary glands, parotid, sublingual, and submandibular. This images shows the position of each gland and its duct emptying into the oral cavity.

Parotid duct
Parotid gland
Submandibular duct
Submandibular gland
Tongue
Sublingual duct
Sublingual gland

Gallbladder

common bile duct

cystic duct (SIS-tik)

hepatic duct (hep-PAT-tik)

Bile produced by the liver is stored in the gallbladder (GB). As the liver produces bile, it travels down the **hepatic duct** and up the **cystic duct** into the gallbladder (see Figure 9). In response to the presence of fat in the chyme, the muscular wall of the gallbladder contracts and sends bile back down the cystic duct and into the **common bile duct** (CBD), which carries bile to the duodenum where it is able to emulsify the fat in chyme.

Pancreas

buffers

pancreatic duct (pan-kree-AT-ik)

pancreatic enzymes
(pan-kree-AT-ik EN-zimes)

The pancreas, connected to the duodenum by the **pancreatic duct,** produces two important secretions for digestion—**buffers** and **pancreatic enzymes** (see Figure 9). Buffers neutralize acidic chyme that has just left the stomach, and pancreatic enzymes chemically digest carbohydrates, fats, and proteins. The pancreas is also an endocrine gland that produces the hormones insulin and glucagon, which play a role in regulating the level of glucose in the blood.

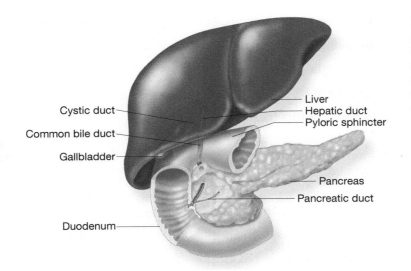

■ **Figure 9** The accessory organs of the digestive system: the liver, gallbladder, and pancreas. Image shows the relationship of these three organs and their ducts to the duodenum.

Cystic duct
Common bile duct
Gallbladder
Duodenum
Liver
Hepatic duct
Pyloric sphincter
Pancreas
Pancreatic duct

Word Building

The following list contains examples of medical terms built directly from word parts. The definitions for these terms can be determined by a straightforward translation of the word parts.

COMBINING FORM	COMBINED WITH	MEDICAL TERM	DEFINITION
an/o	-al	**anal**	pertaining to the anus

Med Term Tip

Word watch—Be careful when using the combining form *an/o* meaning "anus" and the prefix *an* meaning "none."

COMBINING FORM	COMBINED WITH	MEDICAL TERM	DEFINITION
append/o	-ectomy	**appendectomy** (ap-en-DEK-toh-mee)	removal of the appendix
appendic/o	-itis	**appendicitis** (ah-pen-dih-SIGH-tis)	inflammation of the appendix
bucc/o	-al	**buccal** (BYOO-kal)	pertaining to cheeks
	labi/o -al	**buccolabial** (BYOO-koh-labe-ee-all)	pertaining to cheeks and lips
cholecyst/o	-ectomy	**cholecystectomy** (koh-lee-sis-TEK-toh-mee)	removal of the gallbladder
	-gram	**cholecystogram** (koh-lee-SIS-toh-gram)	record of the gallbladder
	-ic	**cholecystic** (koh-lee-SIS-tik)	pertaining to the gallbladder
	-algia	**cholecystalgia** (koh-lee-sis-TAL-jee-ah)	gallbladder pain
col/o	-ectomy	**colectomy** (koh-LEK-toh-mee)	removal of the colon
	-ostomy	**colostomy** (koh-LOSS-toh-mee)	create an opening in the colon
	rect/o -al	**colorectal** (kohl-oh-REK-tall)	pertaining to the colon and rectum
colon/o	-scope	**colonoscope** (koh-LON-oh-scope)	instrument to view colon
	-ic	**colonic** (koh-LON-ik)	pertaining to the colon
dent/o	-al	**dental** (DENT-al)	pertaining to teeth
	-algia	**dentalgia** (dent-AL-gee-ah)	tooth pain
duoden/o	-al	**duodenal** (duo-DEN-all / do-ODD-in-all)	pertaining to the duodenum
enter/o	-ic	**enteric** (en-TARE-ik)	pertaining to the small intestine
	-itis	**enteritis** (en-ter-EYE-tis)	small intestine inflammation
esophag/o	-eal	**esophageal** (eh-soff-ah-JEE-al)	pertaining to the esophagus
	-ectasis	**esophagectasis** (eh-soff-ah-JEK-tah-sis)	dilated esophagus
gastr/o	-algia	**gastralgia** (gas-TRAL-jee-ah)	stomach pain
	-ic	**gastric** (GAS-trik)	pertaining to the stomach
	enter/o -itis	**gastroenteritis** (gas-troh-en-ter-EYE-tis)	inflammation of stomach and small intestine
	enter/o -ologist	**gastroenterologist** (gas-troh-en-ter-ALL-oh-jist)	specialist in the stomach and small intestine
	-malacia	**gastromalacia** (gas-troh-mah-LAY-she-ah)	softening of the stomach
	nas/o -ic	**nasogastric** (nay-zoh-GAS-trik)	pertaining to the nose and stomach
	-ostomy	**gastrostomy** (gas-TROSS-toh-mee)	create an opening in the stomach

Word Building *(continued)*

COMBINING FORM	COMBINED WITH	MEDICAL TERM	DEFINITION
	-scope	**gastroscope** (GAS-troh-scope)	instrument to view inside the stomach
	-itis	**gastritis** (gas-TRY-tis)	stomach inflammation
	-ectomy	**gastrectomy** (gas-TREK-toh-mee)	removal of the stomach
gingiv/o	-al	**gingival** (JIN-jih-vul)	pertaining to the gums
	-itis	**gingivitis** (jin-jih-VIGH-tis)	inflammation of the gums
gloss/o	-al	**glossal** (GLOSS-all)	pertaining to the tongue
	hypo- -al	**hypoglossal** (high-poe-GLOSS-all)	pertaining to under the tongue
hepat/o	-itis	**hepatitis** (hep-ah-TYE-tis)	inflammation of the liver
	-oma	**hepatoma** (hep-ah-TOH-mah)	liver tumor
	-ic	**hepatic** (hep-AT-ik)	pertaining to the liver
ile/o	-al	**ileal** (ILL-ee-all)	pertaining to the ileum
	-ostomy	**ileostomy** (ill-ee-OSS-toh-mee)	create an opening in the ileum
jejun/o	-al	**jejunal** (jih-JUNE-all)	pertaining to the jejunum
lapar/o	-otomy	**laparotomy** (lap-ah-ROT-oh-mee)	incision into the abdomen
	-scope	**laparoscope** (LAP-ah-roh-scope)	instrument to view inside the abdomen
lingu/o	sub- -al	**sublingual** (sub-LING-gwal)	pertaining to under the tongue
odont/o	orth/o -ic	**orthodontic** (or-thoh-DON-tik)	pertaining to straight teeth
	peri- -ic	**periodontic** (pair-ee-oh-DON-tik)	pertaining to around the teeth
or/o	-al	**oral** (OR-ral)	pertaining to the mouth
palat/o	-plasty	**palatoplasty** (pa-LOT-toh-plas-tee)	surgical repair of the palate
pancreat/o	-itis	**pancreatitis** (pan-kree-ah-TYE-tis)	inflammation of the pancreas
	-ic	**pancreatic** (pan-kree-AT-ik)	pertaining to the pancreas
pharyng/o	-eal	**pharyngeal** (fair-in-JEE-all)	pertaining to the throat
	-plegia	**pharyngoplegia** (fair-in-goh-PLEE-jee-ah)	paralysis of the throat
	-plasty	**pharyngoplasty** (fair-ING-oh-plas-tee)	surgical repair of the throat
proct/o	-ptosis	**proctoptosis** (prok-top-TOH-sis)	drooping rectum and anus
	-logist	**proctologist** (prok-TOL-oh-jist)	specialist in the rectum and anus
	-pexy	**proctopexy** (PROK-toh-pek-see)	surgical fixation of the rectum and anus
pylor/o	-ic	**pyloric** (pie-LORE-ik)	pertaining to the pylorus
rect/o	-al	**rectal** (RECK-tall)	pertaining to the rectum
sialaden/o	-itis	**sialadenitis** (sigh-al-add-eh-NIGH-tis)	inflammation of a salivary gland
sigmoid/o	-scope	**sigmoidoscope** (sig-MOYD-oh-scope)	instrument to view inside the sigmoid colon
	-al	**sigmoidal** (sig-MOYD-all)	pertaining to the sigmoid colon

Word Building (continued)

SUFFIX	COMBINED WITH	MEDICAL TERM	DEFINITION
-emesis	hemat/o	**hematemesis** (hee-mah-TEM-eh-sis)	vomiting blood
	hyper-	**hyperemesis** (high-per-EM-eh-sis)	excessive vomiting
-orexia	an-	**anorexia** (an-oh-REK-see-ah)	absence of an appetite
	dys-	**dysorexia** (dis-oh-REKS-ee-ah)	abnormal appetite
-pepsia	brady-	**bradypepsia** (brad-ee-PEP-see-ah)	slow digestion
	dys-	**dyspepsia** (dis-PEP-see-ah)	difficult digestion
-phagia	a-	**aphagia** (ah-FAY-jee-ah)	unable to swallow/eat
	dys-	**dysphagia** (dis-FAY-jee-ah)	difficulty swallowing/eating
	poly-	**polyphagia** (pall-ee-FAY-jee-ah)	many (excessive) eating
-prandial	post-	**postprandial** (post-PRAN-dee-all)	after a meal

Vocabulary

TERM	DEFINITION
anorexia (an-oh-REK-see-ah)	A general term meaning loss of appetite that may accompany other conditions. Also used to refer to *anorexia nervosa*, which is a personality disorder involving refusal to eat.
ascites (ah-SIGH-teez)	Collection or accumulation of fluid in the peritoneal cavity.
bowel incontinence (in-CON-tih-nence)	Inability to control defecation.
bridge	Dental appliance that is attached to adjacent teeth for support to replace missing teeth.
cachexia (ka-KEK-see-ah)	Loss of weight and generalized wasting that occurs during a chronic disease.
constipation (kon-stih-PAY-shun)	Experiencing difficulty in defecation or infrequent defecation.
crown	Artificial covering for the tooth created to replace the original crown.
dental caries (KAIR-eez)	Gradual decay and disintegration of teeth caused by bacteria; may lead to abscessed teeth. Commonly called a *tooth cavity*.
dentistry	Branch of healthcare involved with the prevention, diagnosis, and treatment of conditions involving the teeth, jaw, and mouth. Dentistry is practiced by a *dentist* or *oral surgeon*.
denture (DEN-chur)	Partial or complete set of artificial teeth that are set in plastic materials. Acts as a substitute for the natural teeth and related structures.
diarrhea (dye-ah-REE-ah)	Passing of frequent, watery bowel movements. Usually accompanies gastrointestinal (GI) disorders.

Vocabulary *(continued)*

TERM	DEFINITION
emesis (EM-eh-sis)	Vomiting.
gastroenterology (gas-troh-en-ter-ALL-oh-jee)	Branch of medicine involved in diagnosis and treatment of diseases and disorders of the digestive system. Physician is a *gastroenterologist*.
hematochezia (he-mat-oh-KEY-zee-ah)	Passing bright red blood in the stools.
implant (IM-plant)	Prosthetic device placed in the jaw to which a tooth or denture may be anchored.
internal medicine	Branch of medicine involving the diagnosis and treatment of diseases and conditions of internal organs such as the digestive system. The physician is an *internist*.
jaundice (JAWN-diss)	Yellow cast to the skin, mucous membranes, and the whites of the eyes caused by the deposit of bile pigment from too much bilirubin in the blood. Bilirubin is a waste product produced when worn-out red blood cells are broken down. May be a symptom of a disorder such as gallstones blocking the common bile duct or carcinoma of the liver.
melena (me-LEE-nah)	Passage of dark tarry stools. Color is the result of digestive enzymes working on blood in the gastrointestinal tract.
nausea (NAW-see-ah)	The urge to vomit. **Med Term Tip** The term *nausea* comes from the Greek word for "seasickness."
obesity	Body weight that is above a healthy level. A person whose overweight interferes with normal activity and body function has *morbid obesity*.
orthodontics (or-thoh-DON-tiks)	Branch of dentistry concerned with correction of problems with tooth alignment. A specialist is an *orthodontist*.
periodontics (pair-ee-oh-DON-tiks)	Branch of dentistry concerned with treating conditions involving the gums and tissues surrounding the teeth. A specialist is a *periodontist*.
polyp (POLL-ip)	Small tumor with a pedicle or stem attachment. Commonly found on mucous membranes such as those lining the colon or nasal cavity. Colon polyps may be precancerous.
proctology (prok-TOL-oh-jee)	Branch of medicine involved in diagnosis and treatment of diseases and disorders of the anus and rectum. Physician is a *proctologist*.
pyrosis (pie-ROW-sis)	Pain and burning sensation usually caused by stomach acid splashing up into the esophagus. Commonly called *heartburn*.
regurgitation (ree-gur-jih-TAY-shun)	Return of fluids and solids from the stomach into the mouth.

Pathology

TERM	DEFINITION
■ Oral Cavity	
aphthous ulcers (AF-thus)	Painful ulcers in the mouth of unknown cause. Commonly called *canker sores*.
cleft lip (CLEFT)	Congenital anomaly in which the upper lip and jaw bone fail to fuse in the midline leaving an open gap. Often seen along with a cleft palate. Corrected with surgery.
cleft palate (CLEFT-PAL-at)	Congenital anomaly in which the roof of the mouth has a split or fissure. Corrected with surgery.
herpes labialis (HER-peez lay-bee-AL-iz)	Infection of the lip by the herpes simplex virus type 1 (HSV-1). Also called *fever blisters* or *cold sores*.
periodontal disease (pair-ee-oh-DON-tal dih-ZEEZ)	Disease of the supporting structures of the teeth, including the gums and bones; the most common cause of tooth loss.
■ Esophagus	
esophageal varices (eh-soff-ah-JEE-al VAIR-ih-seez)	Enlarged and swollen varicose veins in the lower end of the esophagus. If these rupture, serious hemorrhage results; often related to liver disease.
gastroesophageal reflux disease (GERD) (gas-troh-ee-sof-ah-GEE-all REE-fluks)	Acid from the stomach flows backward up into the esophagus causing inflammation and pain.
■ Stomach	
gastric carcinoma (GAS-trik car-si-NOH-mah)	Cancerous tumor in the stomach.
hiatal hernia (high-AY-tal HER-nee-ah)	Protrusion of the stomach through the diaphragm (also called a *diaphragmatocele*) and extending into the thoracic cavity; gastroesophageal reflux disease is a common symptom.

■ Figure 10 A hiatal hernia or diaphragmatocele. A portion of the stomach protrudes through the diaphragm into the thoracic cavity.

Esophagus

Herniation of the stomach through the hiatal opening

Diaphragm

Stomach

Pathology *(continued)*

TERM	DEFINITION
peptic ulcer disease (PUD) (PEP-tik ULL-sir)	Ulcer occurring in the lower portion of the esophagus, stomach, and/or duodenum; thought to be caused by the acid of gastric juices. Initial damage to the protective lining of the stomach may be caused by a *Helicobacter pylori* (*H. pylori*) bacterial infection. If the ulcer extends all the way through the wall of the stomach, it is called a *perforated ulcer* which requires immediate surgery to repair.

Gastric juices are released into the stomach

Gastric juices (acidic)

Duodenal ulcer

Acid secretions further break down the lining of the stomach, forming an ulcer

Gastric ulcer

A.

B.

■ **Figure 11** A) Figure illustrating the location and appearance of a peptic ulcer in both the stomach and the duodenum. B) Photomicrograph illustrating a gastric ulcer. *(Dr. E. Walker/Science Photo Library/Photo Researchers, Inc.)*

■ *Small Intestine and Colon*

anal fistula (FIH-styoo-lah)	Abnormal tubelike passage from the surface around the anal opening directly into the rectum.
colorectal carcinoma (kohl-oh-REK-tall car-ci-NOH-mah)	Cancerous tumor along the length of the colon and rectum.
Crohn's disease (KROHNZ dih-ZEEZ)	Form of chronic inflammatory bowel disease affecting primarily the ileum and/or colon. Also called *regional ileitis.* This autoimmune condition affects all the layers of the bowel wall and results in scarring and thickening of the gut wall.
diverticulitis (dye-ver-tik-yoo-LYE-tis)	Inflammation of a *diverticulum* (an outpouching off the gut), especially in the colon. Inflammation often results when food becomes trapped within the pouch.

■ **Figure 12** Diverticulosis. Figure illustrates external and internal appearance of diverticula.

Diverticulum

Infection in diverticulum

Pathology *(continued)*

TERM	DEFINITION
diverticulosis (dye-ver-tik-yoo-LOW-sis)	Condition of having diverticula (outpouches off the gut). May lead to *diverticulitis* if one becomes inflamed.
dysentery (dis-in-TARE-ee)	Disease characterized by diarrhea, often with mucus and blood, severe abdominal pain, fever, and dehydration. Caused by ingesting food or water contaminated by chemicals, bacteria, protozoans, or parasites.
hemorrhoids (HEM-oh-roydz)	Varicose veins in the rectum.
ileus (ILL-ee-us)	Severe abdominal pain, inability to pass stools, vomiting, and abdominal distension as a result of an intestinal blockage. May require surgery to reverse the blockage.
inguinal hernia (ING-gwih-nal HER-nee-ah)	Hernia or protrusion of a loop of small intestines into the inguinal (groin) region through a weak spot in the abdominal muscle wall that develops into a hole. May become *incarcerated* or *strangulated* if the muscle tightens down around the loop of intestines and cuts off its blood flow.

■ **Figure 13** An inguinal hernia. A portion of the small intestine is protruding through the abdominal muscles into the groin region.

Loop of intestine protruding through opening in abdominal muscles

intussusception (in-tuh-suh-SEP-shun)	Result of the intestine slipping or telescoping into another section of intestine just below it. More common in children.

■ **Figure 14** Intussusception. A short length of small intestine has telescoped into itself.

Pathology *(continued)*

TERM	DEFINITION
irritable bowel syndrome (IBS)	Disturbance in the functions of the intestine from unknown causes. Symptoms generally include abdominal discomfort and an alteration in bowel activity. Also called *spastic colon* or *functional bowel syndrome*.
polyposis (pall-ee-POH-sis)	Small tumors that contain a pedicle or stemlike attachment in the mucous membranes of the large intestine (colon); may be precancerous.

■ **Figure 15** Photograph showing a polyp in the colon. Note the mushroom-like shape, an enlarged top growing at the end of a stem. *(ISM/Phototake NYC)*

TERM	DEFINITION
ulcerative colitis (ULL-sir-ah-tiv koh-LYE-tis)	Chronic inflammatory condition that produces numerous ulcers to form on the mucous membrane lining of the colon; the cause is unknown. Also known as *inflammatory bowel disease* (IBD).
volvulus (VOL-vyoo-lus)	Condition in which the bowel twists upon itself and causes an obstruction. Painful and requires immediate surgery.

■ **Figure 16** Volvulus. A length of small intestine has twisted around itself, cutting off blood circulation to the twisted loop.

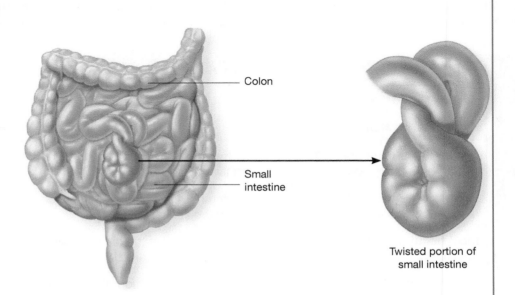

Colon

Small intestine

Twisted portion of small intestine

Pathology *(continued)*

TERM	DEFINITION
■ *Accessory Organs*	
cholecystitis (koh-lee-sis-TYE-tis)	Inflammation of the gallbladder; most commonly caused by gallstones in the gallbladder or common bile duct that block the flow of bile.
cholelithiasis (koh-lee-lih-THIGH-ah-sis)	Presence of gallstones; may or may not cause symptoms such as *cholecystalgia*.

■ **Figure 17** A) Cholelithiasis, red circles indicate common sites for gallstones including the gallbladder, cystic duct, hepatic duct, and common bile duct. B) Photograph of a gallbladder specimen with multiple gallstones. *(Martin Rotker/Phototake NYC)*

TERM	DEFINITION
cirrhosis (sih-ROH-sis)	Chronic disease of the liver associated with failure of the liver to function properly.
hepatitis (hep-ah-TYE-tis)	Inflammation of the liver, usually due to a viral infection. Different viruses are transmitted by different routes, such as sexual contact or from exposure to blood or fecally contaminated water or food.

Diagnostic Procedures

TERM	DEFINITION
■ *Clinical Laboratory Tests*	
alanine transaminase (ALT) (AL-ah-neen trans-AM-in-nase)	Enzyme normally present in the blood. Blood levels are increased in persons with liver disease.
aspartate transaminase (AST) (ass-PAR-tate trans-AM-in-nase)	Enzyme normally present in the blood. Blood levels are increased in persons with liver disease.
fecal occult blood test (FOBT) (uh-CULT)	Laboratory test on the feces to determine if microscopic amounts of blood are present. Also called *hemoccult* or *stool guaiac*.
ova and parasites (O&P) (OH-vah and PAR-ah-sights)	Laboratory examination of feces with a microscope for the presence of parasites or their eggs.
serum bilirubin (SEE-rum BILLY-rubin)	Blood test to determine the amount of the waste product bilirubin in the bloodstream. Elevated levels indicate liver disease.

Diagnostic Procedures *(continued)*

TERM	DEFINITION
stool culture	Laboratory test of feces to determine if any pathogenic bacteria are present.

■ *Diagnostic Imaging*

TERM	DEFINITION
bite-wing x-ray	X-ray taken with a part of the film holder held between the teeth and parallel to the teeth.
intravenous cholecystography (in-trah-VEE-nus koh-lee-sis-TOG-rah-fee)	Dye is administered intravenously to the patient, which allows for x-ray visualization of the gallbladder and bile ducts.
lower gastrointestinal series (lower GI series)	X-ray image of the colon and rectum is taken after the administration of barium (a radiopaque dye) by enema. Also called a *barium enema (BE)*.

■ **Figure 18** Color enhanced x-ray of the colon taken during a barium enema. *(CNRI/Science Photo Library/Photo Researchers, Inc.)*

TERM	DEFINITION
percutaneous transhepatic cholangiography (PTC) (per-kyoo-TAY-nee-us trans-heh-PAT-ik koh-lan-jee-OG-rah-fee)	Procedure in which contrast medium is injected directly into the liver to visualize the bile ducts. Used to detect obstructions.
upper gastrointestinal (UGI) **series**	Administering of a barium contrast material orally and then taking an x-ray to visualize the esophagus, stomach, and duodenum. Also called a *barium swallow*.

■ *Endoscopic Procedures*

TERM	DEFINITION
colonoscopy (koh-lon-OSS-koh-pee)	Flexible fiberscope called a *colonoscope* is passed through the anus, rectum, and colon; used to examine the upper portion of the colon. Polyps and small growths can be removed during this procedure (see Figure 15).
endoscopic retrograde cholangiopancreatography (ERCP) (en-doh-SKOP-ik RET-roh-grayd koh-lan-jee-oh-pan-kree-ah-TOG-rah-fee)	Procedure using an endoscope to visually examine the hepatic duct, common bile duct, and pancreatic duct. Retrograde means to go in the backwards direction. In this case the endoscope is inserted through the anus and worked backwards to the area where the pancreatic and common bile ducts empty into the duodenum.

Diagnostic Procedures *(continued)*

TERM	DEFINITION
esophagogastroduodenoscopy (EGD) (eh-soff-ah-go-gas-troh-duo-den-OS-koh-pee)	Use of a flexible fiberoptic endoscope to visually examine the esophagus, stomach, and beginning of the duodenum.
gastroscopy (gas-TROS-koh-pee)	Procedure in which a flexible *gastroscope* is passed through the mouth and down the esophagus in order to visualize inside the stomach. Used to diagnose peptic ulcers and gastric carcinoma.
laparoscopy (lap-ar-OSS-koh-pee)	*Laparoscope* is passed into the abdominal wall through a small incision. The abdominal cavity is then visually examined for tumors and other conditions with this lighted instrument. Also called *peritoneoscopy*.
sigmoidoscopy (sig-moid-OS-koh-pee)	Procedure using a flexible *sigmoidoscope* to visually examine the sigmoid colon. Commonly done to diagnose cancer and polyps.
■ *Additional Diagnostic Procedures*	
paracentesis (pair-ah-sin-TEE-sis)	Insertion of a needle into the abdominal cavity to withdraw fluid. Tests to diagnose diseases may be conducted on the fluid.

Therapeutic Procedures

TERM	DEFINITION
■ *Dental Procedures*	
extraction	Removing or "pulling" of teeth.
root canal	Dental treatment involving the pulp cavity of the root of a tooth. Procedure is used to save a tooth that is badly infected or abscessed.
■ *Medical Procedures*	
gavage	Using a nasogastric (NG) tube to place liquid nourishment directly into the stomach.
lavage	Using a nasogastric (NG) tube to wash out the stomach. For example, after ingestion of dangerous substances.
nasogastric intubation (NG tube) (NAY-zo-gas-trik in-two-BAY-shun)	Flexible catheter is inserted into the nose and down the esophagus to the stomach. May be used for feeding or to suction out stomach fluids.
total parenteral nutrition (TPN) (pair-in-TARE-all)	Providing 100% of a patient's nutrition intravenously. Used when a patient is unable to eat.
■ *Surgical Procedures*	
anastomosis (ah-nas-toh-MOH-sis)	To surgically create a connection between two organs or vessels. For example, joining together two cut ends of the intestines after a section is removed.

Therapeutic Procedures *(continued)*

TERM	DEFINITION
bariatric surgery (bear-ee-AT-rik)	A group of surgical procedures such as stomach stapling and restrictive banding to reduce the size of the stomach. A treatment for morbid (extreme) obesity.
choledocholithotripsy (koh-led-oh-koh-LITH-oh-trip-see)	Crushing of a gallstone in the common bile duct.
colostomy (koh-LOSS-toh-mee)	Surgical creation of an opening of some portion of the colon through the abdominal wall to the outside surface. Fecal material (stool) drains into a bag worn on the abdomen.

■ **Figure 19** A) The colon illustrating various ostomy sites. B) Colostomy in the descending colon, illustrating functioning stoma and nonfunctioning distal sigmoid colon and rectum.

Transverse colostomy
Ascending colostomy
Descending colostomy
Ileostomy
Cecostomy
Sigmoid colostomy

A

B
Functioning stoma
Non-functioning remaining colon

TERM	DEFINITION
diverticulectomy (dye-ver-tik-yoo-LEK-toh-mee)	Surgical removal of a diverticulum.
exploratory laparotomy (ek-SPLOR-ah-tor-ee lap-ah-ROT-oh-mee)	Abdominal operation for the purpose of examining the abdominal organs and tissues for signs of disease or other abnormalities.
fistulectomy (fis-tyoo-LEK-toh-mee)	Removal of a fistula.
gastric stapling	Procedure that closes off a large section of the stomach with rows of staples. Results in a much smaller stomach to assist very obese patients to lose weight.
hemorrhoidectomy (hem-oh-royd-EK-toh-mee)	Surgical removal of hemorrhoids from the anorectal area.
hernioplasty (her-nee-oh-PLAS-tee)	Surgical repair of a hernia. Also called *herniorrhaphy*.
laparoscopic cholecystectomy (lap-ar-oh-SKOP-ik koh-lee-sis-TEK-toh-mee)	Surgical removal of the gallbladder through a very small abdominal incision with the assistance of a laparoscope.
liver transplant	Transplant of a liver from a donor.

Pharmacology

CLASSIFICATION	ACTION	GENERIC AND BRAND NAMES
anorexiant (an-oh-REKS-ee-ant)	Treats obesity by suppressing appetite.	phendimetrazine, Adipost, Obezine; phentermine, Zantryl, Adipex
antacid	Used to neutralize stomach acids.	calcium carbonate, Tums; aluminum hydroxide and magnesium hydroxide, Maalox, Mylanta
antidiarrheal	Used to control diarrhea.	loperamide, Imodium; diphenoxylate, Lomotil; kaolin/pectin, Kaopectate
antiemetic (an-tye-ee-MEH-tik)	Treats nausea, vomiting, and motion sickness.	prochlorperazine, Compazine; promethazine, Phenergan
emetic (ee-MEH-tik)	Induces vomiting.	Ipecac syrup
H₂-receptor antagonist	Used to treat peptic ulcers and gastroesophageal reflux disease. When stimulated, H$_2$-receptors increase the production of stomach acid. Using an antagonist to block these receptors results in a low acid level in the stomach.	ranitidine, Zantac; cimetidine, Tagamet; famotidine, Pepcid
laxative	Treats constipation by stimulating a bowel movement.	senosides, Senokot; psyllium, Metamucil

> **Med Term Tip**
> The term *laxative* that refers to a medication to stimulate a bowel movement comes from the Latin term meaning "to relax."

proton pump inhibitors	Used to treat peptic ulcers and gastroesophageal reflux disease. Blocks the stomach's ability to secrete acid.	esomeprazole, Nexium; omeprazole, Prilosec

Abbreviations

ac	before meals		**HCV**	hepatitis C virus
ALT	alanine transaminase		**HDV**	hepatitis D virus
AST	aspartate transaminase		**HEV**	hepatitis E virus
Ba	barium		**HSV-1**	herpes simplex virus type 1
BE	barium enema		**IBD**	inflammatory bowel disease
BM	bowel movement		**IBS**	irritable bowel syndrome
BS	bowel sounds		**IVC**	intravenous cholangiography
CBD	common bile duct		**NG**	nasogastric (tube)
EGD	esophagogastroduodenoscopy		**NPO**	nothing by mouth
ERCP	endoscopic retrograde cholangio-pancreatography		**n&v**	nausea and vomiting
FOBT	fecal occult blood test		**O&P**	ova and parasites
GB	gallbladder		**pc**	after meals
GERD	gastroesophageal reflux disease		**PO**	by mouth
GI	gastrointestinal		**pp**	postprandial
HAV	hepatitis A virus		**PTC**	percutaneous transhepatic cholangiography
HBV	hepatitis B virus		**PUD**	peptic ulcer disease
HCl	hydrochloric acid		**TPN**	total parenteral nutrition
			UGI	upper gastrointestinal series

Chapter Review

Terminology Checklist

Below are all Anatomy and Physiology key terms, Word Building, Vocabulary, Pathology, Diagnostic, Therapeutic, and Pharmacology terms presented in this chapter. Use this list as a study tool by placing a check in the box in front of each term as you master its meaning.

- ☐ accessory organs
- ☐ alanine transaminase
- ☐ alimentary canal
- ☐ amylase
- ☐ anal
- ☐ anal fistula
- ☐ anal sphincter
- ☐ anastomosis
- ☐ anorexia
- ☐ anorexiant
- ☐ antacid
- ☐ antidiarrheal
- ☐ antiemetic
- ☐ antrum
- ☐ anus
- ☐ aphagia
- ☐ aphthous ulcers
- ☐ appendectomy
- ☐ appendicitis
- ☐ ascending colon
- ☐ ascites
- ☐ aspartate transaminase
- ☐ bariatric surgery
- ☐ bicuspids
- ☐ bile
- ☐ bite-wing x-ray
- ☐ body
- ☐ bolus
- ☐ bowel incontinence
- ☐ bradypepsia
- ☐ bridge
- ☐ buccal
- ☐ buccolabial
- ☐ buffers
- ☐ cachexia
- ☐ canines
- ☐ cardiac sphincter
- ☐ cecum
- ☐ cementum

- ☐ cheeks
- ☐ cholecystalgia
- ☐ cholecystectomy
- ☐ cholecystic
- ☐ cholecystitis
- ☐ cholecystogram
- ☐ choledocholithotripsy
- ☐ cholelithiasis
- ☐ chyme
- ☐ cirrhosis
- ☐ cleft lip
- ☐ cleft palate
- ☐ colectomy
- ☐ colon
- ☐ colonic
- ☐ colonoscope
- ☐ colonoscopy
- ☐ colorectal
- ☐ colorectal carcinoma
- ☐ colostomy
- ☐ common bile duct
- ☐ constipation
- ☐ Crohn's disease
- ☐ crown
- ☐ cuspids
- ☐ cystic duct
- ☐ deciduous teeth
- ☐ defecation
- ☐ dental
- ☐ dental caries
- ☐ dentalgia
- ☐ dentin
- ☐ dentistry
- ☐ denture
- ☐ descending colon
- ☐ diarrhea
- ☐ diverticulectomy
- ☐ diverticulitis
- ☐ diverticulosis

- ☐ duodenal
- ☐ duodenum
- ☐ dysentery
- ☐ dysorexia
- ☐ dyspepsia
- ☐ dysphagia
- ☐ emesis
- ☐ emetic
- ☐ emulsification
- ☐ enamel
- ☐ endoscopic retrograde cholangiopancreatography
- ☐ enteric
- ☐ enteritis
- ☐ epiglottis
- ☐ esophageal
- ☐ esophageal varices
- ☐ esophagectasis
- ☐ esophagogastroduodenoscopy
- ☐ esophagus
- ☐ exploratory laparotomy
- ☐ extraction
- ☐ fecal occult blood test
- ☐ feces
- ☐ fistulectomy
- ☐ fundus
- ☐ gallbladder
- ☐ gastralgia
- ☐ gastrectomy
- ☐ gastric
- ☐ gastric carcinoma
- ☐ gastric stapling
- ☐ gastritis
- ☐ gastroenteritis
- ☐ gastroenterologist
- ☐ gastroenterology
- ☐ gastroesophageal reflux disease
- ☐ gastrointestinal system

Digestive System

- gastrointestinal tract
- gastromalacia
- gastroscope
- gastroscopy
- gastrostomy
- gavage
- gingiva
- gingival
- gingivitis
- glossal
- gums
- gut
- H$_2$-receptor antagonist
- hematemesis
- hematochezia
- hemorrhoidectomy
- hemorrhoids
- hepatic
- hepatic duct
- hepatitis
- hepatoma
- hernioplasty
- herpes labialis
- hiatal hernia
- hydrochloric acid
- hyperemesis
- hypoglossal
- ileal
- ileocecal valve
- ileostomy
- ileum
- ileus
- implant
- incisors
- inguinal hernia
- internal medicine
- intravenous cholecystography
- intussusception
- irritable bowel syndrome
- jaundice
- jejunal
- jejunum
- laparoscope
- laparoscopic cholecystectomy
- laparoscopy
- laparotomy
- laryngopharynx
- lavage
- laxative
- lips
- liver
- liver transplant
- lower esophageal sphincter
- lower gastrointestinal series
- melena
- molars
- nasogastric
- nasogastric intubation
- nausea
- obesity
- oral
- oral cavity
- oropharynx
- orthodontic
- orthodontics
- ova and parasites
- palate
- palatoplasty
- pancreas
- pancreatic
- pancreatic duct
- pancreatic enzymes
- pancreatitis
- paracentesis
- parotid glands
- peptic ulcer disease
- percutaneous transhepatic cholangiography
- periodontal disease
- periodontal ligaments
- periodontic
- periodontics
- peristalsis
- permanent teeth
- pharyngeal
- pharyngoplasty
- pharyngoplegia
- pharynx
- polyp
- polyphagia
- polyposis
- postprandial
- premolar
- proctologist
- proctology
- proctopexy
- proctoptosis
- proton pump inhibitor
- pulp cavity
- pyloric
- pyloric sphincter
- pyrosis
- rectal
- rectum
- regurgitation
- root
- root canal
- rugae
- saliva
- salivary glands
- serum bilirubin
- sialadenitis
- sigmoidal
- sigmoid colon
- sigmoidoscope
- sigmoidoscopy
- small intestine
- sphincter
- stomach
- stool culture
- sublingual
- sublingual glands
- submandibular glands
- taste buds
- teeth
- tongue
- total parenteral nutrition
- transverse colon
- ulcerative colitis
- upper gastrointestinal series
- uvula
- vermiform appendix
- volvulus

Practice Exercises

A. Complete the following statements.

1. The digestive system is also known as the _gastrointestinal_ system. (GI)

2. The continuous muscular tube of the digestive system is called the _alimentary canal_ or _gastrointestinal tract_ and stretches between the _mouth_ and _anus_.

3. The accessory organs of the digestive system are the _liver_, _pancreas_, _gallbladder_, and _salivary glands_

4. The three main functions of the digestive system are: _digesting food_, _absorbing nutrients_ and _eliminating waste_.

5. The incisors are examples of _cutting_ teeth and the molars are examples of _grinding_ teeth.

6. Food is propelled through the gut by wavelike muscular contractions called _peristalsis_.

7. Food in the stomach is mixed with _hydrochloric acid_ and other gastric juices to form a watery mixture called _chyme_.

8. The three sections of small intestine in order are the _duodenum_, _jejunum_, and _ileum_.

9. The S-shaped section of colon that curves back towards the rectum is called the _sigmoid_ colon.

10. _Bile_ produced by the liver is responsible for the _amulsification_ of fats. It is stored in the _gallbladder_.

B. Define the following combining forms and use them to form digestive terms.

	Definition	Digestive Term
1. esophag/o	esophagus	esophageal
2. hepat/o	liver	hepatitis
3. ile/o	ileum	ileal
4. proct/o	anus and rectum	proctoptosis
5. gloss/o	tongue	glossal
6. labi/o	lip	buccolabial
7. jejun/o	jejunum	jejunal
8. sigmoid/o	sigmoid colon	sigmoidoscope
9. rect/o	rectum	rectal
10. gingiv/o	gums	gingivitis

Digestive System

11. cholecyst/o ___gallbladder___   cholecystectomy

12. duoden/o ___duodenum___   duodenal

13. an/o ___anus___   anal

14. enter/o ___small intestine___   enteritis

15. dent/o ___tooth___   dentalgia

C. State the terms described using the combining forms provided.

The combining form *gastr/o* refers to the stomach. Use it to write a term that means:

1. inflammation of the stomach ___gastritis___

2. study of the stomach and small intestines ___gastroenterology___

3. removal of the stomach ___gastrectomy___

4. visual exam of the stomach ___gastroscopy___

5. stomach pain ___gastralgia___

6. enlargement of the stomach ___gastromegaly___

7. incision into the stomach ___gastrotomy___

The combining form *esophag/o* refers to the esophagus. Use it to write a term that means:

8. inflammation of the esophagus ___esophagitis___

9. visual examination of the esophagus ___esophagoscopy___

10. surgical repair of the esophagus ___esophagoplasty___

11. pertaining to the esophagus ___esophageal___

12. stretched out esophagus ___esophagactasis___

The combining form *proct/o* refers to the rectum and anus. Use it to write a term that means:

13. surgical fixation of the rectum and anus ___proctopexy___

14. drooping of the rectum and anus ___proctoptosis___

15. inflammation of the rectum and anus ___proctitis___

16. specialist in the study of the rectum and anus ___proctologist___

The combining form *cholecyst/o* refers to the gallbladder. Use it to write a term that means:

17. removal of the gallbladder ___cholecystectomy___

18. condition of having gallbladder stones ___cholecystolithiasis___

19. gallbladder stone surgical crushing ___cholecystolithiatripsy___

20. gallbladder inflammation ___cholecystitis___

Digestive System

The combining form *lapar/o* refers to the abdomen. Use it to write a term that means:

21. instrument to view inside the abdomen _____ laparoscope _____

22. incision into the abdomen _____ laparotomy _____

23. visual examination of the abdomen _____ laparoscopy _____

The combining form *hepat/o* refers to the liver. Use it to write a term that means:

24. liver tumor _____ hepatoma _____

25. enlargement of the liver _____ hepatomegaly _____

26. pertaining to the liver _____ hepatic _____

27. inflammation of the liver _____ hepatitis _____

The combining form *pancreat/o* refers to the pancreas. Use it to write a term that means:

28. inflammation of the pancreas _____ pancreatitis _____

29. pertaining to the pancreas _____ pancreatic _____

The combining form *col/o* refers to the colon. Use it to write a term that means:

30. create an opening in the colon _____ colotomy _____

31. inflammation of the colon _____ colitis _____

D. Use the following suffixes to create a medical term for each definition relating to the digestive system.

-orexia   -phagia   -pepsia   -prandial

-emesis   -lithiasis

1. taken after meals _____ postprandial _____

2. gallstones _____ cholecystolithiasis _____

3. no appetite _____ anorexia _____

4. difficulty swallowing _____ dysphagia _____

5. vomiting blood _____ hematemesis _____

6. slow digestion _____ bradypepsia _____

E. Identify the following abbreviations.

1. BM _____ bowel movement _____

2. UGI _____ upper gastrointestinal series _____

3. BE _____ barium enema _____

4. BS _____ bowel sounds _____

Digestive System

5. n & v _____ nausea and vomiting _____

6. O & P _____ ova and parasites _____

7. PO _____ by mouth _____

8. CBD _____ common bile duct _____

9. NPO _____ nothing by mouth _____

10. pp _____ postprandial _____

F. Write the abbreviation for the following terms.

1. nasogastric _____ NG _____

2. gastrointestinal _____ GI _____

3. hepatitis B virus _____ HBV _____

4. fecal occult blood test _____ FOBT _____

5. inflammatory bowel disease _____ IBD _____

6. herpes simplex virus type 1 _____ HSV-1 _____

7. aspartate transaminase _____ AST _____

8. after meals _____ pc _____

9. peptic ulcer disease _____ PUD _____

10. gastroesophageal reflux disease _____ GERD _____

G. Define the following terms.

1. colonoscopy _____ visual examination of the colon _____

2. bite-wing x-ray _____ x-ray taken with a part of the film holder held between the teeth & parallel to the teeth _____

3. hematochezia _____ passing bright red blood in the stools _____

4. serum bilirubin _____ blood test to determine the amount of the waste product billirubin in the bloodstream. Elevated levels indicate liver disease. _____

5. cachexia _____ loss of weight & generalized wasting that occurs during a chronic disease. _____

6. lavage _____ using an NG tube to wash out the stomach. _____

7. hernioplasty _____ surgical repair of a hernia _____

8. extraction _____ removing or "pulling" of teeth _____

9. choledocholithotripsy _____ crushing of a gall stone in the common bile duct. _____

10. anastomosis _____ to surgically create a connection between 2 organs or vessels. _____

H. Match each term to its definition.

1. __h__ dentures

2. __i__ anorexia

3. __f__ hematemesis

4. __c__ pyrosis

5. __a__ obesity

a.   excess body weight

b.   chronic liver disease

c.   heart burn

d.   small colon tumors

e.   fluid accumulation in abdominal cavity

Digestive System

270

6. ___j___ constipation
7. ___l___ melena
8. ___e___ ascites
9. ___b___ cirrhosis
10. ___k___ spastic colon
11. ___d___ polyposis
12. ___g___ volvulus
13. ___o___ hiatal hernia
14. ___p___ ulcerative colitis
15. ___n___ dysentery
16. ___m___ jaundice

f. vomit blood
g. bowel twists on self
h. set of artificial teeth
i. loss of appetite
j. difficulty having BM
k. irritable bowel syndrome
l. black tarry stool
m. yellow skin color
n. bloody diarrhea
o. diaphragmatocele
p. inflammatory bowel disease

I. Use the following terms in the sentences below.

colonoscopy

gastric stapling

total parenteral nutrition

ileostomy

barium swallow

colostomy

choledocholithotripsy

fecal occult blood test

lower GI series

colectomy

liver biopsy

intravenous cholecystography

1. Excising a small piece of hepatic tissue for microscopic examination is called a(n) _liver biopsy_.

2. When a surgeon performs a total or partial colectomy for cancer, she may have to create an opening on the surface of the skin for fecal matter to leave the body. This procedure is called a(n) _colostomy_.

3. Another name for an upper GI series is a(n) _barium swallow_

4. Mr. White has had a radiopaque material placed into his large bowel by means of an enema for the purpose of viewing his colon. This procedure is called a(n) _barium enema_ or _lower GI series_.

5. A(n) _colectomy_ is the surgical removal of the colon.

6. Jessica has been on a red-meat-free diet in preparation for a test of her feces for the presence of hidden blood. This test is called a(n) _fecal occult blood test_.

7. Dr. Mendez uses equipment to crush gallstones in the common bile duct. This procedure is called a(n) _choledocholithotripsy_.

8. Mrs. Alcazar required _total parenteral nutrition_ because she could not eat following her intestinal surgery.

9. Mr. Bright had a _gastric stapling_ to treat his morbid obesity.

10. Visualizing the gallbladder and bile ducts by injecting a dye into the patient's arm is called an _intravenous cholecystography_.

Digestive System

271

11. Passing an instrument into the anus and rectum in order to see the colon is called a(n) _colonoscopy_.

12. Ms. Fayne suffers from Crohn's disease, which has necessitated the removal of much of her small intestine. She has had a surgical passage created for the external disposal of waste material from the ileum. This is called a(n) _ileostomy_.

J. Match each term to its definition.

1. _d_ dentures
2. _g_ cementum
3. _h_ root canal
4. _e_ crown
5. _f_ bridge
6. _b_ implant
7. _c_ gingivitis
8. _a_ dental caries

a. tooth decay
b. prosthetic device used to anchor a tooth
c. inflammation of the gums
d. full set of artificial teeth
e. portion of the tooth covered by enamel
f. replacement for missing teeth
g. anchors root in bony socket of jaw
h. surgery on the tooth pulp

K. Fill in the classification for each drug description, then match the brand name.

Drug Description	Classification	Brand Name
1. _____ Controls diarrhea	_____	a. Pepcid
2. _____ Blocks stomach's ability to secrete acid	_____	b. Obezine
3. _____ Induces vomiting	_____	c. Metamucil
4. _____ Treats motion sickness	_____	d. Compazine
5. _____ Blocks acid-producing receptors	_____	e. Maalox
6. _____ Suppresses appetite	_____	f. Ipecac syrup
7. _____ Stimulates a bowel movement	_____	g. Imodium
8. _____ Neutralizes stomach acid	_____	h. Nexium

Medical Record Analysis

Below is an item from a patient's medical record. Read it carefully, make sure you understand all the medical terms used, and then answer the questions that follow.

Gastroenterology Consultation Report

Reason for Consultation:	Evaluation of recurrent epigastric and LUQ pain with anemia.
History of Present Illness:	Patient is a 56-year-old male. He reports a long history of mild dyspepsia characterized by burning epigastric pain, especially when his stomach is empty. This pain has been relieved by over-the-counter antacids. Approximately two weeks ago, the pain became significantly worse; he is also nauseated and has vomited several times.
Past Medical History:	Patient's history is not significant for other digestive system disorders. He had a tonsillectomy at age 8. He sustained a compound fracture of the left ankle in a bicycle accident at age 11 that required surgical fixation. More recently he has been diagnosed with an enlarged prostate gland, and surgery has been recommended. However, he would like to resolve this epigastric pain before going forward with the TUR.
Results of Physical Examination:	CBC indicates anemia, and a fecal occult blood test is positive for blood in the feces. A blood test for *Helicobacter pylori* is positive. Erosion in the gastric lining was visualized on an upper GI. Follow-up gastroscopy found evidence of mild reflux esophagitis and an ulcerated lesion in the lining of the pyloric section of the stomach. This ulcer is 1.5 cm in diameter and deep. There is evidence of active bleeding from the ulcer. Multiple biopsies were taken, and they were negative for gastric cancer. IV Tagamet relieved the painful symptoms in two days.
Assessment:	Peptic ulcer. Gastric cancer has been ruled out in light of the negative biopsies.
Recommendations:	A gastrectomy to remove the ulcerated portion of stomach is indicated because the ulcer is already bleeding. Patient should continue on Tagamet to reduce stomach acid. Two medications will be added: Keflex to treat the bacterial infection and iron pills to reverse the anemia. Patient was instructed to eat frequent small meals and avoid alcohol and irritating foods.

Critical Thinking Questions

1. This patient reports LUQ pain. What does LUQ stand for and what organs do you find there? Left Upper Quadrant - sm. portion of liver, spleen, lft kidney, stomach, colon, pancreas, small intestines

2. This patient had two diagnostic tests that indicated he was losing blood. Name these two tests and then describe them in your own words. CBC - complete blood count - tests for counts of all blood cells/levels. C & S - blood culture & sensitivity - to test for bacteria.

3. This patient had a procedure to visually examine the ulcer. Name the procedure and then describe in your own words what the physician observed. Gastroscopy - mild raflux inflammation of the esophagus & a bleeding ulcer in the stomach.

4. Name the serious pathological condition that was ruled out. _gastric cancer_

5. Which of the following is NOT a recommendation of the consulting physician?
   a. medication to reduce stomach acid
   b. surgical removal of a portion of the stomach
   c. an antibiotic
   d. blood transfusion

6. Briefly describe this patient's past medical history in your own words. _No serious health issues or past digestive issues. Recent diagnosis of enlarged prostate gland._

Chart Note Transcription

The chart note below contains twelve phrases that can be reworded with a medical term that you learned in this chapter. Each phrase is identified with an underline. Determine the medical term and write your answers in the space provided.

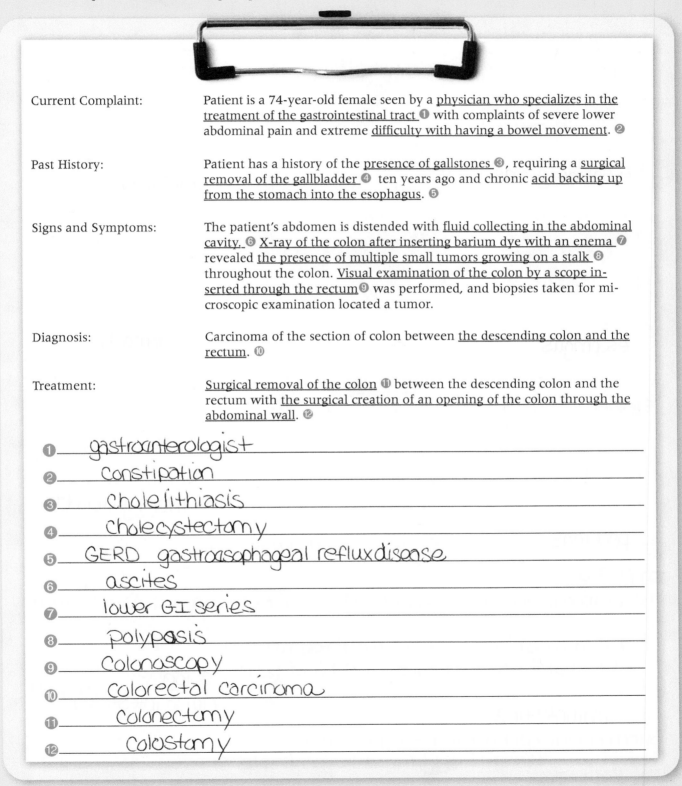

Current Complaint: Patient is a 74-year-old female seen by a <u>physician who specializes in the treatment of the gastrointestinal tract</u> ❶ with complaints of severe lower abdominal pain and extreme <u>difficulty with having a bowel movement.</u> ❷

Past History: Patient has a history of the <u>presence of gallstones</u> ❸, requiring a <u>surgical removal of the gallbladder</u> ❹ ten years ago and chronic <u>acid backing up from the stomach into the esophagus.</u> ❺

Signs and Symptoms: The patient's abdomen is distended with <u>fluid collecting in the abdominal cavity.</u> ❻ <u>X-ray of the colon after inserting barium dye with an enema</u> ❼ revealed <u>the presence of multiple small tumors growing on a stalk</u> ❽ throughout the colon. <u>Visual examination of the colon by a scope inserted through the rectum</u> ❾ was performed, and biopsies taken for microscopic examination located a tumor.

Diagnosis: Carcinoma of the section of colon between <u>the descending colon and the rectum.</u> ❿

Treatment: <u>Surgical removal of the colon</u> ⓫ between the descending colon and the rectum with <u>the surgical creation of an opening of the colon through the abdominal wall.</u> ⓬

❶ gastroenterologist

❷ constipation

❸ cholelithiasis

❹ cholecystectomy

❺ GERD gastroesophageal reflux disease

❻ ascites

❼ lower GI series

❽ polyposis

❾ colonoscopy

❿ colorectal carcinoma

⓫ colonectomy

⓬ colostomy

Labeling Exercise

A. System Review

Write the labels for this figure on the numbered lines provided.

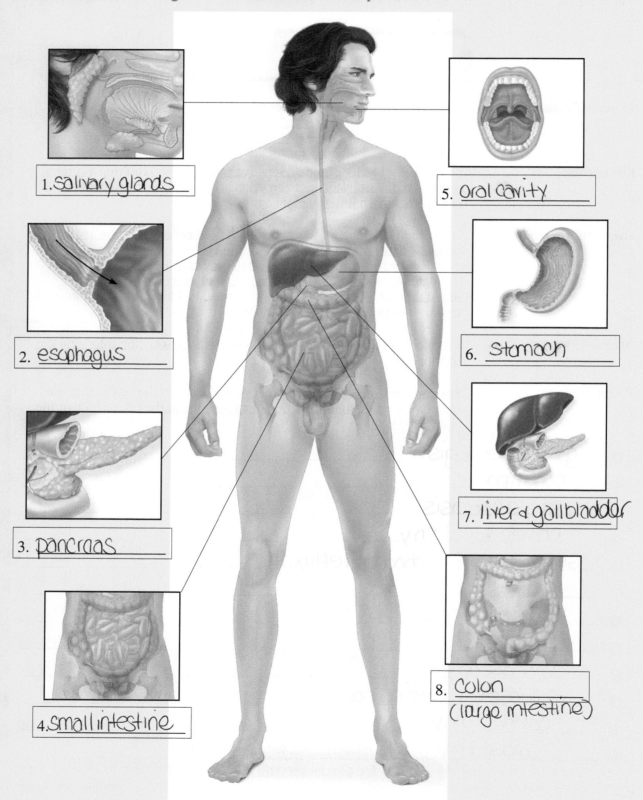

1. salivary glands

2. esophagus

3. pancreas

4. small intestine

5. oral cavity

6. stomach

7. liver & gallbladder

8. colon (large intestine)

B. Anatomy Challenge

1. Write the labels for this figure on the numbered lines provided.

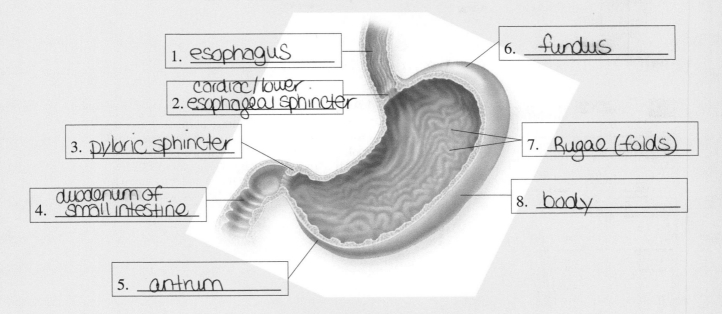

1. esophagus
2. cardiac/lower esophageal sphincter
3. pyloric sphincter
4. duodenum of small intestine
5. antrum
6. fundus
7. Rugae (folds)
8. body

2. Write the labels for this figure on the numbered lines provided.

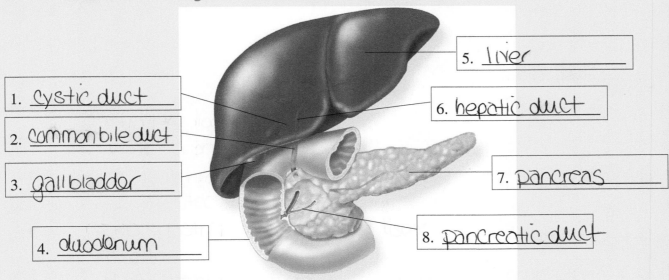

1. cystic duct
2. common bile duct
3. gall bladder
4. duodenum
5. liver
6. hepatic duct
7. pancreas
8. pancreatic duct

Multimedia Preview

Additional interactive resources and activities for this chapter can be found on the Companion Website.

Website Highlights—www.prenhall.com/fremgen

LABELING EXERCISE

Click here and take advantage of the free-access on-line study guide that accompanies your textbook. You'll find a figure labeling quiz that corresponds to this chapter. By clicking on this URL you'll also access links to download mp3 audio reviews, current news articles, and an audio glossary.

Urinary System

Learning Objectives

Upon completion of this chapter, you will be able to:

- Identify and define the combining forms and suffixes introduced in this chapter.
- Correctly spell and pronounce medical terms and major anatomical structures relating to the urinary system.
- Locate and describe the major organs of the urinary system and their functions.
- Describe the nephron and the mechanisms of urine production.
- Identify the characteristics of urine and a urinalysis.
- Build and define urinary system medical terms from word parts.
- Identify and define urinary system vocabulary terms.
- Identify and define selected urinary system pathology terms.
- Identify and define selected urinary system diagnostic procedures.
- Identify and define selected urinary system therapeutic procedures.
- Identify and define selected medications relating to the urinary system.
- Define selected abbreviations associated with the urinary system.

From Chapter 9 of *Medical Terminology: A Living Language*, 4/e. Bonnie F. Fremgen. Suzanne S. Frucht. Copyright © 2009 by Pearson Education. Published by Prentice Hall. All rights reserved.

Urinary System at a Glance

Function

The urinary system is responsible for maintaining a stable internal environment for the body. In order to achieve this state, the urinary system removes waste products, adjusts water and electrolyte levels, and maintains the correct pH.

Organs

kidneys
ureters
urethra
urinary bladder

Combining Forms

azot/o	nitrogenous waste	**noct/i**	night
bacteri/o	bacteria	**olig/o**	scanty
cyst/o	urinary bladder	**pyel/o**	renal pelvis
glomerul/o	glomerulus	**ren/o**	kidney
glycos/o	sugar, glucose	**ur/o**	urine
keton/o	ketones	**ureter/o**	ureter
lith/o	stone	**urethr/o**	urethra
meat/o	meatus	**urin/o**	urine
nephr/o	kidney		

Suffixes

-lith	stone
-lithiasis	condition of stones
-ptosis	drooping
-tripsy	surgical crushing
-uria	condition of the urine

Urinary System Illustrated

kidney

Filters blood and
produces urine

ureter

Transports urine to the bladder

urinary bladder

Stores urine

male urethra

Transports urine to exterior

female urethra

Transports urine to exterior

Anatomy and Physiology of the Urinary System

genitourinary system
  (jen-ih-toh-YOO-rih-nair-ee)
kidneys
nephrons (NEF-ronz)
uremia (yoo-REE-mee-ah)

ureters (yoo-REE-ters)
urethra (yoo-REE-thrah)
urinary bladder (YOO-rih-nair-ee)
urine (YOO-rin)

Think of the urinary system, sometimes referred to as the **genitourinary** (GU) **system**, as similar to a water filtration plant. Its main function is to filter and remove waste products from the blood. These waste materials result in the production and excretion of **urine** from the body.

The urinary system is one of the hardest working systems of the body. All the body's metabolic processes result in the production of waste products. These waste products are a natural part of life but quickly become toxic if they are allowed to build up in the blood, resulting in a condition called **uremia**. Waste products in the body are removed through a very complicated system of blood vessels and kidney tubules. The actual filtration of wastes from the blood takes place in millions of **nephrons**, which make up each of your two **kidneys**. As urine drains from each kidney, the **ureters** transport it to the **urinary bladder**. We are constantly producing urine, and our bladders can hold about one quart of this liquid. When the urinary bladder empties, urine moves from the bladder down the **urethra** to the outside of the body.

Kidneys

calyx (KAY-liks)
cortex (KOR-teks)
hilum (HIGH-lum)
medulla (meh-DULL-ah)
renal artery

renal papilla (pah-PILL-ah)
renal pelvis
renal pyramids
renal vein
retroperitoneal (ret-roh-pair-ih-toh-NEE-al)

The two kidneys are located in the lumbar region of the back above the waist on either side of the vertebral column. They are not inside the peritoneal sac, a location referred to as **retroperitoneal**. Each kidney has a concave or indented area on the edge toward the center that gives the kidney its bean shape. The center of this concave area is called the **hilum**. The hilum is where the **renal artery** enters and the **renal vein** leaves the kidney (see Figure 1 ■). The renal artery delivers the blood that is full of waste products to the kidney and the renal vein returns the now cleansed blood to the general circulation. The ureters also leave the kidneys at the hilum. The ureters are narrow tubes that lead from the kidneys to the bladder.

When a surgeon cuts into a kidney, several structures or areas are visible. The outer portion, called the **cortex**, is much like a shell for the kidney. The inner area is called the **medulla**. Within the medulla are a dozen or so triangular-shaped areas, the **renal pyramids**, which resemble their namesake, the Egyptian pyramids. The tip of each pyramid points inward toward the hilum. At its tip, called the **renal papilla**, each pyramid opens into a **calyx** (plural is *calyces*), which is continuous with the **renal pelvis**. The calyces and ultimately the renal pelvis collect urine as it is formed. The ureter for each kidney arises from the renal pelvis (see Figure 2 ■).

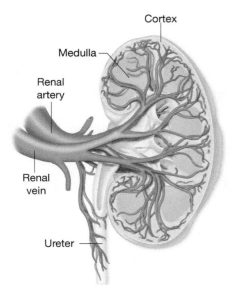

Cortex

Medulla

Renal artery

Renal vein

Ureter

■ Figure 1 Kidney structure. Longitudinal section showing the renal artery entering and the renal vein and ureter exiting at the hilum of the kidney.

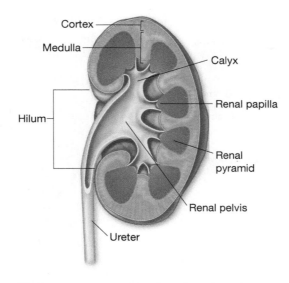

Cortex

Medulla

Hilum

Calyx

Renal papilla

Renal pyramid

Renal pelvis

Ureter

■ Figure 2 Longitudinal section of a kidney illustrating the internal structures.

Nephrons

afferent arteriole (AFF-er-ent)

Bowman's capsule

collecting tubule

distal convoluted tubule
  (DISS-tall con-voh-LOOT-ed)

efferent arteriole (EF-er-ent)

glomerular capsule (glom-AIR-yoo-lar)

glomerulus (glom-AIR-yoo-lus)

loop of Henle

proximal convoluted tubule
  (PROK-sim-al con-voh-LOOT-ed)

renal corpuscle (KOR-pus-ehl)

renal tubule

The functional or working unit of the kidney is the nephron. There are more than one million of these microscopic structures in each human kidney.

Each nephron consists of the **renal corpuscle** and the **renal tubule** (see Figure 3 ■). The renal corpuscle is the blood-filtering portion of the nephron. It has a double-walled cuplike structure called the **glomerular** or **Bowman's capsule** (also called the *glomerular capsule*) that encases a ball of capillaries called the **glomerulus**. An **afferent arteriole** carries blood to the glomerulus, and an **efferent arteriole** carries blood away from the glomerulus.

Water and substances that were removed from the bloodstream in the renal corpuscle flow into the renal tubules to finish the urine production process. This continuous tubule is divided into four sections: the **proximal convoluted tubule**, followed by the narrow **loop of Henle** (also called the *nephron loop*), then the **distal convoluted tubule**, and finally the **collecting tubule.**

Ureters

As urine drains out of the renal pelvis it enters the ureter, which carries it down to the urinary bladder (see Figure 4 ■). Ureters are very narrow tubes measuring less than 1/4 inch wide and 10 to 12 inches long that extend from the renal pelvis to the urinary bladder. Mucous membrane lines the ureters just as it lines most passages that open to the external environment.

Med Term Tip

Afferent, meaning moving toward, and *efferent*, meaning moving away from, are terms used when discussing moving either toward or away from the central point in many systems. For example, there are afferent and efferent nerves in the nervous system.

Med Term Tip

The terms *ureter* and *urethra* are frequently confused. Remember that there are two ureters carrying urine from the kidneys into the bladder. There is only one urethra, and it carries urine from the bladder to the outside of the body.

■ **Figure 3** The structure of a nephron, illustrating the nephron structure in relation to the circulatory system.

Distal convoluted tubule

Efferent arteriole

Glomerular (Bowman's) capsule

Glomerulus

Afferent arteriole

Proximal convoluted tubule

Descending loop of Henle

Collecting tubule

Ascending loop of Henle

Peritubular capillaries

Urinary Bladder

external sphincter (SFINGK-ter)
internal sphincter

rugae (ROO-gay)
urination

The urinary bladder is an elastic muscular sac that lies in the base of the pelvis just behind the pubic symphysis (see Figure 5 ■). It is composed of three layers of smooth muscle tissue lined with mucous membrane containing **rugae** or folds that allow it to stretch. The bladder receives the urine directly from the ureters, stores it, and excretes it by **urination** through the urethra.

Generally, an adult bladder will hold 250 mL of urine. This amount then creates an urge to void or empty the bladder. Involuntary muscle action causes the bladder to contract and the **internal sphincter** to relax. The internal sphincter protects us from having our bladder empty at the wrong time. Voluntary action controls the **external sphincter**, which opens on demand to allow the intentional emptying of the bladder. The act of controlling the emptying of urine is developed sometime after a child is 2 years of age.

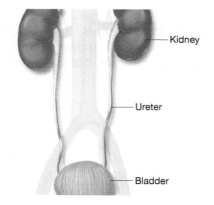

Kidney

Ureter

Bladder

■ **Figure 4** The ureters extend from the kidneys to the urinary bladder.

Ureter

Bladder

Prostate

Urethra

■ **Figure 5** The structure of the urinary bladder in a male. (Note the prostate gland.)

Urethra

urinary meatus (mee-AY-tus)

The urethra is a tubular canal that carries the flow of urine from the bladder to the outside of the body (see Figure 6 ■ for the male urethra). The external opening through which urine passes out of the body is called the **urinary meatus**. Mucous membrane also lines the urethra as it does other structures of the urinary system. This is one of the reasons that infection spreads up the urinary tract. The urethra is 1½ inches long in the female and 8 inches long in the male. In a woman it functions only as the outlet for urine and is in front of the vagina. In the male, however, it has two functions: an outlet for urine and the passageway for semen to leave the body.

Med Term Tip

Mucous membranes will carry infections up the urinary tract from the urinary meatus and urethra into the bladder and eventually up the ureters and the kidneys if not stopped. It is never wise to ignore a simple bladder infection or what is called *cystitis*.

Role of Kidneys in Homeostasis

electrolytes (ee-LEK-troh-lites)   **homeostasis** (hoh-mee-oh-STAY-sis)

The kidneys are responsible for **homeostasis** or balance in your body. They continually adjust the chemical conditions in the body that allow you to survive. Because of its interaction with the bloodstream and its ability to excrete substances from the body, the urinary system maintains the body's proper balance of water and chemicals. If the body is low on water, the kidneys conserve it, or in the opposite case, if there is excess water in the body, the kidneys excrete the excess. In addition to water, the kidneys regulate the level of **electrolytes**—small biologically important molecules such as sodium (Na^+), potassium (K^+), chloride (Cl^-), and bicarbonate (HCO_3^-). Finally, the kidneys play an important role in maintaining the correct pH range within the body, making sure we do not become too acidic or too alkaline. The kidneys accomplish these important tasks through the production of urine.

Stages of Urine Production

filtration   **reabsorption**
glomerular filtrate   **secretion**
peritubular capillaries

As wastes and unnecessary substances are removed from the bloodstream by the nephrons, many desirable molecules are also removed initially. Waste products are eliminated from the body, but other substances such as water, electrolytes, and nutrients must be returned to the bloodstream. Urine, in its final form ready for elimination from the body, is the ultimate product of this entire process.

Med Term Tip

The amount of water and other fluids processed by the kidneys each day is astonishing. Approximately 190 quarts of fluid are filtered out of the glomerular blood every day. Most of this fluid returns to the body through the reabsorption process. About 99 percent of the water that leaves the blood each day through the filtration process returns to the blood by proximal tubule reabsorption.

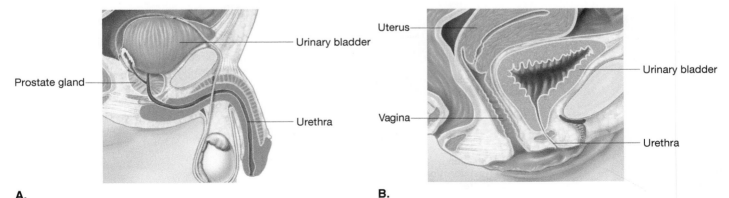

A.   B.

■ **Figure 6** A) The male urethra extends from the urinary bladder in the floor of the pelvis through the prostate gland and penis to the urinary meatus. B) The much shorter female urethra extends from the urinary bladder to the floor of the pelvis and exits just in front of the vaginal opening.

Urine production occurs in three stages: **filtration**, **reabsorption**, and **secretion**. Each of these steps is performed by a different section of the nephrons (see Figure 7 ■).

1. **Filtration.** The first stage is the filtering of particles, which occurs in the renal corpuscle. The pressure of blood flowing through the glomerulus forces material out of the bloodstream, through the wall of Bowman's capsule, and into the renal tubules. This fluid in the tubules is called the **glomerular filtrate** and consists of water, electrolytes, nutrients such as glucose and amino acids, wastes, and toxins.

2. **Reabsorption.** After filtration, the filtrate passes through the four sections of the tubule. As the filtrate moves along its twisted journey, most of the water and much of the electrolytes and nutrients are reabsorbed into the **peritubular capillaries**, a capillary bed that surrounds the renal tubules. They can then reenter the circulating blood.

3. **Secretion.** The final stage of urine production occurs when the special cells of the renal tubules secrete ammonia, uric acid, and other waste substances directly into the renal tubule. Urine formation is now finished; it passes into the collecting tubules, renal papilla, calyx, renal pelvis, and ultimately into the ureter.

Urine

albumin (al-BEW-min)   **specific gravity**
nitrogenous wastes (nigh-TROJ-eh-nus)   **urinalysis** (yoo-rih-NAL-ih-sis)

Urine is normally straw colored to clear, and sterile. Although it is 95 percent water, it also contains many dissolved substances, such as electrolytes, toxins, and **nitrogenous wastes**, the byproducts of muscle metabolism. At times the urine also contains substances that should not be there, such as glucose, blood, or **albumin**, a protein that should remain in the blood. This is the reason for performing a **urinalysis**, a physical and chemical analysis of urine, which gives medical personnel important information regarding disease processes occurring in a patient.

■ **Figure 7** The three stages of urine production: filtration, reabsorption, and secretion.

Normally, during a 24-hour period the output of urine will be 1,000 to 2,000 mL, depending on the amount of fluid consumed and the general health of the person. Normal urine is acidic because this is one way our bodies dispose of excess acids. **Specific gravity** indicates the amount of dissolved substances in urine. The specific gravity of pure water is 1.000. The specific gravity of urine varies from 1.001 to 1.030. Highly concentrated urine has a higher specific gravity, while the specific gravity of very dilute urine is close to that of water. See Table 1 ■ for the normal values for urine testing and Table 2 ■ for abnormal findings.

Med Term Tip

The color, odor, volume, and sugar content of urine have been examined for centuries. Color charts for urine were developed by 1140, and "taste testing" was common in the late seventeenth century. By the nineteenth century, urinalysis was a routine part of a physical examination.

Table 1	**Values for Urinalysis Testing**
ELEMENT	**NORMAL FINDINGS**
Color	Straw colored, pale yellow to deep gold
Odor	Aromatic
Appearance	Clear
Specific gravity	1.005–1.030
pH	5.0–8.0
Protein	Negative to trace
Glucose	None
Ketones	None
Blood	Negative

Table 2	**Abnormal Urinalysis Findings**
ELEMENT	**IMPLICATIONS**
Color	Color varies depending on the patient's fluid intake and output or medication. Brown or black urine color indicates a serious disease process.
Odor	A fetid or foul odor may indicate infection. For instance, a fruity odor may be found in diabetes mellitus, dehydration, or starvation. Other odors may be due to medication or foods.
Appearance	Cloudiness may mean that an infection is present.
Specific gravity	Concentrated urine has a higher specific gravity. Dilute urine, such as can be found with diabetes insipidus, acute tubular necrosis, or salt-restricted diets, has a lower specific gravity.
pH	A pH value below 7.0 (acidic) is common in urinary tract infections, metabolic or respiratory acidosis, diets high in fruits or vegetables, or administration of some drugs. A pH higher than 7.0 (basic or alkaline) is common in metabolic or respiratory alkalosis, fever, high-protein diets, and taking ascorbic acid.
Protein	Protein may indicate glomerulonephritis or preeclampsia in a pregnant woman.
Glucose	Small amounts of glucose may be present as the result of eating a high-carbohydrate meal, stress, pregnancy, and taking some medications, such as aspirin or corticosteroids. Higher levels may indicate poorly controlled diabetes, Cushing's syndrome, or infection.
Ketones	The presence of ketones may indicate poorly controlled diabetes, dehydration, starvation, or ingestion of large amounts of aspirin.
Blood	Blood may indicate some types of anemia, taking of some medications (such as blood thinners), arsenic poisoning, reactions to transfusion, trauma, burns, and convulsions.

Word Building

The following list contains examples of medical terms built directly from word parts. The definition for these terms can be determined by a straightforward translation of the word parts.

COMBINING FORM	COMBINED WITH	MEDICAL TERM	DEFINITION
cyst/o	-algia	**cystalgia** (sis-TAL-jee-ah)	bladder pain

Med Term Tip

Word watch—Be careful using the combining forms *cyst/o* meaning "bladder" and *cyt/o* meaning "cell."

	-ectomy	**cystectomy** (sis-TEK-toh-me)	removal of the bladder
	-gram	**cystogram** (SIS-toh-gram)	record of the bladder
	-ic	**cystic** (SIS-tik)	pertaining to the bladder
	-itis	**cystitis** (sis-TYE-tis)	bladder inflammation
	-lith	**cystolith** (SIS-toh-lith)	bladder stone
	-ostomy	**cystostomy** (sis-TOSS-toh-mee)	create a new opening into the bladder
	-otomy	**cystotomy** (sis-TOT-oh-mee)	incision into the bladder
	-pexy	**cystopexy** (SIS-toh-pek-see)	surgical fixation of the bladder
	-plasty	**cystoplasty** (SIS-toh-plas-tee)	surgical repair of the bladder
	-rrhagia	**cystorrhagia** (sis-toh-RAH-jee-ah)	rapid bleeding from the bladder
	-scope	**cystoscope** (SIS-toh-scope)	instrument used to visually examine the bladder
lith/o	-tripsy	**lithotripsy** (LITH-oh-trip-see)	surgical crushing of a stone
	-otomy	**lithotomy** (lith-OT-oh-me)	incision to remove a stone
nephr/o	-ectomy	**nephrectomy** (ne-FREK-toh-mee)	removal of a kidney
	-gram	**nephrogram** (NEH-fro-gram)	x-ray of the kidney
	-itis	**nephritis** (neh-FRYE-tis)	kidney inflammation
	-lith	**nephrolith** (NEF-roh-lith)	kidney stone
	-logist	**nephrologist** (neh-FROL-oh-jist)	specialist in the kidney
	-malacia	**nephromalacia** (nef-roh-mah-LAY-she-ah)	softening of the kidney
	-megaly	**nephromegaly** (nef-roh-MEG-ah-lee)	enlarged kidney
	-oma	**nephroma** (neh-FROH-ma)	kidney tumor
	-osis	**nephrosis** (neh-FROH-sis)	abnormal kidney condition
	-ptosis	**nephroptosis** (nef-rop-TOH-sis)	drooping kidney
	-ostomy	**nephrostomy** (neh-FROS-toh-mee)	create a new opening into the kidney
	-otomy	**nephrotomy** (neh-FROT-oh-mee)	incision into a kidney

Word Building *(continued)*

COMBINING FORM	COMBINED WITH	MEDICAL TERM	DEFINITION
	-pathy	**nephropathy** (neh-FROP-ah-thee)	kidney disease
	-pexy	**nephropexy** (NEF-roh-pek-see)	surgical fixation of kidney
	-lithiasis	**nephrolithiasis** (nef-roh-lith-EE-a-sis)	condition of kidney stones
	-sclerosis	**nephrosclerosis** (nef-roh-skleh-ROH-sis)	hardening of the kidney
pyel/o	-gram	**pyelogram** (PYE-eh-loh-gram)	x-ray record of the renal pelvis
	-itis	**pyelitis** (pye-eh-LYE-tis)	renal pelvis inflammation
	-plasty	**pyeloplasty** (PIE-ah-loh-plas-tee)	surgical repair of the renal pelvis
ren/o	-al	**renal** (REE-nal)	pertaining to the kidney
ur/o	-logist	**urologist** (yoo-RALL-oh-jist)	specialist in urine
	-emia	**uremia** (yoo-REE-mee-ah)	blood condition of urine
ureter/o	-al	**ureteral** (yoo-REE-ter-all)	pertaining to the ureter

Med Term Tip

Word watch—Be particularly careful when using the three very similar combining forms: *uter/o* meaning "uterus," *ureter/o* meaning "ureter," and *urethr/o* meaning "urethra."

COMBINING FORM	COMBINED WITH	MEDICAL TERM	DEFINITION
	-ectasis	**ureterectasis** (yoo-ree-ter-EK-tah-sis)	ureter dilation
	-lith	**ureterolith** (yoo-REE-teh-roh-lith)	ureter stone
	-stenosis	**ureterostenosis** (yoo-ree-ter-oh-sten-OH-sis)	narrowing of a ureter
urethr/o	-al	**urethral** (yoo-REE-thral)	pertaining to the urethra
	-algia	**urethralgia** (yoo-ree-THRAL-jee-ah)	urethra pain
	-itis	**urethritis** (yoo-ree-THRIGH-tis)	urethra inflammation
	-rrhagia	**urethrorrhagia** (yoo-ree-throh-RAH-jee-ah)	rapid bleeding from the urethra
	-scope	**urethroscope** (yoo-REE-throh-scope)	instrument to visually examine the urethra
	-stenosis	**urethrostenosis** (yoo-ree-throh-steh-NOH-sis)	narrowing of the urethra
urin/o	-meter	**urinometer** (yoo-rin-OH-meter)	instrument to measure urine
	-ary	**urinary** (yoo-rih-NAIR-ee)	pertaining to urine

SUFFIX	COMBINED WITH	MEDICAL TERM	DEFINITION
-uria	an-	**anuria** (an-YOO-ree-ah)	condition of no urine
	bacteri/o	**bacteriuria** (back-teer-ree-YOO-ree-ah)	bacteria in the urine

Word Building (continued)

SUFFIX	COMBINED WITH	MEDICAL TERM	DEFINITION
	dys-	**dysuria** (dis-YOO-ree-ah)	condition of difficult or painful urination
	glycos/o	**glycosuria** (glye-kohs-YOO-ree-ah)	condition of sugar in the urine
	hemat/o	**hematuria** (hee-mah-TOO-ree-ah)	condition of blood in the urine
	keton/o	**ketonuria** (key-tone-YOO-ree-ah)	ketones in the urine
	noct/i	**nocturia** (nok-TOO-ree-ah)	condition of frequent nighttime urination
	olig/o	**oliguria** (ol-ig-YOO-ree-ah)	condition of scanty amount of urine
	poly-	**polyuria** (pol-ee-YOO-ree-ah)	condition of (too) much urine
	protein	**proteinuria** (pro-ten-YOO-ree-ah)	protein in the urine
	py/o	**pyuria** (pye-YOO-ree-ah)	condition of pus in the urine

Vocabulary

TERM	DEFINITION
anuria (an-YOO-ree-ah)	Complete suppression of urine formed by the kidneys and a complete lack of urine excretion.
azotemia (a-zo-TEE-mee-ah)	Accumulation of nitrogenous waste in the bloodstream. Occurs when the kidney fails to filter these wastes from the blood.
calculus (KAL-kew-lus)	Stone formed within an organ by an accumulation of mineral salts. Found in the kidney, renal pelvis, ureters, bladder, or urethra. Plural is *calculi* (see Figure 8 ■).
catheter (KATH-eh-ter)	Flexible tube inserted into the body for the purpose of moving fluids into or out of the body. Most commonly used to refer to a tube threaded through the urethra into the bladder to withdraw urine (see Figure 9 ■).

■ **Figure 8** Photograph of sectioned kidney specimen illustrating extensive renal calculi.
(Dr. E. Walker/Science Photo Library/Photo Researchers, Inc.)

■ **Figure 9** Healthcare worker draining urine from a urinary catheter bag.

Vocabulary (*continued*)

TERM	DEFINITION
diuresis (dye-yoo-REE-sis)	Increased formation and secretion of urine.
enuresis (en-yoo-REE-sis)	Involuntary discharge of urine after the age by which bladder control should have been established. This usually occurs by the age of 5. *Nocturnal enuresis* refers to bed-wetting at night.
frequency	Greater-than-normal occurrence in the urge to urinate, without an increase in the total daily volume of urine. Frequency is an indication of inflammation of the bladder or urethra.
hesitancy	Decrease in the force of the urine stream, often with difficulty initiating the flow. It is often a symptom of a blockage along the urethra, such as an enlarged prostate gland.
micturition (mik-too-RIH-shun)	Another term for urination. **Med Term Tip** Terms such as *micturition*, *voiding*, and *urination* all mean basically the same thing—the process of releasing urine from the body.
nephrology (neh-FROL-oh-jee)	Branch of medicine involved in diagnosis and treatment of diseases and disorders of the kidney. Physician is a *nephrologist*.
renal colic (KOL-ik)	Pain caused by a kidney stone. Can be an excruciating pain and generally requires medical treatment.
stricture (STRIK-chur)	Narrowing of a passageway in the urinary system.
uremia (yoo-REE-me-ah)	Accumulation of waste products (especially nitrogenous wastes) in the bloodstream. Associated with renal failure.
urgency (ER-jen-see)	Feeling the need to urinate immediately.
urinary incontinence (in-CON-tin-ens)	Involuntary release of urine. In some patients an indwelling catheter is inserted into the bladder for continuous urine drainage (see Figure 9).
urinary retention	Inability to fully empty the bladder, often indicates a blockage in the urethra.
urology (yoo-RAL-oh-jee)	Branch of medicine involved in diagnosis and treatment of diseases and disorders of the urinary system (and male reproductive system). Physician is a *urologist*.
voiding	Another term for urination.

Pathology

TERM	DEFINITION
■ *Kidney*	
acute tubular necrosis (ATN) (ne-KROH-sis)	Damage to the renal tubules due to presence of toxins in the urine or to ischemia. Results in oliguria.
diabetic nephropathy (ne-FROH-path-ee)	Accumulation of damage to the glomerulus capillaries due to the chronic high blood sugars of diabetes mellitus.

Pathology *(continued)*

TERM	DEFINITION
glomerulonephritis (gloh-mair-yoo-loh-neh-FRYE-tis)	Inflammation of the kidney (primarily of the glomerulus). Since the glomerular membrane is inflamed, it becomes more permeable and will allow protein and blood cells to enter the filtrate. Results in protein in the urine (proteinuria) and hematuria.
hydronephrosis (high-droh-neh-FROH-sis)	Distention of the renal pelvis due to urine collecting in the kidney; often a result of the obstruction of a ureter.
nephrolithiasis (nef-roh-lith-EE-a-sis)	Presence of calculi in the kidney. Usually begins with the solidification of salts present in the urine.
nephrotic syndrome (NS)	Damage to the glomerulus resulting in protein appearing in the urine, proteinuria, and the corresponding decrease in protein in the bloodstream.
nephroptosis (nef-rop-TOH-sis)	Downward displacement of the kidney out of its normal location; commonly called a *floating kidney*.
polycystic kidneys (POL-ee-sis-tik)	Formation of multiple cysts within the kidney tissue. Results in the destruction of normal kidney tissue and uremia.

■ **Figure 10** Photograph of a polycystic kidney on the left compared to a normal kidney on the right.

(Simon Fraser/Royal Victoria Infirmary, Newcastle/ Science Photo Library/Photo Researchers, Inc.)

TERM	DEFINITION
pyelonephritis (pye-eh-loh-neh-FRYE-tis)	Inflammation of the renal pelvis and the kidney. One of the most common types of kidney disease. It may be the result of a lower urinary tract infection that moved up to the kidney by way of the ureters. There may be large quantities of white blood cells and bacteria in the urine. Blood (hematuria) may even be present in the urine in this condition. Can occur with any untreated or persistent case of cystitis.
renal cell carcinoma	Cancerous tumor that arises from kidney tubule cells.
renal failure	Inability of the kidneys to filter wastes from the blood resulting in uremia. May be acute or chronic. Major reason for a patient being placed on dialysis.
Wilm's tumor (VILMZ TOO-mor)	Malignant kidney tumor found most often in children.

■ *Urinary Bladder*

TERM	DEFINITION
bladder cancer	Cancerous tumor that arises from the cells lining the bladder; major sign is hematuria.
bladder neck obstruction (BNO)	Blockage of the bladder outlet. Often caused by an enlarged prostate gland in males.

Pathology *(continued)*

TERM	DEFINITION
cystocele (SIS-toh-seel)	Hernia or protrusion of the urinary bladder into the wall of the vagina.
interstitial cystitis (in-ter-STISH-al sis-TYE-tis)	Disease of unknown cause in which there is inflammation and irritation of the bladder. Most commonly seen in middle-aged women.
neurogenic bladder (noo-roh-JEN-ik)	Loss of nervous control that leads to retention; may be caused by spinal cord injury or multiple sclerosis.
urinary tract infection (UTI)	Infection, usually from bacteria, of any organ of the urinary system. Most often begins with cystitis and may ascend into the ureters and kidneys. Most common in women because of their shorter urethra.

Diagnostic Procedures

TERM	DEFINITION
■ *Clinical Laboratory Tests*	
blood urea nitrogen (BUN) (BLUD yoo-REE-ah NIGH-troh-jen)	Blood test to measure kidney function by the level of nitrogenous waste (urea) that is in the blood.
clean catch specimen (CC)	Urine sample obtained after cleaning off the urinary opening and catching or collecting a urine sample in midstream (halfway through the urination process) to minimize contamination from the genitalia.
creatinine clearance (kree-AT-tih-neen)	Test of kidney function. Creatinine is a waste product cleared from the bloodstream by the kidneys. For this test, urine is collected for 24 hours, and the amount of creatinine in the urine is compared to the amount of creatinine that remains in the bloodstream.
urinalysis (U/A, UA) (yoo-rih-NAL-ih-sis)	Laboratory test that consists of the physical, chemical, and microscopic examination of urine.
urine culture and sensitivity (C&S)	Laboratory test of urine for bacterial infection. Attempt to grow bacteria on a culture medium in order to identify it and determine which antibiotics it is sensitive to.
■ *Diagnostic Imaging*	
cystography (sis-TOG-rah-fee)	Process of instilling a contrast material or dye into the bladder by catheter to visualize the urinary bladder on x-ray.
excretory urography (EU) (EKS-kreh-tor-ee yoo-ROG-rah-fee)	Injecting dye into the bloodstream and then taking an x-ray to trace the action of the kidney as it excretes the dye.
intravenous pyelogram (IVP) (in-trah-VEE-nus PYE-eh-loh-gram)	Injecting a contrast medium into a vein and then taking an x-ray to visualize the renal pelvis.
kidneys, ureters, bladder (KUB)	X-ray taken of the abdomen demonstrating the kidneys, ureters, and bladder without using any contrast dye. Also called a *flat-plate abdomen*.

Diagnostic Prodedures *(continued)*

TERM	DEFINITION
retrograde pyelogram (RP) (RET-roh-grayd PYE-eh-loh-gram)	Diagnostic X-ray in which dye is inserted through the urethra to outline the bladder, ureters, and renal pelvis.

■ **Figure 11** Color enhanced retrograde pyelogram X-ray. Radiopaque dye outlines urinary bladder, ureters, and renal pelves. *(Clinique Ste. Catherine/CNRI/Science Photo Library/Photo Researchers, Inc.)*

TERM	DEFINITION
voiding cystourethrography (VCUG) (sis-toh-yoo-ree-THROG-rah-fee)	X-ray taken to visualize the urethra while the patient is voiding after a contrast dye has been placed in the bladder.

■ *Endoscopic Procedure*

TERM	DEFINITION
cystoscopy (cysto) (sis-TOSS-koh-pee)	Visual examination of the urinary bladder using an instrument called a *cystoscope*.

Therapeutic Procedures

TERM	DEFINITION
■ *Medical Treatments*	
catheterization (cath) (kath-eh-ter-ih-ZAY-shun)	Insertion of a tube through the urethra and into the urinary bladder for the purpose of withdrawing urine or inserting dye.
extracorporeal shockwave lithotripsy (ESWL) (eks-trah-cor-POR-ee-al shock-wave LITH-oh-trip-see)	Use of ultrasound waves to break up stones. Process does not require invasive surgery (see Figure 12 ■).
hemodialysis (HD) (hee-moh-dye-AL-ih-sis)	Use of an artificial kidney machine that filters the blood of a person to remove waste products. Use of this technique in patients who have defective kidneys is lifesaving (see Figure 13 ■).

■ **Figure 12** Extracorporeal shockwave lithotripsy, a non-invasive procedure using high frequency sound waves to shatter kidney stones.

- Beam focused on kidney stones
- Shockwave generator
- Reflector

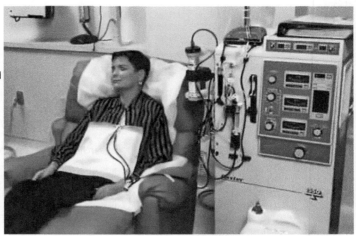

■ **Figure 13** Patient undergoing hemodialysis. Patient's blood passes through hemodialysis machine for cleansing and is then returned to her body.

 Therapeutic Procedures *(continued)*

TERM	DEFINITION
peritoneal dialysis (pair-ih-TOH-nee-al dye-AL-ih-sis)	Removal of toxic waste substances from the body by placing warm chemically balanced solutions into the peritoneal cavity. Wastes are filtered out of the blood across the peritoneum. Used in treating renal failure and certain poisonings.

■ **Figure 14** Peritoneal dialysis. Chemically balanced solution is placed into the abdominal cavity to draw impurities out of the bloodstream. It is removed after several hours.

- Collecting tube
- Peritoneal cavity
- Position of bag to receive used dialysis fluid

Therapeutic Procedures *(continued)*

TERM	DEFINITION
Surgical Treatments	
lithotripsy (LITH-oh-trip-see)	Destroying or crushing stones in the bladder or urethra.
meatotomy (mee-ah-TOT-oh-me)	Incision into the meatus in order to enlarge the opening of the urethra.
nephrolithotomy (nef-roh-lith-OT-oh-mee)	Surgical incision to directly remove stones from the kidney.
renal transplant	Surgical placement of a donor kidney.

■ **Figure 15** Figure illustrates location of transplanted donor kidney.

Transplanted kidney

Internal iliac artery and vein

Grafted ureter

External iliac artery and vein

Pharmacology

CLASSIFICATION	ACTION	GENERIC AND BRAND NAMES
antibiotic	Used to treat bacterial infections of the urinary tract.	ciprofloxacin, Cipro; nitrofurantoin, Macrobid
antispasmodic (an-tye-spaz-MAH-dik)	Medication to prevent or reduce bladder muscle spasms.	oxybutynin, Ditropan; neostigmine, Prostigmine
diuretic (dye-yoo-REH-tiks)	Medication that increases the volume of urine produced by the kidneys. Useful in the treatment of edema, kidney failure, heart failure, and hypertension.	furosemide, Lasix; spironolactone, Aldactone

Abbreviations

AGN	acute glomerulonephritis		**HD**	hemodialysis
ARF	acute renal failure		**H$_2$O**	water
ATN	acute tubular necrosis		**I&O**	intake and output
BNO	bladder neck obstruction		**IPD**	intermittent peritoneal dialysis
BUN	blood urea nitrogen		**IVP**	intravenous pyelogram
CAPD	continuous ambulatory peritoneal dialysis		**K$^+$**	potassium
cath	catheterization		**KUB**	kidney, ureter, bladder
CC	clean catch urine specimen		**mL**	milliliter
Cl$^-$	chloride		**Na$^+$**	sodium
CRF	chronic renal failure		**NS**	nephrotic syndrome
C&S	culture and sensitivity		**pH**	acidity or alkalinity of urine
cysto	cystoscopy		**RP**	retrograde pyelogram
ESRD	end-stage renal disease		**SG, sp. gr.**	specific gravity
ESWL	extracorporeal shockwave lithotripsy		**U/A, UA**	urinalysis
EU	excretory urography		**UC**	urine culture
GU	genitourinary		**UTI**	urinary tract infection
HCO$_3^-$	bicarbonate		**VCUG**	voiding cystourethrography

Chapter Review

Terminology Checklist

Below are all Anatomy and Physiology key terms, Word Building, Vocabulary, Pathology, Diagnostic, Therapeutic, and Pharmacology terms presented in this chapter. Use this list as a study tool by placing a check in the box in front of each term as you master its meaning.

- □ acute tubular necrosis
- □ afferent arteriole
- □ albumin
- □ antibiotic
- □ antispasmodic
- □ anuria
- □ azotemia
- □ bacteriuria
- □ bladder cancer
- □ bladder neck obstruction
- □ blood urea nitrogen
- □ Bowman's capsule
- □ calculus
- □ calyx
- □ catheter
- □ catheterization
- □ clean catch specimen
- □ collecting tubule
- □ cortex
- □ creatinine clearance
- □ cystalgia
- □ cystectomy
- □ cystic
- □ cystitis
- □ cystocele
- □ cystogram
- □ cystography
- □ cystolith
- □ cystopexy
- □ cystoplasty
- □ cystorrhagia
- □ cystoscope
- □ cystoscopy
- □ cystostomy
- □ cystotomy
- □ diabetic nephropathy
- □ distal convoluted tubule
- □ diuresis

- □ diuretic
- □ dysuria
- □ efferent arteriole
- □ electrolyte
- □ enuresis
- □ excretory urography
- □ external sphincter
- □ extracorporeal shockwave lithotripsy
- □ filtration
- □ frequency
- □ genitourinary system
- □ glomerular capsule
- □ glomerular filtrate
- □ glomerulonephritis
- □ glomerulus
- □ glycosuria
- □ hematuria
- □ hemodialysis
- □ hesitancy
- □ hilum
- □ homeostasis
- □ hydronephrosis
- □ internal sphincter
- □ interstitial cystitis
- □ intravenous pyelogram
- □ ketonuria
- □ kidneys
- □ kidneys, ureters, bladder
- □ lithotomy
- □ lithotripsy
- □ loop of Henle
- □ meatotomy
- □ medulla
- □ micturition
- □ nephrectomy
- □ nephritis
- □ nephrogram
- □ nephrolith

- □ nephrolithiasis
- □ nephrolithotomy
- □ nephrologist
- □ nephrology
- □ nephroma
- □ nephromalacia
- □ nephromegaly
- □ nephron
- □ nephropathy
- □ nephropexy
- □ nephroptosis
- □ nephrosclerosis
- □ nephrosis
- □ nephrostomy
- □ nephrotic syndrome
- □ nephrotomy
- □ neurogenic bladder
- □ nitrogenous wastes
- □ nocturia
- □ oliguria
- □ peritoneal dialysis
- □ peritubular capillaries
- □ polycystic kidneys
- □ polyuria
- □ proteinuria
- □ proximal convoluted tubule
- □ pyelitis
- □ pyelogram
- □ pyelonephritis
- □ pyeloplasty
- □ pyuria
- □ reabsorption
- □ renal
- □ renal artery
- □ renal cell carcinoma
- □ renal colic
- □ renal corpuscle
- □ renal failure

- □ renal papilla
- □ renal pelvis
- □ renal pyramid
- □ renal transplant
- □ renal tubule
- □ renal vein
- □ retrograde pyelogram
- □ retroperitoneal
- □ rugae
- □ secretion
- □ specific gravity
- □ stricture
- □ uremia
- □ ureteral

- □ ureterectasis
- □ ureterolith
- □ ureterostenosis
- □ ureters
- □ urethra
- □ urethral
- □ urethralgia
- □ urethritis
- □ urethrorrhagia
- □ urethroscope
- □ urethrostenosis
- □ urgency
- □ urinalysis
- □ urinary

- □ urinary bladder
- □ urinary incontinence
- □ urinary meatus
- □ urinary retention
- □ urinary tract infection
- □ urination
- □ urine
- □ urine culture and sensitivity
- □ urinometer
- □ urologist
- □ urology
- □ voiding
- □ voiding cystourethrography
- □ Wilm's tumor

Practice Exercises

A. Complete the following statements.

1. The functional or working units of the kidneys are the _nephrons_.

2. The three stages of urine production are _filtration_, _reabsorption_, and _secretion_.

3. Na⁺, K⁺, and Cl⁻ are collectively known as _electrolytes_.

4. The term that describes the location of the kidneys is _retroperitoneal_

5. The center of the concave side of the kidney is the _hilum_.

6. Bowman's capsule surrounds the _glomerulus_.

7. The tip of each renal pyramid opens into a(n) _calyx_.

8. There are _two_ ureters and _one_ urethra.

9. Urination can also be referred to as _voiding_ or _micturition_.

10. A(n) _urinalysis_ is the physical and chemical analysis of urine.

B. State the terms described using the combining forms indicated.

The combining form *nephr/o* refers to the kidney. Use it to write a term that means:

1. surgical fixation of the kidney _nephropexy_

2. x-ray record of the kidney _nephrogram_

3. condition of kidney stones _nephrolithiasis_

4. removal of a kidney _nephrectomy_

5. inflammation of the kidney _nephritis_

6. kidney disease ___nephropathy___

7. hardening of the kidney ___nephrosclerosis___

The combining form *cyst/o* refers to the urinary bladder. Use it to write a term that means:

8. inflammation of the bladder ___cystitis___

9. rapid bleeding from the bladder ___cystorrhagia___

10. surgical repair of the bladder ___cystoplasty___

11. instrument to view inside the bladder ___cystoscope___

12. bladder pain ___cystalgia___

The combining form *pyel/o* refers to the renal pelvis. Use it to write a term that means:

13. surgical repair of the renal pelvis ___pyelactomy___

14. inflammation of the renal pelvis ___pyelitis___

15. X-ray record of the renal pelvis ___pyelogram___

The combining form *ureter/o* refers to one or both of the ureters. Use it to write a term that means:

16. a ureteral stone ___ureterolith___

17. ureter dilation ___ureteractasis___

18. ureter narrowing ___ureterostenosis___

The combining form *urethr/o* refers to the urethra. Use it to write a term that means:

19. urethra inflammation ___urethritis___

20. instrument to view inside the urethra ___urethroscope___

C. Define the following combining forms and use them to form urinary terms.

	Definition	Urinary Term
1. ur/o	urine	urologist
2. meat/o	maatus	maatomy
3. cyst/o	urinary bladder	cystalgia
4. ren/o	kidney	renal
5. pyel/o	ranal pelvis	pyelogram
6. glycos/o	sugar, glucose	glycosuria
7. noct/i	night	nocturia
8. olig/o	scanty	oliguria

9. ureter/o   ureter   ureteral

10. glomerul/o   glomerulus   glomerulonephritis

D. Define each suffix and use it to form urinary terms.

	Meaning	Urinary Term
1. -ptosis	drooping	nephroptosis
2. -uria	condition of the urine	anuria
3. -lith	stone	ureterolith
4. -tripsy	surgical crushing	lithotripsy
5. -lithiasis	condition of stones	nephrolithiasis

E. Define the following terms.

1. micturition   another term for urination

2. diuretic   medication that increases the volume of urine produced by the kidneys.

3. renal colic   pain caused by a kidney stone

4. catheterization   insertion of a tube through the urethra & in the urinary bladder to withdraw urine or insert dye

5. pyelitis   renal pelvis inflammation

6. glomerulonephritis   inflammation of the kidney (primarily the glomerulus) - results in protein in the urine & hematuria

7. lithotomy   incision to remove a stone

8. enuresis   involuntary discharge of urine after the age by which bladder control should have been established

9. meatotomy   incision into the meatus

10. diabetic nephropathy   accumulation of damage to the glomerulus capillaries due to the chronic high blood sugars of diabetes mellitus.

11. urinalysis   lab test that consists of the physical, chemical & microscopic examination of urine

12. hesitancy   decrease of the force of the urine stream, often w/difficulty initiating the flow

F. Write the medical term that means:

1. absence of urine   anuria

2. blood in the urine   hematuria

3. kidney stone   nephrolith

4. crushing a stone   lithotripsy

5. inflammation of the urethra   urethritis

6. pus in the urine   pyuria

7. bacteria in the urine __bacteruria__

8. painful urination __dysuria__

9. ketones in the urine __ketonuria__

10. protein in the urine __proteinuria__

11. (too) much urine __polyuria__

G. Write the abbreviation for the following terms.

1. potassium __K+__

2. sodium __Na+__

3. urinalysis __U/A, UA__

4. blood urea nitrogen __BUN__

5. specific gravity __SG, sp.gr.__

6. intravenous pyelogram __IVP__

7. bladder neck obstruction __BNO__

8. intake and output __I&O__

9. acute tubular necrosis __ATN__

10. end stage renal disease __ESRD__

H. Identify the following abbreviations.

1. KUB __kidney, ureter, bladder__

2. cath __catheterization__

3. cysto __cystoscopy__

4. GU __genitourinary__

5. ESWL __extracorporeal shockwave lithotripsy__

6. UTI __urinary tract infection__

7. UC __urine culture__

8. RP __retrograde pyelogram__

9. ARF __acute renal failure__

10. BUN __blood urea nitrogen__

11. CRF __chronic renal failure__

12. H_2O __water__

I. Match each term to its definition.

1. __C__ Wilm's tumor

2. __g__ electrolytes

3. __h__ nephrons

a. kidney stones

b. feeling the need to urinate immediately

c. childhood malignant kidney tumor

4. ___i___ loop of Henle

5. ___f___ calyx

6. ___e___ incontinence

7. ___d___ hydronephrosis

8. ___b___ urgency

9. ___a___ nephrolithiasis

10. ___j___ polycystic kidneys

d. swelling of the kidney due to urine collecting in the renal pelvis

e. involuntary release of urine

f. collects urine as it is produced

g. sodium and potassium

h. functional unit of the kidneys

i. part of the renal tubule

j. multiple cysts in the kidneys

J. Use the following terms in the sentences below.

renal transplant   ureterectomy   intravenous pyelogram (IVP)

cystostomy   pyelolithectomy   nephropexy

renal biopsy   cystoscopy   urinary tract infection

1. Juan suffered from chronic renal failure. His sister, Maria, donated one of her normal kidneys to him, and he had a(n)
   renal transparent

2. Anesha's floating kidney needed surgical fixation. Her physician performed a surgical procedure known as
   nephropexy .

3. Kenya's physician stated that she had a general infection that he referred to as a UTI. The full name for this infection is
   urinary tract infection

4. The surgeons operated on Robert to remove calculi from his renal pelvis. The name of this surgery is
   pyelolithectomy

5. Charles had to have a small piece of his kidney tissue removed so that the physician could perform a microscopic evaluation. This procedure is called a(n) renal biopsy .

6. Naomi had to have one of her ureters removed due to a stricture. This procedure is called ureterectomy.

7. The physician had to create a temporary opening between Eric's bladder and his abdominal wall. This procedure is called
   cystostomy .

8. Sally's bladder was visually examined using a special instrument. This procedure is called a(n) cystoscopy .

9. The doctors believe that Jacob has a tumor of the right kidney. They are going to do a test called a(n)
   intravenous pyelogram that requires them to inject a radiopaque contrast medium intravenously so that they can see the kidney on x-ray.

K. Fill in the classification for each drug description, then match the brand name.

Drug Description	Classification	Brand Name
1. _____ Reduces bladder muscle spasms	_____	a. Lasix
2. _____ Treats bacterial infections	_____	b. Ditropan
3. _____ Increases volume of urine produced	_____	c. Cipro

Medical Record Analysis

Below is an item from a patient's medical record. Read it carefully, make sure you understand all the medical terms used, and then answer the questions that follow.

Discharge Summary

Admitting Diagnosis:	Severe right side pain, visible blood in his urine.
Final Diagnosis:	Pyelonephritis right kidney, complicated by chronic cystitis.
History of Present Illness:	Patient has long history of frequent bladder infections, but denies any recent lower pelvic pain or dysuria. Earlier today he had rapid onset of severe right side pain and is unable to stand fully erect. His temperature was 101°F, and his skin was sweaty and flushed. He was admitted from the ER for further testing and diagnosis.
Summary of Hospital Course:	Clean catch urinalysis revealed gross hematuria and pyuria, but no albuminuria. A culture and sensitivity was ordered to identify the pathogen, and a broad-spectrum IV antibiotic was started. An intravenous pyelogram indicated no calculi or obstructions in the ureters. Cystoscopy showed evidence of chronic cystitis, bladder irritation, and a bladder neck obstruction. The obstruction appears to be congenital and the probable cause of the chronic cystitis. The patient was catheterized to ensure complete emptying of the bladder, and fluids were encouraged. Patient responded well to the antibiotic therapy and fluids, and his symptoms improved.
Discharge Plans:	Patient was discharged home after three days in the hospital. He was switched to an oral antibiotic for the pyelonephritis and chronic cystitis. A repeat urinalysis is scheduled for next week. After all inflammation is corrected, will repeat cystoscopy to reevaluate bladder neck obstruction. Will discuss urethroplasty if it is indicated at that time.

Critical Thinking Questions

1. This patient has a long history of frequent bladder infections. What did the physician discover that explained this? _a congenital bladder neck obstruction_

2. Describe, in your own words, the patient's condition when he came to the emergency room. _severe right side pain, blood in urine, fever, sweaty & flushed skin_

3. This patient has gross hematuria. What do you think the term *gross* means in this context? _excessive / alot_

4. The following terms are not referred to in this chapter. Define each in your own words, using your text as a dictionary.
   a. congenital _defect present at birth_
   b. chronic _continuing, ongoing_
   c. pathogen _disease causing agent_
   d. oral _pertaining to the mouth_

Urinary System

5. Which of the following substances was not found in the patient's urine?
   a. protein
   b. pus
   c. blood

6. How are pyelonephritis and glomerulonephritis alike? How are they different?

Both are an inflammation of the kidney — pyelonephritis is renal pelvis & kidney while glomerulonephritis is primarily the glomerulus. Pyelonephritis can have white blood cells, bacteria & blood in the urine while glomerulonephritis results in blood & protein in the urine.

Chart Note Transcription

The chart note below contains eleven phrases that can be reworded with a medical term that you learned in this chapter. Each phrase is identified with an underline. Determine the medical term and write your answers in the space provided.

Current Complaint: A 36-year-old male was seen by the <u>specialist in the treatment of diseases of the urinary system</u> ❶ because of right flank pain and <u>blood in the urine</u>. ❷

Past History: Patient has a history of <u>bladder infection</u>; ❸ denies experiencing any symptoms for two years.

Signs and Symptoms: A <u>technique used to obtain an uncontaminated urine sample</u> ❹ obtained for <u>laboratory analysis of the urine</u> ❺ revealed blood in the urine, but no <u>pus in the urine</u>. ❻ A <u>kidney x-ray made after inserting dye into the bladder</u> ❼ was normal on the left, but dye was seen filling the right <u>tube between the kidney and bladder</u> ❽ only halfway to the kidney.

Diagnosis: <u>Stone in the tube between the kidney and the bladder</u> ❾ on the right.

Treatment: Patient underwent <u>the use of ultrasound waves to break up stones</u>.❿ Pieces of dissolved <u>kidney stones</u> ⓫ were flushed out, after which symptoms resolved.

❶ urologist

❷ hematuria

❸ cystitis

❹ clean catch

❺ urinalysis

❻ pyuria

❼ cystography

❽ ureter

❾ ureterolith

❿ extracorporeal shockwave lithotripsy (ESWL)

⓫ nephroliths

Labeling Exercise

A. System Review

Write the labels for this figure on the numbered lines provided.

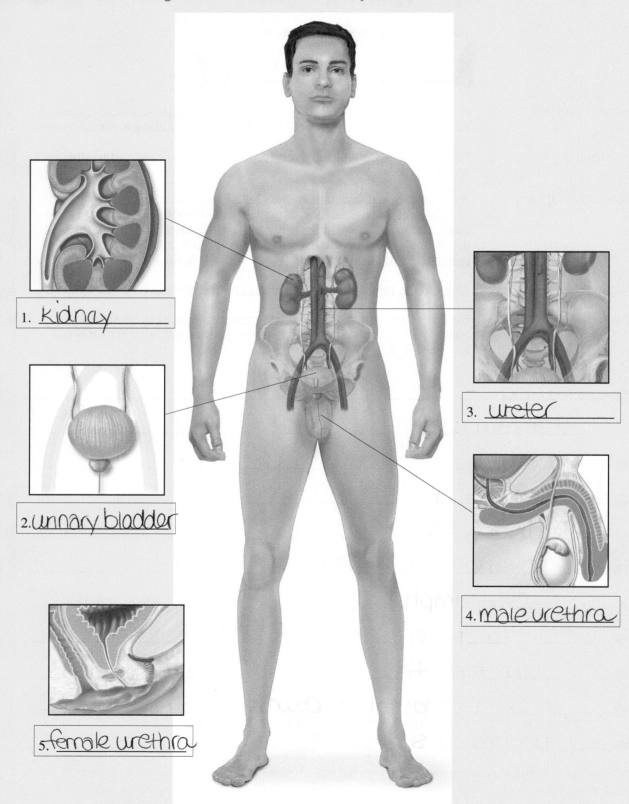

1. kidney

2. urinary bladder

3. ureter

4. male urethra

5. female urethra

B. Anatomy Challenge

1. Write the labels for this figure on the numbered lines provided.

1. Cortex
2. medulla
3. Calyx
4. renal pelvis
5. renal papilla
6. renal pyramid
7. ureter

2. Write the labels for this figure on the numbered lines provided.

7. distal convoluted tubule
1. efferent arteriole
2. Glomerular (Bowman's) Capsule
3. Glomerulus
4. afferent arteriole
5. proximal convoluted tubule
6. descending loop of Henle
8. collecting tubule
9. ascending loop of Henle
10. peritubular capillaries

Urinary System

Multimedia Preview

Additional interactive resources and activities for this chapter can be found on the Companion Website.

Website Highlights—www.prenhall.com/fremgen

DRUG UPDATES

Click here and take advantage of the free-access on-line study guide that accompanies your textbook. You'll find a feature that allows you to search for current information on the drugs discussed in this chapter. By clicking on this URL you'll also access links to download mp3 audio reviews, current news articles, review questions, and an audio glossary.

Reproductive System

Learning Objectives

Upon completion of this chapter, you will be able to:

- Identify and define the combining forms and suffixes introduced in this chapter.
- Correctly spell and pronounce medical terms and major anatomical structures relating to the reproductive systems.
- Locate and describe the major organs of the reproductive systems and their functions.
- Use medical terms to describe circumstances relating to pregnancy.
- Identify the symptoms and origin of sexually transmitted diseases.
- Build and define reproductive system medical terms from word parts.
- Identify and define reproductive system vocabulary terms.
- Identify and define selected reproductive system pathology terms.
- Identify and define selected reproductive system diagnostic procedures.
- Identify and define selected reproductive system therapeutic procedures.
- Identify and define selected medications relating to the reproductive systems.
- Define selected abbreviations associated with the reproductive systems.

From Chapter 10 of *Medical Terminology: A Living Language,* 4/e. Bonnie F. Fremgen. Suzanne S. Frucht. Copyright © 2009 by Pearson Education. Published by Prentice Hall. All rights reserved.

Section I: Female Reproductive System at a Glance

Function

The female reproductive system produces ova (the female reproductive cell), provides a location for fertilization and growth of a baby, and secretes female sex hormones. In addition, the breasts produce milk to nourish the newborn.

Organs

breasts
fallopian tubes
ovaries
uterus
vagina
vulva

Combining Forms

amni/o	amnion	mast/o	breast
cervic/o	neck, cervix	men/o	menses, menstruation
chori/o	chorion	metr/o	uterus
colp/o	vagina	nat/o	birth
culd/o	cul-de-sac	oophor/o	ovary
embry/o	embryo	ov/o	egg
episi/o	vulva	ovari/o	ovary
fet/o	fetus	perine/o	perineum
gynec/o	woman, female	salping/o	fallopian tubes, uterine tubes
hymen/o	hymen	uter/o	uterus
hyster/o	uterus	vagin/o	vagina
lact/o	milk	vulv/o	vulva
mamm/o	breast		

Suffixes Relating

-arche	beginning
-cyesis	state of pregnancy
-gravida	pregnancy
-para	to bear (offspring)
-partum	childbirth
-salpinx	fallopian tube
-tocia	labor, childbirth

Female Reproductive System Illustrated

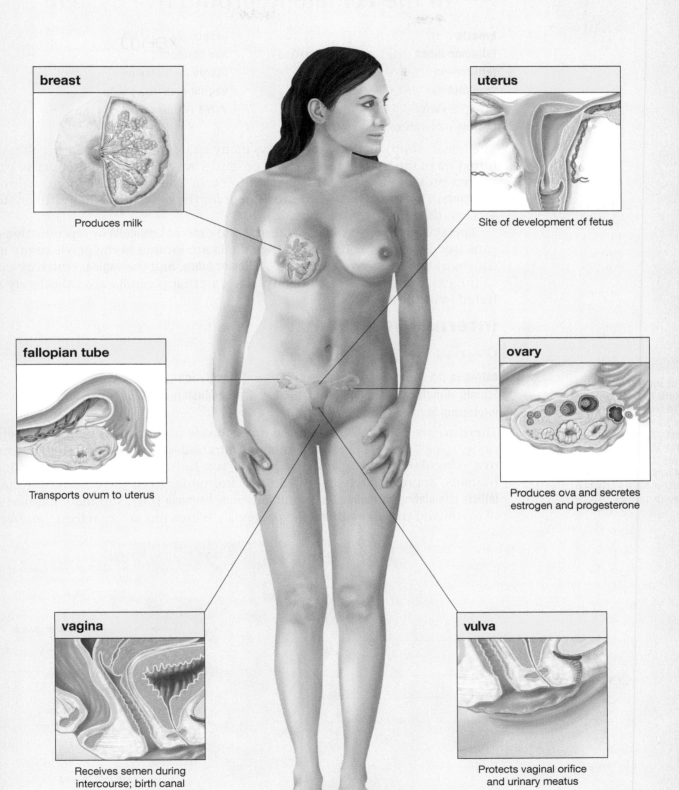

breast

Produces milk

uterus

Site of development of fetus

fallopian tube

Transports ovum to uterus

ovary

Produces ova and secretes estrogen and progesterone

vagina

Receives semen during intercourse; birth canal

vulva

Protects vaginal orifice and urinary meatus

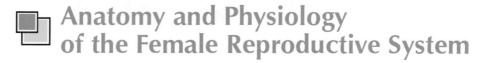

Anatomy and Physiology of the Female Reproductive System

breasts
fallopian tubes (fah-LOH-pee-an TOOBS)
fertilization
genitalia (jen-ih-TAY-lee-ah)
ova (OH-vah)
ovaries (OH-vah-reez)

pregnancy
sex hormones
uterus (YOO-ter-us)
vagina (vah-JIGH-nah)
vulva (VULL-vah)

The female reproductive system plays many vital functions that ensure the continuation of the human race. First, it produces **ova**, the female reproductive cells. It then provides a place for **fertilization** to occur and for a baby to grow during **pregnancy**. The **breasts** provide nourishment for the newborn. Finally, this system secretes the female **sex hormones**.

This system consists of both internal and external **genitalia** or reproductive organs (see Figure 1 ■). The internal genitalia are located in the pelvic cavity and consist of the **uterus**, two **ovaries**, two **fallopian tubes**, and the **vagina**, which extends to the external surface of the body. The external genitalia are collectively referred to as the **vulva**.

Internal Genitalia

Ovaries

estrogen (ESS-troh-jen)
follicle stimulating hormone (FOLL-ih-kl)
luteinizing hormone (loo-teh-NIGH-zing)

ovulation (ov-yoo-LAY-shun)
progesterone (proh-JES-ter-ohn)

There are two ovaries, one located on each side of the uterus within the pelvic cavity (see Figure 1). These are small almond-shaped glands that produce ova (singular is *ovum*) and the female sex hormones (see Figure 2 ■). In humans, approximately every 28 days, hormones from the anterior pituitary, **follicle stimulating hormone** (FSH) and **luteinizing hormone** (LH), stimulate maturation of ovum and trigger **ovulation**, the process by which one ovary releases an ovum

> **Med Term Tip**
>
> The singular for egg is *ovum*. The plural term for many eggs is *ova*. The term *ova* is not used exclusively when discussing the human reproductive system. For instance, testing the stool for ova and parasites is used to detect the presence of parasites or their ova in the digestive tract, a common cause for severe diarrhea.

■ Figure 1 The female reproductive system, sagittal view showing organs of the system in relation to the urinary bladder and rectum.

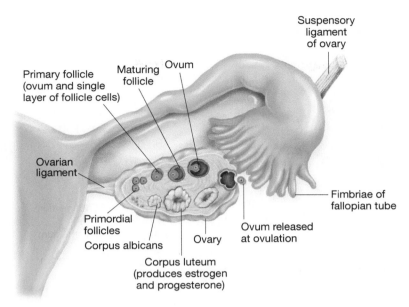

■ **Figure 2** Structure of the ovary and fallopian (uterine) tube. Figure illustrates stages of ovum development and the relationship of the ovary to the fallopian tube.

(see Figure 3 ■). The principal female sex hormones produced by the ovaries, **estrogen** and **progesterone**, stimulate the lining of the uterus to be prepared to receive a fertilized ovum. These hormones are also responsible for the female secondary sexual characteristics.

Fallopian Tubes

conception (con-SEP-shun)	**oviducts** (OH-vih-ducts)
fimbriae (FIM-bree-ay)	**uterine tubes** (YOO-ter-in)

The fallopian tubes, also called the **uterine tubes** or **oviducts**, are approximately 5½ inches long and run from the area around each ovary to either side of the upper portion of the uterus (see Figures 4 ■ and 5 ■). As they near the ovaries, the unattached ends of these two tubes expand into finger-like projections called

Med Term Tip

When the fertilized egg adheres or implants to the fallopian tube instead of moving into the uterus, a condition called *tubal pregnancy* exists. There is not enough room in the fallopian tube for the fetus to grow normally. Implantation of the fertilized egg in any location other than the uterus is called an *ectopic pregnancy*. *Ectopic* is a general term meaning "in the wrong place."

■ **Figure 3** Enhanced color scanning electron micrograph showing an ovum (pink) released by the ovary at ovulation surrounded by follicle (white) tissue. The external surface of the ovary is brown in this photo. *(P.M. Motta and J. Van Blekrom/Science Photo Library/Photo Researchers, Inc.)*

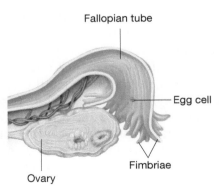

■ **Figure 4** Fallopian (uterine) tube, longitudinal view showing released ovum within the fallopian tube.

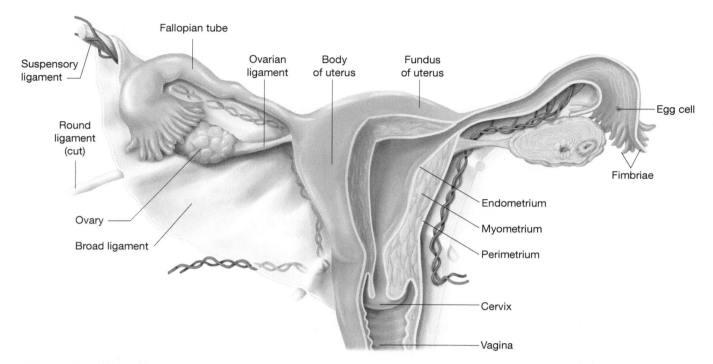

Suspensory ligament

Fallopian tube

Ovarian ligament

Body of uterus

Fundus of uterus

Egg cell

Round ligament (cut)

Fimbriae

Endometrium

Myometrium

Perimetrium

Ovary

Broad ligament

Cervix

Vagina

■ **Figure 5** The uterus. Cutaway view shows regions of the uterus and cervix and its relationship to the fallopian (uterine) tubes and vagina.

fimbriae. The fimbriae catch an ovum after ovulation and direct it into the fallopian tube. The fallopian tube can then propel the ovum from the ovary to the uterus so that it can implant. The meeting of the egg and sperm, called fertilization or **conception**, normally takes place within the upper one-half of the fallopian tubes.

Uterus

anteflexion (an-tee-FLEK-shun)
cervix (SER-viks)
corpus (KOR-pus)
endometrium (en-doh-MEE-tre-um)
fundus (FUN-dus)
menarche (men-AR-kee)

menopause (MEN-oh-pawz)
menstrual period (MEN-stroo-all)
menstruation (men-stroo-AY-shun)
myometrium (my-oh-MEE-tre-um)
perimetrium (pear-ee-MEE-tre-um)

The uterus is a hollow, pear-shaped organ that contains a thick muscular wall, a mucous membrane lining, and a rich supply of blood (see Figure 5). It lies in the center of the pelvic cavity between the bladder and the rectum. It is normally bent slightly forward, which is called **anteflexion**, and is held in position by strong fibrous ligaments anchored in the outer layer of the uterus, called the **perimetrium** (see Figure 1). The uterus has three sections: the **fundus** or upper portion, between where the fallopian tubes connect to the uterus; **corpus** or body, which is the central portion; and **cervix** (Cx), or lower portion, also called the neck of the uterus, which opens into the vagina.

The inner layer, or **endometrium**, of the uterine wall contains a rich blood supply. The endometrium reacts to hormonal changes every month that prepare it to receive a fertilized ovum. In a normal pregnancy the fertilized ovum implants in the endometrium, which can then provide nourishment and protection for the developing baby. Contractions of the thick muscular walls of the uterus, called the **myometrium**, assist in propelling the fetus through the birth canal at delivery.

Med Term Tip

During pregnancy, the height of the fundus is an important measurement for estimating the stage of pregnancy and the size of the fetus. Following birth, massaging the fundus with pressure applied in a circular pattern stimulates the uterine muscle to contract to help stop bleeding. Patients may be more familiar with a common term for uterus, *womb*. However, the correct medical term is uterus.

If a pregnancy is not established, the endometrium is sloughed off, resulting in **menstruation** or the **menstrual period.** During a pregnancy, the lining of the uterus does not leave the body but remains to nourish the unborn child. A girl's first menstrual period (usually during her early teenage years) is called **menarche**, while the ending of menstrual activity and childbearing years is called **menopause**. This generally occurs between the ages of 40 and 55.

Vagina

Bartholin's glands (BAR-toh-linz)   **vaginal orifice** (VAJ-ih-nal OR-ih-fis)
hymen (HIGH-men)

The vagina is a muscular tube, lined with mucous membrane that extends from the cervix of the uterus to the outside of the body (see Figure 6 ■). The vagina allows for the passage of the menstrual flow. In addition, during intercourse, it receives the male's penis and semen, which is the fluid containing sperm. The vagina also serves as the birth canal through which the baby passes during a normal vaginal birth.

The **hymen** is a thin membranous tissue that partially covers the external vaginal opening or **vaginal orifice**. This membrane is broken by the use of tampons, during physical activity, or during sexual intercourse. A pair of glands, called **Bartholin's glands**, are located on either side of the vaginal orifice and secrete mucus for lubrication during intercourse.

Vulva

clitoris (KLIT-oh-ris)   **labia minora** (LAY-bee-ah min-NOR-ah)
erectile tissue (ee-REK-tile)   **perineum** (pair-ih-NEE-um)
labia majora (LAY-bee-ah mah-JOR-ah)   **urinary meatus** (YOO-rih-nair-ee mee-AY-tus)

The vulva is a general term that refers to the group of structures that make up the female external genitalia. The **labia majora** and **labia minora** are folds of skin that serve as protection for the genitalia, the vaginal orifice, and the **urinary meatus** (see Figure 7 ■). Since the urinary tract and the reproductive organs are located in proximity to one another and each contains mucous membranes that can transport infection, there is a danger of infection entering the urinary tract. The **clitoris** is a small organ containing sensitive **erectile tissue** that is aroused during sexual stimulation and corresponds to the penis in the male. The region between the vaginal orifice and the anus is referred to as the **perineum**.

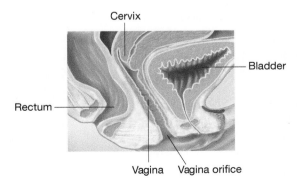

■ **Figure 6** The vagina, sagittal section showing the location of the vagina and its relationship to the cervix, uterus, rectum, and bladder.

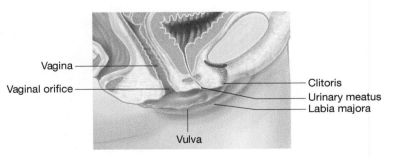

■ **Figure 7** The vulva, sagittal section illustrating how the labia major and labia minora cover and protect the vaginal orifice, clitoris, and urinary meatus.

Breast

areola (ah-REE-oh-la)	**mammary glands** (MAM-ah-ree)
lactation (lak-TAY-shun)	**nipple**
lactiferous ducts (lak-TIF-er-us)	**nurse**
lactiferous glands (lak-TIF-er-us)	

The breasts, or **mammary glands**, play a vital role in the reproductive process because they produce milk, a process called **lactation**, to nourish the newborn. The size of the breasts, which varies greatly from woman to woman, has no bearing on the ability to **nurse** or feed a baby. Milk is produced by the **lactiferous glands** and is carried to the **nipple** by the **lactiferous ducts** (see Figure 8 ■). The **areola** is the pigmented area around the nipple. As long as the breast is stimulated by the nursing infant, the breast will continue to secrete milk.

Pregnancy

amnion (AM-nee-on)	**gestation** (jess-TAY-shun)
amniotic fluid (am-nee-OT-ik)	**placenta** (plah-SEN-tah)
chorion (KOR-ree-on)	**premature**
embryo (EM-bree-oh)	**umbilical cord** (um-BILL-ih-kal KORD)
fetus (FEE-tus)	

Pregnancy refers to the period of time during which a baby grows and develops in its mother's uterus (see Figure 9 ■). The normal length of time for a pregnancy, **gestation**, is 40 weeks. If a baby is born before completing at least 37 weeks of gestation, it is considered **premature**.

Mid Term Tip

The term *abortion* (AB) has different meanings for medical professionals and the general population. The general population equates the term *abortion* specifically with the planned termination of a pregnancy. However, to the medical community, abortion is a broader medical term meaning that a pregnancy has ended before a fetus is *viable*, meaning before it can live on its own.

■ **Figure 8** The breast, cutaway view showing both internal and external features.

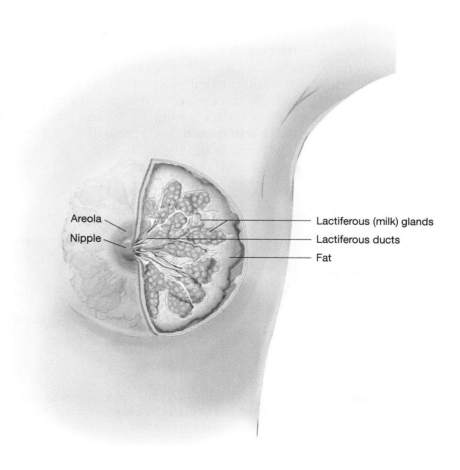

Areola
Nipple
Lactiferous (milk) glands
Lactiferous ducts
Fat

Uterus

Placenta

Fundus
of uterus

Umbilical
cord

Amniotic
fluid

Cervix
of uterus

Rectum

Symphysis pubis

Urinary bladder

Vagina (birth canal)

Perineum

■ **Figure 9** A full-term
pregnancy. Images illustrates
position of the fetus and the
structures associated with
pregnancy.

During pregnancy the female body undergoes many changes. In fact, all of the body systems become involved in the development of a healthy infant. From the time the fertilized egg implants in the uterus until approximately the end of the eighth week, the infant is referred to as an **embryo** (see Figure 10 ■). During this period all the major organs and body systems are formed. Following the embryo stage and lasting until birth, the infant is called a **fetus** (see Figure 11 ■). During this time, the longest period of gestation, the organs mature and begin to function.

The fetus receives nourishment from its mother by way of the **placenta**, which is a spongy, blood-filled organ that forms in the uterus next to the fetus. The placenta is commonly referred to as the afterbirth. The fetus is attached to the

Med Term Tip

During the embryo stage of gestation, the organs and organ systems of the body are formed. Therefore, this is a very common time for *congenital anomalies*, or birth defects, to occur. This may happen before the woman is even aware of being pregnant.

■ **Figure 10** Photograph illustrating the development of an embryo. *(Petit Format/Nestle/Photo Researchers, Inc.)*

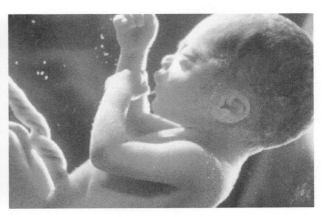

■ **Figure 11** Photograph illustrating the development of a fetus. *(Petit Format/Nestle/Photo Researchers, Inc.)*

placenta by way of the **umbilical cord** and is surrounded by two membranous sacs, the **amnion** and the **chorion**. The amnion is the innermost sac, and it holds the **amniotic fluid** in which the fetus floats. The chorion is an outer, protective sac and also forms part of the placenta.

Labor and Delivery

breech presentation	**effacement** (eh-FACE-ment)
crowning	**expulsion stage** (ex-PULL-shun)
delivery	**labor**
dilation stage (dye-LAY-shun)	**placental stage** (plah-SEN-tal)

Labor is the actual process of expelling the fetus from the uterus and through the vagina. The first stage is referred to as the **dilation stage**, in which the uterine muscle contracts strongly to expel the fetus (see Figure 12A ■). During this

A

DILATION STAGE:
Uterine contractions dilate cervix

B

EXPULSION STAGE:
Birth of baby or expulsion

C

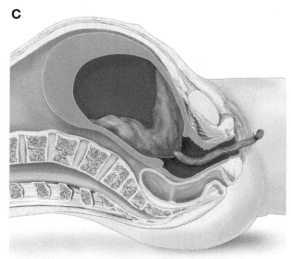

PLACENTAL STAGE:
Delivery of placenta

■ **Figure 12** The stages of labor and delivery. A) During the dilation stage the cervix thins and dilates to 10 cm. B) During the expulsion stage the infant is delivered. C) During the placental stage the placenta is delivered.

■ **Figure 13** A breech birth. This image illustrates a newborn that has been delivered buttocks first.

process the fetus presses on the cervix and causes it to dilate or expand. As the cervix dilates, it also becomes thinner, referred to as **effacement**. When the cervix is completely dilated to 10 centimeters, the second stage of labor begins (see Figure 12B ■). This is the **expulsion stage** and ends with **delivery** of the baby. Generally, the head of the baby appears first, which is referred to as **crowning** (see Figure 10). In some cases the baby's buttocks will appear first, and this is referred to as a **breech presentation** (see Figure 13 ■). The last stage of labor is the **placental stage** (see Figure 12C ■). Immediately after childbirth, the uterus continues to contract, causing the placenta to be expelled through the vagina.

Word Building

The following list contains examples of medical terms built directly from word parts. The definition for these terms can be determined by a straightforward translation of the word parts.

COMBINING FORM	COMBINED WITH	MEDICAL TERM	DEFINITION
amni/o	-otomy	**amniotomy** (am-nee-OT-oh-mee)	incision into amnion
	-tic	**amniotic** (am-nee-OT-ik)	pertaining to the amnion
	-rrhea	**amniorrhea** (am-nee-oh-REE-ah)	flow of fluid from amnion
cervic/o	-ectomy	**cervicectomy** (ser-vih-SEK-toh-mee)	removal of cervix
	-al	**cervical** (SER-vih-kal)	pertaining to the cervix
	endo- -itis	**endocervicitis** (en-doh-ser-vih-SIGH-tis)	inflammation within cervix
chori/o	-nic	**chorionic** (koh-ree-ON-ik)	pertaining to the chorion
colp/o	-scope	**colposcope** (KOL-poh-scope)	instrument to view inside vagina

Word Building *(continued)*

COMBINING FORM	COMBINED WITH	MEDICAL TERM	DEFINITION
embry/o	-nic	**embryonic** (em-bree-ON-ik)	pertaining to the embryo
episi/o	-rrhaphy	**episiorrhaphy** (eh-peez-ee-OR-ah-fee)	suture of vulva
fet/o	-al	**fetal** (FEE-tall)	pertaining to the fetus
gynec/o	-ologist	**gynecologist** (gigh-neh-KOL-oh-jist)	specialist in female reproductive system
hymen/o	-ectomy	**hymenectomy** (high-men-EK-toh-mee)	removal of the hymen
hyster/o	-pexy	**hysteropexy** (HISS-ter-oh-pek-see)	surgical fixation of the uterus
	-rrhexis	**hysterorrhexis** (hiss-ter-oh-REK-sis)	ruptured uterus
	-ectomy	**hysterectomy** (hiss-ter-EK-toh-mee)	surgical removal of the uterus
lact/o	-ic	**lactic** (LAK-tik)	pertaining to milk
	-rrhea	**lactorrhea** (lak-toh-REE-ah)	milk discharge
lapar/o	-otomy	**laparotomy** (lap-ah-ROT-oh-mee)	incision into the abdomen
	-scope	**laparoscope** (LAP-ah-row-scope)	instrument to view inside the abdomen
mamm/o	-gram	**mammogram** (MAM-moh-gram)	record of the breast
	-ary	**mammary** (MAM-mah-ree)	pertaining to the breast
	-plasty	**mammoplasty** (MAM-moh-plas-tee)	surgical repair of breast
mast/o	-algia	**mastalgia** (mas-TAL-jee-ah)	breast pain
	-itis	**mastitis** (mas-TYE-tis)	inflammation of the breast
	-ectomy	**mastectomy** (mass-TEK-toh-mee)	removal of the breast
men/o	a- -rrhea	**amenorrhea** (ah-men-oh-REE-ah)	no menstrual flow
	dys- -rrhea	**dysmenorrhea** (dis-men-oh-REE-ah)	painful menstrual flow
	oligo- -rrhea	**oligomenorrhea** (ol-lih-goh-men-oh-REE-ah)	scanty menstrual flow
	-rrhagia	**menorrhagia** (men-oh-RAY-jee-ah)	abnormal, rapid menstrual flow
metr/o	endo- -itis	**endometritis** (en-doh-meh-TRY-tis)	inflammation within the uterus

> **Med Term Tip**
>
> Word watch—Be careful when using the combining form *metr/o* meaning "uterus" and the suffix *–metry* meaning "process of measuring."

	peri- -itis	**perimetritis** (pair-ih-meh-TRY-tis)	inflammation around the uterus
	-rrhea	**metrorrhea** (meh-troh-REE-ah)	flow from uterus
	-rrhagia	**metrorrhagia** (meh-troh-RAY-jee-ah)	rapid (menstrual) blood flow from uterus
nat/o	neo-	**neonate** (NEE-oh-nayt)	newborn
	neo- -ologist	**neonatologist** (nee-oh-nay-TALL-oh-jist)	specialist in the study of the newborn
oophor/o	-ectomy	**oophorectomy** (oh-off-oh-REK-toh-mee)	removal of the ovary
	-itis	**oophoritis** (oh-off-oh-RIGH-tis)	inflammation of the ovary

Word Building (continued)

COMBINING FORM	COMBINED WITH	MEDICAL TERM	DEFINITION
ovari/o	-an	**ovarian** (oh-VAIR-ee-an)	pertaining to the ovary
salping/o	-cyesis	**salpingocyesis** (sal-ping-goh-sigh-EE-sis)	tubal pregnancy
	-ectomy	**salpingectomy** (sal-ping-JECK-toh-mee)	removal of the fallopian tube
	-itis	**salpingitis** (sal-ping-JIGH-tis)	inflammation of the fallopian tubes
uter/o	-ine	**uterine** (YOO-ter-in)	pertaining to the uterus
vagin/o	-al	**vaginal** (VAJ-ih-nal)	pertaining to the vagina
	-itis	**vaginitis** (vaj-ih-NIGH-tis)	inflammation of the vagina

PREFIX	SUFFIX	MEDICAL TERM	DEFINITION
pseudo-	-cyesis	**pseudocyesis** (soo-doh-sigh-EE-sis)	false pregnancy
nulli-	-gravida	**nulligravida** (null-ih-GRAV-ih-dah)	no pregnancies
primi-		**primigravida** (prem-ih-GRAV-ih-dah)	first pregnancy
multi-		**multigravida** (mull-tih-GRAV-ih-dah)	multiple pregnancies
nulli-	-para	**nullipara** (null-IP-ah-rah)	no births
primi-		**primipara** (prem-IP-ah-rah)	first birth
multi-		**multipara** (mull-TIP-ah-rah)	multiple births
ante-	-partum	**antepartum** (an-tee-PAR-tum)	before birth
post-		**postpartum** (post-PAR-tum)	after birth
hemato-	-salpinx	**hematosalpinx** (hee-mah-toh-SAL-pinks)	blood in fallopian tube
pyo-		**pyosalpinx** (pie-oh-SAL-pinks)	pus in fallopian tube
dys-	-tocia	**dystocia** (dis-TOH-she-ah)	difficult labor and childbirth

Vocabulary

TERM	DEFINITION
atresia (ah-TREE-she-ah)	Congenital lack of a normal body opening.
barrier contraception (kon-trah-SEP-shun)	Prevention of a pregnancy using a device to prevent sperm from meeting an ovum. Examples include condoms, diaphragms, and cervical caps.
colostrum (kuh-LOS-trum)	Thin fluid first secreted by the breast after delivery. It does not contain much protein, but is rich in antibodies.
fraternal twins	Twins that develop from two different ova fertilized by two different sperm. Although twins, these siblings do not have identical DNA.
gynecology (GYN) (gigh-neh-KOL-oh-jee)	Branch of medicine specializing in the diagnosis and treatment of conditions of the female reproductive system. Physician is called a *gynecologist*.
hormonal contraception	Use of hormones to block ovulation and prevent contraception. May be in the form of a pill, a patch, an implant under the skin, or injection.
identical twins	Twins that develop from the splitting of one fertilized ovum. These siblings have identical DNA.

Vocabulary *(continued)*

TERM	DEFINITION
infertility	Inability to produce children. Generally defined as no pregnancy after properly timed intercourse for 1 year.
intrauterine device (IUD) (in-trah-YOO-ter-in)	Device that is inserted into the uterus by a physician for the purpose of contraception.
■ **Figure 14** Photographs illustrating the shape of two different intrauterine devices (IUDs). *(Jules Selmes and Debi Treloar/Dorling Kindersley Media Library)*	
meconium (meh-KOH-nee-um)	First bowel movement of a newborn. It is greenish-black in color and consists of mucus and bile.
neonatology (nee-oh-nay-TALL-oh-jee)	Branch of medicine specializing in the diagnosis and treatment of conditions involving newborns. Physician is called a *neonatologist*.
obstetrics (OB) (ob-STET-riks)	Branch of medicine specializing in the diagnosis and treatment of women during pregnancy and childbirth, and immediately after childbirth. Physician is called an *obstetrician*.
premenstrual syndrome (PMS) (pre-MEN-stroo-al SIN-drohm)	Symptoms that develop just prior to the onset of a menstrual period, which can include irritability, headache, tender breasts, and anxiety.
puberty (PEW-ber-tee)	Beginning of menstruation and the ability to reproduce.

■ Pathology

TERM	DEFINITION
■ *Ovary*	
ovarian carcinoma (oh-VAY-ree-an kar-sih-NOH-mah)	Cancer of the ovary.
ovarian cyst (oh-VAY-ree-an SIST)	Cyst that develops within the ovary. These may be multiple cysts and may rupture, causing pain and bleeding.
■ *Uterus*	
cervical cancer (SER-vih-kal CAN-ser)	Malignant growth in the cervix. Some cases are caused by the *human papilloma virus* (HPV), a sexually transmitted virus for which there is now a vaccine. An especially difficult type of cancer to treat that causes 5 percent of the cancer deaths in women. Pap smear tests have helped to detect early cervical cancer.
endometrial cancer (en-doh-MEE-tree-al CAN-ser)	Cancer of the endometrial lining of the uterus.

Pathology *(continued)*

TERM	DEFINITION
fibroid tumor (FIGH-broyd TOO-mor) ■ Figure 15 Common sites for the development of fibroid tumors.	Benign tumor or growth that contains fiber-like tissue. Uterine fibroid tumors are the most common tumors in women. Under the perimetrium Within the myometrium Under the endometrium
menometrorrhagia (men-oh-met-thro-RAY-jee-ah)	Excessive bleeding during the menstrual period and at intervals between menstrual periods.
prolapsed uterus (pro-LAPS'D YOO-ter-us)	Fallen uterus that can cause the cervix to protrude through the vaginal opening. Generally caused by weakened muscles from vaginal delivery or as the result of pelvic tumors pressing down.

■ Vagina

TERM	DEFINITION
candidiasis (kan-dih-DYE-ah-sis)	Yeast infection of the skin and mucous membranes that can result in white plaques on the tongue and vagina.

Med Term Tip

The term *candida* comes from a Latin term meaning "dazzling white." Candida is the scientific name for yeast and refers to the very white discharge that is the hallmark of a yeast infection.

TERM	DEFINITION
cystocele (SIS-toh-seel)	Hernia or outpouching of the bladder that protrudes into the vagina. This may cause urinary frequency and urgency.
rectocele (REK-toh-seel)	Protrusion or herniation of the rectum into the vagina.
toxic shock syndrome (TSS)	Rare and sometimes fatal staphylococcus infection that generally occurs in menstruating women. Initial infection of the vagina is associated with prolonged wearing of a super-absorbent tampon.

■ Pelvic Cavity

TERM	DEFINITION
endometriosis (en-doh-mee-tree-OH-sis)	Abnormal condition of endometrium tissue appearing throughout the pelvis or on the abdominal wall. This tissue is normally found within the uterus.
pelvic inflammatory disease (PID) (PELL-vik in-FLAM-mah-toh-ree dih-ZEEZ)	Chronic or acute infection, usually bacterial, that has ascended through the female reproductive organs and out into the pelvic cavity. May result in scarring that interferes with fertility.

■ Breast

TERM	DEFINITION
breast cancer	Malignant tumor of the breast. Usually forms in the milk-producing gland tissue or the lining of the milk ducts (see Figure 16A ■).

Figure 16
Comparison of breast
cancer and fibrocystic
disease. A) Breast with
a malignant tumor
growing in the
lactiferous gland
and duct. B) The
location of a fibrocystic
lump in the adipose
tissue
covering the breast.

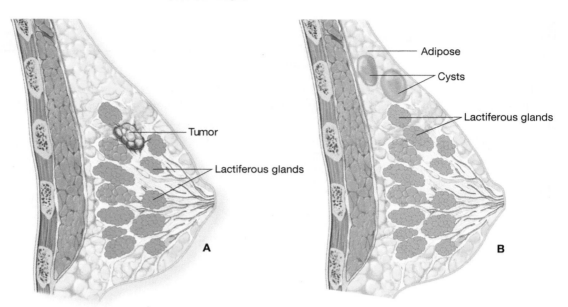

Pathology *(continued)*

TERM	DEFINITION
fibrocystic breast disease (figh-bro-SIS-tik)	Benign cysts forming in the breast (see Figure 16B ■).
■ *Pregnancy*	
abruptio placentae (ah-BRUP-tee-oh plah-SEN-tee)	Emergency condition in which the placenta tears away from the uterine wall prior to delivery of the infant. Requires immediate delivery of the baby.
eclampsia (eh-KLAMP-see-ah)	Convulsive seizures and coma occurring in the woman between the twentieth week of pregnancy and the first week of postpartum. Preceded by preeclampsia.
hemolytic disease of the newborn (HDN) (hee-moh-LIT-ik)	Condition developing in the baby when the mother's blood type is Rh-negative and the baby's blood is Rh-positive. Antibodies in the mother's blood enter the fetus's bloodstream through the placenta and destroy fetus's red blood cells causing anemia, jaundice, and enlargement of the spleen. Treatment is early diagnosis and blood transfusion. Also called *erythroblastosis fetalis.*
placenta previa (plah-SEN-tah PREE-vee-ah)	A placenta that is implanted in the lower portion of the uterus and, in turn, blocks the birth canal.

■ Figure 17 Placenta previa,
longitudinal section showing the
placenta growing over the opening
into the cervix.

Pathology *(continued)*

TERM	DEFINITION
preeclampsia (pre-eh-KLAMP-see-ah)	Metabolic disease of pregnancy. If untreated, it may result in true eclampsia. Symptoms include hypertension, headaches, albumin in the urine, and edema. Also called *toxemia.*
prolapsed umbilical cord (pro-LAPS'D um-BILL-ih-kal)	When the umbilical cord of the baby is expelled first during delivery and is squeezed between the baby's head and the vaginal wall. This presents an emergency situation since the baby's circulation is compromised.
spontaneous abortion	Unplanned loss of a pregnancy due to the death of the embryo or fetus before the time it is viable, commonly referred to as a *miscarriage.*
stillbirth	Birth in which a viable-aged fetus dies shortly before or at the time of delivery.

 # Diagnostic Procedures

TERM	DEFINITION
■ *Clinical Laboratory Tests*	
Pap (Papanicolaou) **smear** (pap-ah-NIK-oh-low)	Test for the early detection of cancer of the cervix named after the developer of the test, George Papanicolaou, a Greek physician. A scraping of cells is removed from the cervix for examination under a microscope.
pregnancy test (PREG-nan-see)	Chemical test that can determine a pregnancy during the first few weeks. Can be performed in a physician's office or with a home-testing kit.
■ *Diagnostic Imaging*	
hysterosalpingography (HSG) (hiss-ter-oh-sal-pin-GOG-rah-fee)	Taking of an X-ray after injecting radiopaque material into the uterus and fallopian tubes.
mammography (mam-OG-rah-fee)	Using X-ray to diagnose breast disease, especially breast cancer.
pelvic ultrasonography (PELL-vik-ull-trah-son-OG-rah-fee)	Use of ultrasound waves to produce an image or photograph of an organ, such as the uterus, ovaries, or fetus.
■ *Endoscopic Procedures*	
colposcopy	Examination of vagina using an instrument called a *colposcope.*
culdoscopy (kul-DOS-koh-pee)	Examination of the female pelvic cavity, particularly behind the uterus, by introducing an endoscope through the wall of the vagina.
laparoscopy (lap-ar-OS-koh-pee)	Examination of the peritoneal cavity using an instrument called a *laparoscope.* The instrument is passed through a small incision made by the surgeon into the abdominopelvic cavity.

■ **Figure 18** Photograph taken during a laparoscopic procedure. The fundus of the uterus is visible below the probe, the ovary is at the tip of the probe, and the fallopian tube extends along the left side of the photo. *(Southern Illinois University/Photo Researchers, Inc.)*

Diagnostic Procedures *(continued)*

TERM	DEFINITION
■ *Obstetrical Diagnostic Procedures*	
amniocentesis (am-nee-oh-sen-TEE-sis)	Puncturing of the amniotic sac using a needle and syringe for the purpose of withdrawing amniotic fluid for testing. Can assist in determining fetal maturity, development, and genetic disorders.
Apgar score (AP-gar)	Evaluation of a neonate's adjustment to the outside world. Observes color, heart rate, muscle tone, respiratory rate, and response to stimulus at one minute and five minutes after birth.
chorionic villus sampling (CVS) (kor-ree-ON-ik vill-us)	Removal of a small piece of the chorion for genetic analysis. May be done at an earlier stage of pregnancy than amniocentesis.
fetal monitoring (FEE-tal)	Using electronic equipment placed on the mother's abdomen or the fetus' scalp to check the fetal heart rate (FHR) and fetal heart tone (FHT) during labor. The normal heart rate of the fetus is rapid, ranging from 120 to 160 beats per minute. A drop in the fetal heart rate indicates the fetus is in distress.
■ *Additional Diagnostic Procedures*	
cervical biopsy (SER-vih-kal BYE-op-see)	Taking a sample of tissue from the cervix to test for the presence of cancer cells.
endometrial biopsy (EMB) (en-doh-MEE-tre-al BYE-op-see)	Taking a sample of tissue from the lining of the uterus to test for abnormalities.
pelvic examination (PELL-vik)	Physical examination of the vagina and adjacent organs performed by a physician placing the fingers of one hand into the vagina. An instrument called a *speculum* is used to open the vagina.

■ **Figure 19** A speculum used to hold the vagina open in order to visualize the cervix.

Therapeutic Procedures

TERM	DEFINITION
■ *Surgical Procedures*	
cesarean section (CS, C-section) (see-SAYR-ee-an)	Surgical delivery of a baby through an incision into the abdominal and uterine walls. Legend has it that the Roman emperor, Julius Caesar, was the first person born by this method.
conization (kon-ih-ZAY-shun)	Surgical removal of a core of cervical tissue. Also refers to partial removal of the cervix.

Therapeutic Procedures *(continued)*

TERM	DEFINITION
dilation and curettage (D & C) (dye-LAY-shun and koo-reh-TAHZ)	Surgical procedure in which the opening of the cervix is dilated and the uterus is scraped or suctioned of its lining or tissue. Often performed after a spontaneous abortion and to stop excessive bleeding from other causes.
elective abortion	Legal termination of a pregnancy for nonmedical reasons.
episiotomy (eh-peez-ee-OT-oh-mee)	Surgical incision of the perineum to facilitate the delivery process. Can prevent an irregular tearing of tissue during birth.
lumpectomy (lump-EK-toh-mee)	Removal of only a breast tumor and the tissue immediately surrounding it.
radical mastectomy (mast-EK-toh-mee)	Surgical removal of the breast tissue plus chest muscles and axillary lymph nodes.
simple mastectomy (mast-EK-toh-mee)	Surgical removal of the breast tissue.
therapeutic abortion	Termination of a pregnancy for the health of the mother or another medical reason.
total abdominal hysterectomy— bilateral salpingo-oophorectomy (TAH-BSO) (hiss-ter-EK-toh-me sal-ping-goh oh-oh-foe-REK-toh-mee)	Removal of the entire uterus, cervix, both ovaries, and both fallopian tubes.
tubal ligation (TOO-bal lye-GAY-shun)	Surgical tying off of the fallopian tubes to prevent conception from taking place. Results in sterilization of the female.
vaginal hysterectomy (VAJ-ih-nal hiss-ter-EK-toh-me)	Removal of the uterus through the vagina rather than through an abdominal incision.

Pharmacology

CLASSIFICATION	ACTION	GENERIC AND BRAND NAMES
abortifacient (ah-bore-tih-FAY-shee-ent)	Medication that terminates a pregnancy.	mifepristone, Mifeprex; dinoprostone, Prostin E2
fertility drug	Medication that triggers ovulation. Also called *ovulation stimulant*.	clomiphene, Clomid; follitropin alfa, Gonal-F
hormone replacement therapy (HRT)	Menopause or the surgical loss of the ovaries results in the lack of estrogen production. Replacing this hormone may prevent some of the consequences of menopause, especially in younger women who have surgically lost their ovaries.	conjugated estrogens, Cenestin, Premarin
oral contraceptive pills (OCPs) (kon-trah-SEP-tive)	Birth control medication that uses low doses of female hormones to prevent conception by blocking ovulation.	desogestrel/ethinyl estradiol, Ortho-Cept; ethinyl estradiol/norgestrel, Lo/Ovral
oxytocin (ox-ee-TOH-sin)	Oxytocin is a natural hormone that begins or improves uterine contractions during labor and delivery.	oxytocin, Pitocin, Syntocinon

Abbreviations

AB	abortion	**HPV**	human papilloma virus
AI	artificial insemination	**HRT**	hormone replacement therapy
BSE	breast self-examination	**HSG**	hysterosalpingography
CS, C-section	cesarean section	**IUD**	intrauterine device
CVS	chorionic villus sampling	**IVF**	*in vitro* fertilization
Cx	cervix	**LBW**	low birth weight
D & C	dilation and curettage	**LH**	luteinizing hormone
EDC	estimated date of confinement	**LMP**	last menstrual period
EMB	endometrial biopsy	**NB**	newborn
ERT	estrogen replacement therapy	**OB**	obstetrics
FEKG	fetal electrocardiogram	**OCPs**	oral contraceptive pills
FHR	fetal heart rate	**PAP**	Papanicolaou test
FHT	fetal heart tone	**PI, para I**	first delivery
FSH	follicle-stimulating hormone	**PID**	pelvic inflammatory disease
FTND	full-term normal delivery	**PMS**	premenstrual syndrome
GI, grav I	first pregnancy	**TAH-BSO**	total abdominal hysterectomy–
GYN, gyn	gynecology		bilateral salpingo-oophorectomy
HCG, hCG	human chorionic gonadotropin	**TSS**	toxic shock syndrome
HDN	hemolytic disease of the newborn	**UC**	uterine contractions

Section II: Male Reproductive System at a Glance

Function

Similar to the female reproductive system, the male reproductive system is responsible for producing sperm, the male reproductive cell, secreting the male sex hormones, and delivering sperm to the female reproductive tract.

Organs

bulbourethral glands
epididymis
penis
prostate gland
seminal vesicles
testes
vas deferens

Combining Forms

andr/o	male	**prostat/o**	prostate
balan/o	glans penis	**spermat/o**	sperm
crypt/o	hidden	**testicul/o**	testes
epididym/o	epididymis	**varic/o**	varicose veins
orch/o	testes	**vas/o**	vas deferens
orchi/o	testes	**vesicul/o**	seminal vesicle
orchid/o	testes		

Suffixes Relating

-spermia	condition of sperm

Male Reproductive System Illustrated

testes

Produces sperm and secretes testosterone

vas deferens

Transports sperm to urethra

prostate gland

Secretes fluid for semen

penis

Delivers semen during intercourse

epididymis

Stores sperm

seminal vesicles

Secretes fluid for semen

bulbourethral gland

Secretes fluid for semen

Anatomy and Physiology of the Male Reproductive System

bulbourethral glands
  (buhl-boh-yoo-REE-thral)
epididymis (ep-ih-DID-ih-mis)
genitourinary system
  (jen-ih-toh-YOO-rih-nair-ee)
penis (PEE-nis)
prostate gland (PROSS-tayt)

semen (SEE-men)
seminal vesicles (SEM-ih-nal VESS-ih-kls)
sex hormones
sperm
testes (TESS-teez)
vas deferens (VAS DEF-er-enz)

The male reproductive system has two main functions. The first is to produce **sperm**, the male reproductive cell. The second is to secrete the male **sex hormones**. In the male, the major organs of reproduction are located outside the body: the **penis**, and the two **testes**, each with an **epididymis** (see Figure 20 ■). The penis contains the urethra, which carries both urine and **semen** to the outside of the body. For this reason, this system is sometimes referred to as the **genitourinary system** (GU).

The internal organs of reproduction include two **seminal vesicles**, two **vas deferens**, the **prostate gland,** and two **bulbourethral glands.**

External Organs of Reproduction

Testes

perineum
scrotum (SKROH-tum)
seminiferous tubules
  (sem-ih-NIF-er-us TOO-byools)

spermatogenesis (sper-mat-oh-JEN-eh-sis)
testicles (test-IH-kles)
testosterone (tess-TOSS-ter-ohn)

The testes (singular is *testis*) or **testicles** are oval in shape and are responsible for the production of sperm (see Figure 20). This process, called **spermatogenesis,**

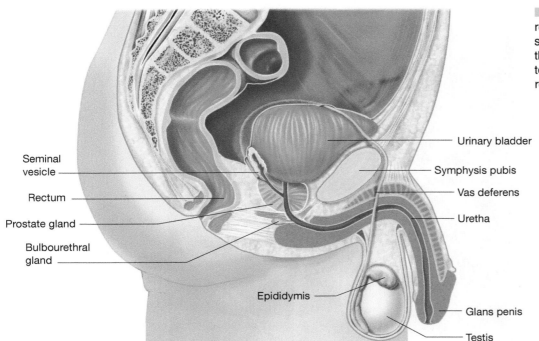

■ **Figure 20** The male reproductive system, sagittal section showing the organs of the system and their relation to the urinary bladder and rectum.

Seminal vesicle

Rectum

Prostate gland

Bulbourethral gland

Epididymis

Urinary bladder

Symphysis pubis

Vas deferens

Uretha

Glans penis

Testis

333

takes place within the **seminiferous tubules** that make up the insides of the testes (see Figure 21 ■). The testes must be maintained at the proper temperature for the sperm to survive. This lower temperature level is achieved by the placement of the testes suspended in the **scrotum**, a sac outside the body. The **perineum** of the male is similar to that in the female. It is the area between the scrotum and the anus. The male sex hormone **testosterone**, which is responsible for the development of the male reproductive organs, sperm, and secondary sex characteristics, is also produced by the testes.

Epididymis

Each epididymis is a coiled tubule that lies on top of the testes within the scrotum (see Figure 20). This elongated structure serves as the location for sperm maturation and storage until they are ready to be released into the vas deferens.

Penis

circumcision (ser-kum-SIH-zhun)
ejaculation (ee-jak-yoo-LAY-shun)
erectile tissue (ee-REK-tile)
glans penis (GLANS PEE-nis)

prepuce (PREE-pyoos)
sphincter (SFINGK-ter)
urinary meatus (YOO-rih-nair-ee me-AY-tus)

The penis is the male sex organ containing **erectile tissue** that is encased in skin (see Figure 20). This organ delivers semen into the female vagina. The soft tip of the penis is referred to as the **glans penis**. It is protected by a covering called the **prepuce** or foreskin. It is this covering of skin that is removed during the procedure known as **circumcision**. The penis becomes erect during sexual stimulation, which allows it to be placed within the female for the **ejaculation** of semen. The male urethra extends from the urinary bladder to the external opening in the penis, the **urinary meatus**, and serves a dual function: the elimination of urine and the ejaculation of semen. During the ejaculation process, a **sphincter** closes to keep urine from escaping.

Med Term Tip

Spermatozoon and its plural form, *spermatozoa*, are other terms that mean "sperm." You have no doubt realized that there can be several terms with the same meaning in medical terminology. You must continue to remain flexible when working with these terms in your career. In some cases, one term will be more commonly used, depending on the type of medical specialty or even what part of the country you are in.

Med Term Tip

During sexual intercourse, which is also referred to as *coitus*, the male can eject up to 100 million sperm cells. The adult male produces nearly 200 million sperm daily.

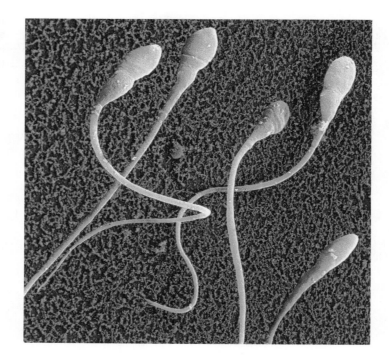

■ Figure 21
Electronmicrograph of human sperm. *(Juergen Berger, Max-Planck Institute/Science Photo Library/Photo Researchers, Inc.)*

Internal Organs of Reproduction

Vas Deferens

spermatic cord (sper-MAT-ik)

Each vas deferens carries sperm from the epididymis up into the pelvic cavity. They travel up in front of the urinary bladder, over the top, and then back down the posterior side of the bladder to empty into the urethra (see Figure 20). They, along with nerves, arteries, veins, and lymphatic vessels running between the pelvic cavity and the testes, form the **spermatic cord**.

Seminal Vesicles

The two seminal vesicles are small glands located at the base of the urinary bladder (see Figure 20). These vesicles are connected to the vas deferens just before it empties into the urethra. The seminal vesicles secrete a glucose-rich fluid that nourishes the sperm. This liquid, along with the sperm, constitutes semen, the fluid that is eventually ejaculated during sexual intercourse.

Prostate Gland

The single prostate gland is located just below the urinary bladder (see Figure 20). It surrounds the urethra and when enlarged can cause difficulty in urination. The prostate is important for the reproductive process since it secretes an alkaline fluid that assists in keeping the sperm alive by neutralizing the pH of the urethra and vagina.

Bulbourethral Glands

Cowper's glands (KOW-perz)

The bulbourethral glands, also known as **Cowper's glands**, are two small glands located on either side of the urethra just below the prostate (see Figure 20). They produce a mucuslike lubricating fluid that joins with semen to become a part of the ejaculate.

 # Word Building

The following list contains examples of medical terms built directly from word parts. The definition for these terms can be determined by a straightforward translation of the word parts.

COMBINING FORM	COMBINED WITH	MEDICAL TERM	DEFINITION
andr/o	-gen	**androgen** (AN-droh-jen)	male producing
	-pathy	**andropathy** (an-DROP-ah-thee)	male disease
balan/o	-itis	**balanitis** (bal-ah-NYE-tis)	inflammation of glans penis
	-plasty	**balanoplasty** (BAL-ah-noh-plas-tee)	surgical repair of glans penis
	-rrhea	**balanorrhea** (bah-lah-noh-REE-ah)	discharge from glans penis
epididym/o	-ectomy	**epididymectomy** (ep-ih-did-ih-MEK-toh-mee)	removal of epididymis
	-al	**epididymal** (ep-ih-DID-ih-mal)	pertaining to the epididymis
	-itis	**epididymitis** (ep-ih-did-ih-MYE-tis)	inflammation of the epididymis

Word Building (continued)

COMBINING FORMS	COMBINED WITH	MEDICAL TERM	DEFINITION
orch/o	an- -ism	**anorchism** (an-OR-kizm)	condition of no testes
orchi/o	-ectomy	**orchiectomy** (or-kee-EK-toh-mee)	removal of testes
	-otomy	**orchiotomy** (or-kee-OT-oh-mee)	incision into testes
	-plasty	**orchioplasty** (OR-kee-oh-plas-tee)	surgical repair of testes
orchid/o	-ectomy	**orchidectomy** (or-kid-EK-toh-mee)	removal of the testes
	-pexy	**orchidopexy** (OR-kid-oh-peck-see)	surgical fixation of testes
prostat/o	-itis	**prostatitis** (pross-tah-TYE-tis)	prostate inflammation
	-ectomy	**prostatectomy** (pross-tah-TEK-toh-mee)	removal of prostate
	-ic	**prostatic** (pross-TAT-ik)	pertaining to the prostate
spermat/o	-ic	**spermatic** (sper-MAT-ik)	pertaining to sperm
	-lysis	**spermatolysis** (sper-mah-TOL-ih-sis)	sperm destruction
testicul/o	-ar	**testicular** (tes-TIK-yoo-lar)	pertaining to the testes
vesicul/o	-ar	**vesicular** (veh-SIC-yoo-lar)	pertaining to the seminal vesicle

Med Term Tip

Word watch—Be careful using the combining forms *vesic/o* meaning "bladder" and *vesicul/o* meaning "seminal vesicle."

PREFIX	SUFFIX	MEDICAL TERM	DEFINITION
a-	-spermia	**aspermia** (ah-SPER-mee-ah)	condition of no sperm
oligo-		**oligospermia** (ol-ih-goh-SPER-mee-ah)	condition of scanty (few) sperm

Vocabulary

TERM	DEFINITION
erectile dysfunction (ED) (ee-REK-tile)	Inability to engage in sexual intercourse due to inability to maintain an erection. Also called *impotence*.
sterility	Inability to father children due to a problem with spermatogenesis.

Pathology

TERM	DEFINITION
■ Testes	
cryptorchidism (kript-OR-kid-izm)	Failure of the testes to descend into the scrotal sac before birth. Usually, the testes will descend before birth. A surgical procedure called orchidopexy may be required to bring the testes down into the scrotum permanently. Failure of the testes to descend could result in sterility in the male or an increased risk of testicular cancer.
hydrocele (HIGH-droh-seel)	Accumulation of fluid around the testes or along the spermatic cord. Common in infants.

Pathology (continued)

TERM	DEFINITION
testicular carcinoma (kar-sih-NOH-mah)	Cancer of one or both testicles; most common cancer in men under age 40.
testicular torsion	A twisting of the spermatic cord.
varicocele (VAIR-ih-koh-seel)	Enlargement of the veins of the spermatic cord that commonly occurs on the left side of adolescent males.

■ Prostate Gland

benign prostatic hypertrophy (BPH) (bee-NINE pross-TAT-ik high-PER-troh-fee)	Noncancerous enlargement of the prostate gland commonly seen in males over age 50.
prostate cancer (PROSS-tayt CAN-ser)	Slow-growing cancer that affects a large number of males after age 50. The prostate-specific antigen (PSA) test is used to assist in early detection of this disease.

■ Penis

epispadias (ep-ih-SPAY-dee-as)	Congenital opening of the urethra on the dorsal surface of the penis.
hypospadias (high-poh-SPAY-dee-as)	Congenital opening of the male urethra on the underside of the penis.
phimosis (fih-MOH-sis)	Narrowing of the foreskin over the glans penis resulting in difficulty with hygiene. This condition can lead to infection or difficulty with urination. The condition is treated with circumcision, the surgical removal of the foreskin.
priapism (pri-ah-pizm)	A persistent and painful erection due to pathological causes, not sexual arousal.

■ Sexually Transmitted Diseases

chancroid (SHANG-kroyd)	Highly infectious nonsyphilitic venereal ulcer.

■ **Figure 22** Photograph showing a chancroid on the glans penis. *(Joe Miller/Centers for Disease Control and Prevention [CDC])*

chlamydia (klah-MID-ee-ah)	Bacterial infection causing genital inflammation in males and females. Can lead to pelvic inflammatory disease in females and eventual infertility.
genital herpes (JEN-ih-tal HER-peez)	Creeping skin disease that can appear like a blister or vesicle, caused by a sexually transmitted virus.

Pathology *(continued)*

TERM	DEFINITION
genital warts (JEN-ih-tal)	Growth of warts on the genitalia of both males and females that can lead to cancer of the cervix in females. Caused by the sexual transmission of the human papilloma virus (HPV).
gonorrhea (GC) (gon-oh-REE-ah)	Sexually transmitted bacterial infection of the mucous membranes of either sex. Can be passed on to an infant during the birth process.
human immunodeficiency virus (HIV)	Sexually transmitted virus that attacks the immune system.
sexually transmitted disease (STD)	Disease usually acquired as the result of sexual intercourse. Formerly referred to as *venereal disease* (VD).
syphilis (SIF-ih-lis)	Infectious, chronic, bacterial venereal disease that can involve any organ. May exist for years without symptoms, but is fatal if untreated. Treated with the antibiotic penicillin.
trichomoniasis (trik-oh-moh-NYE-ah-sis)	Genitourinary infection caused by a single-cell protist that is usually without symptoms (asymptomatic) in both males and females. In women the disease can produce itching and/or burning, a foul-smelling discharge, and result in vaginitis.

Diagnostic Procedures

TERM	DEFINITION
■ *Clinical Laboratory Tests*	
prostate-specific antigen (PSA) (PROSS-tayt-specific AN-tih-jen)	A blood test to screen for prostate cancer. Elevated blood levels of PSA are associated with prostate cancer.
semen analysis (SEE-men ah-NAL-ih-sis)	Procedure used when performing a fertility workup to determine if the male is able to produce sperm. Semen is collected by the patient after abstaining from sexual intercourse for a period of three to five days. The sperm in the semen are analyzed for number, swimming strength, and shape. Also used to determine if a vasectomy has been successful. After a period of six weeks, no further sperm should be present in a sample from the patient.
■ *Additional Diagnostic Procedures*	
digital rectal exam (DRE) (DIJ-ih-tal REK-tal)	Manual examination for an enlarged prostate gland performed by palpating (feeling) the prostate gland through the wall of the rectum.

Therapeutic Procedures

TERM	DEFINITION
■ *Surgical Procedures*	
castration (kass-TRAY-shun)	Removal of the testicles in the male or the ovaries in the female.
circumcision (ser-kum-SIH-zhun)	Surgical removal of the end of the prepuce or foreskin of the penis. Generally performed on the newborn male at the request of the parents. The primary reason is for ease of hygiene. Circumcision is also a ritual practice in some religions.

Therapeutic Procedures *(continued)*

TERM	DEFINITION
orchidopexy (OR-kid-oh-peck-see)	Surgical fixation to move undescended testes into the scrotum and to attach them to prevent retraction. Used to treat cryptorchidism.
sterilization (ster-ih-lih-ZAY-shun)	Process of rendering a male or female sterile or unable to conceive children.
transurethral resection of the prostate (TUR, TURP) (trans-yoo-REE-thrall REE-sek-shun of the PROSS-tayt)	Surgical removal of the prostate gland by inserting a device through the urethra and removing prostate tissue.
vasectomy (vas-EK-toh-mee)	Removal of a segment or all of the vas deferens to prevent sperm from leaving the male body. Used for contraception purposes.

Med Term Tip

The vas deferens is the tubing that is severed during a procedure called a *vasectomy*. A vasectomy results in the sterilization of the male since the sperm are no longer able to travel into the urethra and out of the penis during sexual intercourse. The surgical procedure to reverse a vasectomy is a *vasovasostomy*. A new opening is created in order to reconnect one section of the vas deferens to another section of the vas deferens, thereby reestablishing an open tube for sperm to travel through.

Figure 23 A vasectomy, showing how each vas deferens is tied off in two places and then a section is removed from the middle. This prevents sperm from traveling through the vas deferens during ejaculation.

vasovasostomy (vas-oh-vay-ZOS-toh-mee)	Surgical procedure to reconnect the vas deferens to reverse a vasectomy.

Pharmacology

CLASSIFICATION	ACTION	GENERIC AND BRAND NAME
androgen therapy (AN-droh-jen)	Replacement of male hormones to treat patients who produce insufficient hormone naturally.	testosterone cypionate, Andronate, depAndro
antiprostatic agents (an-tye-pross-TAT-ik)	Medication to treat early cases of benign prostatic hypertrophy. May prevent surgery for mild cases.	finasteride, Proscar; dutasteride, Avodart
erectile dysfunction agents (ee-REK-tile)	Medication that temporarily produces an erection in patients with erectile dysfunction.	sildenafil citrate, Viagra; tadalafil, Cialis
spermatocide (sper-mah-toh-LIT-ik)	Destruction of sperm. One form of birth control is the use of spermatolytic creams.	nonoxynol 9, Semicid, Ortho-Gynol

Abbreviations

BPH	benign prostatic hypertrophy	**RPR**	rapid plasma reagin (test for syphilis)
DRE	digital rectal exam	**SPP**	suprapubic prostatectomy
ED	erectile dysfunction	**STD**	sexually transmitted disease
GC	gonorrhea	**TUR**	transurethral resection
GU	genitourinary	**TURP**	transurethral resection of the prostate
PSA	prostate-specific antigen	**VD**	venereal disease

Chapter Review

Terminology Checklist

 Below are all Anatomy and Physiology key terms, Word Building, Vocabulary, Pathology, Diagnostic, Therapeutic, and Pharmacology terms presented in this chapter. Use this list as a study tool by placing a check in the box in front of each term as you master its meaning.

- ☐ abortifacient
- ☐ abruptio placentae
- ☐ amenorrhea
- ☐ amniocentesis
- ☐ amnion
- ☐ amniorrhea
- ☐ amniotic
- ☐ amniotic fluid
- ☐ amniotomy
- ☐ androgen
- ☐ androgen therapy
- ☐ andropathy
- ☐ anorchism
- ☐ anteflexion
- ☐ antepartum
- ☐ antiprostatic agents
- ☐ Apgar score
- ☐ areola
- ☐ aspermia
- ☐ atresia
- ☐ balanitis
- ☐ balanoplasty
- ☐ balanorrhea
- ☐ barrier contraception
- ☐ Bartholin's glands
- ☐ benign prostatic hypertrophy
- ☐ breast cancer
- ☐ breasts
- ☐ breech presentation
- ☐ bulbourethral gland
- ☐ candidiasis
- ☐ castration
- ☐ cervical
- ☐ cervical biopsy
- ☐ cervical cancer
- ☐ cervicectomy
- ☐ cervix
- ☐ cesarean section

- ☐ chancroid
- ☐ chlamydia
- ☐ chorion
- ☐ chorionic
- ☐ chorionic villus sampling
- ☐ circumcision
- ☐ clitoris
- ☐ colostrum
- ☐ colposcope
- ☐ colposcopy
- ☐ conception
- ☐ conization
- ☐ corpus
- ☐ Cowper's glands
- ☐ crowning
- ☐ cryptorchidism
- ☐ culdoscopy
- ☐ cystocele
- ☐ delivery
- ☐ digital rectal exam
- ☐ dilation and curettage
- ☐ dilation stage
- ☐ dysmenorrhea
- ☐ dystocia
- ☐ eclampsia
- ☐ effacement
- ☐ ejaculation
- ☐ elective abortion
- ☐ embryo
- ☐ embryonic
- ☐ endocervicitis
- ☐ endometrial biopsy
- ☐ endometrial cancer
- ☐ endometriosis
- ☐ endometritis
- ☐ endometrium
- ☐ epididymal
- ☐ epididymectomy

- ☐ epididymis
- ☐ epididymitis
- ☐ episiorrhaphy
- ☐ episiotomy
- ☐ epispadias
- ☐ erectile dysfunction
- ☐ erectile dysfunction agents
- ☐ erectile tissue
- ☐ estrogen
- ☐ expulsion stage
- ☐ fallopian tubes
- ☐ fertility drug
- ☐ fertilization
- ☐ fetal
- ☐ fetal monitoring
- ☐ fetus
- ☐ fibrocystic breast disease
- ☐ fibroid tumor
- ☐ fimbriae
- ☐ follicle stimulating hormone
- ☐ fraternal twins
- ☐ fundus
- ☐ genital herpes
- ☐ genitalia
- ☐ genital warts
- ☐ genitourinary system
- ☐ gestation
- ☐ glans penis
- ☐ gonorrhea
- ☐ gynecologist
- ☐ gynecology
- ☐ hematosalpinx
- ☐ hemolytic disease of the newborn
- ☐ hormonal contraception
- ☐ hormone replacement therapy
- ☐ human immunodeficiency virus
- ☐ hydrocele

- hymen
- hymenectomy
- hypospadias
- hysterectomy
- hysteropexy
- hysterorrhexis
- hysterosalpingography
- identical twins
- infertility
- intrauterine device
- labia majora
- labia minora
- labor
- lactation
- lactic
- lactiferous ducts
- lactiferous glands
- lactorrhea
- laparoscope
- laparoscopy
- laparotomy
- lumpectomy
- luteinizing hormone
- mammary
- mammary glands
- mammogram
- mammography
- mammoplasty
- mastalgia
- mastectomy
- mastitis
- meconium
- menarche
- menometrorrhagia
- menopause
- menorrhagia
- menstrual period
- menstruation
- metrorrhagia
- metrorrhea
- multigravida
- multipara
- myometrium
- neonate
- neonatologist
- neonatology
- nipple
- nulligravida
- nullipara
- nurse
- obstetrics
- oligomenorrhea
- oligospermia
- oophorectomy
- oophoritis
- oral contraceptive pills
- orchidectomy
- orchidopexy
- orchiectomy
- orchioplasty
- orchiotomy
- ova
- ovarian
- ovarian carcinoma
- ovarian cyst
- ovaries
- oviducts
- ovulation
- oxytocin
- Pap (Papanicolaou) smear
- pelvic examination
- pelvic inflammatory disease
- pelvic ultrasonography
- penis
- perimetritis
- perimetrium
- perineum
- phimosis
- placenta
- placenta previa
- placental stage
- postpartum
- preeclampsia
- pregnancy
- pregnancy test
- premature
- premenstrual syndrome
- prepuce
- priapism
- primigravida
- primipara
- progesterone
- prolapsed umbilical cord
- prolapsed uterus
- prostate cancer
- prostate gland
- prostatectomy
- prostate-specific antigen
- prostatic
- prostatitis
- pseudocyesis
- puberty
- pyosalpinx
- radical mastectomy
- rectocele
- salpingectomy
- salpingitis
- salpingocyesis
- scrotum
- semen
- semen analysis
- seminal vesicles
- seminiferous tubules
- sex hormones
- sexually transmitted disease
- simple mastectomy
- sperm
- spermatic
- spermatic cord
- spermatocide
- spermatogenesis
- spermatolysis
- sphincter
- spontaneous abortion
- sterility
- sterilization
- stillbirth
- syphilis
- testes
- testicles
- testicular
- testicular carcinoma
- testicular torsion
- testosterone
- therapeutic abortion

Reproductive System

- ☐ total abdominal hysterectomy–bilateral salpingo-oophorectomy
- ☐ toxic shock syndrome
- ☐ transurethral resection of the prostate
- ☐ trichomoniasis
- ☐ tubal ligation
- ☐ umbilical cord
- ☐ urinary meatus
- ☐ uterine
- ☐ uterine tubes
- ☐ uterus
- ☐ vagina
- ☐ vaginal
- ☐ vaginal hysterectomy
- ☐ vaginal orifice
- ☐ vaginitis
- ☐ varicocele
- ☐ vas deferens
- ☐ vasectomy
- ☐ vasovasostomy
- ☐ vesicular
- ☐ vulva

Practice Exercises

A. Complete the following statements.

1. The study of the female reproductive system is the medical specialty of _____.

2. A physician who specializes in the treatment of women is called a(n) _____.

3. The three stages of labor and delivery are the _____ stage, the _____ stage, and the _____ stage.

4. The time required for the development of a fetus is called _____.

5. The cessation of menstruation is called _____.

6. The female sex cell is a(n) _____.

7. The inner lining of the uterus is called the _____.

8. The organ in which the developing fetus resides is called the _____.

9. The tubes that extend from the outer edges of the uterus and assist in transporting the ova and sperm are called _____.

10. One of the longest terms used in medical terminology refers to the removal of the uterus, cervix, ovaries, and fallopian tubes. This term is _____.

B. State the terms described using the combining forms provided.

The combining form *colp/o* refers to the vagina. Use it to write a term that means:

1. visual examination of the vagina _____

2. instrument used to examine the vagina _____

The combining form *cervic/o* refers to the cervix. Use it to write a term that means:

3. removal of the cervix _____

4. inflammation of the cervix _____

5. pertaining to the cervix _____

The combining form *hyster/o* also refers to the uterus. Use it to write a term that means:

6. surgical fixation of the uterus _____

7. removal of the uterus _____

8. rupture of the uterus _____

The combining form *oophor/o* refers to the ovaries. Use it to write a term that means:

9. inflammation of an ovary _____

10. removal of an ovary _____

The combining form *mamm/o* refers to the breasts. Use it to write a term that means:

11. pertaining to the breasts _____

12. record of breast _____

13. surgical repair of breast _____

The combining form *amni/o* refers to the amnion. Use it to write a term that means:

14. pertaining to the amnion _____

15. incision into amnion _____

16. flow from amnion _____

C. Identify the following abbreviations.

1. Cx _____

2. LMP _____

3. FHR _____

4. PID _____

5. GYN _____

6. CS _____

7. NB _____

8. PMS _____

9. TSS _____

10. LBW _____

D. Write the abbreviations for the following terms.

1. first pregnancy _____   4. full-term normal delivery _____

2. artificial insemination _____   5. intrauterine device _____

3. uterine contractions _____   6. dilation and curettage _____

7. hormone replacement therapy _____   9. abortion _____

8. gynecology _____   10. oral contraception pills _____

E. Define the following combining forms and use them to form female reproductive terms.

	Definition	Female Reproductive Term
1. metr/o	_____	_____
2. hyster/o	_____	_____
3. gynec/o	_____	_____
4. episi/o	_____	_____
5. oophor/o	_____	_____
6. ovari/o	_____	_____
7. salping/o	_____	_____
8. men/o	_____	_____
9. vagin/o	_____	_____
10. mast/o	_____	_____

F. Match each term to its definition.

1. _____ hemolytic disease of the newborn   a.   lack of a normal body opening

2. _____ ovary   b.   erythroblastosis fetalis

3. _____ vagina   c.   detached placenta

4. _____ abruption placentae   d.   female erectile tissue

5. _____ placenta   e.   produces eggs

6. _____ endometrium   f.   normal place for fertilization

7. _____ clitoris   g.   buttocks first to appear in birth canal

8. _____ candidiasis   h.   birth canal

9. _____ Pap smear   i.   nourishes fetus

10. _____ fallopian tube   j.   uterine lining

11. _____ dysmenorrhea   k.   measures newborn's adjustment to outside world

12. _____ breech presentation   l.   test for cervical cancer

13. _____ Apgar   m.   newborn

14. _____ neonate   n.   yeast infection

15. _____ atresia   o.   painful menstruation

G. Use the following terms in the sentences below.

premenstrual syndrome   stillbirth   conization   laparoscopy

D & C   puberty   endometriosis   eclampsia

fibroid tumor   cesarean section

1. Kesha had a core of tissue from her cervix removed for testing. This is called _____.

2. Joan delivered a baby that had died while still in the uterus. She had a(n) _____.

3. Ashley has just started her first menstrual cycle. She is said to have entered _____.

4. Kimberly is experiencing tender breasts, headaches, and some irritability just prior to her monthly menstrual cycle. This may be _____.

5. Ana has been scheduled for an examination in which her physician will use an instrument to observe her abdominal cavity to rule out the diagnosis of severe endometriosis. The physician will insert the instrument through a small incision. This procedure is called a(n) _____.

6. Lenora is scheduled to have a hysterectomy as a result of a long history of large benign growths in her uterus that have caused pain and bleeding. Lenora has a(n) _____.

7. Tiffany's physician has recommended that she have a uterine scraping to stop excessive bleeding after a miscarriage. She will be scheduled for a _____.

8. Stacey is having frequent prenatal checkups to prevent the serious condition of pregnancy called _____.

9. Marion has experienced painful menstrual periods as a result of the lining of her uterus being displaced into her pelvic cavity. This is called _____.

10. Because her cervix was not dilating, Shataundra was informed that she will probably require a(n) _____ for her baby's delivery.

H. Define the following suffixes and use them to form reproductive system terms.

	Definition	Reproductive Term
1. -tocia	_____	_____
2. -gravida	_____	_____
3. -arche	_____	_____
4. -cyesis	_____	_____
5. -partum	_____	_____
6. -para	_____	_____
7. -salpinx	_____	_____
8. -spermia	_____	_____

I. Match each term to its definition.

1. _____ gonorrhea

2. _____ genital herpes

3. _____ human immunodeficiency virus

4. _____ syphilis

5. _____ venereal disease

6. _____ genital warts

7. _____ chancroid

8. _____ chlamydia

9. _____ trichomoniasis

a. also called STD

b. caused by parasitic microorganism

c. treated with penicillin

d. caused by human papilloma virus

e. can pass to infant during birth

f. genitourinary infection

g. venereal ulcer

h. attacks the immune system

i. skin disease with vesicles

J. Complete the following statements.

1. The male reproductive system is a combination of the _____ and _____ systems.

2. The male's external organs of reproduction consist of the _____, _____, and the _____.

3. Another term for the prepuce is the _____.

4. The organs responsible for developing the sperm cells are the _____.

5. The glands of lubrication and fluid production at each side of the male urethra are the _____.

6. The male sex hormone is _____.

7. The area between the scrotum and the anus is called the _____.

K. State the terms described using the combining forms provided.

The combining form *prostat/o* refers to the prostate. Use this to write a term that means:

1. removal of prostate _____

2. pertaining to the prostate _____

3. inflammation of the prostate _____

The combining form *orchi/o* refers to the testes. Use this to write a term that means:

4. removal of the testes _____

5. surgical repair of the testes _____

6. incision into the testes _____

The combining form *andr/o* refers to male. Use this to write a term that means:

7. disease of the male _____

8. male producing _____

Reproductive System

The combining form *spermat/o* refers to sperm. Use this to write a term that means:

9. sperm forming _____

10. sperm destruction _____

L. Identify the following abbreviations.

1. SPP _____

2. TUR _____

3. GU _____

4. BPH _____

5. DRE _____

6. PSA _____

M. Define the following terms.

1. spermatogenesis _____

2. hydrocele _____

3. transurethral resection of the prostate (TURP) _____

4. aspermia _____

5. orchiectomy _____

6. vasectomy _____

7. castration _____

N. Fill in the classification for each drug description, then match the brand name.

Drug Description	Classification	Brand Name
1. _____ replacement male hormone	_____	a. Pitocin
2. _____ improves uterine contractions	_____	b. Avodart
3. _____ treats early BPH	_____	c. Clomid
4. _____ blocks ovulation	_____	d. nonoxynol 9
5. _____ kills sperm	_____	e. Mifeprex
6. _____ produces an erection	_____	f. Andronate
7. _____ replaces estrogen	_____	g. Ortho-Cept
8. _____ terminates a pregnancy	_____	h. Viagra
9. _____ triggers ovulation	_____	i. Premarin

Medical Record Analysis

Below is an item from a patient's medical record. Read it carefully, make sure you understand all the medical terms used, and then answer the questions that follow.

High-Risk Obstetrics Consultation Report

Reason for Consultation:	High-risk pregnancy with late-term bleeding
History of Present Illness:	Patient is 23 years old. She is currently estimated to be at 175 days of gestation. She has had a 23-lb weight gain with this pregnancy. Amniocentesis at 20 weeks indicated male fetus with no evidence of genetic or developmental disorders. She noticed a moderate degree of vaginal bleeding this morning but denies any cramping or pelvic pain. She immediately saw her obstetrician who referred her for high-risk evaluation.
Past Medical History:	This patient is multigravida but nullipara with three early miscarriages without obvious cause. She was diagnosed with cancer of the left ovary four years ago. It was treated with a left oophorectomy and chemotherapy. She continues to undergo full-body CT scan every six months, and there has been no evidence of metastasis since that time. Menarche was at age 13, and her menstrual history is significant for menorrhagia resulting in chronic anemia.
Results of Physical Examination:	Patient appears well nourished and abdominal girth appears consistent with length of gestation. She is understandably quite anxious regarding the sudden spotting. Pelvic ultrasound indicates placenta previa with placenta almost completely overlying cervix. However, there is no evidence of abruptio placentae at this time. Fetal size estimate is consistent with 25 weeks of gestation. The fetus is turned head down, and the umbilical cord is not around the neck. The fetal heart tones are strong with a rate of 130 beats/minute. There is no evidence of cervical effacement or dilation at this time.
Recommendations:	Fetus appears to be developing well and in no distress at this time. The placenta appears to be well attached on ultrasound, but the bleeding is cause for concern. With the extremely low position of the placenta, this patient is at very high risk for abruptio placentae when cervix begins effacement and dilation. She may require early delivery by cesarean section at that time. She will definitely require C-section at onset of labor. At this time, recommend bed rest with bathroom privileges. She is to return every other day for two weeks and every day after that for evaluation of cervix and fetal condition. She is to call immediately if she notes any further bleeding or change in activity level of the fetus.

Critical Thinking Questions

1. Describe in your own words the treatment this patient received for her ovarian cancer. What procedure does she continue to have every six months?

_____

_____

2. Describe in your own words this patient's menstrual history. _____

_____

Reproductive System

3. Which of the following choices describes this patient (choose all that apply)?

    a. She has never been pregnant.
    b. She has several live children.
    c. She has no live children.
    d. She has been pregnant several times.

4. This patient has placenta previa. What procedure discovered this condition? The physician, however, is much more concerned about abruptio placentae. Explain why.

    _____

    _____

5. Describe the condition of the fetus. _____

    _____

6. The following two phrases are not specifically defined by your text. Explain what you believe them to mean based on the context of this consultation report.

    a. high-risk pregnancy _____

    _____

    b. abdominal girth appears consistent with length of gestation _____

    _____

Chart Note Transcription

The chart note below contains ten phrases that can be reworded with a medical term that you learned in this chapter. Each phrase is identified with an underline. Determine the medical term and write your answers in the space provided.

Current Complaint:	Patient is a 77-year-old male seen by the urologist with complaints of nocturia and difficulty with <u>the release of semen from the urethra</u>. ❶
Past History:	Medical history revealed that the patient had <u>failure of the testes to descend into the scrotum</u> ❷ at birth, which was repaired by <u>surgical fixation of the testes</u>. ❸ He had also undergone elective sterilization <u>by removal of a segment of the vas deferens</u> ❹ at the age of 41.
Signs and Symptoms:	Patient states he first noted these symptoms about five years ago. They have become increasingly severe and now he is not able to sleep without waking to urinate up to 20 times a night. He has difficulty with <u>release of semen</u>. ❺ <u>Palpation of the prostate gland through the rectum</u> ❻ revealed multiple round firm nodules in prostate gland. A needle biopsy was negative for <u>slow-growing cancer that frequently affects males over 50</u> ❼ and a <u>blood test for prostate cancer</u> ❽ was normal.
Diagnosis:	<u>Noncancerous enlargement of the prostate gland</u>. ❾
Treatment:	Patient was scheduled for a <u>surgical removal of prostate tissue through the urethra</u>. ❿

❶ _____

❷ _____

❸ _____

❹ _____

❺ _____

❻ _____

❼ _____

❽ _____

❾ _____

❿ _____

Labeling Exercise

A. System Review

1. Write the labels for this figure on the numbered lines provided.

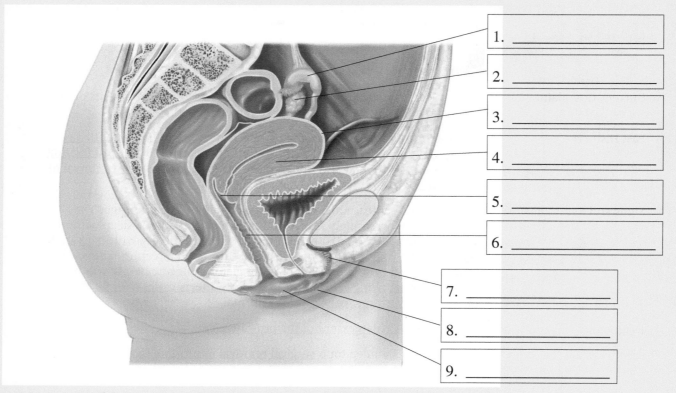

1. _____
2. _____
3. _____
4. _____
5. _____
6. _____
7. _____
8. _____
9. _____

2. Write the labels for this figure on the numbered lines provided.

1. _____
2. _____
3. _____
4. _____
5. _____
6. _____
7. _____
8. _____

Reproductive System

B. Anatomy Challenge

Write the labels for this figure on the numbered lines provided.

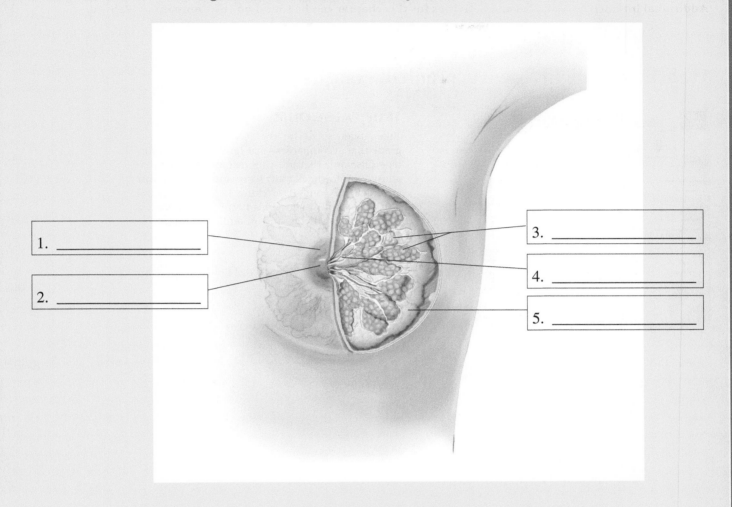

1. _____

2. _____

3. _____

4. _____

5. _____

Multimedia Preview

Additional interactive resources and activities for this chapter can be found on the Companion Website.

Website Highlights—www.prenhall.com/fremgen

TRUE/FALSE QUIZ

Take advantage of the free-access on-line study guide that accompanies your textbook. You'll find a true/false quiz that provides instant feedback that allows you to check your score and see what you got right or wrong. By clicking on this URL you'll also access links to download mp3 audio reviews, current news articles, and an audio glossary.

Endocrine System

Learning Objectives

Upon completion of this chapter, you will be able to:

- Identify and define the combining forms and suffixes introduced in this chapter.
- Correctly spell and pronounce medical terms and major anatomical structures relating to the endocrine system.
- Locate and describe the major organs of the endocrine system and their functions.
- List the major hormones secreted by each endocrine gland and describe their functions.
- Build and define endocrine system medical terms from word parts.
- Identify and define endocrine system vocabulary terms.
- Identify and define selected endocrine system pathology terms.
- Identify and define selected endocrine system diagnostic procedures.
- Identify and define selected endocrine system therapeutic procedures.
- Identify and define selected medications relating to the endocrine system.
- Define selected abbreviations associated with the endocrine system.

From Chapter 11 of *Medical Terminology: A Living Language*, 4/e. Bonnie F. Fremgen. Suzanne S. Frucht. Copyright © 2009 by Pearson Education. Published by Prentice Hall. All rights reserved.

Endocrine System at a Glance

Function

Endocrine glands secrete hormones that regulate many body activities such as metabolic rate, water and mineral balance, immune system reactions, and sexual functioning.

Organs

adrenal glands
ovaries
pancreas (islets of Langerhans)
parathyroid glands
pineal gland
pituitary gland
testes
thymus gland
thyroid gland

Combining Forms

acr/o	extremities	**kal/i**	potassium
adren/o	adrenal glands	**natr/o**	sodium
adrenal/o	adrenal glands	**ophthalm/o**	eye
andr/o	male	**pancreat/o**	pancreas
calc/o	calcium	**parathyroid/o**	parathyroid gland
crin/o	secrete	**pineal/o**	pineal gland
estr/o	female	**pituitar/o**	pituitary gland
glyc/o	sugar	**thym/o**	thymus gland
glycos/o	sugar	**thyr/o**	thyroid gland
gonad/o	sex glands	**thyroid/o**	thyroid gland
home/o	sameness	**toxic/o**	poison

Suffixes

-crine	to secrete
-dipsia	thirst
-prandial	relating to a meal
-tropin	stimulate

Endocrine System Illustrated

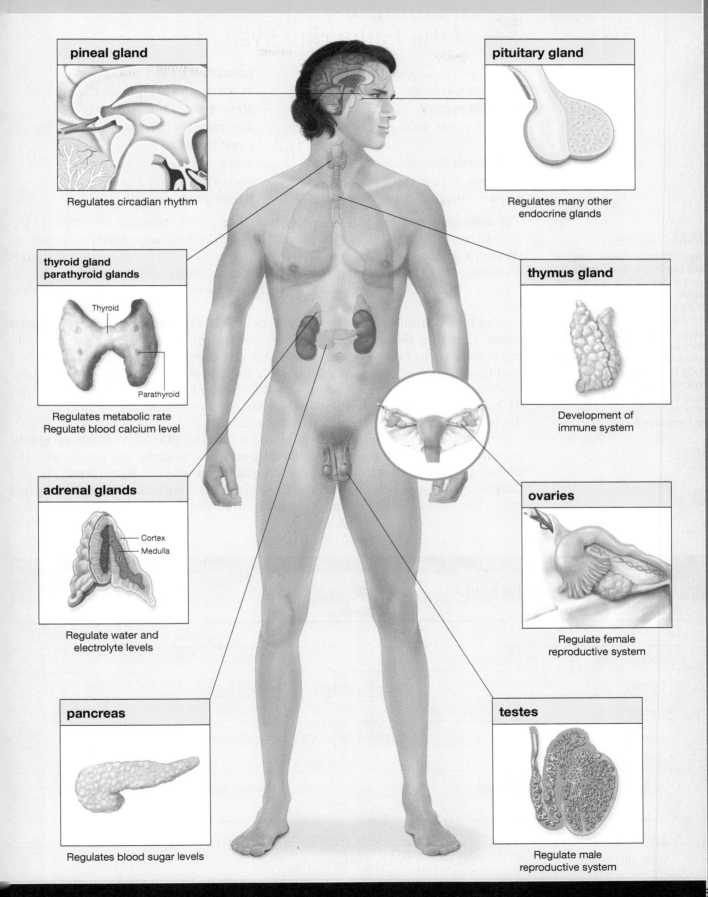

pineal gland

Regulates circadian rhythm

pituitary gland

Regulates many other endocrine glands

thyroid gland parathyroid glands

Thyroid

Parathyroid

Regulates metabolic rate
Regulate blood calcium level

thymus gland

Development of immune system

adrenal glands

Cortex
Medulla

Regulate water and electrolyte levels

ovaries

Regulate female reproductive system

pancreas

Regulates blood sugar levels

testes

Regulate male reproductive system

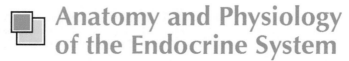

Anatomy and Physiology of the Endocrine System

adrenal glands (ad-REE-nal)

endocrine glands (EN-doh-krin)

endocrine system

exocrine glands (EKS-oh-krin)

glands

homeostasis (hoe-me-oh-STAY-sis)

hormones (HOR-mohnz)

ovaries (OH-vah-reez)

pancreas (PAN-kree-ass)

parathyroid glands (pair-ah-THIGH-royd)

pineal gland (pih-NEAL)

pituitary gland (pih-TOO-ih-tair-ee)

target organs

testes (TESS-teez)

thymus gland (THIGH-mus)

thyroid gland (THIGH-royd)

Med Term Tip

The terms *endocrine* and *exocrine* were constructed to reflect the function of each type of gland. As glands, they both secrete, indicated by the combining form *crin/o*. The prefix *exo-*, meaning "external" or "outward," tells us that exocrine gland secretions are carried to the outside of the body. However, the prefix *endo-*, meaning "within" or "internal," indicates that endocrine gland secretions are carried to other internal body structures by the bloodstream.

The **endocrine system** is a collection of **glands** that secrete **hormones** directly into the bloodstream. Hormones are chemicals that act on their **target organs** to either increase or decrease the target's activity level. In this way the endocrine system is instrumental in maintaining **homeostasis**—that is, adjusting the activity level of most of the tissues and organs of the body to maintain a stable internal environment.

The body actually has two distinct types of glands: **exocrine glands** and **endocrine glands**. Exocrine glands release their secretions into a duct that carries them to the outside of the body. For example, sweat glands release sweat into a sweat duct that travels to the surface of the body. Endocrine glands, however, release hormones directly into the bloodstream. For example, the thyroid gland secretes its hormones directly into the bloodstream. Because endocrine glands have no ducts, they are also referred to as *ductless glands*.

The endocrine system consists of the following glands: two **adrenal glands**, two **ovaries** in the female, four **parathyroid glands**, the **pancreas**, the **pineal gland**, the **pituitary gland**, two **testes** in the male, the **thymus gland**, and the **thyroid gland**. The endocrine glands as a whole affect the functions of the entire body. Table 1 ■ presents a description of the endocrine glands, their hormones, and their functions.

Table 1	Endocrine Glands and Their Hormones
GLAND AND HORMONE	**FUNCTION**
Adrenal cortex	
Glucocorticoids	
Cortisol	Regulates carbohydrate levels in the body
Mineralocorticoids	
Aldosterone	Regulates electrolytes and fluid volume in body
Steroid sex hormones	
Androgen, estrogen, progesterone	Responsible for reproduction and secondary sexual characteristics
Adrenal medulla	
Epinephrine (adrenaline)	Intensifies response during stress; "fight or flight" response
Norepinephrine	Chiefly a vasoconstrictor

Table 1   Endocrine Glands and Their Hormones *(continued)*

GLAND AND HORMONE	FUNCTION
Ovaries	
Estrogen	Stimulates development of secondary sex characteristics in females; regulates menstrual cycle
Progesterone	Prepares for conditions of pregnancy
Pancreas	
Glucagon	Stimulates liver to release glucose into the blood
Insulin	Regulates and promotes entry of glucose into cells
Parathyroid glands	
Parathyroid hormone (PTH)	Stimulates bone breakdown; regulates calcium level in the blood
Pituitary anterior lobe	
Adrenocorticotropin hormone (ACTH)	Regulates function of adrenal cortex
Follicle-stimulating hormone (FSH)	Stimulates growth of eggs in female and sperm in males
Growth hormone (GH)	Stimulates growth of the body
Luteinizing hormone (LH)	Regulates function of male and female gonads and plays a role in releasing ova in females
Melanocyte-stimulating hormone (MSH)	Stimulates pigment in skin
Prolactin	Stimulates milk production
Thyroid-stimulating hormone (TSH)	Regulates function of thyroid gland
Pituitary posterior lobe	
Antidiuretic hormone (ADH)	Stimulates reabsorption of water by the kidneys
Oxytocin	Stimulates uterine contractions and releases milk into ducts
Testes	
Testosterone	Promotes sperm production and development of secondary sex characteristics in males
Thymus	
Thymosin	Promotes development of cells in immune system
Thyroid gland	
Calcitonin	Stimulates deposition of calcium into bone
Thyroxine (T_4)	Stimulates metabolism in cells
Triiodothyronine (T_3)	Stimulates metabolism in cells

Adrenal Glands

adrenal cortex (KOR-tex)
adrenal medulla (meh-DOOL-lah)
adrenaline (ah-DREN-ah-lin)
aldosterone (al-DOSS-ter-ohn)
androgens (AN-druh-jenz)
corticosteroids (kor-tih-koh-STAIR-oydz)
cortisol (KOR-tih-sal)
epinephrine (ep-ih-NEF-rin)

estrogen (ESS-troh-jen)
glucocorticoids (gloo-koh-KOR-tih-koydz)
mineralocorticoids
  (min-er-al-oh-KOR-tih-koydz)
norepinephrine (nor-ep-ih-NEF-rin)
progesterone (proh-JESS-ter-ohn)
steroid sex hormones (STAIR-oyd)

Med Term Tip

The term *cortex* is frequently used in anatomy to indicate the outer portion of an organ such as the adrenal gland or the kidney. The term *cortex* means "bark," as in the bark of a tree. The term *medulla* means "marrow." Because marrow is found in the inner cavity of bones, the term came to stand for the middle of an organ.

The two adrenal glands are located above each of the kidneys (see Figure 1 ■). Each gland is composed of two sections: **adrenal cortex** and **adrenal medulla**.

The outer adrenal cortex manufactures several different families of hormones: **mineralocorticoids**, **glucocorticoids**, and **steroid sex hormones**. However, because they are all produced by the cortex, they are collectively referred to as **corticosteroids**. The mineralocorticoid hormone, **aldosterone**, regulates sodium (Na^+) and potassium (K^+) levels in the body. The glucocorticoid hormone, **cortisol**, regulates carbohydrates in the body. The adrenal cortex of both men and women secretes steroid sex hormones: **androgens**, **estrogen**, and **progesterone**. These hormones regulate secondary sexual characteristics. All hormones secreted by the adrenal cortex are steroid hormones.

The inner adrenal medulla is responsible for secreting the hormones **epinephrine**, also called **adrenaline**, and **norepinephrine**. These hormones are critical during emergency situations because they increase blood pressure, heart rate, and respiration levels. This helps the body perform better during emergencies or otherwise stressful times.

Ovaries

estrogen
gametes (gam-EATS)
gonads (GOH-nadz)

menstrual cycle (men-STROO-all)
ova
progesterone

The two ovaries are located in the lower abdominopelvic cavity of the female (see Figure 2 ■). They are the female **gonads**. Gonads are organs that produce **gametes** or the reproductive sex cells. In the case of females, the gametes are the **ova**. Of importance to the endocrine system, the ovaries produce the female sex hormones, **estrogen** and **progesterone**. Estrogen is responsible for the appearance of the female sexual characteristics and regulation of the **menstrual cycle**. Progesterone helps to maintain a suitable uterine environment for pregnancy.

■ **Figure 1** The adrenal glands. These glands sit on top of each kidney. Each adrenal is subdivided into an outer cortex and an inner medulla. Each region secretes different hormones.

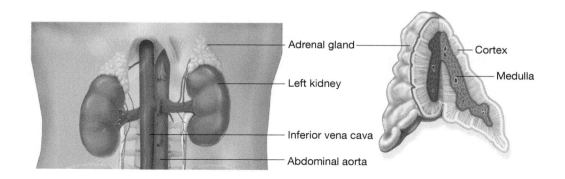

Adrenal gland

Left kidney

Inferior vena cava

Abdominal aorta

Cortex

Medulla

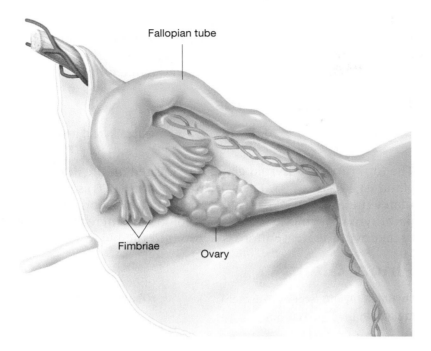

Fallopian tube

Fimbriae

Ovary

■ **Figure 2** The ovaries. In addition to producing ova, the ovaries secrete the female sex hormones, estrogen and progesterone.

Pancreas

glucagon (GLOO-koh-gon)
insulin (IN-suh-lin)

islets of Langerhans
(EYE-lets of LAHNG-er-hahnz)

The pancreas is located along the lower curvature of the stomach (see Figure 3A ■). It is the only organ in the body that has both endocrine and exocrine functions. The exocrine portion of the pancreas releases digestive enzymes through a duct into the duodenum of the small intestine. The endocrine sections of the pancreas, **islets of Langerhans**, are named after Dr. Paul Langerhans, a German anatomist. The islets cells produce two different hormones: **insulin** and **glucagon** (see Figure 3B ■). Insulin, produced by beta (β) islet cells, stimulates the cells of the body to take in glucose from the bloodstream, lowering your blood sugar level. This occurs after you have eaten a meal and absorbed the carbohydrates into your bloodstream. In this way the cells obtain the glucose they need for cellular respiration.

Another set of islet cells, the alpha (α) cells, secrete a different hormone, glucagon, which stimulates the liver to release glucose, thereby raising the blood

A

Liver

Stomach

Pancreas

BETA CELL
Insulin-secreting cell

ALPHA CELL
Glucagon-secreting cell

Islet of Langerhans in pancreas

B

Glucagon-raises blood glucose level
Insulin-lowers blood glucose level

■ **Figure 3** The pancreas. This organ sits just below the stomach and is both an exocrine and an endocrine gland. The endocrine regions of the pancreas are called the islets of Langerhans and they secrete insulin and glucagon.

glucose level. Glucagon is released when the body needs more sugar, such as at the beginning of strenuous activity or several hours after the last meal has been digested. Insulin and glucagon have opposite effects on blood sugar level. Insulin will reduce the blood sugar level, while glucagon will increase it.

Parathyroid Glands

calcium   **parathyroid hormone**
                                                                               (pair-ah-THIGH-royd HOR-mohn)

The four tiny parathyroid glands are located on the dorsal surface of the thyroid gland (see Figure 4 ■). The **parathyroid hormone** (PTH) secreted by these glands regulates the amount of **calcium** in the blood. If blood calcium levels fall too low, parathyroid hormone levels in the blood are increased and will stimulate bone breakdown to release more calcium into the blood.

Pineal Gland

circadian rhythm (seer-KAY-dee-an)   **thalamus** (THALL-mus)
melatonin (mel-ah-TOH-nin)

The pineal gland is a small pine-cone-shaped gland that is part of the **thalamus** region of the brain (see Figure 5 ■). The pineal gland secretes **melatonin**, a hormone not well understood, but that plays a role in regulating the body's **circadian rhythm**. This is the 24-hour clock that governs our periods of wakefulness and sleepiness.

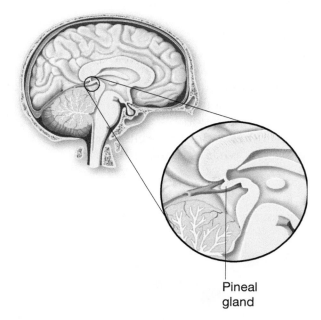

■ **Figure 4** The parathyroid glands. These four glands are located on the posterior side of the thyroid gland. They secrete parathyroid hormone.

■ **Figure 5** The pineal gland is a part of the thalamus region of the brain. It secretes melatonin.

Pituitary Gland

adrenocorticotropin hormone
(ah-dree-noh-kor-tih-koh-TROH-pin)
anterior lobe
antidiuretic hormone (an-tye-dye-yoo-RET-ik)
follicle-stimulating hormone
(FOLL-ih-kl STIM-yoo-lay-ting)
gonadotropins (go-nad-oh-TROH-pins)
growth hormone
hypothalamus (high-poh-THAL-ah-mus)

luteinizing hormone (LOO-tee-in-eye-zing)
melanocyte-stimulating hormone
oxytocin (ok-see-TOH-sin)
posterior lobe
prolactin (proh-LAK-tin)
somatotropin (so-mat-oh-TROH-pin)
thyroid-stimulating hormone

The pituitary gland is located underneath the brain (see Figure 6 ■). The small marble-shaped gland is divided into an **anterior lobe** and a **posterior lobe**. Both lobes are controlled by the **hypothalamus**, a region of the brain active in regulating automatic body responses.

The anterior pituitary secretes several different hormones (see Figure 7 ■). **Growth hormone** (GH), also called **somatotropin**, promotes growth of the body by stimulating cells to rapidly increase in size and divide. **Thyroid-stimulating hormone** (TSH) regulates the function of the thyroid gland. **Adrenocorticotropin hormone** (ACTH) regulates the function of the adrenal cortex. **Prolactin** (PRL) stimulates milk production in the breast following pregnancy and birth. **Follicle-stimulating hormone** (FSH) and **luteinizing hormone** (LH) both exert their influence on the male and female gonads. Therefore, these two hormones together are referred to as the **gonadotropins**. Follicle-stimulating hormone is responsible for the develop-

Med Term Tip

The pituitary gland is sometimes referred to as the "master gland" because several of its secretions regulate other endocrine glands.

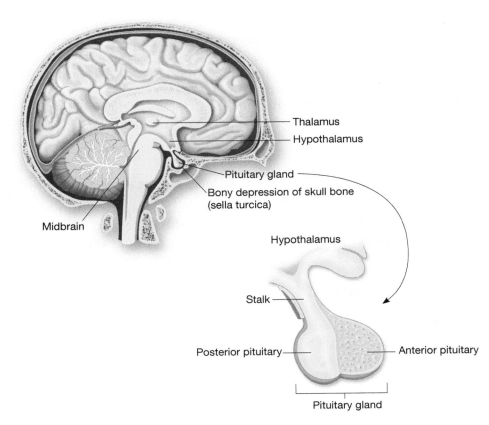

■ **Figure 6** The pituitary gland lies just underneath the brain. It is subdivided into anterior and posterior lobes. Each lobe secretes different hormones.

Thalamus
Hypothalamus
Pituitary gland
Bony depression of skull bone (sella turcica)
Midbrain
Hypothalamus
Stalk
Posterior pituitary
Anterior pituitary
Pituitary gland

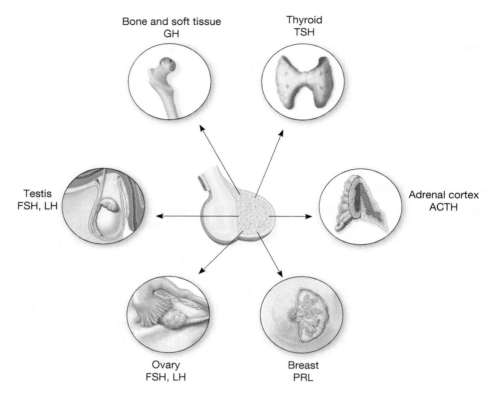

Bone and soft tissue
GH

Thyroid
TSH

Testis
FSH, LH

Adrenal cortex
ACTH

Ovary
FSH, LH

Breast
PRL

■ **Figure 7** The anterior pituitary is sometimes called the master gland because it secretes many hormones that regulate other glands. This figure illustrates the different hormones and target tissues for the anterior pituitary.

Med Term Tip

Many people use the term *diabetes* to refer to diabetes mellitus (DM). But there is another type of diabetes, called *diabetes insipidus* (DI) that is a result of the inadequate secretion of the antidiuretic hormone (ADH) from the pituitary gland.

ment of ova in ovaries and sperm in testes. It also stimulates the ovary to secrete estrogen. Luteinizing hormone stimulates secretion of sex hormones in both males and females and plays a role in releasing ova in females. **Melanocyte-stimulating hormone** (MSH) stimulates melanocytes to produce more melanin, thereby darkening the skin.

The posterior pituitary secretes two hormones, **antidiuretic hormone** (ADH) and **oxytocin**. Antidiuretic hormone promotes water reabsorption by the kidney tubules. Oxytocin stimulates uterine contractions during labor and delivery, and after birth the release of milk from the mammary glands.

Testes

sperm   **testosterone** (tess-TOSS-ter-own)

The testes are two oval glands located in the scrotal sac of the male (see Figure 8 ■). They are the male gonads, which produce the male gametes, **sperm**, and the male sex hormone, **testosterone**. Testosterone produces the male secondary sexual characteristics and regulates sperm production.

Thymus Gland

T cells   **thymosin** (thigh-MOH-sin)

In addition to its role as part of the immune system, the thymus is also one of the endocrine glands because it secretes the hormone **thymosin**. Thymosin, like the rest of the thymus gland, is important for proper development of the immune system. The thymus gland is located in the mediastinal cavity anterior and superior to the heart (see Figure 9 ■). The thymus is present at birth and grows to its largest size during puberty. At puberty it begins to shrink and eventually is replaced with connective and adipose tissue.

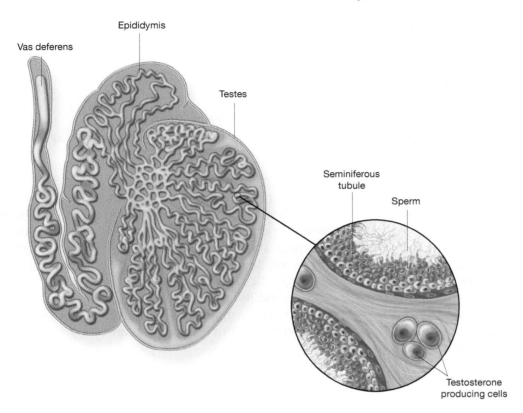

Vas deferens

Epididymis

Testes

Seminiferous tubule

Sperm

Testosterone producing cells

■ **Figure 8** The testes. In addition to producing sperm, the testes secrete the male sex hormones, primarily testosterone.

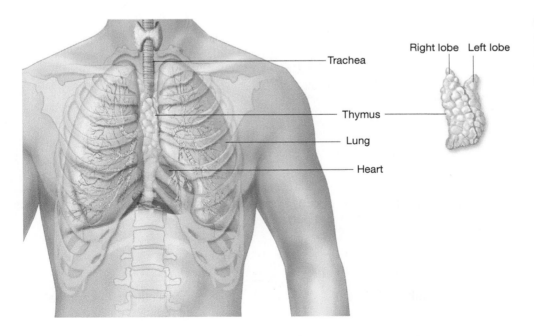

Trachea

Thymus

Lung

Heart

Right lobe   Left lobe

■ **Figure 9** The thymus gland. This gland lies in the mediastinum of the thoracic cavity, just above the heart. It secretes thymosin.

The most important function of the thymus is the development of the immune system in the newborn. It is essential to the growth and development of thymic lymphocytes or **T cells**, which are critical for the body's immune system.

Thyroid Gland

calcitonin (kal-sih-TOH-nin)
iodine
thyroxine (thigh-ROKS-in)

triiodothyronine
(try-eye-oh-doh-THIGH-roh-neen)

Med Term Tip

Iodine is found in many foods, including vegetables and seafood. It is also present in iodized salt, which is one of the best sources of iodine for people living in the goiter belt, composed of states located away from saltwater. A lack of iodine in the diet can lead to thyroid disorders, including *goiter*.

The thyroid gland, which resembles a butterfly in shape, has right and left lobes (see Figure 10 ■). It is located on either side of the trachea and larynx. The thyroid cartilage, or Adam's apple, is located just above the thyroid gland. This gland produces the hormones **thyroxine** (T_4) and **triiodothyronine** (T_3). These hormones are produced in the thyroid gland from the mineral **iodine** (**EYE** oh dine). Thyroxine and triiodothyronine help to regulate the production of energy and heat in the body to adjust the body's metabolic rate.

The thyroid gland also secretes **calcitonin** in response to hypercalcemia (too high blood calcium level). Its action is the opposite of parathyroid hormone and stimulates the increased deposition of calcium into bone, thereby lowering blood levels of calcium.

■ **Figure 10** The thyroid gland is subdivided into two lobes, one on each side of the trachea.

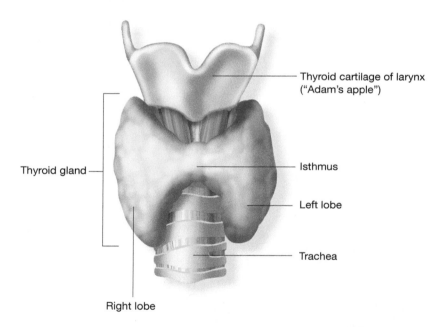

Thyroid cartilage of larynx ("Adam's apple")

Thyroid gland

Isthmus

Left lobe

Trachea

Right lobe

Word Building

The following list contains examples of medical terms built directly from word parts. The definitions of these terms can be determined by a straightforward translation of the word parts.

COMBINING FORM	COMBINED WITH	MEDICAL TERM	DEFINITION
adren/o	-al	**adrenal** (ah-DREE-nall)	pertaining to the adrenal glands
	-megaly	**adrenomegaly** (ad-ree-noh-MEG-ah-lee)	enlarged adrenal gland
	-pathy	**adrenopathy** (ad-ren-OP-ah-thee)	adrenal gland disease

Word Building (continued)

COMBINING FORM	COMBINED WITH	MEDICAL TERM	DEFINITION
adrenal/o	-ectomy	**adrenalectomy** (ad-ree-nal-EK-toh-mee)	removal of adrenal glands
	-itis	**adrenalitis** (ad-ree-nal-EYE-tis)	inflammation of an adrenal gland
calc/o	hyper- -emia	**hypercalcemia** (high-per-kal-SEE-mee-ah)	excessive calcium in the blood
	hypo- -emia	**hypocalcemia** (high-poh-kal-SEE-mee-ah)	low calcium in the blood
crin/o	endo- -ologist	**endocrinologist** (en-doh-krin-ALL-oh-jist)	specialist in the endocrine system
	endo- -pathy	**endocrinopathy** (en-doh-krin-OP-ah-thee)	endocrine system disease
glyc/o	hyper- -emia	**hyperglycemia** (high-per-glye-SEE-mee-ah)	excessive sugar in the blood
	hypo- -emia	**hypoglycemia** (high-poh-glye-SEE-mee-ah)	low sugar in the blood
kal/i	hyper- -emia	**hyperkalemia** (high-per-kal-EE-mee-ah)	excessive potassium in the blood
natr/o	hypo- -emia	**hyponatremia** (high-poh-nah-TREE-mee-ah)	low sodium in the blood
pancreat/o	-ic	**pancreatic** (pan-kree-AT-ik)	pertaining to the pancreas
parathyroid/o	-al	**parathyroidal** (pair-ah-THIGH-roy-dall)	pertaining to the parathyroid gland
	-ectomy	**parathyroidectomy** (pair-ah-thigh-royd-EK-toh-mee)	removal of the parathyroid gland
	hyper- -ism	**hyperparathyroidism** (HIGH-per-pair-ah-THIGH-royd-izm)	state of excessive parathyroid
	hypo- -ism	**hypoparathyroidism** (HIGH-poh-pair-ah-THIGH-royd-izm)	state of insufficient parathyroid
pituitar/o	-ary	**pituitary** (pih-TOO-ih-tair-ee)	pertaining to the pituitary gland
	hypo- -ism	**hypopituitarism** (HIGH-poh-pih-TOO-ih-tuh-rizm)	state of insufficient pituitary
	hyper- -ism	**hyperpituitarism** (HIGH-per-pih-TOO-ih-tuh-rizm)	state of excessive pituitary
thym/o	-ic	**thymic** (THIGH-mik)	pertaining to the thymus gland
	-ectomy	**thymectomy** (thigh-MEK-toh-mee)	removal of the thymus
	-itis	**thymitis** (thigh-MY-tis)	thymus inflammation
	-oma	**thymoma** (thigh-MOH-mah)	thymus tumor
thyr/o	-megaly	**thyromegaly** (thigh-roh-MEG-ah-lee)	enlarged thyroid
thyroid/o	-al	**thyroidal** (thigh-ROYD-all)	pertaining to the thyroid gland

Word Building *(continued)*

COMBINING FORM	COMBINED WITH	MEDICAL TERM	DEFINITION
	-ectomy	**thyroidectomy** (thigh-royd-EK-toh-mee)	removal of the thyroid
	hyper- -ism	**hyperthyroidism** (hi-per-THIGH-royd-izm)	state of excessive thyroid
	hypo- -ism	**hypothyroidism** (high-poh-THIGH-royd-izm)	state of insufficient thyroid

SUFFIX	COMBINED WITH	MEDICAL TERM	DEFINITION
-dipsia	poly-	**polydipsia** (pall-ee-DIP-see-ah)	many (excessive) thirst
-uria	poly-	**polyuria** (pall-ee-YOO-ree-ah)	condition of (too) much urine
	glycos/o	**glycosuria** (glye-kohs-YOO-ree-ah)	sugar in the urine

Vocabulary

TERM	DEFINITION
acidosis (as-ih-DOH-sis)	Excessive acidity of body fluids due to the accumulation of acids, as in diabetic acidosis.
edema (eh-DEE-mah)	Condition in which the body tissues contain excessive amounts of fluid.
endocrinology (en-doh-krin-ALL-oh-jee)	Branch of medicine involving diagnosis and treatment of conditions and diseases of endocrine glands. Physician is an *endocrinologist*.
exophthalmos (eks-off-THAL-mohs)	Condition in which the eyeballs protrude, such as in Graves' disease. This is generally caused by an overproduction of thyroid hormone.

■ **Figure 11** A photograph of a woman with exophthalmos. This condition is associated with hypersecretion of the thyroid gland. *(Custom Medical Stock Photo, Inc.)*

TERM	DEFINITION
gynecomastia (gigh-neh-koh-MAST-ee-ah)	Development of breast tissue in males. May be a symptom of adrenal feminization (see Pathology table).
hirsutism (HER-soot-izm)	Condition of having an excessive amount of hair. Term generally used to describe females who have the adult male pattern of hair growth. Can be the result of a hormonal imbalance.
hypersecretion	Excessive hormone production by an endocrine gland.
hyposecretion	Deficient hormone production by an endocrine gland.
obesity (oh-BEE-sih-tee)	Having an abnormal amount of fat in the body.
syndrome (SIN-drohm)	Group of symptoms and signs that, when combined, present a clinical picture of a disease or condition.

Pathology

TERM	DEFINITION
■ Adrenal Glands	
Addison's disease (AD-ih-sons dih-ZEEZ)	Disease named for British physician Thomas Addison that results from a deficiency in adrenocortical hormones. There may be an increased pigmentation of the skin, generalized weakness, and weight loss.
adrenal feminization (ad-REE-nal fem-ih-nigh-ZAY-shun)	Development of female secondary sexual characteristics (such as breasts) in a male. Often as a result of increased estrogen secretion by the adrenal cortex.
adrenal virilism (ad-REE-nal VIR-ill-izm)	Development of male secondary sexual characteristics (such as deeper voice and facial hair) in a female. Often as a result of increased androgen secretion by the adrenal cortex.
Cushing's syndrome (CUSH-ings SIN-drohm)	Set of symptoms, named after U.S. neurosurgeon Harvey Cushing, that result from hypersecretion of the adrenal cortex. This may be the result of a tumor of the adrenal glands. The syndrome may present symptoms of weakness, edema, excess hair growth, skin discoloration, and osteoporosis.

■ **Figure 12** Cushing's syndrome. A photograph of a woman with the characteristic facial features of Cushing's syndrome. *(Biophoto Associates/ Science Source/Photo Researchers, Inc.)*

TERM	DEFINITION
pheochromocytoma (fee-oh-kroh-moh-sigh-TOH-ma)	Usually benign tumor of the adrenal medulla that secretes epinephrine. Symptoms include anxiety, heart palpitations, dyspnea, profuse sweating, headache, and nausea.
■ Pancreas	
diabetes mellitus (DM) (dye-ah-BEE-teez MELL-ih-tus)	Chronic disorder of carbohydrate metabolism that results in hyperglycemia and glycosuria. There are two distinct forms of diabetes mellitus: *insulin-dependent diabetes mellitus* (IDDM) or *type 1*, and *non–insulin-dependent diabetes mellitus* (NIDDM) or *type 2*.
diabetic retinopathy (dye-ah-BET-ik ret-in-OP-ah-thee)	Secondary complication of diabetes that affects the blood vessels of the retina, resulting in visual changes and even blindness.
insulin-dependent diabetes mellitus (IDDM) (dye-ah-BEE-teez MELL-ih-tus)	Also called *type 1 diabetes mellitus.* It develops early in life when the pancreas stops insulin production. Patient must take daily insulin injections.
insulinoma (in-sue-lin-OH-mah)	Tumor of the islets of Langerhans cells of the pancreas that secretes an excessive amount of insulin.
ketoacidosis (kee-toh-ass-ih-DOH-sis)	Acidosis due to an excess of acidic ketone bodies (waste products). A serious condition requiring immediate treatment that can result in death for the diabetic patient if not reversed. Also called *diabetic acidosis.*

Pathology *(continued)*

TERM	DEFINITION
non–insulin-dependent diabetes mellitus (dye-ah-BEE-teez MELL-ih-tus)	Also called *type 2 diabetes mellitus.* It typically develops later in life. The pancreas produces normal to high levels of insulin, but the cells fail to respond to it. Patients may take oral hypoglycemics to improve insulin function, or may eventually have to take insulin.
peripheral neuropathy (per-IF-eh-rall new-ROP-ah-thee)	Damage to the nerves in the lower legs and hands as a result of diabetes mellitus. Symptoms include either extreme sensitivity or numbness and tingling.

■ *Parathyroid Glands*

tetany (TET-ah-nee)	Nerve irritability and painful muscle cramps resulting from hypocalcemia. Hypoparathyroidism is one cause of tetany.
Recklinghausen disease (REK-ling-how-zenz)	Excessive production of parathyroid hormone, which results in degeneration of the bones. Named for German histologist Friedrich von Recklinghausen.

■ *Pituitary Gland*

acromegaly (ak-roh-MEG-ah-lee)	Chronic disease of adults that results in an elongation and enlargement of the bones of the head and extremities. There can also be mood changes. Due to an excessive amount of growth hormone in an adult.

■ Figure 13 Acromegaly. The hand on the right is from an adult with normal levels of growth hormone. The hand on the left is from an adult with excessive levels of growth hormone. This results in an increase in the size of the hands, feet, and jaw. *(Bart's Medical Library/Phototake NYC)*

diabetes insipidus (DI) (dye-ah-BEE-teez in-SIP-ih-dus)	Disorder caused by the inadequate secretion of antidiuretic hormone by the posterior lobe of the pituitary gland. There may be polyuria and polydipsia.
dwarfism (DWARF-izm)	Condition of being abnormally short in height. It may be the result of a hereditary condition or a lack of growth hormone.
gigantism (JYE-gan-tizm)	Excessive development of the body due to the overproduction of the growth hormone by the pituitary gland in a child or teenager. The opposite of *dwarfism.*
panhypopituitarism (pan-high-poh-pih-TOO-ih-tair-izm)	Deficiency in all the hormones secreted by the pituitary gland. Often recognized because of problems with the glands regulated by the pituitary–adrenal cortex, thyroid, ovaries, and testes.

■ *Thyroid Gland*

cretinism (KREE-tin-izm)	Congenital condition in which a lack of thyroid hormones may result in arrested physical and mental development.

Pathology *(continued)*

TERM	DEFINITION
goiter (GOY-ter)	Enlargement of the thyroid gland.

■ **Figure 14** Goiter. A photograph of a male with an extreme goiter or enlarged thyroid gland.

TERM	DEFINITION
Graves' disease	Condition named for Irish physician Robert Graves that results in overactivity of the thyroid gland and can cause a crisis situation. Symptoms include exophthalmos and goiter. A type of *hyperthyroidism*.
Hashimoto's disease (hash-ee-MOH-tohz dih-ZEEZ)	Chronic autoimmune form of thyroiditis, results in hyposecretion of thyroid hormones.
myxedema (miks-eh-DEE-mah)	Condition resulting from a hyposecretion of the thyroid gland in an adult. Symptoms can include anemia, slow speech, swollen facial features, edematous skin, drowsiness, and mental lethargy.
thyrotoxicosis (thigh-roh-toks-ih-KOH-sis)	Condition resulting from marked overproduction of the thyroid gland. Symptoms include rapid heart action, tremors, enlarged thyroid gland, exophthalmos, and weight loss.

■ *All Glands*

TERM	DEFINITION
adenocarcinoma (ad-eh-no-car-sih-NO-mah)	Cancerous tumor in a gland that is capable of producing the hormones secreted by that gland. One cause of hypersecretion pathologies.

Diagnostic Procedures

TERM	DEFINITION

■ *Clinical Laboratory Tests*

TERM	DEFINITION
blood serum test	Blood test to measure the level of substances such as calcium, electrolytes, testosterone, insulin, and glucose. Used to assist in determining the function of various endocrine glands.
fasting blood sugar (FBS)	Blood test to measure the amount of sugar circulating throughout the body after a 12-hour fast.

Diagnostic Procedures *(continued)*

TERM	DEFINITION
glucose tolerance test (GTT) (GLOO-kohs)	Test to determine the blood sugar level. A measured dose of glucose is given to a patient either orally or intravenously. Blood samples are then drawn at certain intervals to determine the ability of the patient to use glucose. Used for diabetic patients to determine their insulin response to glucose.
protein-bound iodine test (PBI)	Blood test to measure the concentration of thyroxine (T_4) circulating in the bloodstream. The iodine becomes bound to the protein in the blood and can be measured. Useful in establishing thyroid function.
radioimmunoassay (RIA) (ray-dee-oh-im-yoo-noh-ASS-ay)	Test used to measure the levels of hormones in the plasma of the blood.
thyroid function test (TFT) (THIGH-royd)	Blood test used to measure the levels of thyroxine, triiodothyronine, and thyroid-stimulating hormone in the bloodstream to assist in determining thyroid function.
total calcium	Blood test to measure the total amount of calcium to assist in detecting parathyroid and bone disorders.
two-hour postprandial glucose tolerance test (post-PRAN-dee-al)	Blood test to assist in evaluating glucose metabolism. The patient eats a high carbohydrate diet and then fasts overnight before the test. Then the blood sample is taken two hours after a meal.
■ *Diagnostic Imaging*	
thyroid echogram (THIGH-royd EK-oh-gram)	Ultrasound examination of the thyroid that can assist in distinguishing a thyroid nodule from a cyst.
thyroid scan (THIGH-royd)	Test in which radioactive iodine is administered that localizes in the thyroid gland. The gland can then be visualized with a scanning device to detect pathology such as tumors.

Therapeutic Procedures

TERM	DEFINITION
■ *Medical Procedures*	
chemical thyroidectomy (thigh-royd-EK-toh-mee)	Large dose of radioactive iodine is given in order to kill thyroid gland cells without having to actually do surgery.
hormone replacement therapy	Artificial replacement of hormones in patients with hyposecretion disorders. May be oral pills, injections, or adhesive skin patches.
■ *Surgical Procedures*	
laparoscopic adrenalectomy (lap-row-SKOP-ik ad-ree-nal-EK-toh-mee)	Removal of the adrenal gland through a small incision in the abdomen and using endoscopic instruments.
lobectomy (lobe-EK-toh-mee)	Removal of a lobe from an organ. In this case, one lobe of the thyroid gland.

Pharmacology

CLASSIFICATION	ACTION	GENERIC AND BRAND NAMES
antithyroid agents	Medication given to block production of thyroid hormones in patients with hypersecretion disorders.	methimazole, Tapazole; propylthiouracil
corticosteroids (kor-tih-koh-STAIR-oydz)	Although the function of these hormones in the body is to regulate carbohydrate metabolism, they also have a strong anti-inflammatory action. Therefore they are used to treat severe chronic inflammatory diseases such as rheumatoid arthritis. Long-term use of corticosteroids has adverse side effects such as osteoporosis and the symptoms of Cushing's disease. Also used to treat adrenal cortex hyposecretion disorders such as Addison's disease.	prednisone, Deltasone
human growth hormone therapy	Hormone replacement therapy with human growth hormone in order to stimulate skeletal growth. Used to treat children with abnormally short stature.	somatropin, Genotropin; somatrem, Protropin
insulin (IN-suh-lin)	Administered to replace insulin for type 1 diabetics or to treat severe type 2 diabetics.	human insulin, Humulin L
oral hypoglycemic agents (high-poh-glye-SEE-mik)	Medications taken by mouth that cause a decrease in blood sugar; not used for insulin-dependent patients.	metformin, Glucophage; glipizide, Glucotrol
thyroid replacement hormone	Hormone replacement therapy for patients with hypothyroidism or who have had a thyroidectomy.	levothyroxine, Levo-T; liothyronine, Cytomel
vasopressin (vaz-oh-PRESS-in)	Given to control diabetes insipidus and promote reabsorption of water in the kidney tubules.	desmopressin acetate, Desmopressin; conivaptan, Vaprisol

Abbreviations

α	alpha		MSH	melanocyte-stimulating hormone
ACTH	adrenocorticotropin hormone		Na$^+$	sodium
ADH	antidiuretic hormone		NIDDM	non–insulin-dependent diabetes mellitus
β	beta		NPH	neutral protamine Hagedorn (insulin)
BMR	basal metabolic rate		PBI	protein-bound iodine
DI	diabetes insipidus		PRL	prolactin
DM	diabetes mellitus		PTH	parathyroid hormone
FBS	fasting blood sugar		RAI	radioactive iodine
FSH	follicle-stimulating hormone		RIA	radioimmunoassay
GH	growth hormone		T$_3$	triiodothyronine
GTT	glucose tolerance test		T$_4$	thyroxine
IDDM	insulin-dependent diabetes mellitus		TFT	thyroid function test
K$^+$	potassium		TSH	thyroid-stimulating hormone
LH	luteinizing hormone			

Chapter Review

Terminology Checklist

Below are all Anatomy and Physiology key terms, Word Building, Vocabulary, Pathology, Diagnostic, Therapeutic, and Pharmacology terms presented in this chapter. Use this list as a study tool by placing a check in the box in front of each term as you master its meaning.

☐ acidosis
☐ acromegaly
☐ Addison's disease
☐ adenocarcinoma
☐ adrenal
☐ adrenal cortex
☐ adrenalectomy
☐ adrenal feminization
☐ adrenal glands
☐ adrenaline
☐ adrenalitis
☐ adrenal medulla
☐ adrenal virilism
☐ adrenocorticotropin hormone
☐ adrenomegaly
☐ adrenopathy
☐ aldosterone
☐ androgen
☐ anterior lobe
☐ antidiuretic hormone
☐ antithyroid agents
☐ blood serum test
☐ calcitonin
☐ calcium
☐ chemical thyroidectomy
☐ circadian rhythm
☐ corticosteroids
☐ cortisol
☐ cretinism
☐ Cushing's syndrome
☐ diabetes insipidus
☐ diabetes mellitus
☐ diabetic retinopathy
☐ dwarfism
☐ edema
☐ endocrine glands
☐ endocrine system
☐ endocrinologist
☐ endocrinology

☐ endocrinopathy
☐ epinephrine
☐ estrogen
☐ exocrine glands
☐ exophthalmos
☐ fasting blood sugar
☐ follicle-stimulating hormone
☐ gametes
☐ gigantism
☐ glands
☐ glucagon
☐ glucocorticoids
☐ glucose tolerance test
☐ glycosuria
☐ goiter
☐ gonadotropins
☐ gonads
☐ Graves' disease
☐ growth hormone
☐ gynecomastia
☐ Hashimoto's disease
☐ hirsutism
☐ homeostasis
☐ hormone
☐ hormone replacement therapy
☐ human growth hormone therapy
☐ hypercalcemia
☐ hyperglycemia
☐ hyperkalemia
☐ hyperparathyroidism
☐ hyperpituitarism
☐ hypersecretion
☐ hyperthyroidism
☐ hypocalcemia
☐ hypoglycemia
☐ hyponatremia
☐ hypoparathyroidism
☐ hypopituitarism

☐ hyposecretion
☐ hypothalamus
☐ hypothyroidism
☐ insulin
☐ insulin-dependent diabetes mellitus
☐ insulinoma
☐ iodine
☐ islets of Langerhans
☐ ketoacidosis
☐ laparoscopic adrenalectomy
☐ lobectomy
☐ luteinizing hormone
☐ melanocyte-stimulating hormone
☐ melatonin
☐ menstrual cycle
☐ mineralocorticoids
☐ myxedema
☐ non–insulin-dependent diabetes mellitus
☐ norepinephrine
☐ obesity
☐ oral hypoglycemic agent
☐ ova
☐ ovaries
☐ oxytocin
☐ pancreas
☐ pancreatic
☐ panhypopituitarism
☐ parathyroid glands
☐ parathyroidal
☐ parathyroidectomy
☐ parathyroid hormone
☐ peripheral neuropathy
☐ pheochromocytoma
☐ pineal gland
☐ pituitary
☐ pituitary gland
☐ polydipsia

- polyuria
- posterior lobe
- progesterone
- prolactin
- protein-bound iodine test
- radioimmunoassay
- Recklinghausen disease
- somatotropin
- sperm
- steroid sex hormones
- syndrome
- target organs
- T cells
- testes
- testosterone
- tetany
- thalamus
- thymectomy
- thymic
- thymitis
- thymoma
- thymosin
- thymus gland
- thyroidal
- thyroid echogram
- thyroidectomy
- thyroid function tests
- thyroid gland
- thyroid replacement hormone
- thyroid scan
- thyroid-stimulating hormone
- thyromegaly
- thyrotoxicosis
- thyroxine
- total calcium
- triiodothyronine
- two-hour postprandial glucose tolerance test
- vasopressin

Practice Exercises

A. Complete the following statements.

1. The study of the endocrine system is called _endocrinology_

2. The master endocrine gland is the _pituitary gland_.

3. _Gonads_ is a general term for the sexual organs that produce gametes.

4. The term for the hormones produced by the outer portion of the adrenal cortex is _corticosteroids_

5. The hormone produced by the testes is _testosterone_

6. The two hormones produced by the ovaries are _estrogen_ and _progesterone_

7. An inadequate supply of the hormone _ADH (antidiuretic hormone)_ causes diabetes insipidus.

8. The endocrine gland associated with the immune system is the _thymus_.

9. The term for a protrusion of the eyeballs in Graves' disease is _exophthalmos_

10. A general medical term for a hormone-secreting cancerous tumor is _adenocarcinoma_

B. State the terms described using the combining forms provided.

The combining form *thyroid/o* refers to the thyroid. Use it to write a term that means:

1. removal of the thyroid _thyroidectomy_

2. pertaining to the thyroid _thyroidal_

3. state of excessive thyroid _hyperthyroidism_

The combining form *pancreat/o* refers to the pancreas. Use it to write a term that means:

4. pertaining to the pancreas _pancreatic_

5. inflammation of the pancreas _pancreatitis_

Endocrine System

6. removal of the pancreas ___pancreatactomy___

7. incision into the pancreas ___pancreatotomy___

The combining form *adren/o* refers to the adrenal glands. Use it to write a term that means:

8. pertaining to the adrenal gland ___adrenal___

9. enlargement of the adrenal glands ___adrenomagaly___

10. adrenal gland disease ___adrenopathy___

The combining form *thym/o* refers to the thymus glands. Use it to write a term that means:

11. tumor of the thymus gland ___thymoma___

12. removal of the thymus gland ___thymactomy___

13. pertaining to the thymus gland ___thymic___

14. inflammation of the thymus gland ___thymitis___

C. Match each term to its definition.

1. _b_ Cushing's disease   a. enlarged thyroid

2. _a_ goiter   b. overactive adrenal cortex

3. _e_ acidosis   c. hyperthyroidism

4. _k_ gigantism   d. underactive adrenal cortex

5. _h_ cretinism   e. associated with diabetes

6. _j_ myxedema   f. causes polyuria and polydipsia

7. _i_ diabetes mellitus   g. thyroiditis

8. _f_ diabetes insipidus   h. arrested growth

9. _g_ Hashimoto's disease   i. poor carbohydrate metabolism

10. _c_ Graves' disease   j. enlarged facial features and edematous skin

11. _d_ Addison's disease   k. excessive growth hormone

D. Identify the following abbreviations.

1. PBI ___protein-bound iodine___

2. K^+ ___potassium___

3. T_4 ___thyroxine___

4. GTT ___glucose tolerance test___

5. DM _____ diabetes mellitus

6. BMR _____ basal metabolic rate

7. Na⁺ _____ sodium

8. ADH _____ antidiuretic hormone

E. Write the abbreviations for the following terms.

1. non–insulin-dependent diabetes mellitus _____ NIDDM

2. insulin-dependent diabetes mellitus _____ IDDM

3. adrenocorticotropin hormone _____ ACTH

4. parathyroid hormone _____ PTH

5. triiodothyronine _____ T3

6. thyroid stimulating hormone _____ TSH

7. fasting blood sugar _____ FBS

8. prolactin _____ PRL

F. Build an endocrine system term using one of the following suffixes.

-crine	-uria	-tropin
-dipsia	-emia	-prandial

1. the presence of sugar or glucose in the urine _____ glycosuria

2. the glandular system that secretes directly into the bloodstream _____ endocrine

3. excessive urination _____ polyuria

4. condition of excessive calcium in the blood _____ hyparcalcamia

5. excessive thirst _____ polydipsia

6. stimulate adrenal cortex _____ adranocorticotropin

7. after a meal _____ postprandial

G. Define the following terms.

1. corticosteroid _____ hormonas that raguate carbohydrate matabolism & have anti-inflammatory action

2. hirsutism _____ condition of having an axcessive amount of hair

3. tetany _____ narve irritability & painful muscle cramps rasulting from hypocalcamia

4. diabetic retinopathy _____ Secondary complication of diabetes -affacts blood vessels of the retina

5. hyperglycemia _____ axcassive sugar in the blood

Endocrine System

6. hypoglycemia _low sugar in the blood_

7. adrenaline _a hormone produced by the adrenal medulla - aka epinephrine_

8. insulin _hormone secreted by the pancreas, regulates level of sugar in the blood_

9. thyrotoxicosis _condition that results from overproduction of the thyroid gland_

10. hypersecretion _excessive hormone production by an endocrine gland_

H. Define the following combining forms and use them to form endocrine terms.

	Definition	Endocrine System Term
1. natr/o	sodium	hyponatremia
2. estr/o	female	estrogen
3. pineal/o	pineal gland	pineal gland
4. pituitar/o	pituitary gland	hypopituitarism
5. kal/i	potassium	hyperkalemia
6. calc/o	calcium	hypocalcemia
7. parathyroid/o	parathyroid gland	parathyroidal
8. acr/o	extremities	acromegaly
9. glyc/o	sugar	hypoglycemia
10. gonad/o	sex glands	gonadotropins

I. Match each term to its definition.

1. _e_ protein bound iodine test

2. _d_ fasting blood sugar

3. _a_ radioimmunoassay

4. _f_ thyroid scan

5. _c_ 2-hour postprandial glucose tolerance test

6. _b_ gluose tolerance test

a. measures levels of hormones in the blood

b. determines glucose metabolism after patient receives a measure dose of glucose

c. test of glucose metabolism two hours after eating a meal

d. measures blood sugar level after 12-hour fast

e. measures T4 concentration in the blood

f. uses radioactive iodine

J. Use the following terms in the sentences below.

insulinoma   ketoacidosis   pheochromocytoma

gynecomastia   panhypopituitarinism   Hashimoto's disease

1. The doctor found that Marsha's high level of insulin and hypoglycemia was caused by a(n) *insulinoma*.

2. Kevin developed *ketoacidosis* as a result of his diabetes mellitus and required emergency treatment.

3. It was determined that Karen had *panhypopituitarinism* when doctors realized she had problems with her thyroid gland, adrenal cortex, and ovaries.

4. Luke's high epinephrine level was caused by a(n) *pheochromocytoma*

5. When it was determined that Carl's thyroiditis was an autoimmune condition, it became obvious that he had *Hashimoto's disease*.

6. Excessive sex hormones caused Jack to develop *gynecomastia*

K. Fill in the classification for each drug description, then match the brand name.

Drug Description	Classification	Brand Name
1. _____ strong anti-inflammatory	_____	a. genotropin
2. _____ stimulates skeletal growth	_____	b. Desmopressin
3. _____ treats type 1 diabetes mellitus	_____	c. Tapazole
4. _____ blocks production of thyroid hormone	_____	d. glucophage
5. _____ treats type 1 diabetes mellitus	_____	e. Deltasone
6. _____ controls diabetes insipidus	_____	f. Humulin L

Medical Record Analysis

Below is an item from a patient's medical record. Read it carefully, make sure you understand all the medical terms used, and then answer the questions that follow.

Discharge Summary

Admitting Diagnosis:	Hyperglycemia, ketoacidosis, glycosuria
Final Diagnosis:	New-onset type 1 diabetes mellitus
History of Present Illness:	Patient presented to pediatrician's office with a two-month history of weight loss, fatigue, polyuria, and polydipsia. Her family history is significant for a grandfather, mother, and older brother with type 1 diabetes mellitus. The pediatrician found hyperglycemia with a fasting blood sugar and glycosuria with a urine dipstick. Patient was also noted to be dehydrated and extremely lethargic. She is being admitted at this time for management of new-onset diabetes mellitus.
Summary of Hospital Course:	At the time of admission, the FBS was 300 mg/100 mL and she was in ketoacidosis. She rapidly improved after receiving insulin; her serum glucose level normalized, and her lethargy disappeared. The next day a two-hour postprandial glucose tolerance test confirmed the diagnosis of diabetes mellitus while an abdominal x-ray and a pancreas CT scan were normal. There was no evidence of diabetic retinopathy. The patient was started on insulin injections. She was discharged three days later on a protocol of b.i.d. (twice a day) insulin injections. The patient and her family were instructed in diet, exercise, symptoms of hypoglycemic coma, insulin shock, and long-term complications of diabetes mellitus.
Discharge Plans:	Patient was discharged to home with her parents. She is on a 2,000-calorie ADA diet with three meals and two snacks. She may engage in any activity and may return to school next Monday. Her parents are to check her serum glucose levels b.i.d. and call the office for insulin dosage. She is to return to the office in two weeks.

Critical Thinking Questions

1. The patient's admitting diagnosis is three symptoms related to her final diagnosis. List the three symptoms and describe each in your own words.

   a. hyperglycemia - excessive sugar in the blood

   b. ketoacidosis - excess of acidic ketone bodies (waste products)

   c. glycosuria - sugar in the urine

2. This patient has type 1 diabetes mellitus. Use your text or other resource, such as the Internet, to explain the difference between type 1 and type 2.

   Diabetes mellitus is a chronic disorder of carbohydrate metabolism that results in hyperglycemia & glycosuria. Diabetes insipidus is a result of the inadequate secretion of the antidiuretic hormone ADH from the pituitary gland.

Endocrine System

3. This discharge summary contains four medical terms that have not been introduced yet. Describe each of these terms in your own words. Use your text as a dictionary.

a. retinopathy   retinal disease

b. protocol the actual plan of care, medications, surgeries, treatments for the care of the patient.

c. coma profound unconsciousness resulting from an illness or injury

d. b.i.d.   twice a day

4. This patient had three different types of blood tests during her hospital stay. List the three blood tests and describe the differences among them in your own words.

a. fasting blood sugar - measure amount of sugar in blood after 12hr fast

b. blood serum test - measures substances such as calcium, electrolytes, testosterone, insulin & glucose

c. two hour post prandial glucose tolerance test - assists in evaluating glucose metabolism

5. This patient had two imaging procedures conducted by the radiology department while she was in the hospital. List them and describe the differences between the two.

a. abdominal x-ray - picture of the whole abdomen

b. pancreas CT scan - scan of the pancreas

6. Describe the patient's discharge instructions in your own words. Patient must follow 2,000 calorie ADA diet w/3 meals & 2 snacks. May resume normal activities & return to school. Parents need to check her serum glucose levels twice a day & call doctor's office for her insulin dosage. She should come back for a follow up visit in 2 weeks.

Chart Note Transcription

The chart note below contains eleven phrases that can be reworded with a medical term that you learned in this chapter. Each phrase is identified with an underline. Determine the medical term and write your answers in the space provided.

Current Complaint: A 56-year-old female was referred to the specialist in the treatment of diseases of the endocrine glands ❶ for evaluation of weakness, edema, an abnormal amount of fat in the body, ❷ and an excessive amount of hair for a female. ❸

Past History: Patient reports she has been overweight most of her life in spite of a healthy diet and regular exercise. She was diagnosed with osteoporosis after incurring a pathological rib fracture following a coughing attack.

Signs and Symptoms: Patient has moderate edema in bilateral feet and lower legs as well as a puffy face and an upper lip moustache. She is 100 lbs. over normal body weight for her age and height. She moves slowly and appears generally lethargic. A test to measure the hormone levels in the blood plasma ❹ reports increased steroid hormone that regulates carbohydrates in the body ❺ levels in the blood. A CT scan demonstrates a gland tumor ❻ in the right outer layer of the adrenal gland. ❼

Diagnosis: A group of symptoms associated with hypersecretion of the adrenal cortex ❽ secondary to a gland tumor ❾ in the right outer layer of the adrenal gland ❿

Treatment: Surgical removal of the right adrenal gland. ⓫

1. endicrinologist
2. obesity
3. hirsutism
4. radioimmunoassay (RIA)
5. cortisol
6. adanocarcinoma
7. adranal cortex
8. Adranal virilism
9. adanocarcinoma
10. adrenal cortex
11. adranalectomy

Labeling Exercise

A. System Review

Write the labels for this figure on the numbered lines provided.

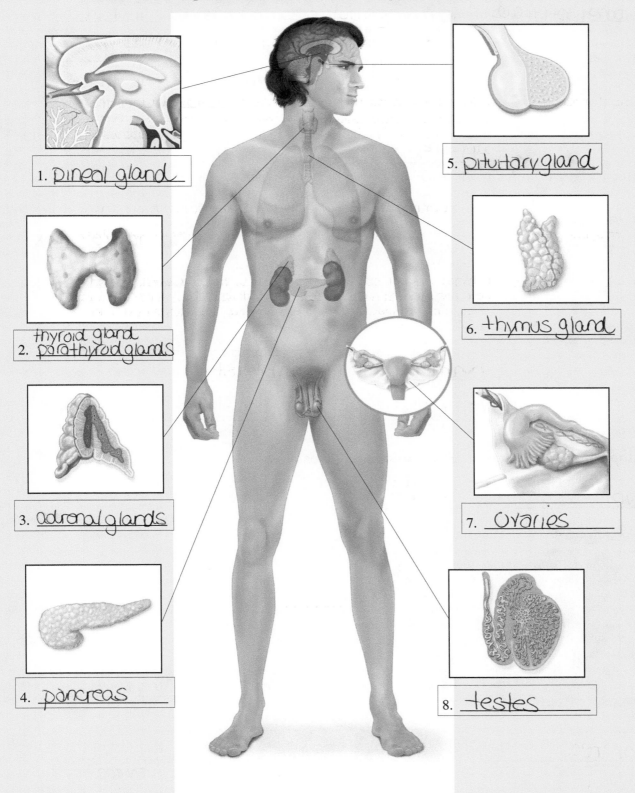

1. pineal gland

2. thyroid gland
   parathyroid glands

3. adrenal glands

4. pancreas

5. pituitary gland

6. thymus gland

7. ovaries

8. testes

Endocrine System

B. Anatomy Challenge

1. Write the labels for this figure on the numbered lines provided.

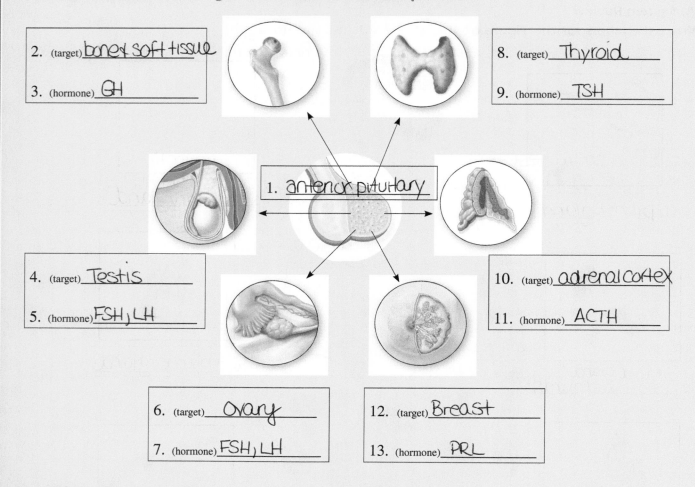

2. (target) bone & soft tissue

3. (hormone) GH

8. (target) Thyroid

9. (hormone) TSH

1. anterior pituitary

4. (target) Testis

5. (hormone) FSH, LH

10. (target) adrenal cortex

11. (hormone) ACTH

6. (target) Ovary

7. (hormone) FSH, LH

12. (target) Breast

13. (hormone) PRL

2. Write the labels for this figure on the numbered lines provided.

1. Liver

2. Stomach

4. Insulin-secreting cell
Beta cell

3. Pancreas

5. Glucagon-secreting cell
Alpha cell

6. Islet of Langerhans in pancreas

Endocrine System

Multimedia Preview

Additional interactive resources and activities for this chapter can be found on the Companion Website.

DVD-ROM Highlights

Website Highlights—www.prenhall.com/fremgen

FILL-IN-THE-BLANKS EXERCISE

Take advantage of the free-access on-line study guide that accompanies your textbook. You'll find a fill-in-the-blank quiz that provides instant feedback that allows you to check your score and see what you got right or wrong. By clicking on this URL you'll also access links to download mp3 audio reviews, current news articles, and an audio glossary.

386

Nervous System

Learning Objectives

Upon completion of this chapter, you will be able to:

- Identify and define the combining forms and suffixes introduced in this chapter.
- Correctly spell and pronounce medical terms and major anatomical structures relating to the nervous system.
- Locate and describe the major organs of the nervous system and their functions.
- Describe the components of a neuron.
- Distinguish between the central nervous system, peripheral nervous system, and autonomic nervous system.
- Build and define nervous system medical terms from word parts.
- Identify and define nervous system vocabulary terms.
- Identify and define selected nervous system pathology terms.
- Identify and define selected nervous system diagnostic procedures.
- Identify and define selected nervous system therapeutic procedures.
- Identify and define selected medications relating to the nervous system.
- Define selected abbreviations associated with the nervous system.

From Chapter 12 of *Medical Terminology: A Living Language*, 4/e. Bonnie F. Fremgen. Suzanne S. Frucht. Copyright © 2009 by Pearson Education. Published by Prentice Hall. All rights reserved.

Nervous System at a Glance

Function

The nervous system coordinates and controls body function. It receives sensory input, makes decisions, and then orders body responses.

Organs

brain
nerves
spinal cord

Combining Forms

cephal/o	head
cerebell/o	cerebellum
cerebr/o	cerebrum
encephal/o	brain
gli/o	glue
medull/o	medulla oblongata
mening/o	meninges
meningi/o	meninges
myel/o	spinal cord
neur/o	nerve
phas/o	speech
poli/o	gray matter
pont/o	pons
radicul/o	nerve root
thalam/o	thalamus
thec/o	sheath (meninges)
ventricul/o	brain ventricle

Suffixes

-algesia	pain, sensitivity
-esthesia	feeling, sensation
-paresis	weakness
-phasia	speech
-plegia	paralysis
-taxia	muscle coordination

Nervous System Illustrated

brain

Coordinates body functions

spinal cord

Transmits messages to and from the brain

nerves

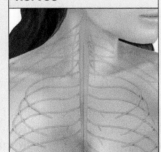

Transmit messages to and from the central nervous system

Anatomy and Physiology of the Nervous System

brain	nerves
central nervous system	peripheral nervous system (per-IF-er-al)
cranial nerves (KRAY-nee-al)	sensory receptors
glands	spinal cord
muscles	spinal nerves

The nervous system is responsible for coordinating all the activity of the body. To do this, it first receives information from both external and internal **sensory receptors** and then uses that information to adjust the activity of **muscles** and **glands** to match the needs of the body.

The nervous system can be subdivided into the **central nervous system** (CNS) and the **peripheral nervous system** (PNS). The central nervous system consists of the **brain** and **spinal cord**. Sensory information comes into the central nervous system, where it is processed. Motor messages then exit the central nervous system carrying commands to muscles and glands. The **nerves** of the peripheral nervous system are **cranial nerves** and **spinal nerves**. Sensory nerves carry information to the central nervous system, and motor nerves carry commands away from the central nervous system. All portions of the nervous system are composed of nervous tissue.

Nervous Tissue

axon (AK-son)	neuron (NOO-ron)
dendrites (DEN-drights)	neurotransmitter (noo-roh-TRANS-mit-ter)
myelin (MY-eh-lin)	synapse (sih-NAPSE)
nerve cell body	synaptic cleft (sih-NAP-tik)
neuroglial cells (noo-ROH-glee-all)	

Nervous tissue consists of two basic types of cells: **neurons** and **neuroglial cells**. Neurons are individual nerve cells. These are the cells that are capable of conducting electrical impulses in response to a stimulus. Neurons have three basic parts: **dendrites**, a **nerve cell body**, and an **axon** (see Figure 1A ■). Dendrites are highly branched projections that receive impulses. The nerve cell body contains the nucleus and many of the other organelles of the cell (see Figure 1B ■). A neuron has only a single axon, a projection from the nerve cell body that conducts the electrical impulse toward its destination. The point at which the axon of one neuron meets the dendrite of the next neuron is called a **synapse**. Electrical impulses cannot pass directly across the gap between two neurons, called the **synaptic cleft**. They instead require the help of a chemical messenger, called a **neurotransmitter**.

A variety of neuroglial cells are found in nervous tissue. Each has a different support function for the neurons. For example, some neuroglial cells produce **myelin**, a fatty substance that acts as insulation for many axons so that they conduct electrical impulses faster. Neuroglial cells *do not* conduct electrical impulses.

Central Nervous System

gray matter	tract
meninges (men-IN-jeez)	white matter
myelinated (MY-eh-lih-nayt-ed)	

Because the central nervous system is a combination of the brain and spinal cord, it is able to receive impulses from all over the body, process this informa-

A

B

■**Figure 1** A) The structure of a neuron, showing the dendrites, nerve cell body, and axon. B) Photomicrograph of typical neuron showing the nerve cell body, nucleus, and dendrites.

tion, and then respond with an action. This system consists of both **gray** and **white matter.** Gray matter is comprised of unsheathed or uncovered cell bodies and dendrites. White matter is **myelinated** nerve fibers (see Figure 2 ■). The myelin sheath makes the nervous tissue appear white. Bundles of nerve fibers inter-

■**Figure 2**
Electronmicrograph
illustrating an axon (red)
wrapped in its myelin sheath
(blue). *(Quest/Science Photo
Library/Photo Researchers, Inc.)*

connecting different parts of the central nervous system are called **tracts**. The central nervous system is encased and protected by three membranes known as the **meninges**.

The Brain

brain stem
cerebellum (ser-eh-BELL-um)
cerebral cortex (seh-REE-bral KOR-teks)
cerebral hemisphere
cerebrospinal fluid (ser-eh-broh-SPY-nal)
cerebrum (SER-eh-brum)
diencephalon (dye-en-SEFF-ah-lon)
frontal lobe
gyri (JYE-rye)
hypothalamus (high-poh-THAL-ah-mus)

medulla oblongata
    (meh-DULL-ah ob-long-GAH-tah)
midbrain
occipital lobe (ock-SIP-ih-tal)
parietal lobe (pah-RYE-eh-tal)
pons (PONZ)
sulci (SULL-kye)
temporal lobe (TEM-por-al)
thalamus (THAL-ah-mus)
ventricles (VEN-trik-lz)

The brain is one of the largest organs in the body and coordinates most body activities. It is the center for all thought, memory, judgment, and emotion. Each part of the brain is responsible for controlling different body functions, such as temperature regulation, blood pressure, and breathing. There are four sections to the brain: **cerebrum**, **cerebellum**, **diencephalon**, and **brain stem** (see Figure 3 ■).

The largest section of the brain is the cerebrum. It is located in the upper portion of the brain and is the area that processes thoughts, judgment, memory, problem solving, and language. The outer layer of the cerebrum is the **cerebral cortex**, which is composed of folds of gray matter. The elevated portions of the cerebrum, or convolutions, are called **gyri** and are separated by fissures, or valleys, called **sulci**. The cerebrum is subdivided into left and right halves called **cerebral hemispheres**. Each hemisphere has four lobes. The lobes and their locations and functions are as follows (see Figure 4 ■):

■ **Figure 3** The regions of the brain.

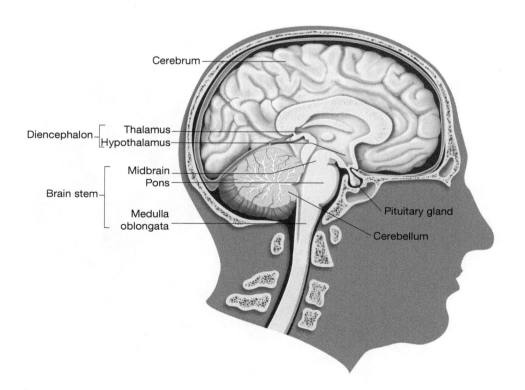

Cerebrum

Diencephalon — Thalamus
          Hypothalamus

Midbrain
Pons
Brain stem
Medulla oblongata

Pituitary gland
Cerebellum

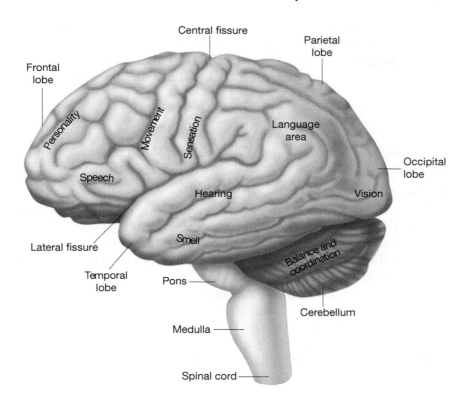

Central fissure

Parietal lobe

Frontal lobe

Personality

Movement

Sensation

Language area

Occipital lobe

Speech

Hearing

Vision

Lateral fissure

Smell

Balance and coordination

Temporal lobe

Pons

Cerebellum

Medulla

Spinal cord

Figure 4 The functional regions of the cerebrum.

1. **Frontal lobe:** Most anterior portion of the cerebrum; controls motor function, personality, and speech
2. **Parietal lobe:** Most superior portion of the cerebrum; receives and interprets nerve impulses from sensory receptors and interprets language
3. **Occipital lobe:** Most posterior portion of the cerebrum; controls vision
4. **Temporal lobe:** Left and right lateral portion of the cerebrum; controls hearing and smell

The diencephalon, located below the cerebrum, contains two of the most critical areas of the brain, the **thalamus** and the **hypothalamus**. The thalamus is composed of gray matter and acts as a center for relaying impulses from the eyes, ears, and skin to the cerebrum. Our pain perception is controlled by the thalamus. The hypothalamus located just below the thalamus controls body temperature, appetite, sleep, sexual desire, and emotions. The hypothalamus is actually responsible for controlling the autonomic nervous system, cardiovascular system, digestive system, and the release of hormones from the pituitary gland.

The cerebellum, the second largest portion of the brain, is located beneath the posterior part of the cerebrum. This part of the brain aids in coordinating voluntary body movements and maintaining balance and equilibrium. The cerebellum refines the muscular movement that is initiated in the cerebrum.

The final portion of the brain is the brain stem. This area has three components: **midbrain, pons,** and **medulla oblongata**. The midbrain acts as a pathway for impulses to be conducted between the brain and the spinal cord. The pons—a term meaning bridge—connects the cerebellum to the rest of the brain. The medulla oblongata is the most inferior positioned portion of the brain; it connects the brain to the spinal cord. However, this vital area contains the centers that control respiration, heart rate, temperature, and blood pressure. Additionally, this is the site where nerve tracts cross from one side of the brain to control functions and movement on the other side of the body. In other words, with few exceptions, the left side of the brain controls the right side of the body and vice versa.

The brain has four interconnected cavities called **ventricles**: one in each cerebral hemisphere, one in the thalamus, and one in front of the cerebellum. These contain **cerebrospinal fluid** (CSF), which is the watery, clear fluid that provides protection from shock or sudden motion to the brain and spinal cord.

Spinal Cord

ascending tracts	**spinal cavity**
central canal	**vertebral canal**
descending tracts	**vertebral column**

The function of the spinal cord is to provide a pathway for impulses traveling to and from the brain. The spinal cord is actually a column of nervous tissue that extends from the medulla oblongata of the brain down to the level of the second lumbar vertebra within the **vertebral column**. The thirty-three vertebrae of the backbone line up to form a continuous canal for the spinal cord called the **spinal cavity** or **vertebral canal** (see Figure 5 ■).

Similar to the brain, the spinal cord is also protected by cerebrospinal fluid. It flows down the center of the spinal cord within the **central canal**. The inner core of the spinal cord consists of cell bodies and dendrites of peripheral nerves and therefore is gray matter. The outer portion of the spinal cord is myelinated white matter. The white matter is either **ascending tracts** carrying sensory information up to the brain or **descending tracts** carrying motor commands down from the brain to a peripheral nerve.

Med Term Tip

Certain disease processes attack the gray matter and the white matter of the central nervous system. For instance, *poliomyelitis* is a viral infection of the gray matter of the spinal cord. The combining term *poli/o* means "gray matter." This disease has almost been eradicated, due to the polio vaccine.

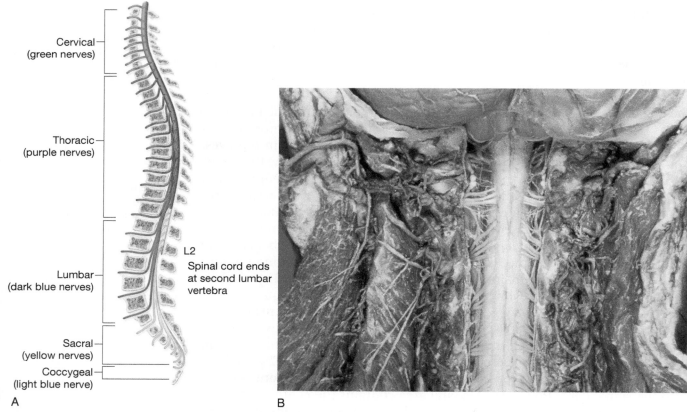

Cervical (green nerves)

Thoracic (purple nerves)

Lumbar (dark blue nerves)

Sacral (yellow nerves)

Coccygeal (light blue nerve)

L2
Spinal cord ends at second lumbar vertebra

A

B

■ **Figure 5** A) The levels of the spinal cord and spinal nerves. B) Photograph of the spinal cord as it descends from the brain. The spinal nerve roots are clearly visible branching off from the spinal cord. *(Video Surgery/Photo Researchers, Inc.)*

Meninges

arachnoid layer (ah-RAK-noyd)

dura mater (DOO-rah MATE-er)

pia mater (PEE-ah MATE-er)

subarachnoid space (sub-ah-RAK-noyd)

subdural space (sub-DOO-ral)

The meninges are three layers of connective tissue membranes that surround the brain and spinal cord (see Figure 6 ■). Moving from external to internal, the meninges are:

1. **Dura mater**: Meaning *tough mother*; it forms a tough, fibrous sac around the central nervous system
2. **Subdural space**: Actual space between the dura mater and arachnoid layers
3. **Arachnoid layer**: Meaning *spiderlike*; it is a thin, delicate layer attached to the pia mater by weblike filaments
4. **Subarachnoid space**: Space between the arachnoid layer and the pia mater; it contains cerebrospinal fluid that cushions the brain from the outside
5. **Pia mater**: Meaning *soft mother*; it is the innermost membrane layer and is applied directly to the surface of the brain and spinal cord

Peripheral Nervous System

afferent neurons (AFF-er-ent)

autonomic nervous system (aw-toh-NOM-ik)

efferent neurons (EFF-er-ent)

ganglion (GANG-lee-on)

motor neurons

nerve root

sensory neurons

somatic nerves

The peripheral nervous system (PNS) includes both the twelve pairs of cranial nerves and the thirty-one pairs of spinal nerves. A nerve is a group or bundle of axon fibers located outside the central nervous system that carries messages between the central nervous system and the various parts of the body. Whether a nerve is cranial or spinal is determined by where the nerve originates. Cranial nerves arise from the brain, mainly at the medulla oblongata. Spinal nerves split off from the spinal cord, and one pair (a left and a right) exits between each pair of vertebrae. The point where either type of nerve is attached to the central nervous system is called the **nerve root**. The names of most nerves reflect either

■ **Figure 6** The meninges. This figure illustrates the location and structure of each layer of the meninges and their relationship to the skull and brain.

Med Term Tip

Because nerve tracts cross from one side of the body to the other side of the brain, damage to one side of the brain results in symptoms appearing on the opposite side of the body. Since nerve cells that control the movement of the right side of the body are located in the left side of the medulla oblongata, a stroke that paralyzed the right side of the body would actually have occurred in the left side of the brain.

the organ the nerve serves or the portion of the body the nerve is traveling through. The entire list of cranial nerves is found in Table 1 ■. Figure 7 ■ illustrates some of the major spinal nerves in the human body.

Although most nerves carry information to and from the central nervous system, individual neurons carry information in only one direction. **Afferent neurons**, also called **sensory neurons**, carry sensory information from a sensory receptor to the central nervous system. **Efferent neurons**, also called **motor neurons**, carry activity instructions from the central nervous system to muscles or glands out in the body (see Figure 8 ■). The nerve cell bodies of the neurons forming the nerve are grouped together in a knot-like mass, called a **ganglion**, located outside the central nervous system.

The nerves of the peripheral nervous system are subdivided into two divisions, the **autonomic nervous system** (ANS) and **somatic nerves**, each serving a different area of the body.

Autonomic Nervous System

parasympathetic branch (pair-ah-sim-pah-THET-ik)

sympathetic branch (sim-pah-THET-ik)

The autonomic nervous system is involved with the control of involuntary or unconscious bodily functions. It may increase or decrease the activity of the smooth muscle found in viscera and blood vessels, cardiac muscle, and glands. The autonomic nervous system is divided into two branches: **sympathetic branch** and **parasympathetic branch**. The sympathetic nerves control the "fight or flight" reaction during times of stress and crisis. These nerves increase heart rate, dilate airways, increase blood pressure, inhibit digestion, and stimulate the production of adrenaline during a crisis. The parasympathetic nerves serve as a counterbalance for the sympathetic nerves, the "rest and digest" reaction. Therefore, they cause heart rate to slow down, lower blood pressure, and stimulate digestion.

Table 1	Cranial Nerves	
NUMBER	**NAME**	**FUNCTION**
I	Olfactory	Transports impulses for sense of smell
II	Optic	Carries impulses for sense of sight
III	Oculomotor	Motor impulses for eye muscle movement and the pupil of eye
IV	Trochlear	Controls oblique muscle of eye on each side
V	Trigeminal	Carries sensory facial impulses and controls muscles for chewing; branches into eyes, forehead, upper and lower jaw
VI	Abducens	Controls an eyeball muscle to turn eye to side
VII	Facial	Controls facial muscles for expression, salivation, and taste on two-thirds of tongue (anterior)
VIII	Vestibulocochlear	Responsible for impulses of equilibrium and hearing; also called auditory nerve
IX	Glossopharyngeal	Carries sensory impulses from pharynx (swallowing) and taste on one-third of tongue
X	Vagus	Supplies most organs in abdominal and thoracic cavities
XI	Accessory	Controls the neck and shoulder muscles
XII	Hypoglossal	Controls tongue muscles

Nervous System

Brachial plexus

Cervical nerve

Radial nerve
Median nerve
Ulnar nerve

Intercostal nerve

Lumbosacral plexus

Sciatic nerve

Common
peroneal nerve

■ **Figure 7** The major spinal nerves.

Sensory (afferent) neuron

Spinal cord

A

B

Motor (efferent) neuron

C

■ **Figure 8** The functional structure of the peripheral nervous system. A) Afferent or sensory neurons carry sensory information to the spinal cord. B) The spinal cord receives incoming sensory information and delivers motor messages. C) Efferent or motor neurons deliver motor commands to muscles and glands.

Somatic Nerves

Somatic nerves serve the skin and skeletal muscles and are mainly involved with the conscious and voluntary activities of the body. The large variety of sensory receptors found in the dermis layer of the skin use somatic nerves to send their information, such as touch, temperature, pressure, and pain, to the brain. These are also the nerves that carry motor commands to skeletal muscles.

Word Building

The following list contains examples of medical terms built directly from word parts. The definition for these terms can be determined by a straightforward translation of the word parts.

COMBINING FORM	COMBINED WITH	MEDICAL TERM	DEFINITION
cephal/o	-algia	**cephalalgia** (seff-al-AL-jee-ah)	head pain (headache)
cerebell/o	-ar	**cerebellar** (ser-eh-BELL-ar)	pertaining to the cerebellum
	-itis	**cerebellitis** (ser-eh-bell-EYE-tis)	cerebellum inflammation
cerebr/o	-al	**cerebral** (seh-REE-bral)	pertaining to the cerebrum
	spin/o -al	**cerebrospinal** (ser-eh-broh-SPY-nal)	pertaining to the cerebrum and spine
encephal/o	electr/o -gram	**electroencephalogram** (EEG) (ee-lek-troh-en-SEFF-ah-loh-gram)	record of brain's electricity
	-itis	**encephalitis** (en-seff-ah-LYE-tis)	brain inflammation
meningi/o	-oma	**meningioma** (meh-nin-jee-OH-mah)	meninges tumor
mening/o	-eal	**meningeal** (meh-NIN-jee-all)	pertaining to the meninges
	-itis	**meningitis** (men-in-JYE-tis)	meninges inflammation
myel/o	-gram	**myelogram** (MY-eh-loh-gram)	record of spinal cord

Med Term Tip

The combining form *myel/o* means "marrow" and is used for both the spinal cord and bone marrow. To the ancient Greek philosophers and physicians, the spinal cord appeared to be much like the marrow found in the medullary cavity of a long bone.

	-itis	**myelitis** (my-eh-LYE-tis)	spinal cord inflammation
neur/o	-al	**neural** (NOO-rall)	pertaining to nerves
	-algia	**neuralgia** (noo-RAL-jee-ah)	nerve pain
	-ectomy	**neurectomy** (noo-REK-toh-mee)	removal of nerve
	-ologist	**neurologist** (noo-RAL-oh-jist)	specialist in nerves
	-oma	**neuroma** (noo-ROH-mah)	nerve tumor
	-pathy	**neuropathy** (noo-ROP-ah-thee)	nerve disease
	-plasty	**neuroplasty** (NOOR-oh-plas-tee)s	surgical repair of nerves
	poly- -itis	**polyneuritis** (pol-ee-noo-RYE-tis)	inflammation of many nerves

Word Building *(continued)*

COMBINING FORM	COMBINED WITH	MEDICAL TERM	DEFINITION
	-rrhaphy	**neurorrhaphy** (noo-ROR-ah-fee)	suture of nerve
pont/o	-ine	**pontine** (pon-TEEN)	pertaining to the pons
radicul/o	-itis	**radiculitis** (rah-dick-yoo-LYE-tis)	nerve root inflammation
	-pathy	**radiculopathy** (rah-dick-yoo-LOP-ah-thee)	nerve root disease
thalam/o	-ic	**thalamic** (tha-LAM-ik)	pertaining to the thalamus
thec/o	intra- -al	**intrathecal** (in-tra-THEE-kal)	pertaining to within the meninges

SUFFIX	COMBINED WITH	MEDICAL TERM	DEFINITION
-algesia	an-	**analgesia** (an-al-JEE-zee-ah)	absence of pain or sensation
-esthesia	an-	**anesthesia** (an-ess-THEE-zee-ah)	lack of sensations
	hyper-	**hyperesthesia** (high-per-ess-THEE-zee-ah)	excessive sensations
-paresis	mono-	**monoparesis** (mon-oh-pah-REE-sis)	weakness of one
-phasia	a-	**aphasia** (ah-FAY-zee-ah)	lack of speech
	dys-	**dysphasia** (dis-FAY-zee-ah)	difficult speech
-plegia	mono-	**monoplegia** (mon-oh-PLEE-jee-ah)	paralysis of one
	quadri-	**quadriplegia** (kwod-rih-PLEE-jee-ah)	paralysis of four
-taxia	a-	**ataxia** (ah-TAK-see-ah)	lack of muscle coordination

Vocabulary

TERM	DEFINITION
anesthesiology (an-es-thee-zee-ol-oh-jee)	Branch of medicine specializing in all aspects of anesthesia, including for surgical procedures, resuscitation measures, and the management of acute and chronic pain. Physician is an *anesthesiologist*.
aura (AW-ruh)	Sensations, such as seeing colors or smelling an unusual odor, that occur just prior to an epileptic seizure or migraine headache.
coma (COH-mah)	Profound unconsciousness or stupor resulting from an illness or injury.
conscious (KON-shus)	Condition of being awake and aware of surroundings.
convulsion (kon-VULL-shun)	Severe involuntary muscle contractions and relaxations. These have a variety of causes, such as epilepsy, fever, and toxic conditions.
delirium (dee-LEER-ee-um)	Abnormal mental state characterized by confusion, disorientation, and agitation.

Vocabulary *(continued)*

TERM	DEFINITION
dementia (dee-MEN-she-ah)	Progressive impairment of intellectual function that interferes with performing activities of daily living. Patients have little awareness of their condition. Found in disorders such as Alzheimer's.
focal seizure (FOE-kal)	Localized seizure often affecting one limb.
hemiparesis (hem-ee-par-EE-sis)	Weakness or loss of motion on one side of the body.
hemiplegia (hem-ee-PLEE-jee-ah)	Paralysis on only one side of the body.
neurology (noo-rol-oh-jee)	Branch of medicine concerned with diagnosis and treatment of diseases and conditions of the nervous system. Physician is a *neurologist*.
neurosurgery (noo-roh-SIR-jury)	Branch of medicine concerned with treating conditions and diseases of the nervous systems by surgical means. Physician is a *neurosurgeon*.
palsy (PAWL-zee)	Temporary or permanent loss of the ability to control movement.
paralysis (pah-RAL-ih-sis)	Temporary or permanent loss of function or voluntary movement.
paraplegia (pair-ah-PLEE-jee-ah)	Paralysis of the lower portion of the body and both legs.
paresthesia (par-es-THEE-zee-ah)	Abnormal sensation such as burning or tingling.
seizure (SEE-zyoor)	Sudden, uncontrollable onset of symptoms; such as in an epileptic seizure.
syncope (SIN-koh-pee)	Fainting.
tremor (TREM-or)	Involuntary repetitive alternating movement of a part of the body.
unconscious (un-KON-shus)	Condition or state of being unaware of surroundings, with the inability to respond to stimuli.

Pathology

TERM	DEFINITION
■ *Brain*	
absence seizure	Type of epileptic seizure that lasts only a few seconds to half a minute, characterized by a loss of awareness and an absence of activity. It is also called a *petit mal seizure*.
Alzheimer's disease (ALTS-high-merz)	Chronic, organic mental disorder consisting of dementia, which is more prevalent in adults between ages 40 and 60. Involves progressive disorientation, apathy, speech and gait disturbances, and loss of memory. Named for German neurologist Alois Alzheimer.
astrocytoma (ass-troh-sigh-TOH-mah)	Tumor of the brain or spinal cord that is composed of astrocytes, one of the types of neuroglial cells.

TERM	DEFINITION
brain tumor	Intracranial mass, either benign or malignant. A benign tumor of the brain can still be fatal since it will grow and cause pressure on normal brain tissue.

■ **Figure 9** Color enhanced CT-scan showing two malignant tumors in the brain. (*Scott Camazine/Photo Researchers, Inc.*)

| **cerebral aneurysm** (AN-yoo-rizm) | Localized abnormal dilation of a blood vessel, usually an artery; the result of a congenital defect or weakness in the wall of the vessel. A ruptured aneurysm is a common cause of a hemorrhagic cerebrovascular accident. |

■ **Figure 10** Common locations for cerebral artery aneurysms in the Circle of Willis.

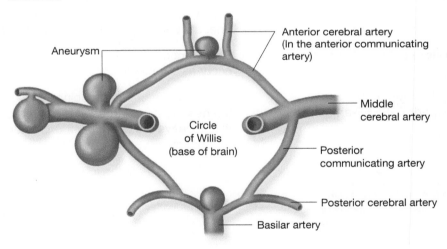

cerebral contusion (kon-TOO-shun)	Bruising of the brain from a blow or impact. Symptoms last longer than 24 hours and include unconsciousness, dizziness, vomiting, unequal pupil size, and shock.
cerebral palsy (CP) (ser-REE-bral PAWL-zee)	Nonprogressive brain damage resulting from a defect, trauma, or oxygen deprivation at the time of birth.
cerebrovascular accident (CVA) (ser-eh-broh-VASS-kyoo-lar AK-sih-dent)	The development of an infarct due to loss in the blood supply to an area of the brain. Blood flow can be interrupted by a ruptured blood vessel (hemorrhage), a floating clot (embolus), a stationary clot (thrombosis), or compression (see Figure 11 ■). The extent of damage depends on the size and location of the infarct and often includes dysphasia and hemiplegia. Commonly called a *stroke.*

Figure 11 The four common causes for cerebrovascular accidents.

Cerebral hemorrhage: Cerebral artery ruptures and bleeds into brain tissue.

Cerebral embolism: Embolus from another area lodges in cerebral artery and blocks blood flow.

Cerebral thrombosis: Blood clot forms in cerebral artery and blocks blood flow.

Compression: Pressure from tumor squeezes adjacent blood vessel and blocks blood flow.

 ## Pathology (continued)

TERM	DEFINITION
concussion (kon-KUSH-un)	Injury to the brain resulting from the brain being shaken inside the skull from a blow or impact. Can result in unconsciousness, dizziness, vomiting, unequal pupil size, and shock. Symptoms last 24 hours or less.
epilepsy (EP-ih-lep-see)	Recurrent disorder of the brain in which seizures and loss of consciousness occur as a result of uncontrolled electrical activity of the neurons in the brain.
hydrocephalus (high-droh-SEFF-ah-lus)	Accumulation of cerebrospinal fluid within the ventricles of the brain, causing the head to be enlarged. It is treated by creating an artificial shunt for the fluid to leave the brain. If left untreated, it may lead to seizures and mental retardation.

Figure 12 Hydrocephalus. The figure on the left is a child with the enlarged ventricles of hydrocephalus. The figure on the right is the same child with a shunt to send the excess cerebrospinal fluid to the abdominal cavity.

Bulging fontanel

Enlarged ventricles

Catheter tip in ventricle

Valve

Blocked aqueduct

Shunt

■ Pathology *(continued)*

TERM	DEFINITION
migraine (MY-grain)	Specific type of headache characterized by severe head pain, sensitivity to light, dizziness, and nausea.
Parkinson's disease (PARK-in-sons dih-ZEEZ)	Chronic disorder of the nervous system with fine tremors, muscular weakness, rigidity, and a shuffling gait. Named for British physician Sir James Parkinson.
Reye syndrome (RISE SIN-drohm)	Combination of symptoms first recognized by Australian pathologist R. D. K. Reye that includes acute encephalopathy and damage to various organs, especially the liver. This occurs in children under age 15 who have had a viral infection. It is also associated with taking aspirin. For this reason, it's not recommended for children to use aspirin.
tonic-clonic seizure	Type of severe epileptic seizure characterized by a loss of consciousness and convulsions. The seizure alternates between strong continuous muscle spasms (tonic) and rhythmic muscle contraction and relaxation (clonic). It is also called a *grand mal seizure.*
transient ischemic attack (TIA) (TRAN-shent iss-KEM-ik)	Temporary interference with blood supply to the brain, causing neurological symptoms such as dizziness, numbness, and hemiparesis. May eventually lead to a full-blown stroke (cerebrovascular accident).

■ *Spinal Cord*

amyotrophic lateral sclerosis (ALS) (ah-my-oh-TROFF-ik LAT-er-al skleh-ROH-sis)	Disease with muscular weakness and atrophy due to degeneration of motor neurons of the spinal cord. Also called *Lou Gehrig's disease,* after the New York Yankees baseball player who died from the disease.
meningocele (men-IN-goh-seel)	Congenital condition in which the meninges protrude through an opening in the vertebral column (see Figure 13B ■). See *spina bifida.*

■ **Figure 13** Spina bifida. A) Spina bifica occulta, the vertebra is not complete, but there is not protrusion of nervous system structures. B) Meningocele, the meninges sac protrudes through the opening in the vertebra. C) Myelomeningocele, the meninges sac and spinal cord protrude through the opening in the vertebra.

A. Spina bifida

B. Meningocele

C. Myelomeningocele

Pathology *(continued)*

TERM	DEFINITION
myelomeningocele (my-eh-loh-meh-NIN-goh-seel)	Congenital condition in which the meninges and spinal cord protrude through an opening in the vertebral column (see Figure 13C ■). See *spina bifida*.
poliomyelitis (poh-lee-oh-my-eh-lye-tis)	Viral inflammation of the gray matter of the spinal cord. Results in varying degrees of paralysis, may be mild and reversible or may be severe and permanent. This disease has been almost eliminated due to the discovery of a vaccine in the 1950s.
spina bifida (SPY-nah BIFF-ih-dah)	Congenital defect in the walls of the spinal canal in which the laminae of the vertebra do not meet or close (see Figure 13A ■). May result in a meningocele or a myelomeningocele—meninges or the spinal cord being pushed through the opening.
spinal cord injury (SCI)	Damage to the spinal cord as a result of trauma. Spinal cord may be bruised or completely severed.

■ *Nerves*

TERM	DEFINITION
Bell's palsy (BELLZ PAWL-zee)	One-sided facial paralysis due to inflammation of the facial nerve, probably viral in nature. The patient cannot control salivation, tearing of the eyes, or expression, but most will eventually recover.
Guillain-Barré syndrome (GHEE-yan bah-RAY)	Disease of the nervous system in which nerves lose their myelin covering. May be caused by an autoimmune reaction. Characterized by loss of sensation and/or muscle control starting in the legs. Symptoms then move toward the trunk and may even result in paralysis of the diaphragm.
multiple sclerosis (MS) (MULL-tih-pl skleh-ROH-sis)	Inflammatory disease of the central nervous system in which there is extreme weakness and numbness due to loss of myelin insulation from nerves.
myasthenia gravis (my-ass-THEE-nee-ah GRAV-iss)	Disease with severe muscular weakness and fatigue due to insufficient neurotransmitter at a synapse.
shingles (SHING-lz) ■ Figure 14 Photograph of the skin eruptions associated with shingles.	Eruption of painful blisters on the body along a nerve path. Thought to be caused by a *Herpes zoster* virus infection of the nerve root.

■ *Meninges*

TERM	DEFINITION
epidural hematoma (ep-ih-DOO-ral hee-mah-TOH-mah)	Mass of blood in the space outside the dura mater of the brain and spinal cord.

Pathology *(continued)*

TERM	DEFINITION
subdural hematoma (sub-DOO-ral hee-mah-TOH-mah)	Mass of blood forming beneath the dura mater if the meninges are torn by trauma. May exert fatal pressure on the brain if the hematoma is not drained by surgery.

■ **Figure 15** A subdural hematoma. A meningeal vein is ruptured and blood has accumulated in the subdural space producing pressure on the brain.

Torn cerebral vein

Subdural hematoma

Compressed brain tissue

Dura mater

Arachnoid layer

Diagnostic Procedures

TERM	DEFINITION
■ *Clinical Laboratory Tests*	
cerebrospinal fluid analysis (ser-eh-broh-SPY-nal FLOO-id an-NAL-ih-sis)	Laboratory examination of the clear, watery, colorless fluid from within the brain and spinal cord. Infections and the abnormal presence of blood can be detected in this test.
■ *Diagnostic Imaging*	
brain scan	Image of the brain taken after injection of radioactive isotopes into the circulation.
cerebral angiography (seh-REE-bral-an-jee-OG-rah-fee)	X-ray of the blood vessels of the brain after the injection of radiopaque dye.
echoencephalography (ek-oh-en-SEFF-ah-log-rah-fee)	Recording of the ultrasonic echoes of the brain. Useful in determining abnormal patterns of shifting in the brain.
myelography (my-eh-LOG-rah-fee)	Injection of radiopaque dye into the spinal canal. An X-ray is then taken to examine the normal and abnormal outlines made by the dye.

Diagnostic Procedures *(continued)*

TERM	DEFINITION
positron emission tomography (PET) (PAHZ-ih-tron ee-MISH-un toh-MOG-rah-fee)	Use of positive radionuclides to reconstruct brain sections. Measurement can be taken of oxygen and glucose uptake, cerebral blood flow, and blood volume. The amount of glucose the brain uses indicates how metabolically active the tissue is.

■ *Additional Diagnostic Tests*

Babinski reflex (bah-BIN-skeez)	Reflex test developed by French neurologist Joseph Babinski to determine lesions and abnormalities in the nervous system. The Babinski reflex is present if the great toe extends instead of flexes when the lateral sole of the foot is stroked. The normal response to this stimulation is flexion of the toe.
electroencephalography (EEG) (ee-lek-troh-en-SEFF-ah-LOG-rah-fee)	Recording the electrical activity of the brain by placing electrodes at various positions on the scalp. Also used in sleep studies to determine if there is a normal pattern of activity during sleep.
lumbar puncture (LP) (LUM-bar PUNK-chur)	Puncture with a needle into the lumbar area (usually the fourth intervertebral space) to withdraw fluid for examination and for the injection of anesthesia. Also called *spinal puncture* or *spinal tap*.

■ **Figure 16** A lumbar puncture. The needle is inserted between the lumbar vertebrae and into the spinal canal.

L1 vertebra

Lumbar puncture needle

Coccyx

Skin

Fat

Interspinous ligament

L4

L5

Extradural "space"

Tip end of spinal cord

CSF in lumbar cistern

Dura mater

Sacrum

| **nerve conduction velocity** | Test that measures how fast an impulse travels along a nerve. Can pinpoint an area of nerve damage. |

Therapeutic Procedures

TERM	DEFINITION
Medical Procedures	
nerve block	Injection of regional anesthetic to stop the passage of sensory or pain impulses along a nerve path.
Surgical Procedures	
carotid endarterectomy (kah-ROT-id end-ar-ter-EK-toh-mee)	Surgical procedure for removing an obstruction within the carotid artery, a major artery in the neck that carries oxygenated blood to the brain. Developed to prevent strokes, but is found to be useful only in severe stenosis with transient ischemic attack.
cerebrospinal fluid shunts (ser-eh-broh SPY-nal FLOO-id)	Surgical procedure in which a bypass is created to drain cerebrospinal fluid. It is used to treat hydrocephalus by draining the excess cerebrospinal fluid from the brain and diverting it to the abdominal cavity.
laminectomy (lam-ih-NEK-toh-mee)	Removal of a portion of a vertebra in order to relieve pressure on the spinal nerve.
tractotomy (track-OT-oh-mee)	Surgical interruption of a nerve tract in the spinal cord. Used to treat intractable pain or muscle spasms.

Pharmacology

CLASSIFICATION	ACTION	GENERIC AND BRAND NAMES
analgesic (an-al-JEE-zik)	Non-narcotic medication to treat minor to moderate pain. Includes aspirin, acetaminophen, and ibuprofen.	aspirin, Bayer, Ecotrin; acetaminophen, Tylenol; ibuprofen, Aleve
anesthetic (an-ess-THET-ik)	Drug that produces a loss of sensation or a loss of consciousness.	lidocaine, Xylocaine; pentobarbital, Nembutal; propofol, Diprivan; procaine, Novocain
anticonvulsant (an-tye-kon-VULL-sant)	Substance that reduces the excitability of neurons and therefore prevents the uncontrolled neuron activity associated with seizures.	carbamazepine, Tegretol; phenobarbital, Nembutal
dopaminergic drugs (dope-ah-men-ER-gik)	Group of medications to treat Parkinson's disease by either replacing the dopamine that is lacking or increasing the strength of the dopamine that is present.	levodopa; L-dopa, Larodopa; levodopa/carbidopa, Sinemet
hypnotic (hip-NOT-tik)	Drug that promotes sleep.	secobarbital, Seconal; temazepam, Restoril
narcotic analgesic (nar-KOT-tik)	Drug used to treat severe pain; has the potential to be habit forming if taken for a prolonged time. Also called *opiates*.	morphine, MS Contin; oxycodone, OxyContin; meperidine, Demerol
sedative (SED-ah-tiv)	Drug that has a relaxing or calming effect.	amobarbital, Amytal; butabarbital, Butisol

Abbreviations

ALS	amyotrophic lateral sclerosis	**HA**	headache
ANS	autonomic nervous system	**ICP**	intracranial pressure
CNS	central nervous system	**LP**	lumbar puncture
CP	cerebral palsy	**MS**	multiple sclerosis
CSF	cerebrospinal fluid	**PET**	positron emission tomography
CVA	cerebrovascular accident	**PNS**	peripheral nervous system
CVD	cerebrovascular disease	**SCI**	spinal cord injury
EEG	electroencephalogram, electroencephalography	**TIA**	transient ischemic attack

Chapter Review

Terminology Checklist

Below are all Anatomy and Physiology key terms, Word Building, Vocabulary, Pathology, Diagnostic, Therapeutic, and Pharmacology terms presented in this chapter. Use this list as a study tool by placing a check in the box in front of each term as you master its meaning.

☐ absence seizure
☐ afferent neurons
☐ Alzheimer's disease
☐ amyotrophic lateral sclerosis
☐ analgesia
☐ analgesic
☐ anesthesia
☐ anesthesiology
☐ anesthetic
☐ anticonvulsant
☐ aphasia
☐ arachnoid layer
☐ ascending tracts
☐ astrocytoma
☐ ataxia
☐ aura
☐ autonomic nervous system
☐ axon
☐ Babinski reflex
☐ Bell's palsy
☐ brain
☐ brain scan
☐ brain stem
☐ brain tumor
☐ carotid endarterectomy
☐ central canal
☐ central nervous system
☐ cephalalgia
☐ cerebellar
☐ cerebellitis
☐ cerebellum
☐ cerebral
☐ cerebral aneurysm
☐ cerebral angiography
☐ cerebral contusion
☐ cerebral cortex
☐ cerebral hemispheres
☐ cerebral palsy
☐ cerebrospinal

☐ cerebrospinal fluid
☐ cerebrospinal fluid analysis
☐ cerebrospinal fluid shunts
☐ cerebrovascular accident
☐ cerebrum
☐ coma
☐ concussion
☐ conscious
☐ convulsion
☐ cranial nerves
☐ delirium
☐ dementia
☐ dendrite
☐ descending tracts
☐ diencephalon
☐ dopaminergic drugs
☐ dura mater
☐ dysphasia
☐ echoencephalography
☐ efferent neurons
☐ electroencephalogram
☐ electroencephalography
☐ encephalitis
☐ epidural hematoma
☐ epilepsy
☐ focal seizure
☐ frontal lobe
☐ ganglion
☐ glands
☐ gray matter
☐ Guillain-Barré syndrome
☐ gyri
☐ hemiparesis
☐ hemiplegia
☐ hydrocephalus
☐ hyperesthesia
☐ hypnotic
☐ hypothalamus
☐ intrathecal

☐ laminectomy
☐ lumbar puncture
☐ medulla oblongata
☐ meningeal
☐ meninges
☐ meningioma
☐ meningitis
☐ meningocele
☐ midbrain
☐ migraine
☐ monoparesis
☐ monoplegia
☐ motor neurons
☐ multiple sclerosis
☐ muscles
☐ myasthenia gravis
☐ myelin
☐ myelinated
☐ myelitis
☐ myelogram
☐ myelography
☐ myelomeningocele
☐ narcotic analgesic
☐ nerve block
☐ nerve cell body
☐ nerve conduction velocity
☐ nerve root
☐ nerves
☐ neural
☐ neuralgia
☐ neurectomy
☐ neuroglial cells
☐ neurologist
☐ neurology
☐ neuroma
☐ neuron
☐ neuropathy
☐ neuroplasty
☐ neurorrhaphy

- ☐ neurosurgery
- ☐ neurotransmitter
- ☐ occipital lobe
- ☐ palsy
- ☐ paralysis
- ☐ paraplegia
- ☐ parasympathetic branch
- ☐ paresthesia
- ☐ parietal lobe
- ☐ Parkinson's disease
- ☐ peripheral nervous system
- ☐ pia mater
- ☐ poliomyelitis
- ☐ polyneuritis
- ☐ pons
- ☐ pontine
- ☐ positron emission tomography
- ☐ quadriplegia

- ☐ radiculitis
- ☐ radiculopathy
- ☐ Reye syndrome
- ☐ sedative
- ☐ seizure
- ☐ sensory neurons
- ☐ sensory receptors
- ☐ shingles
- ☐ somatic nerves
- ☐ spina bifida
- ☐ spinal cavity
- ☐ spinal cord
- ☐ spinal cord injury
- ☐ spinal nerves
- ☐ subarachnoid space
- ☐ subdural hematoma
- ☐ subdural space
- ☐ sulci

- ☐ sympathetic branch
- ☐ synapse
- ☐ synaptic cleft
- ☐ syncope
- ☐ temporal lobe
- ☐ thalamic
- ☐ thalamus
- ☐ tonic-clonic seizure
- ☐ tract
- ☐ tractotomy
- ☐ transient ischemic attack
- ☐ tremor
- ☐ unconscious
- ☐ ventricles
- ☐ vertebral canal
- ☐ vertebral column
- ☐ white matter

Practice Exercises

A. Complete the following statements.

1. The study of the nervous system is called _neurology_.

2. The organs of the nervous system are the _brain_, _nerves_, and _spinal cord_.

3. The two divisions of the nervous system are the _central nervous system_ and _peripheral nervous system_

4. The neurons that carry impulses away from the brain and spinal cord are called _efferent (motor)_ neurons.

5. The neurons that carry impulses to the brain and spinal cord are called _afferent (sensory)_ neurons.

6. The largest portion of the brain is the _cerebrum_.

7. The second largest portion of the brain is the _cerebellum_.

8. The occipital lobe controls _vision_.

9. The temporal lobe controls _hearing_ and _smell_.

10. The two divisions of the autonomic nervous system are the _parasympathetic branch_ and _the sympathetic branch_

B. State the described terms using the combining forms provided.

The combining form *neur/o* refers to the nerve. Use it to write a term that means:

1. inflammation of the nerve _neuritis_

2. specialist in nerves _neurologist_

3. pain in the nerve _neuralgia_

4. inflammation of many nerves ___polyneuritis___

5. removal of a nerve ___neurectomy___

6. surgical repair of a nerve ___neuroplasty___

7. nerve tumor ___neuroma___

8. suture of a nerve ___~~neurorrhaphy~~ neurorrhaphy___

The combining form *mening/o* refers to the meninges or membranes. Use it to write a term that means:

9. inflammation of the meninges ___meningitis___

10. protrusion of the meninges ___meningocele___

11. protrusion of the spinal cord and the meninges ___myelomeningocele___

The combining form *encephal/o* refers to the brain. Use it to write a term that means:

12. X-ray record of the brain ___encephalogram___

13. disease of the brain ___encephalopathy___

14. inflammation of the brain ___encephalitis___

15. protrusion of the brain ___encephalocele___

The combining form *cerebr/o* refers to the cerebrum. Use it to write a term that means:

16. pertaining to the cerebrum and spinal cord ___cerebrospinal___

17. pertaining to the cerebrum ___cerebral___

C. Match each term to its definition.

1. __b__ aura

2. __f__ meningitis

3. __g__ coma

4. __h__ shingles

5. __i__ syncope

6. __a__ palsy

7. __e__ absence seizure

8. __c__ tonic-clonic seizure

9. __d__ meningocele

a. loss of ability to control movement

b. sensations before a seizure

c. seizure with convulsions

d. congenital hernia of meninges

e. form of epilepsy without convulsion

f. inflammation of meninges

g. profound stupor

h. painful virus on nerves

i. fainting

D. Identify the following abbreviations.

1. TIA   transient ischemic attack

2. MS   multiple sclerosis

3. SCI   spinal cord injury

4. CNS   central nervous system

5. PNS   peripheral nervous system

6. HA   headache

7. CP   cerebral palsy

8. LP   lumbar puncture

9. ALS   amyotrophic lateral sclerosis

E. Write the abbreviation for the following terms.

1. cerebrospinal fluid   CSF

2. cerebrovascular disease   CVD

3. electroencephalogram   EEG

4. intracranial pressure   ICP

5. positron emission tomography   PET

6. cerebrovascular accident   CVA

7. subarachnoid hemorrhage

8. autonomic nervous system   ANS

F. Match each cranial nerves to its function.

1. __h__ olfactory   a. carries facial sensory impulses

2. __k__ optic   b. turn eye to side

3. __d__ oculomotor   c. controls tongue muscles

4. __g__ trochlear   d. eye muscles and controls pupils

5. __a__ trigeminal   e. swallowing

6. __b__ abducens   f. controls facial muscles

7. __f__ facial   g. controls oblique eye muscles

8. __j__ vestibulocochlear   h. smell

9. __e__ glossopharyngeal   i.   controls neck and shoulder muscles

10. __l__ vagus   j.   hearing and equilibrium

11. __i__ accessory   k.   vision

12. __c__ hypoglossal   l.   organs in lower body cavities

G. Define the following procedures and tests.

1. myelography _injection of radiopaque dye into the spinal cord w/xray to examine outlines made by the dye_

2. cerebral angiography _X-ray of the blood vessels of the brain after the injection of radiopaque dye_

3. Babinski's reflex _reflex test to determine legions & abnormalities in the nervous system_

4. nerve conduction velocity _test that measures how fast an impulse travels along a nerve_

5. cerebrospinal fluid analysis _lab exam of the clear, watery, colorless fluid from within the brain & spinal cord_

6. PET scan _use of positive radionuclides to reconstruct brain sections. Measures oxygen & glucose uptake, cerebral blood flow & blood volume._

7. echoencephalography _recording the electrical activity of the brain by placing electrodes at various positions on the scalp_

8. lumbar puncture _puncture with a needle into the lumbar area to withdraw fluid for examination & for the injection of anesthesia. aka spinal puncture or spinal tap_

H. Define each suffix and provide an example of its use in the nervous system.

	Meaning	Example
1. -plegia	paralysis	quadriplegia
2. -taxia	muscle coordination	ataxia
3. -algesia	pain, sensitivity	analgesia
4. -paresis	weakness	monoparesis
5. -phasia	speech	dysphasia
6. -esthesia	feeling, sensation	anesthesia

I. Define the following combining forms and use them to form nervous system terms.

	Definition	Nervous System Term
1. mening/o	meninges	meningitis
2. encephal/o	brain	encephalitis
3. cerebell/o	cerebellum	cerebellar
4. myel/o	spinal cord	myelogram
5. cephal/o	head	cephalalgia
6. thalam/o	thalamus	thalamic

Nervous System

7. neur/o _____nerve_____ _____neural_____

8. radicul/o _____narve root_____ _____radiculopathy_____

9. cerebr/o _____carabrum_____ _____carabrospinal_____

10. pont/o _____pons_____ _____pontine_____

J. Define the following terms.

1. astrocytoma _____tumor of the brain or spinal cord that is composed of astrocytes, one of the types of neuroglial cells_____

2. epilepsy _____recurrent disorder of the brain in which seizures & loss of consciousness occur as a result of uncontrolled electrical activity of the neurons in the brain_____

3. anesthesia _____lack of sensations_____

4. hemiparesis _____weakness or loss of motion on one side of the body_____

5. neurosurgeon _____physician specializing in treating conditions & diseases of the nervous system through surgery._____

6. analgesia _____absence of pain or sensation_____

7. focal seizure _____localized seizure often affecting one limb_____

8. quadriplegia _____paralysis of four_____

9. subdural hematoma _____mass of blood forming beneath the dura mater if the maninges are torn by trauma. May exert fatal pressure on the brain if not drained by surgery._____

10. intrathecal _____partaining to within the maninges_____

K. Match each term to its definition.

1. _d_ neurologist

2. _e_ cerebrovascular accident

3. _f_ concussion

4. _g_ aphasia

5. _b_ migraine

6. _a_ seizure

7. _c_ dementia

8. _j_ ataxia

9. _h_ spina bifida

10. _i_ unconscious

a. sudden attack

b. a type of severe headache

c. loss of intellectual ability

d. physician who treats nervous problem

e. stroke

f. brain injury from a blow to the head

g. loss of ability to speak

h. congenital anomaly

i. state of being unaware

j. lack of muscle coordination

L. Use the following terms in the sentences below.

Parkinson's disease   transient ischemic attack   cerebral palsy   cerebrospinal fluid shunt

Bell's palsy   subdural hematoma   amyotrophic lateral sclerosis   nerve conduction velocity

delirium   cerebral aneurysm

1. Dr. Martin noted that the 96-year-old patient suffered from _delirium_ when she determined that he was confused, disoriented, and agitated.

2. Lucinda's _amyotrophic lateral sclerosis_ resulted in increasing muscle weakness as the motor neurons in her spinal cord degenerated.

3. The diagnosis of _Bell's palsy_ was correct because the weakness affected only one side of Charles' face.

4. A cerebral angiogram was ordered because Dr. Larson suspected Mrs. Constantine had a(n) _cerebral aneurysm_

5. Roberta's symptoms included fine tremors, muscular weakness, rigidity, and a shuffling gait, leading to a diagnosis of _Parkinson's disease_

6. Matthew's hydrocephalus required the placement of a(n) _cerebrospinal fluid shunt_.

7. Because Mae's hemiparesis was temporary, the final diagnosis was _transient ischemic attack_

8. Following the car accident, a CT scan showed a(n) _subdural hematoma_ was putting pressure on the brain, necessitating immediate neurosurgery.

9. Birth trauma resulted in the newborn developing _cerebral palsy_

10. A(n) _nerve conduction velocity_ test was performed in order to pinpoint the exact position of the nerve damage.

M. Fill in the classification for each drug description, then match the brand name.

Drug Description	Classification	Brand Name
1. _____ produces loss of sensation	_____	a. L-Dopa
2. _____ treats Parkinson's disease	_____	b. Amytal
3. _____ promotes sleep	_____	c. OxyContin
4. _____ non-narcotic pain medication	_____	d. Seconal
5. _____ produces a calming effect	_____	e. Xylocaine
6. _____ treats severe pain	_____	f. Tegretol
7. _____ treats seizures	_____	g. Aleve

Medical Record Analysis

Below is an item from a patient's medical record. Read it carefully, make sure you understand all the medical terms used, and then answer the questions that follow.

Discharge Summary

Admitting Diagnosis:	Paraplegia following motorcycle accident.
Final Diagnosis:	Comminuted L2 fracture with epidural hematoma and spinal cord damage resulting in complete paraplegia at the L2 level.
History of Present Illness:	Patient is a 23-year-old male who was involved in a motorcycle accident. He was unconscious for 35 minutes but was fully aware of his surroundings upon regaining consciousness. He was immediately aware of total anesthesia and paralysis below the waist.
Summary of Hospital Course:	CT scan revealed extensive bone destruction at the fracture site and that the spinal cord was severed. Lumbar puncture revealed sanguinous cerebrospinal fluid. Patient was unable to voluntarily contract any lower extremity muscles and was not able to feel touch or pinpricks. Lumbar laminectomy with spinal fusion was performed to stabilize the fracture and remove the epidural hematoma. The immediate postoperative recovery period proceeded normally with one incidence of pneumonia due to extended bed rest. It responded to antibiotics and respiratory therapy treatments. Patient began intensive rehabilitation with physical therapy and occupational therapy to strengthen upper extremities, as well as transfer and ADL training. After two months, X-rays indicated full healing of the spinal fusion and patient was transferred to a rehabilitation institute.
Discharge Plans:	Patient was transferred to a rehabilitation institute to continue intensive PT and OT. He will require skilled nursing care to assess his skin for the development of decubitus ulcers and intermittent urinary catheterization for incontinence. Since spinal cord was severed, it is not expected that this patient will regain muscle function and sensation. However, long-term goals include independent transfers, independent mobility with a wheelchair, and independent ADLs.

Critical Thinking Questions

1. The final diagnosis of "paraplegia at the L2 level" is not specifically defined by your text. Explain what you believe it to mean in the context of this discharge summary.

   Paralysis of the lower portion of the body & both legs at the level of the 2nd lumbar vertebra.

2. Is this patient expected to regain use of his muscles? Explain why or why not. _No, because his spinal cord was severed._

3. The following medical terms are not specifically referred to in this chapter. Using your text as a dictionary, define each term in your own words.

   a. comminuted _a fracture in which the bone is shattered, splintered or crushed into many pieces or fragments_

   b. sanguinous _pertaining to blood_

c. decubitus ulcer _bedsore or pressure sore caused by pressure over bony prominences of the body; lack of blood flow_

d. catheterization _insertion of a tube into the urethra & into the urinary bladder for the purpose of withdrawing urine_

4. Which of the following is NOT part of this patient's rehabilitation therapy?

a. arm strengthening

b. transfer training

c. instruction in activities of daily living

(d.) leg strengthening

5. Describe, in your own words, the patient's long-term goals. _Independent transfers, independent mobility w/a wheelchair + independent activities of daily living._

6. Name and describe the complete surgical procedure this patient underwent. Then describe the purpose for this surgery. _Lumbar laminectomy w/ spinal fusion. Removal of a portion of the lumbar vertebra in order to relieve pressure on the spinal nerve & to fuse the spine back together._

Chart Note Transcription

The chart note below contains eleven phrases that can be reworded with a medical term that you learned in this chapter. Each phrase is identified with an underline. Determine the medical term and write your answers in the space provided.

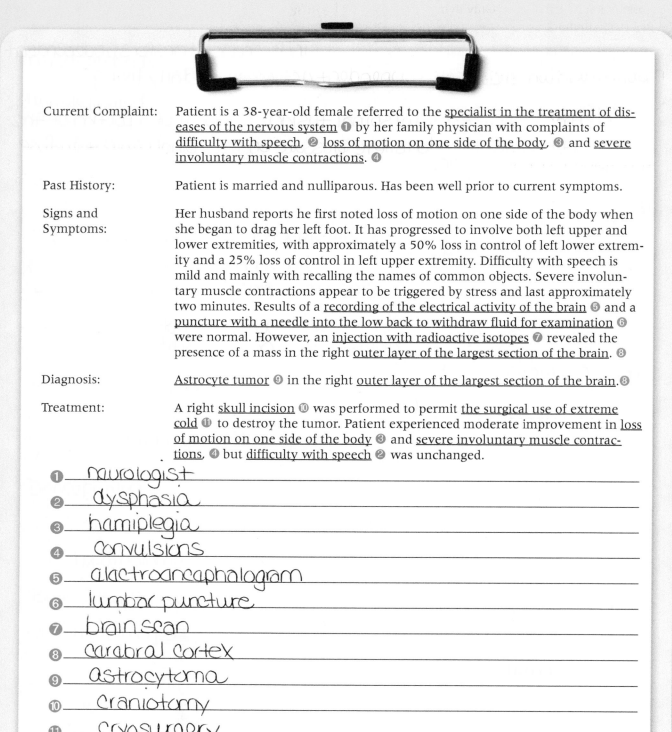

Current Complaint: Patient is a 38-year-old female referred to the <u>specialist in the treatment of diseases of the nervous system</u> ❶ by her family physician with complaints of <u>difficulty with speech</u>, ❷ <u>loss of motion on one side of the body</u>, ❸ and <u>severe involuntary muscle contractions</u>. ❹

Past History: Patient is married and nulliparous. Has been well prior to current symptoms.

Signs and Symptoms: Her husband reports he first noted loss of motion on one side of the body when she began to drag her left foot. It has progressed to involve both left upper and lower extremities, with approximately a 50% loss in control of left lower extremity and a 25% loss of control in left upper extremity. Difficulty with speech is mild and mainly with recalling the names of common objects. Severe involuntary muscle contractions appear to be triggered by stress and last approximately two minutes. Results of a <u>recording of the electrical activity of the brain</u> ❺ and a <u>puncture with a needle into the low back to withdraw fluid for examination</u> ❻ were normal. However, an <u>injection with radioactive isotopes</u> ❼ revealed the presence of a mass in the right <u>outer layer of the largest section of the brain</u>. ❽

Diagnosis: <u>Astrocyte tumor</u> ❾ in the right <u>outer layer of the largest section of the brain</u>.❽

Treatment: A right <u>skull incision</u> ❿ was performed to permit <u>the surgical use of extreme cold</u> ⓫ to destroy the tumor. Patient experienced moderate improvement in <u>loss of motion on one side of the body</u> ❸ and <u>severe involuntary muscle contractions</u>, ❹ but <u>difficulty with speech</u> ❷ was unchanged.

❶ neurologist
❷ dysphasia
❸ hemiplegia
❹ convulsions
❺ electroencephalogram
❻ lumbar puncture
❼ brain scan
❽ cerebral cortex
❾ astrocytoma
❿ craniotomy
⓫ cryosurgery

Labeling Exercise

A. System Review

Write the labels for this figure on the numbered lines provided.

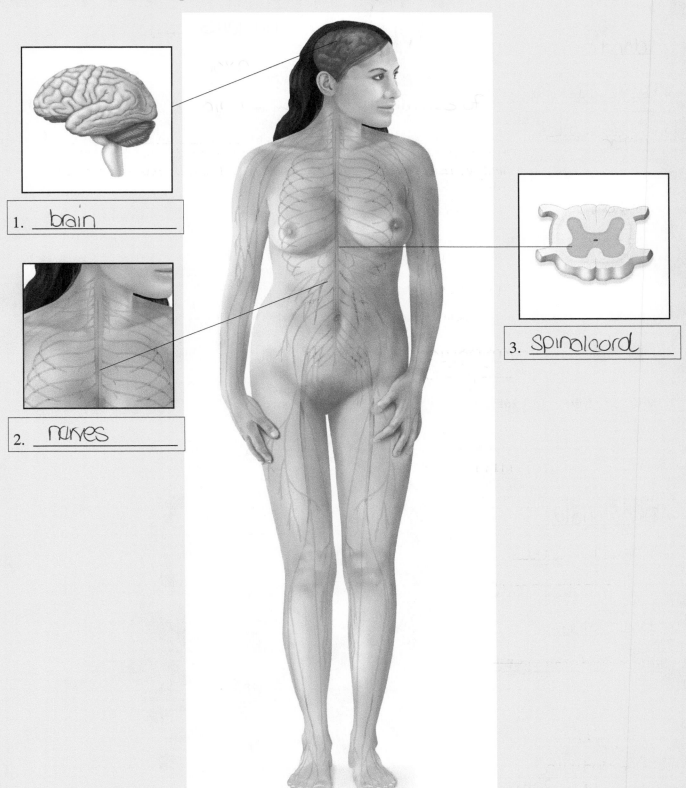

1. brain

2. nerves

3. spinalcord

Nervous System

B. Anatomy Challenge

1. Write the labels for this figure on the numbered lines provided.

1. dendrites
2. nerve cell body
3. unmyelinated region
4. myelinated axon
5. nucleus
6. axon
7. terminal and fibers of axon

2. Write the labels for this figure on the numbered lines provided.

1. Cerebrum
2. Diencephalon
3. thalamus
4. hypothalamus
5. Brain Stem
6. midbrain pons
7. Cerebellum
8. Pons
9. Medulla Oblongata

Multimedia Preview

Additional interactive resources and activities for this chapter can be found on the Companion Website.

Website Highlights—www.prenhall.com/fremgen

MULTIPLE CHOICE QUIZ

Take advantage of the free-access on-line study guide that accompanies your textbook. You'll find a multiple-choice quiz that provides instant feedback that allows you to check your score and see what you got right or wrong. By clicking on this URL you'll also access links to download mp3 audio reviews, current news articles, and an audio glossary.

Special Senses: The Eye and Ear

Learning Objectives

Upon completion of this chapter, you will be able to:

- Identify and define the combining forms and suffixes introduced in this chapter.
- Correctly spell and pronounce medical terms and major anatomical structures relating to the eye and ear.
- Locate and describe the major structures of the eye and ear and their functions.
- Describe how we see.
- Describe the path of sound vibration.
- Build and define eye and ear medical terms from word parts.
- Identify and define eye and ear vocabulary terms.
- Identify and define selected eye and ear pathology terms.
- Identify and define selected eye and ear diagnostic procedures.
- Identify and define selected eye and ear therapeutic procedures.
- Identify and define selected medications relating to the eye and ear.
- Define selected abbreviations associated with the eye and ear.

From Chapter 13 of *Medical Terminology: A Living Language*, 4/e. Bonnie F. Fremgen. Suzanne S. Frucht. Copyright © 2009 by Pearson Education. Published by Prentice Hall. All rights reserved.

Section I: The Eye at a Glance

Function

The eye contains the sensory receptor cells for vision.

Structures

choroid
conjunctiva
eye muscles
eyeball
eyelids
lacrimal apparatus
retina
sclera

Combining Forms

ambly/o	dull, dim	**ocul/o**	eye
aque/o	water	**ophthalm/o**	eye
blephar/o	eyelid	**opt/o**	eye, vision
chrom/o	color	**optic/o**	eye
conjunctiv/o	conjunctiva	**nyctal/o**	night
core/o	pupil	**papill/o**	optic disk
corne/o	cornea	**phac/o**	lens
cycl/o	ciliary muscle	**phot/o**	light
dacry/o	tear, tear duct	**presby/o**	old age
dipl/o	double	**pupill/o**	pupil
glauc/o	gray	**retin/o**	retina
ir/o	iris	**scler/o**	sclera
irid/o	iris	**uve/o**	choroid
kerat/o	cornea	**vitre/o**	glassy
lacrim/o	tears		

Suffixes

-metrist	one who measures
-opia	vision
-tropia	to turn

The Eye Illustrated

retina
contains sensory
receptors for sight

cornea
admits light rays
into the eyeball

iris and pupil
regulate amount of
light entering the
eyebal l

lens
focuses light rays
onto the retina

choroid layer
supplies blood to
eye structures

sclera
tough, protective
outer layer of eyeball

Anatomy and Physiology of the Eye

conjunctiva (kon-JUNK-tih-vah)
eyeball
eyelids
eye muscles

lacrimal apparatus (LAK-rim-al)
ophthalmology (off-thal-MALL-oh-gee)
optic nerve (OP-tik)

The study of the eye is known as **ophthalmology** (Ophth). The **eyeball** is the incredible organ of sight that transmits an external image by way of the nervous system—the **optic nerve**—to the brain. The brain then translates these sensory impulses into an image with computerlike accuracy.

In addition to the eyeball, several external structures play a role in vision. These are the **eye muscles**, **eyelids**, **conjunctiva**, and **lacrimal apparatus**.

The Eyeball

choroid (KOR-oyd)
retina (RET-in-ah)

sclera (SKLAIR-ah)

The actual eyeball is composed of three layers: the **sclera**, the **choroid**, and the **retina**.

Sclera

cornea (COR-nee-ah)

refracts

The outer layer, the sclera, provides a tough protective coating for the inner structures of the eye. Another term for the sclera is the white of the eye.

The anterior portion of the sclera is called the **cornea** (see Figure 1 ■). This clear, transparent area of the sclera allows light to enter the interior of the eyeball. The cornea actually bends, or **refracts**, the light rays.

■ **Figure 1** The internal structures of the eye.

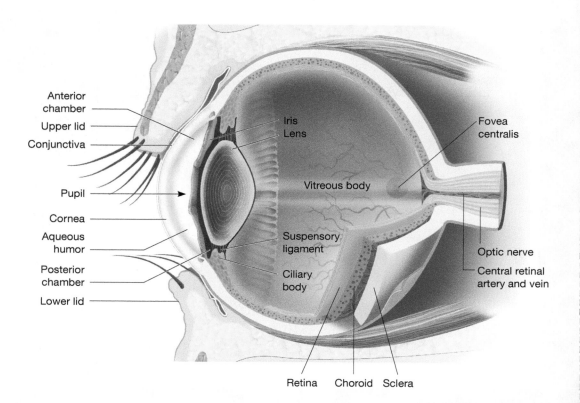

Anterior chamber
Upper lid
Conjunctiva
Pupil
Cornea
Aqueous humor
Posterior chamber
Lower lid
Iris
Lens
Vitreous body
Suspensory ligament
Ciliary body
Fovea centralis
Optic nerve
Central retinal artery and vein
Retina   Choroid   Sclera

Choroid

ciliary body (SIL-ee-ar-ee)   **lens**
iris   **pupil**

The second or middle layer of the eyeball is called the choroid. This opaque layer provides the blood supply for the eye.

The anterior portion of the choroid layer consists of the **iris**, **pupil**, and **ciliary body** (see Figure 1). The iris is the colored portion of the eye and contains smooth muscle. The pupil is the opening in the center of the iris that allows light rays to enter the eyeball. The iris muscle contracts or relaxes to change the size of the pupil, thereby controlling how much light enters the interior of the eyeball. Behind the iris is the **lens.** The lens is not actually part of the choroid layer, but it is attached to the muscular ciliary body. By pulling on the edge of the lens, these muscles change the shape of the lens so it can focus incoming light onto the retina.

Retina

aqueous humor (AY-kwee-us)   **optic disk**
cones   **retinal blood vessels** (RET-in-al)
fovea centralis (FOH-vee-ah sen-TRAH-lis)   **rods**
macula lutea (MAK-yoo-lah loo-TEE-ah)   **vitreous humor** (VIT-ree-us)

The third and innermost layer of the eyeball is the retina. It contains the sensory receptor cells, **rods** and **cones**, that respond to light rays. Rods are active in dim light and help us to see in gray tones. Cones are active only in bright light and are responsible for color vision. When the lens projects an image onto the retina, it strikes an area called the **macula lutea**, or yellow spot (see Figure 1). In the center of the macula lutea is a depression called the **fovea centralis**, meaning central pit. This pit contains a high concentration of sensory receptor cells and, therefore, is the point of clearest vision. Also visible on the retina is the **optic disk**. This is the point where the **retinal blood vessels** enter and exit the eyeball and where the optic nerve leaves the eyeball (see Figure 2 ■). There are no sensory receptor cells in the optic disk and therefore it causes a blind spot in each eye's field of vision. The interior spaces of the eyeball are not empty. The spaces between the cornea and lens are filled with **aqueous humor**, a watery fluid, and the large open area between the lens and retina contains **vitreous humor**, a semisolid gel.

Med Term Tip

The function of the choroid, to provide the rest of the eyeball with blood, is responsible for an alternate name for this layer—*uvea*. The combining form *uve/o* means "vascular."

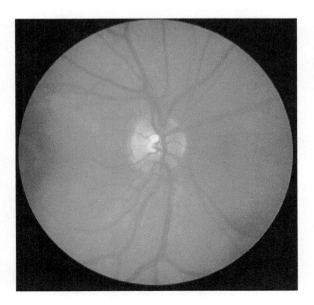

■ **Figure 2** Photograph of the retina of the eye. The optic disk appears yellow and the retinal arteries are clearly visible radiating out from it.

(Rory McClenaghan/Science Photo Library/Photo Researchers, Inc.)

■ **Figure 3** The
arrangement of the external
eye muscles, A) lateral and
B) anterior views.

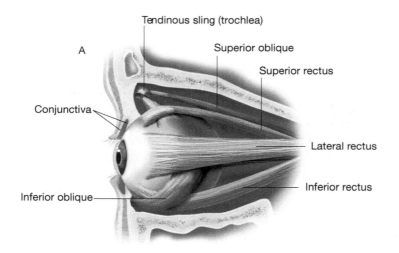

Tendinous sling (trochlea)

Superior oblique

Superior rectus

A

Conjunctiva

Lateral rectus

Inferior rectus

Inferior oblique

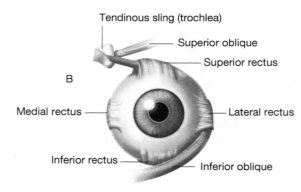

Tendinous sling (trochlea)

Superior oblique

Superior rectus

B

Medial rectus

Lateral rectus

Inferior rectus

Inferior oblique

■ **Figure 3** The
arrangement of the external
eye muscles, A) lateral and
B) anterior views.

Muscles of the Eye

oblique muscles (oh-BLEEK)   **rectus muscles** (REK-tus)

Like many other muscles, the
names *rectus* and *oblique* provide
clues regarding the direction of
their fibers, or their *line of pull*.
Rectus means straight and oblique
means slanted. Rectus muscles
have a straight line of pull. Since
the fibers of an oblique muscle are
slanted on an angle, they produce
rotation.

Six muscles connect the actual eyeball to the skull (see Figure 3 ■). These muscles allow for change in the direction of each eye's sightline. In addition, they provide support for the eyeball in the eye socket. Children may be born with a weakness in some of these muscles and may require treatments such as eye exercises or even surgery to correct this problem commonly referred to as crossed eyes or *strabismus* (see Figure 4 ■). The muscles involved are the four **rectus** and two **oblique muscles**. Rectus muscles (meaning straight) pull the eye up, down, left, or right in a straight line. Oblique muscles are on an angle and produce diagonal eye movement.

■ **Figure 4** Photograph of
an infant with strabismus. The
left eye is turned inward,
called esotropia. *(Bart's Medical
Library/Phototake NYC)*

The Eyelids

cilia (SIL-ee-ah)   **sebaceous glands** (see-BAY-shus)
eyelashes

A pair of eyelids over each eyeball provides protection from foreign particles, injury from the sun and intense light, and trauma (see Figure 1). Both the upper and lower edges of the eyelids have **eyelashes** or **cilia** that protect the eye from foreign particles. In addition, **sebaceous glands** located in the eyelids secrete lubricating oil onto the eyeball.

Conjunctiva

mucous membrane

The conjunctiva of the eye is a **mucous membrane** lining. It forms a continuous covering on the underside of each eyelid and across the anterior surface of each eyeball (see Figure 1). This serves as protection for the eye by sealing off the eyeball in the socket.

Lacrimal Apparatus

lacrimal ducts   **nasolacrimal duct** (naz-oh-LAK-rim-al)
lacrimal gland   **tears**
nasal cavity

The **lacrimal gland** is located under the outer upper corner of each eyelid. These glands produce **tears**. Tears serve the important function of washing and lubricating the anterior surface of the eyeball. **Lacrimal ducts** located in the inner corner of the eye socket then collect the tears and drain them into the **nasolacrimal duct**. This duct ultimately drains the tears into the **nasal cavity** (see Figure 5 ■).

How We See

When light rays strike the eye, they first pass through the cornea, pupil, aqueous humor, lens, and vitreous humor (see Figure 6 ■). They then strike the retina and stimulate the rods and cones. When the light rays hit the retina, an upside-down image is sent along nerve impulses to the optic nerve (see

■ **Figure 5** The structure of the lacrimal apparatus.

Superior lacrimal (tear) gland

Inferior lacrimal (tear) gland

Lacrimal sac

Lacrimal ducts

Nasolacrimal duct
(drains into the nasal cavity)

■ Figure 6 The path of light through the cornea, pupil, lens, and striking the retina.

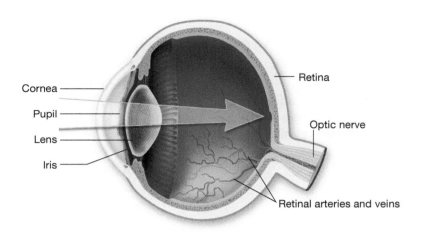

Cornea
Pupil
Lens
Iris
Retina
Optic nerve
Retinal arteries and veins

Figure 7 ■). The optic nerve transmits these impulses to the brain, where the upside-down image is translated into the right-side-up image we are looking at.

Vision requires proper functioning of four mechanisms:

1. Coordination of the external eye muscles so that both eyes move together.
2. The correct amount of light admitted by the pupil.
3. The correct focus of light on the retina by the lens.
4. The optic nerve transmitting sensory images to the brain.

■ Figure 7 The image formed on the retina is inverted. The brain rights the image as part of the interpretation process.

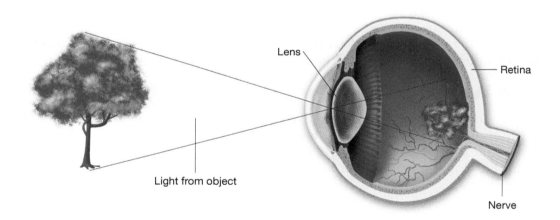

Lens
Retina
Light from object
Nerve

 ## Word Building

The following list contains examples of medical terms built directly from word parts. The definitions of these terms can be determined by a straightforward translation of the word parts.

COMBINING FORM	COMBINED WITH	MEDICAL TERM	DEFINITION
blephar/o	-itis	**blepharitis** (blef-ah-RYE-tis)	eyelid inflammation
	-plasty	**blepharoplasty** (BLEF-ah-roh-plass-tee)	surgical repair of eyelid
	-ptosis	**blepharoptosis** (blef-ah-rop-TOH-sis)	drooping eyelid
	-ectomy	**blepharectomy** (blef-ah-REK-toh-mee)	removal of the eyelid
conjuctiv/o	-al	**conjunctival** (kon-JUNK-tih-vall)	pertaining to the conjunctiva

Word Building *(continued)*

COMBINING FORM	COMBINED WITH	MEDICAL TERM	DEFINITION
	-itis	**conjunctivitis** (kon-junk-tih-VYE-tis)	conjunctiva inflammation (pink eye)
	-plasty	**conjunctivoplasty** (kon-junk-tih-VOH-plas-tee)	surgical repair of the conjunctiva
corne/o	-al	**corneal** (KOR-nee-all)	pertaining to the cornea

Med Term Tip

Word watch — Be careful using the combining forms *core/o* meaning "pupil" and *corne/o* meaning "cornea."

COMBINING FORM	COMBINED WITH	MEDICAL TERM	DEFINITION
cycl/o	-plegia	**cycloplegia** (sigh-kloh-PLEE-jee-ah)	paralysis of the ciliary body
dacry/o	cyst/o -itis	**dacryocystitis** (dak-ree-oh-sis-TYE-tis)	tear bladder inflammation
dipl/o	-opia	**diplopia** (dip-LOH-pee-ah)	double vision
ir/o	-itis	**iritis** (eye-RYE-tis)	iris inflammation
irid/o	-al	**iridal** (ir-id-all)	pertaining to the iris
	-ectomy	**iridectomy** (ir-id-EK-toh-mee)	removal of iris
	-plegia	**iridoplegia** (ir-id-oh-PLEE-jee-ah)	paralysis of iris
	scler/o -otomy	**iridosclerotomy** (ir-ih-doh-skleh-ROT-oh-mee)	incision into iris and sclera
kerat/o	-itis	**keratitis** (kair-ah-TYE-tis)	cornea inflammation

Med Term Tip

Word watch — Be careful using the combining form *kerat/o*, which means both "cornea" and "hard protein keratin."

COMBINING FORM	COMBINED WITH	MEDICAL TERM	DEFINITION
	-meter	**keratometer** (KAIR-ah-toh-mee-ter)	instrument to measure (curve of) cornea
	-otomy	**keratotomy** (kair-ah-TOT-oh-mee)	incision into the cornea
lacrim/o	-al	**lacrimal** (LAK-rim-al)	pertaining to tears
ocul/o	-ar	**ocular** (OCK-yoo-lar)	pertaining to the eye
	intra- -ar	**intraocular** (in-trah-OCK-yoo-lar)	pertaining to within the eye
	myc/o -osis	**oculomycosis** (ok-yoo-loh-my-KOH-sis)	abnormal condition of eye fungus
ophthalm/o	-algia	**ophthalmalgia** (off-thal-MAL-jee-ah)	eye pain
	-ic	**ophthalmic** (off-THAL-mik)	pertaining to the eye
	-ologist	**ophthalmologist** (off-thal-MALL-oh-jist)	specialist in the eye
	-plegia	**ophthalmoplegia** (off-thal-moh-PLEE-jee-ah)	eye paralysis
	-rrhagia	**ophthalmorrhagia** (off-thal-moh-RAH-jee-ah)	rapid bleeding from the eye
	-scope	**ophthalmoscope** (off-THAL-moh-scope)	instrument to view inside the eye
opt/o	-ic	**optic** (OP-tik)	pertaining to the eye or vision
	-meter	**optometer** (op-TOM-eh-ter)	instrument to measure vision
	-metrist	**optometrist** (op-TOM-eh-trist)	one who measures vision

Word Building *(continued)*

COMBINING FORM	COMBINED WITH	MEDICAL TERM	DEFINITION
pupill/o	-ary	**pupillary** (PYOO-pih-lair-ee)	pertaining to the pupil
retin/o	-al	**retinal** (RET-in-al)	pertaining to the retina
	-pathy	**retinopathy** (ret-in-OP-ah-thee)	retina disease
	-pexy	**retinopexy** (ret-ih-noh-PEX-ee)	surgical fixation of the retina
scler/o	-al	**scleral** (SKLAIR-all)	pertaining to the sclera
	-malacia	**scleromalacia** (sklair-oh-mah-LAY-she-ah)	softening of the sclera
	-otomy	**sclerotomy** (skleh-ROT-oh-mee)	incision into the sclera
	-itis	**scleritis** (skler-EYE-tis)	inflammation of the sclera
uve/o	-itis	**uveitis** (yoo-vee-EYE-tis)	inflammation of the choroid

Vocabulary

TERM	DEFINITION
emmetropia (EM) (em-eh-TROH-pee-ah)	State of normal vision.
legally blind	Describes a person who has severely impaired vision. Usually defined as having visual acuity of 20/200 that cannot be improved with corrective lenses or having a visual field of less then 20 degrees.
nyctalopia (nik-tah-LOH-pee-ah)	Difficulty seeing in dim light; also called *night-blindness*. Usually due to damaged rods. **Med Term Tip** The simple translation of *nyctalopia* is "night vision." However, it is used to mean "night blindness."
ophthalmology (opf-thal-MOLL-oh-jee)	Branch of medicine involving the diagnosis and treatment of conditions and diseases of the eye and surrounding structures. The physician is an *ophthalmologist*.
optician (op-TISH-an)	Specialist in grinding corrective lenses.
optometry (op-TOM-eh-tree)	Medical profession specializing in examining the eyes, testing visual acuity, and prescribing corrective lenses. A doctor of optometry is an *optometrist*.
papilledema (pah-pill-eh-DEEM-ah)	Swelling of the optic disk. Often as a result of increased intraocular pressure. Also called *choked disk.*
photophobia (foh-toh-FOH-bee-ah)	Although the term translates into *fear of light,* it actually means a strong sensitivity to bright light.
presbyopia (prez-bee-OH-pee-ah)	Visual loss due to old age, resulting in difficulty in focusing for near vision (such as reading).
xerophthalmia (zee-ROP-thal-mee-ah)	Dry eyes.

Pathology

TERM	DEFINITION
■ *Eyeball*	
achromatopsia (ah-kroh-mah-TOP-see-ah)	Condition of color blindness—unable to perceive one or more colors; more common in males.
amblyopia (am-blee-OH-pee-ah)	Loss of vision not as a result of eye pathology. Usually occurs in patients who see two images. In order to see only one image, the brain will no longer recognize the image being sent to it by one of the eyes. May occur if strabismus is not corrected. This condition is not treatable with a prescription lens. Commonly referred to as *lazy eye*.
astigmatism (Astigm) (ah-STIG-mah-tizm)	Condition in which light rays are focused unevenly on the retina, causing a distorted image, due to an abnormal curvature of the cornea.
cataract (KAT-ah-rakt)	Damage to the lens causing it to become opaque or cloudy, resulting in diminished vision. Treatment is usually surgical removal of the cataract or replacement of the lens.

Med Term Tip

The term *cataract* comes from the Latin word meaning "waterfall." This refers to how a person with a cataract sees the world—as if looking through a waterfall.

■ **Figure 8** Photograph of a person with a cataract in the right eye.

TERM	DEFINITION
corneal abrasion	Scraping injury to the cornea. If it does not heal, it may develop into an ulcer.
glaucoma (glau-KOH-mah)	Increase in intraocular pressure, which, if untreated, may result in atrophy (wasting away) of the optic nerve and blindness. Glaucoma is treated with medication and surgery. There is an increased risk of developing glaucoma in persons over age 60, of African ancestry, who have sustained a serious eye injury, and in anyone with a family history of diabetes or glaucoma.
hyperopia (high-per-OH-pee-ah)	With this condition a person can see things in the distance but has trouble reading material at close range. Also known as *farsightedness*. This condition is corrected with converging or biconvex lenses.

■ **Figure 9** Hyperopia (farsightedness). In the uncorrected top figure, the image would come into focus behind the retina, making the image on the retina blurry. The bottom image shows how a biconvex lens corrects this condition.

Hyperopia (farsightedness)

Corrected with biconvex lens

Pathology *(continued)*

TERM	DEFINITION
macular degeneration (MAK-yoo-lar)	Deterioration of the macular area of the retina of the eye. May be treated with laser surgery to destroy the blood vessels beneath the macula.
monochromatism (mon-oh-KROH-mah-tizm)	Unable to perceive one color.
myopia (MY) (my-OH-pee-ah)	With this condition a person can see things close up but distance vision is blurred. Also known as *nearsightedness.* This condition is corrected with diverging or biconcave lenses.

■ **Figure 10** Myopia (nearsightedness). In the uncorrected top figure, the image comes into focus in front of the lens, making the image on the retina blurry. The bottom image shows how a biconcave lens corrects this condition.

Myopia (nearsightedness)

Corrected with biconcave lens

retinal detachment (RET-in-al)	Occurs when the retina becomes separated from the choroid layer. This separation seriously damages blood vessels and nerves, resulting in blindness. May be treated with surgical or medical procedures to stabilize the retina and prevent separation.
retinitis pigmentosa (ret-in-EYE-tis pig-men-TOH-sah)	Progressive disease of the eye resulting in the retina becoming hard (sclerosed), pigmented (colored), and atrophying (wasting away). There is no known cure for this condition.
retinoblastoma (RET-in-noh-blast-OH-mah)	Malignant eye tumor occurring in children, usually under the age of 3. Requires enucleation.

■ *Conjunctiva*

pterygium (the-RIJ-ee-um)	Hypertrophied conjunctival tissue in the inner corner of the eye.
trachoma (tray-KOH-mah)	Chronic infectious disease of the conjunctiva and cornea caused by bacteria. Occurs more commonly in those living in hot, dry climates. Untreated, it may lead to blindness when the scarring invades the cornea. Trachoma can be treated with antibiotics.

■ *Eyelids*

hordeolum (hor-DEE-oh-lum)	Refers to a *stye* (or *sty*), a small purulent inflammatory infection of a sebaceous gland of the eyelid; treated with hot compresses and/or surgical incision.

Pathology (continued)

TERM	DEFINITION
■ Eye Muscles	
esotropia (ST) (ess-oh-TROH-pee-ah)	Inward turning of the eye; also called *cross-eyed*. An example of a form of strabismus (muscle weakness of the eye).
exotropia (XT) (eks-oh-TROH-pee-ah)	Outward turning of the eye; also called *wall-eyed*. Also an example of strabismus (muscle weakness of the eye).
strabismus (strah-BIZ-mus)	Eye muscle weakness commonly seen in children resulting in the eyes looking in different directions at the same time. May be corrected with glasses, eye exercises, and/or surgery.
■ Brain-Related Vision Pathologies	
hemianopia (hem-ee-ah-NOP-ee-ah)	Loss of vision in half of the visual field. A stroke patient may suffer from this disorder.
nystagmus (niss-TAG-mus)	Jerky-appearing involuntary eye movements, usually left and right. Often an indication of brain injury.

Diagnostic Procedures

TERM	DEFINITION
■ Eye Examination Tests	
color vision tests ■ **Figure 11** An example of color blindness test. A person with red-green color blindness would not be able to distinguish the green 27 from the surrounding red circles.	Use of polychromic (multicolored) charts to determine the ability of the patient to recognize color.
fluorescein angiography (floo-oh-RESS-ee-in an-jee-OG-rah-fee)	Process of injecting a dye (fluorescein) to observe the movement of blood and detect lesions in the macular area of the retina. Used to determine if there is a detachment of the retina.
fluorescein staining (floo-oh-RESS-ee-in)	Applying dye eye drops that are a bright green fluorescent color. Used to look for corneal abrasions or ulcers.
keratometry (kair-ah-TOM-eh-tree)	Measurement of the curvature of the cornea using an instrument called a *keratometer*.
ophthalmoscopy (off-thal-MOSS-koh-pee)	Examination of the interior of the eyes using an instrument called an *ophthalmoscope* (see Figure 12 ■). The physician dilates the pupil in order to see the cornea, lens, and retina. Used to identify abnormalities in the blood vessels of the eye and some systemic diseases.

Figure 12 Examination of the interior of the eye using an ophthalmoscope.

Diagnostic Procedures *(continued)*

TERM	DEFINITION
refractive error test (ree-FRAK-tiv)	Vision test for a defect in the ability of the eye to accurately focus the image that is hitting it. Refractive errors result in myopia and hyperopia.
slit lamp microscopy	Examining the posterior surface of the cornea.
Snellen chart (SNEL-enz)	Chart used for testing distance vision named for Dutch ophthalmologist Hermann Snellen. It contains letters of varying size and is administered from a distance of 20 feet. A person who can read at 20 feet what the average person can read at this distance is said to have 20/20 vision.
tonometry (tohn-OM-eh-tree)	Measurement of the intraocular pressure of the eye using a *tonometer* to check for the condition of glaucoma. The physician places the tonometer lightly on the eyeball and a pressure measurement is taken. Generally part of a normal eye exam for adults.
visual acuity (VA) **test** (VIZH-oo-al ah-KYOO-ih-tee)	Measurement of the sharpness of a patient's vision. Usually, a Snellen chart is used for this test in which the patient identifies letters from a distance of 20 feet.

Therapeutic Procedures

TERMS	DEFINITION
Surgical Procedures	
cryoextraction (cry-oh-eks-TRAK-shun)	Procedure in which cataract is lifted from the lens with an extremely cold probe.
cryoretinopexy (cry-oh-RET-ih-noh-pek-see)	Surgical fixation of the retina by using extreme cold.
enucleation (ee-new-klee-AH-shun)	Surgical removal of an eyeball.
keratoplasty (KAIR-ah-toh-plass-tee)	Surgical repair of the cornea is the simple translation of this term that is utilized to mean corneal transplant.
laser-assisted in-situ keratomileusis (LASIK) (in-SIH-tyoo kair-ah-toh-mih-LOO-sis)	Correction of myopia using laser surgery to remove corneal tissue (see Figure 13 ■).

■ **Figure 13** LASIK surgery. The cornea has been lifted in order to reshape it. *(Chris Barry/Phototake NYC)*

Therapeutic Procedures *(continued)*

TERM	DEFINITION
laser photocoagulation (LAY-zer foh-toh-koh-ag-yoo-LAY-shun)	Use of a laser beam to destroy very small precise areas of the retina. May be used to treat retinal detachment or macular degeneration.
phacoemulsification (fak-oh-ee-mull-sih-fih-KAY-shun)	Use of high-frequency sound waves to emulsify (liquefy) a lens with a cataract, which is then aspirated (removed by suction) with a needle.
photorefractive keratectomy (PRK) (foh-toh-ree-FRAK-tiv kair-ah-TEK-toh-mee)	Use of a laser to reshape the cornea and correct errors of refraction.
radial keratotomy (RK) (RAY-dee-all kair-ah-TOT-oh-mee)	Spokelike incisions around the cornea that result in it becoming flatter. A surgical treatment for myopia.
scleral buckling (SKLAIR-al)	Placing a band of silicone around the outside of the sclera that stabilizes a detaching retina.
strabotomy (strah-BOT-oh-mee)	Incision into the eye muscles in order to correct strabismus.

Pharmacology

CLASSIFICATION	ACTION	GENERIC AND BRAND NAMES
anesthetic ophthalmic solution (off-THAL-mik)	Eye drops for pain relief associated with eye infections, corneal abrasions, or surgery.	proparacain, Ak-Taine, Ocu-Caine; tetracaine, Opticaine, Pontocaine
antibiotic ophthalmic solution (off-THAL-mik)	Eye drops for the treatment of bacterial eye infections.	erythromycin, Del-Mycin, Ilotycin Ophthalmic
antiglaucoma medications (an-tye-glau-KOH-mah)	Group of drugs that reduce intraocular pressure by lowering the amount of aqueous humor in the eyeball. May achieve this by either reducing the production of aqueous humor or increasing its outflow.	timolol, Betimol, Timoptic; acetazolamide, Ak-Zol, Dazamide; prostaglandin analogs, Lumigan, Xalatan

Pharmacology *(continued)*

CLASSIFICATION	ACTION	GENERIC AND BRAND NAMES
artificial tears	Medications, many of them over the counter, to treat dry eyes.	buffered isotonic solutions, Akwa Tears, Refresh Plus, Moisture Eyes
miotic (my-OT-ik)	Any substance that causes the pupil to constrict. These medications may also be used to treat glaucoma.	physostigmine, Eserine Sulfate, Isopto Eserine; carbachol, Carbastat, Miostat
mydriatic (mid-ree-AT-ik)	Any substance that causes the pupil to dilate by paralyzing the iris and/or ciliary body muscles. Particularly useful during eye examinations and eye surgery.	atropine sulfate, Atropine-Care Ophthalmic, Atropisol Ophthalmic
ophthalmic decongestants	Over-the-counter medications that constrict the arterioles of the eye, reduce redness and itching of the conjunctiva.	tetrahydrozoline, Visine, Murine

Abbreviations

ARMD	age-related macular degeneration	**Ophth.**	ophthalmology
Astigm	astigmatism	**OS**	left eye
c.gl.	correction with glasses	**OU**	each eye/both eyes
D	diopter (lens strength)	**PERRLA**	pupils equal, round, react to light and accommodation
DVA	distance visual acuity		
ECCE	extracapsular cataract extraction	**PRK**	photorefractive keratectomy
EENT	eye, ear, nose, and throat	**REM**	rapid eye movement
EM	emmetropia	**s.gl.**	without correction or glasses
EOM	extraocular movement	**SMD**	senile macular degeneration
ICCE	intracapsular cataract extraction	**ST**	esotropia
IOP	intraocular pressure	**VA**	visual acuity
LASIK	laser-assisted in-situ keratomileusis	**VF**	visual field
OD	right eye	**XT**	exotropia

Med Term Tip

The abbreviations for right eye (OD) and left eye (OS) are easy to remember when we know their origins. OD stands for *oculus* (eye) *dexter* (right). OS has its origin in *oculus* (eye) *sinister* (left). At one time in history it was considered to be sinister if a person looked at another from only the left side. Hence the term *oculus sinister* (OS) means left eye.

Section II: The Ear at a Glance

Function

The ear contains the sensory receptors for hearing and equilibrium (balance).

Structures

auricle
external ear
inner ear
middle ear

Combining Forms

acous/o	hearing
audi/o	hearing
audit/o	hearing
aur/o	ear
auricul/o	ear
cerumin/o	cerumen
cochle/o	cochlea
labyrinth/o	labyrinth (inner ear)
myring/o	eardrum
ot/o	ear
salping/o	eustachian tube
staped/o	stapes
tympan/o	eardrum, middle ear

Suffixes

-cusis	hearing
-otia	ear condition

The Ear Illustrated

auricle
directs sound waves into the ear canal

middle ear
transmits sound waves to the inner ear

inner ear
contains sensory receptors for hearing and balance

external ear
transmits sound waves to the middle ear

Anatomy and Physiology of the Ear

audiology (aw-dee-OL-oh-jee)	**middle ear**
cochlear nerve (KOK-lee-ar)	**otology** (oh-TOL-oh-jee)
equilibrium (ee-kwih-LIB-ree-um)	**vestibular nerve** (ves-TIB-yoo-lar)
external ear	**vestibulocochlear nerve**
hearing	(ves-tib-yoo-loh-KOK-lee-ar)
inner ear	

The study of the ear is referred to as **otology** (Oto), and the study of hearing disorders is called **audiology**. While there is a large amount of overlap between these two areas, there are also examples of ear problems that do not affect hearing. The ear is responsible for two senses: **hearing** and **equilibrium**, or our sense of balance. Hearing and equilibrium sensory information is carried to the brain by cranial nerve VIII, the **vestibulocochlear nerve**. This nerve is divided into two major branches. The **cochlear nerve** carries hearing information, and the **vestibular nerve** carries equilibrium information.

The ear is subdivided into three areas:

1. **external ear**
2. **middle ear**
3. **inner ear**

External Ear

auditory canal (AW-dih-tor-ee)	**pinna** (PIN-ah)
auricle (AW-rih-k'l)	**tympanic membrane** (tim-PAN-ik)
cerumen (seh-ROO-men)	
external auditory meatus	
(AW-dih-tor-ee me-A-tus)	

The external ear consists of three parts: the **auricle**, the **auditory canal**, and the **tympanic membrane** (see Figure 14 ▪). The auricle or **pinna** is what is commonly referred to as *the ear* because this is the only visible portion. The auricle with its

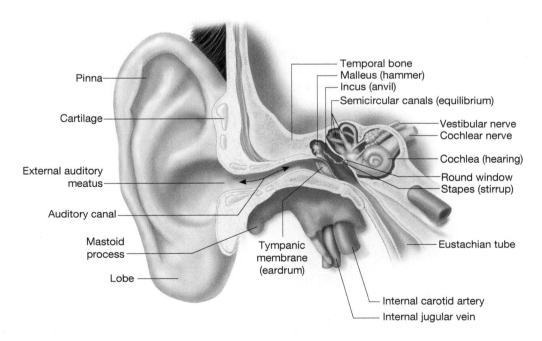

▪ **Figure 14** The internal structures of the outer, middle, and inner ear.

Pinna

Cartilage

External auditory meatus

Auditory canal

Mastoid process

Lobe

Temporal bone
Malleus (hammer)
Incus (anvil)
Semicircular canals (equilibrium)

Vestibular nerve
Cochlear nerve

Cochlea (hearing)

Round window
Stapes (stirrup)

Eustachian tube

Tympanic membrane (eardrum)

Internal carotid artery
Internal jugular vein

441

Med Term Tip

The term *tympanic membrane* comes from the Greek word for "drumhead." The tympanic membrane or eardrum vibrates to sound waves like a drum head.

earlobe has a unique shape in each person and functions like a funnel to capture sound waves as they go past the outer ear and channel them through the **external auditory meatus**. The sound then moves along the auditory canal and causes the tympanic membrane (eardrum) to vibrate. The tympanic membrane actually separates the external ear from the middle ear. Ear wax or **cerumen** is produced in oil glands in the auditory canal. This wax helps to protect and lubricate the ear. It is also just barely liquid at body temperature. This causes cerumen to slowly flow out of the auditory canal, carrying dirt and dust with it. Therefore, the auditory canal is self-cleaning.

Middle Ear

auditory tube (AW-dih-tor-ee)   **ossicles** (OSS-ih-kls)

eustachian tube (yoo-STAY-she-en)   **oval window**

incus (ING-kus)   **stapes** (STAY-peez)

malleus (MAL-ee-us)

Med Term Tip

The three bones in the middle ear are referred to by terms that are similar to their shape. Thus, the malleus is called the hammer, the incus is the anvil, and the stapes is the stirrup (see Figure 15).

The middle ear is located in a small cavity in the temporal bone of the skull. This air-filled cavity contains three tiny bones called **ossicles** (see Figure 15 ■). These three bones, the **malleus**, **incus**, and **stapes**, are vital to the hearing process. They amplify the vibrations in the middle ear and transmit them to the inner ear from the malleus to the incus and finally to the stapes. The stapes, the last of the three ossicles, is attached to a very thin membrane that covers the opening to the inner ear called the **oval window**.

The **eustachian tube** or **auditory tube** connects the nasopharynx with the middle ear (see Figure 14). Each time you swallow the eustachian tube opens. This connection allows pressure to equalize between the middle ear cavity and the atmospheric pressure.

Inner Ear

cochlea (KOK-lee-ah)   **saccule** (SAK-yool)

labyrinth (LAB-ih-rinth)   **semicircular canals**

organs of Corti (KOR-tee)   **utricle** (YOO-trih-k'l)

Med Term Tip

Frequently, children will twirl in circles and fall or stumble from dizziness when they stop. This is caused from a temporary imbalance in the inner ear.

The inner ear is also located in a cavity within the temporal bone (see Figure 14). This fluid-filled cavity is referred to as the **labyrinth** because of its shape. The labyrinth contains the hearing and equilibrium sensory organs: the **cochlea** for hearing and the **semicircular canals**, **utricle**, and **saccule** for equilibrium. Each of these organs contains hair cells, which are the actual sensory receptor cells. In the cochlea, the hair cells are referred to as **organs of Corti**.

■ **Figure 15** Close-up view of the ossicles within the middle ear. These three bones extend from the tympanic membrane to the oval window.

Tympanic membrane

Malleus
Incus
Stapes
Oval window

How We Hear

conductive hearing loss (kon-DUK-tiv)

sensorineural hearing loss (sen-soh-ree-NOO-ral)

Figure 16 ■ outlines the path of sound through the outer ear and middle ear and into the cochlea of the inner ear. Sound waves traveling down the external auditory canal strike the eardrum, causing it to vibrate. The ossicles conduct these vibrations across the middle ear from the eardrum to the oval window. Oval window movements initiate vibrations in the fluid that fills the cochlea. As the fluid vibrations strike a hair cell, they bend the small hairs and stimulate the nerve ending. The nerve ending then sends an electrical impulse to the brain on the cochlear portion of the vestibulocochlear nerve.

Hearing loss can be divided into two main categories: **conductive hearing loss** and **sensorineural hearing loss.** Conductive refers to disease or malformation of the outer or middle ear. All sound is weaker and muffled in conductive hearing loss since it is not conducted correctly to the inner ear. Sensorineural hearing loss is the result of damage or malformation of the inner ear (cochlea) or the cochlear nerve. In this hearing loss, some sounds are distorted and heard incorrectly. There can also be a combination of both conductive and sensorineural hearing loss.

Med Term Tip

Hearing impairment is becoming a greater problem for the general population for several reasons. First, people are living longer. Hearing loss can accompany old age, and there are a greater number of people over 50 years of age requiring hearing assistance. In addition, sound technology has produced music quality that was never available before. However, listening to loud music either naturally or through earphones can cause gradual damage to the hearing mechanism.

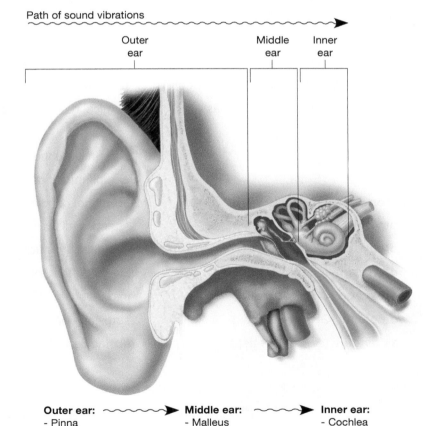

Path of sound vibrations

Outer ear | Middle ear | Inner ear

Outer ear: → **Middle ear:** → **Inner ear:**
- Pinna
- External auditory canal
- Tympanic membrane

- Malleus
- Incus
- Stapes
- Oval window

- Cochlea
- Auditory fluids and
- Organ of Corti
- Auditory nerve fibers
- Cerebral cortex

■ **Figure 16** The path of sound waves through the outer, middle, and inner ear.

Word Building

The following list contains examples of medical terms built directly from word parts. The definitions of these terms can be determined by a straightforward translation of the word parts.

COMBINING FORM	COMBINED WITH	MEDICAL TERM	DEFINITION
acous/o	-tic	**acoustic** (ah-KOOS-tik)	pertaining to hearing
audi/o	-gram	**audiogram** (AW-dee-oh-gram)	record of hearing
	-meter	**audiometer** (aw-dee-OM-eh-ter)	instrument to measure hearing
	-ologist	**audiologist** (aw-dee-OL-oh-jist)	hearing specialist
audit/o	-ory	**auditory** (AW-dih-tor-ee)	pertaining to hearing
aur/o	-al	**aural** (AW-ral)	pertaining to the ear

> **Med Term Tip**
>
> Word watch—Be careful when using two terms that sound the same — *aural* meaning "pertaining to the ear" and *oral* meaning "pertaining to the mouth."

COMBINING FORM	COMBINED WITH	MEDICAL TERM	DEFINITION
auricul/o	-ar	**auricular** (aw-RIK-cu-lar)	pertaining to the ear
cochle/o	-ar	**cochlear** (KOK-lee-ar)	pertaining to the cochlea
labyrinth/o	-ectomy	**labyrinthectomy** (lab-ih-rin-THEK-toh-mee)	removal of the labyrinth
	-otomy	**labyrinthotomy** (lab-ih-rinth-OT-oh-mee)	incision into the labyrinth
myring/o	-itis	**myringitis** (mir-ing-JYE-tis)	eardrum inflammation
	-ectomy	**myringectomy** (mir-in-GEK-toh-mee)	removal of the eardrum
	-plasty	**myringoplasty** (mir-IN-goh-plass-tee)	surgical repair of eardrum
ot/o	-algia	**otalgia** (oh-TAL-jee-ah)	ear pain
	-ic	**otic** (OH-tik)	pertaining to the ear
	-itis	**otitis** (oh-TYE-tis)	ear inflammation
	myc/o -osis	**otomycosis** (oh-toh-my-KOH-sis)	abnormal condition of ear fungus
	-ologist	**otologist** (oh-TOL-oh-jist)	ear specialist
	py/o -rrhea	**otopyorrhea** (oh-toh-pye-oh-REE-ah)	pus discharge from ear
	-rrhagia	**otorrhagia** (oh-toh-RAH-jee-ah)	bleeding from the ear
	-scope	**otoscope** (OH-toh-scope)	instrument to view inside the ear
	-plasty	**otoplasty** (OH-toh-plas-tee)	surgical repair of the (external) ear
salping/o	-itis	**salpingitis** (sal-pin-JIH-tis)	eustachian tube inflammation

> **Med Term Tip**
>
> Word watch—Be careful using the combining form *salping/o*, which can mean either "Eustachian tube" or "fallopian tube."

COMBINING FORM	COMBINED WITH	MEDICAL TERM	DEFINITION
	-otomy	**salpingotomy** (sal-pin-GOT-oh-mee)	incision into eustachian tube
tympan/o	-ic	**tympanic** (tim-PAN-ik)	pertaining to the eardrum
	-itis	**tympanitis** (tim-pan-EYE-tis)	eardrum inflammation
	-meter	**tympanometer** (tim-pah-NOM-eh-ter)	instrument to measure eardrum
	-plasty	**tympanoplasty** (tim-pan-oh-PLASS-tee)	surgical repair of eardrum

Word Building *(continued)*

COMBINING FORM	COMBINED WITH	MEDICAL TERM	DEFINITION
	-rrhexis	**tympanorrhexis** (tim-pan-oh-REK-sis)	eardrum rupture
	-otomy	**tympanotomy** (tim-pan-OT-oh-mee)	incision into the eardrum
	-ectomy	**tympanectomy** (tim-pan-EK-toh-mee)	removal of the eardrum

SUFFIX	COMBINED WITH	MEDICAL TERM	DEFINITION
-otia	micro-	**microtia** (my-KROH-she-ah)	(abnormally) small ears
	macro-	**macrotia** (mah-KROH-she-ah)	(abnormally) large ears

Vocabulary

TERM	DEFINITION
American Sign Language (ASL)	Nonverbal method of communicating in which the hands and fingers are used to indicate words and concepts. Used by both persons who are deaf and persons with speech impairments.

■ **Figure 17** Photograph of a teacher and student communicating using American Sign Language. *(Trevon Baker/Baker Consulting and Design)*

TERM	DEFINITION
binaural (bin-AW-rall)	Referring to both ears.
decibel (dB) (DES-ih-bel)	Measures the intensity or loudness of a sound. Zero decibels is the quietest sound measured and 120 dB is the loudest sound commonly measured.
hertz (Hz)	Measurement of the frequency or pitch of sound. The lowest pitch on an audiogram is 250 Hz. The measurement can go as high as 8000 Hz, which is the highest pitch measured.
monaural (mon-AW-rall)	Referring to one ear.
otorhinolaryngology (ENT) (oh-toh-rye-rye-noh-lair-in-GOL-oh-jee)	Branch of medicine involving the diagnosis and treatment of conditions and diseases of the ear, nose, and throat. Also referred to as *ENT*. Physician is an *otorhinolaryngologist*.
presbycusis (pres-bih-KOO-sis)	Normal loss of hearing that can accompany the aging process.
residual hearing (rih-ZID-yoo-al)	Amount of hearing that is still present after damage has occurred to the auditory mechanism.
tinnitus (tin-EYE-tus)	Ringing in the ears.
vertigo (VER-tih-goh)	Dizziness.

Pathology

TERM	DEFINITION
■ *Hearing Loss*	
anacusis (an-ah-KOO-sis)	Total absence of hearing; inability to perceive sound. Also called *deafness*.
deafness	Inability to hear or having some degree of hearing impairment.
■ *External Ear*	
ceruminoma (seh-roo-men-oh-ma)	Excessive accumulation of ear wax resulting in a hard wax plug. Sound becomes muffled.
otitis externa (OE) (oh-TYE-tis ex-TERN-ah)	External ear infection. Most commonly caused by fungus. Also called *otomycosis* and commonly referred to as *swimmer's ear*.
■ *Middle Ear*	
otitis media (OM) (oh-TYE-tis MEE-dee-ah)	Seen frequently in children; commonly referred to as a *middle ear infection*. Often preceded by an upper respiratory infection during which pathogens move from the pharynx to the middle ear via the eustachian tube. Fluid accumulates in the middle ear cavity. The fluid may be watery, *serous otitis media,* or full of pus, *purulent otitis media.*
otosclerosis (oh-toh-sklair-OH-sis)	Loss of mobility of the stapes bone, leading to progressive hearing loss.
■ *Inner Ear*	
acoustic neuroma (ah-KOOS-tik noor-OH-mah)	Benign tumor of the eighth cranial nerve sheath. The pressure causes symptoms such as tinnitus, headache, dizziness, and progressive hearing loss.
labyrinthitis (lab-ih-rin-THIGH-tis)	May affect both the hearing and equilibrium portions of the inner ear. Also referred to as an *inner ear infection*.
Ménière's disease (may-nee-ARZ dih-ZEEZ)	Abnormal condition within the labyrinth of the inner ear that can lead to a progressive loss of hearing. The symptoms are dizziness or vertigo, hearing loss, and tinnitus (ringing in the ears). Named for French physician Prosper Ménière.

Diagnostic Procedures

TERM	DEFINITION
■ *Audiology Tests*	
audiometry (aw-dee-OM-eh-tree)	Test of hearing ability by determining the lowest and highest intensity (decibels) and frequencies (hertz) that a person can distinguish. The patient may sit in a soundproof booth and receive sounds through earphones as the technician decreases the sound or lowers the tones.

■ **Figure 18** Audiometry exam. Photograph of a young person holding up his hand to indicate in which ear he is able to hear the sound. *(Jorgen Shytte/Peter Arnold, Inc.)*

Diagnostic Procedures (*continued*)

TERM	DEFINITION
Rinne and Weber tuning-fork tests (RIN-eh)	These tests assess both nerve and bone conduction of sound. The physician holds a tuning fork, an instrument that produces a constant pitch when it is struck, against or near the bones on the side of the head. Friedrich Rinne was a German otologist, and Ernst Weber was a German physiologist.

■ *Otology Tests*

otoscopy (oh-TOSS-koh-pee)	Examination of the ear canal, eardrum, and outer ear using an *otoscope*.

> **Med Term Tip**
>
> Small children are prone to placing objects in their ears. In some cases, as with peas and beans, these become moist in the ear canal and swell, which makes removal difficult. *Otoscopy*, or the examination of the ear using an *otoscope*, can aid in identifying and removing the cause of hearing loss if it is due to foreign bodies (see Figure 14).

■ **Figure 19** An otoscope, used to visually examine the external auditory ear canal and tympanic membrane.

tympanometry (tim-pah-NOM-eh-tree)	Measurement of the movement of the tympanic membrane. Can indicate the presence of pressure in the middle ear.

■ *Balance Tests*

falling test	Test used to observe balance and equilibrium. The patient is observed balancing on one foot, then with one foot in front of the other, and then walking forward with eyes open. The same test is conducted with the patient's eyes closed. Swaying and falling with the eyes closed can indicate an ear and equilibrium malfunction.

Therapeutic Procedures

TERM	DEFINITION

■ *Audiology Procedures*

hearing aid	Apparatus or mechanical device used by persons with impaired hearing to amplify sound. Also called an *amplification device*.

■ *Surgical Procedures*

cochlear implant (KOK-lee-ar)	Mechanical device surgically placed under the skin behind the outer ear (pinna) that converts sound signals into magnetic impulses to stimulate the auditory nerve (see Figure 20 ■). Can be beneficial for those with profound sensorineural hearing loss.

■ **Figure 20** Photograph of a child with a cochlear implant. This device sends electrical impulses directly to the brain.

 Therapeutic Procedures *(continued)*

TERM	DEFINITION
myringotomy (mir-in-GOT-oh-mee)	Surgical puncture of the eardrum with removal of fluid and pus from the middle ear to eliminate a persistent ear infection and excessive pressure on the tympanic membrane. A pressure equalizing tube is placed in the tympanic membrane to allow for drainage of the middle ear cavity; this tube typically falls out on its own.
pressure equalizing tube (PE tube)	Small tube surgically placed in a child's eardrum to assist in drainage of trapped fluid and to equalize pressure between the middle ear cavity and the atmosphere.
stapedectomy (stay-pee-DEK-toh-mee)	Removal of the stapes bone to treat otosclerosis (hardening of the bone). A prosthesis or artificial stapes may be implanted.

 # Pharmacology

CLASSIFICATION	ACTION	GENERIC AND BRAND NAMES
antibiotic otic solution (OH-tik)	Eardrops to treat otitis externa.	Neomycin, polymyxin B, and hydrocortisone solution, Otocort, Cortisporin, Otic Care
antiemetics (an-tye-ee-mit-tiks)	Medications that are effective in treating the nausea associated with vertigo.	meclizine, Antivert, Meni-D; phenothiazine, Compazine
anti-inflammatory otic solution (OH-tik)	Reduces inflammation, itching, and edema associated with otitis externa.	antipyrine & benzoaine, Allergan Ear Drops, A/B Otic
wax emulsifiers	Substances used to soften ear wax to prevent buildup within the external ear canal.	carbamide peroxide, Debrox Drops, Murine Ear Drops

 # Abbreviations

AD	right ear	**HEENT**	head, ears, eyes, nose, throat
AS	left ear	**Hz**	hertz
ASL	American Sign Language	**OM**	otitis media
AU	both ears	**Oto**	otology
BC	bone conduction	**PE tube**	pressure tube equalizing
dB	decibel	**PORP**	partial ossicular replacement prosthesis
EENT	eyes, ears, nose, throat	**SOM**	serous otitis media
ENT	ear, nose, and throat	**TORP**	total ossicular replacement prosthesis

Chapter Review

Terminology Checklist

Below are all Anatomy and Physiology key terms, Word Building. Vocabulary, Pathology, Diagnostic, Therapeutic, and Pharmacology terms presented in this chapter. Use this list as a study tool by placing a check in the box in front of each term as you master its meaning.

- [ ] achromatopsia
- [ ] acoustic
- [ ] acoustic neuroma
- [ ] amblyopia
- [ ] American Sign Language
- [ ] anacusis
- [ ] anesthetic ophthalmic solution
- [ ] antibiotic ophthalmic solution
- [ ] antibiotic otic solution
- [ ] antiemetic
- [ ] antiglaucoma medications
- [ ] anti-inflammatory otic solution
- [ ] aqueous humor
- [ ] artificial tears
- [ ] astigmatism
- [ ] audiogram
- [ ] audiologist
- [ ] audiology
- [ ] audiometer
- [ ] audiometry
- [ ] auditory
- [ ] auditory canal
- [ ] auditory tube
- [ ] aural
- [ ] auricle
- [ ] auricular
- [ ] binaural
- [ ] blepharectomy
- [ ] blepharitis
- [ ] blepharoplasty
- [ ] blepharoptosis
- [ ] cataract
- [ ] cerumen
- [ ] ceruminoma
- [ ] choroid
- [ ] cilia
- [ ] ciliary body
- [ ] cochlea
- [ ] cochlear
- [ ] cochlear implant

- [ ] cochlear nerve
- [ ] color vision tests
- [ ] conductive hearing loss
- [ ] cones
- [ ] conjunctiva
- [ ] conjunctival
- [ ] conjunctivitis
- [ ] conjunctivoplasty
- [ ] cornea
- [ ] corneal
- [ ] corneal abrasion
- [ ] cryoextraction
- [ ] cryoretinopexy
- [ ] cycloplegia
- [ ] dacryocystitis
- [ ] deafness
- [ ] decibel
- [ ] diplopia
- [ ] emmetropia
- [ ] enucleation
- [ ] equilibrium
- [ ] esotropia
- [ ] eustachian tube
- [ ] exotropia
- [ ] external auditory meatus
- [ ] external ear
- [ ] eyeball
- [ ] eyelashes
- [ ] eyelids
- [ ] eye muscles
- [ ] falling test
- [ ] fluorescein angiography
- [ ] fluorescein staining
- [ ] fovea centralis
- [ ] glaucoma
- [ ] hearing
- [ ] hearing aid
- [ ] hemianopia
- [ ] hertz
- [ ] hordeolum

- [ ] hyperopia
- [ ] incus
- [ ] inner ear
- [ ] intraocular
- [ ] iridal
- [ ] iridectomy
- [ ] iridoplegia
- [ ] iridosclerotomy
- [ ] iris
- [ ] iritis
- [ ] keratitis
- [ ] keratometer
- [ ] keratometry
- [ ] keratoplasty
- [ ] keratotomy
- [ ] labyrinth
- [ ] labyrinthectomy
- [ ] labyrinthitis
- [ ] labyrinthotomy
- [ ] lacrimal
- [ ] lacrimal apparatus
- [ ] lacrimal ducts
- [ ] lacrimal gland
- [ ] laser-assisted in-situ keratomileusis
- [ ] laser photocoagulation
- [ ] legally blind
- [ ] lens
- [ ] macrotia
- [ ] macula lutea
- [ ] macular degeneration
- [ ] malleus
- [ ] Ménière's disease
- [ ] microtia
- [ ] middle ear
- [ ] miotic
- [ ] monaural
- [ ] monochromatism
- [ ] mucous membrane

- mydriatic
- myopia
- myringectomy
- myringitis
- myringoplasty
- myringotomy
- nasal cavity
- nasolacrimal duct
- nyctalopia
- nystagmus
- oblique muscles
- ocular
- oculomycosis
- ophthalmalgia
- ophthalmic
- ophthalmic decongestants
- ophthalmologist
- ophthalmology
- ophthalmoplegia
- ophthalmorrhagia
- ophthalmoscope
- ophthalmoscopy
- optic
- optic disk
- optician
- optic nerve
- optometer
- optometrist
- optometry
- organs of Corti
- ossicles
- otalgia
- otic
- otitis
- otitis externa
- otitis media
- otologist
- otology

- otomycosis
- otoplasty
- otopyorrhea
- otorhinolaryngology
- otorrhagia
- otosclerosis
- otoscope
- otoscopy
- oval window
- papilledema
- phacoemulsification
- photophobia
- photorefractive keratectomy
- pinna
- pressure equalizing tube
- presbycusis
- presbyopia
- pterygium
- pupil
- pupillary
- radial keratotomy
- rectus muscles
- refractive error test
- refracts
- residual hearing
- retina
- retinal
- retinal blood vessels
- retinal detachment
- retinitis pigmentosa
- retinoblastoma
- retinopathy
- retinopexy
- Rinne and Weber tuning-fork tests
- rods
- saccule
- salpingitis

- salpingotomy
- sclera
- scleral
- scleral buckling
- scleritis
- scleromalacia
- sclerotomy
- sebaceous glands
- semicircular canals
- sensorineural hearing loss
- slit lamp microscopy
- Snellen chart
- stapedectomy
- stapes
- strabismus
- strabotomy
- tears
- tinnitus
- tonometry
- trachoma
- tympanectomy
- tympanic
- tympanic membrane
- tympanitis
- tympanometer
- tympanometry
- tympanoplasty
- tympanorrhexis
- tympanotomy
- utricle
- uveitis
- vertigo
- vestibular nerve
- vestibulocochlear nerve
- visual acuity test
- vitreous humor
- wax emulsifiers
- xerophthalmia

Practice Exercises

A. Complete the following statements.

1. The study of the eye is _____.

2. Another term for eyelashes is _____.

3. The glands responsible for tears are called _____ glands.

4. The clear, transparent portion of the sclera is called the _____.

5. The innermost layer of the eye, which is composed of sensory receptors, is the _____.

6. The pupil of the eye is actually a hole in the _____.

7. The three bones in the middle ear are the _____, _____, and _____.

8. The study of the ear is called _____.

9. Another term for the eardrum is _____.

10. _____ is produced in the oil glands in the auditory canal.

11. The _____ tube connects the nasopharynx with the middle ear.

12. The _____ is responsible for conducting impulses from the ear to the brain.

B. State the terms described using the combining forms provided.

The combining form *blephar/o* refers to the eyelid. Use it to write a term that means:

1. inflammation of the eyelid _____

2. surgical repair of the eyelid _____

3. drooping of the upper eyelid _____

The combining form *retin/o* refers to the retina. Use it to write a term that means:

4. a disease of the retina _____

5. surgical fixation of the retina _____

The combining form *ophthalm/o* refers to the eye. Use it to write a term that means:

6. the study of the eye _____

7. pertaining to the eye _____

8. an eye examination using a scope _____

The combining form *irid/o* refers to the iris. Use it to write a term that means:

9. iris paralysis _____

10. removal of the iris _____

The combining form *ot/o* refers to the ear. Write a word that means:

11. ear surgical repair _____

12. pus flow from the ear _____

13. pain in the ear _____

Special Senses: The Eye and Ear

14. inflammation of the ear _____

The combining form *tympan/o* refers to eardrum. Write a word that means:

15. eardrum rupture _____

16. eardrum incision _____

17. eardrum inflammation _____

The combining form *audi/o* refers to hearing. Write a word that means:

18. record of hearing _____

19. instrument to measure hearing _____

20. study of hearing _____

C. Answer the following questions.

1. Describe the difference between conductive hearing loss and sensorineural hearing loss. _____

_____

_____

2. List in order the eyeball structures light rays pass through: _____, _____,

_____, _____

3. Describe the role of the conjunctiva. _____

_____

_____

4. List the ossicles and what they do. _____

_____

_____

D. Write the suffix for each expression and provide an example of its use from this chapter.

	Suffix	Example
1. to turn	_____	_____
2. vision	_____	_____
3. inflammation of	_____	_____
4. the study of	_____	_____
5. incision into	_____	_____

Special Senses: The Eye and Ear

6. surgical repair   _____   _____

7. surgical fixation   _____   _____

8. pain   _____   _____

9. ear condition   _____   _____

10. hearing   _____   _____

E. Define the following combining forms and use them in words from this chapter.

	Meaning	Example
1. dacry/o	_____	_____
2. uve/o	_____	_____
3. aque/o	_____	_____
4. phot/o	_____	_____
5. kerat/o	_____	_____
6. vitre/o	_____	_____
7. dipl/o	_____	_____
8. glauc/o	_____	_____
9. presby/o	_____	_____
10. ambly/o	_____	_____
11. aur/o	_____	_____
12. staped/o	_____	_____
13. acous/o	_____	_____
14. salping/o	_____	_____
15. myring/o	_____	_____

F. Define the following terms.

1. amblyopia _____

2. diplopia _____

3. mydriatic _____

4. miotic _____

5. presbyopia _____

6. tinnitus _____

7. stapes _____

8. tympanometry _____

9. eustachian tube _____

10. labyrinth _____

11. audiogram _____

12. otitis media _____

G. Match each term to its definition.

1.	_____ emmetropia	a.	opacity of the lens
2.	_____ sclera	b.	muscle regulating size of pupil
3.	_____ cataract	c.	nearsightedness
4.	_____ conjunctiva	d.	protective membrane of eye
5.	_____ iris	e.	blind spot
6.	_____ xerophthalmia	f.	involuntary movements of eye
7.	_____ myopia	g.	white of eye
8.	_____ nystagmus	h.	normal vision
9.	_____ optic disk	i.	dry eyes
10.	_____ vitreous humor	j.	material filling eyeball

H. Match each term to its definition.

1.	_____ myringotomy	a.	removal of stapes bone
2.	_____ tympanoplasty	b.	reconstruction of eardrum
3.	_____ otoplasty	c.	surgical puncture of eardrum
4.	_____ stapedectomy	d.	change size of pinna
5.	_____ anacusis	e.	absence of hearing
6.	_____ falling test	f.	treats sensorineural hearing loss
7.	_____ PE tube	g.	tuning fork tests
8.	_____ cochlear implant	h.	swimmer's ear
9.	_____ otitis externa	i.	drains off fluid
10.	_____ Rinne & Weber	j.	balance test

I. Identify the following abbreviations.

1. Oto _____

2. OU _____

3. REM _____

4. Hz _____

5. SMD _____

6. PERRLA _____

7. IOP _____

8. dB _____

9. OD _____

10. VF _____

J. Write the abbreviation for the following terms.

1. pressure equalizing tube _____

2. eye, ear, nose, and throat _____

3. bone conduction _____

4. both ears _____

5. otitis media _____

6. emmetropia _____

7. exotropia _____

8. left eye _____

9. extraocular movement _____

10. visual acuity _____

K. Use the following terms in the sentences below.

emmetropia   hyperopia   acoustic neuroma   otorhinolaryngologist

conjunctivitis   tonometry   cataract   strabismus

presbycusis   inner ear   Ménière's disease   hordeolum

myopia

1. Cheri is having a regular eye checkup. The pressure reading test that the physician will do to detect glaucoma is

   _____.

2. Carlos's ophthalmologist tells him that he has normal vision. This is called _____.

3. Ana has been given an antibiotic eye ointment for pink eye. The medical term for this condition is _____.

4. Adrian is nearsighted and cannot read signs in the distance. This is called _____.

5. Ivan is scheduled to have surgery to have the opaque lens of his right eye removed. This condition is a(n)

   _____.

6. Roberto has developed a stye on the corner of his left eye. He has been told to treat it with hot compresses. This condition

   is called a(n) _____.

7. Judith has twin boys with crossed eyes that will require surgical correction. The medical term for this condition is

   _____.

8. Beth is farsighted and has difficulty reading textbooks. Her eyeglass correction will be for _____.

9. Grace was told by her physician that her hearing loss was a part of the aging process. The term for this is

   _____.

10. Stacey is having frequent middle ear infections and wishes to be treated by a specialist. She would go to a(n)

    _____.

11. Warren was told that his dizziness may be caused by a problem in the _____ area.

12. Shantel is suffering from an abnormal condition of the inner ear, vertigo, and tinnitus. She may have

    _____.

13. Keisha was told that her tumor of the eighth cranial nerve was benign, but she still experienced a hearing loss as a result

    of the tumor. This tumor is called a(n) _____.

L. Fill in the classification for each drug description, then match the brand name.

Drug Description	Classification	Brand Name
1. _____ treats dry eyes	_____	a. Atropine-Care
2. _____ reduces intraocular pressure	_____	b. Allergan Ear Drops
3. _____ ear drops for ear infection	_____	c. Timoptic
4. _____ dilates pupil	_____	d. Opticaine
5. _____ treats nausea from vertigo	_____	e. Debrox Drops
6. _____ eye drops for bacterial infection	_____	f. Eserine Sulfate
7. _____ treats ear itching	_____	g. Antivert
8. _____ constricts pupil	_____	h. Refresh Plus
9. _____ softens cerumen	_____	i. Otocort
10. _____ eye drops for pain	_____	j. Del-Mycin

Medical Record Analysis

Below is an item from a patient's medical record. Read it carefully, make sure you understand all the medical terms used, and then answer the questions that follow.

Ophthalmology Consultation Report

Reason for Consultation:	Evaluation of progressive loss of vision in right eye.
History of Present Illness:	Patient is a 79-year-old female who has noted gradual deterioration of vision and increasing photophobia during the past year, particularly in the right eye. She states that it feels like there is a film over her right eye. She denies any change in vision in her left eye.
Past Medical History:	Patient has used corrective lenses her entire adult life to correct hyperopia. She is not married and is nulligravida. Past medical history includes left breast cancer successfully treated with left breast mastectomy ten years ago and cholelithiasis necessitating a cholecystectomy two years ago. She has no history of cardiac problems or hypertension.
Results of Physical Examination:	Visual acuity test showed no change in this patient's long-standing hyperopia. The eye muscles function properly, and there is no evidence of conjunctivitis or nystagmus. The pupils react properly to light. Intraocular pressure is normal. Ophthalmoscopy after application of mydriatic drops revealed presence of large opaque cataract in lens of right eye. There is a very small cataract forming in the left eye. There is no evidence of retinopathy, macular degeneration, or keratitis.
Assessment:	Diminished vision in OD secondary to cataract.
Recommendations:	Phacoemulsification of cataract followed by aspiration of lens and prosthetic lens implant.

Critical Thinking Questions

1. The results of the physical exam state that the patient's pupils react properly to light. What does this mean? How do pupils react in bright and dim light? Why is this important? _____ _____ _____

2. Carefully read the results of the physical examination and list the eye structures that do not have any problems. _____ _____

3. Briefly describe the pathologies that form the patient's past medical history that required surgery, and the surgeries. _____ _____

4. The ophthalmologist placed mydriatic drops in her eyes. For what purpose? What is the general name for drops with the opposite effect? _____ _____

5. This patient wears corrective lenses for which condition?
   a. farsightedness
   b. nearsightedness
   c. abnormal curvature of the cornea

6. Her cataract was removed by phacoemulsification. Using your text as a reference, what other procedure could have been used to remove a cataract? _____ _____

Chart Note Transcription

The chart note below contains ten phrases that can be reworded with a medical term that you learned in this chapter. Each phrase is identified with an underline. Determine the medical term and write your answers in the space provided.

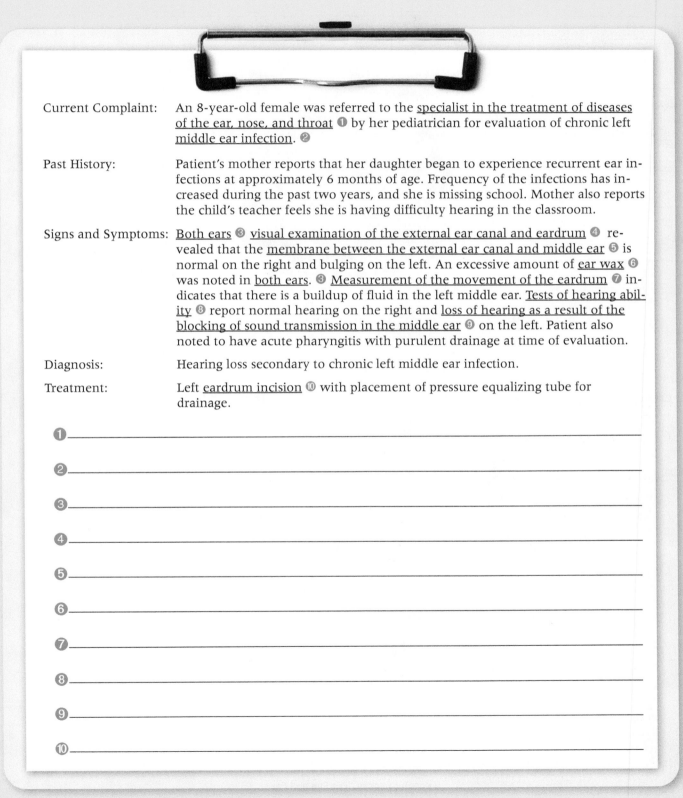

Current Complaint: An 8-year-old female was referred to the <u>specialist in the treatment of diseases of the ear, nose, and throat</u> ❶ by her pediatrician for evaluation of chronic left <u>middle ear infection</u>. ❷

Past History: Patient's mother reports that her daughter began to experience recurrent ear infections at approximately 6 months of age. Frequency of the infections has increased during the past two years, and she is missing school. Mother also reports the child's teacher feels she is having difficulty hearing in the classroom.

Signs and Symptoms: <u>Both ears</u> ❸ <u>visual examination of the external ear canal and eardrum</u> ❹ revealed that the <u>membrane between the external ear canal and middle ear</u> ❺ is normal on the right and bulging on the left. An excessive amount of <u>ear wax</u> ❻ was noted in <u>both ears</u>. ❸ <u>Measurement of the movement of the eardrum</u> ❼ indicates that there is a buildup of fluid in the left middle ear. <u>Tests of hearing ability</u> ❽ report normal hearing on the right and <u>loss of hearing as a result of the blocking of sound transmission in the middle ear</u> ❾ on the left. Patient also noted to have acute pharyngitis with purulent drainage at time of evaluation.

Diagnosis: Hearing loss secondary to chronic left middle ear infection.

Treatment: Left <u>eardrum incision</u> ❿ with placement of pressure equalizing tube for drainage.

❶ _____

❷ _____

❸ _____

❹ _____

❺ _____

❻ _____

❼ _____

❽ _____

❾ _____

❿ _____

Labeling Exercise

A. System Review

1. Write the labels for this figure on the numbered lines provided.

8. _____

9. _____

1. _____

2. _____

3. _____

4. _____

5. _____

6. _____

7. _____

10. _____

11. _____

12. _____

2. Write the labels for this figure on the numbered lines provided.

1. _____

5. _____

6. _____

7. _____

8. _____

9. _____

10. _____

11. _____

12. _____

13. _____

2. _____

4. _____

3. _____

Special Senses: The Eye and Ear

B. Anatomy Challenge
Write the labels for this figure on the numbered lines provided.

1. _____

2. _____

3. _____

4. _____

5. _____

Multimedia Preview

Additional interactive resources and activities for this chapter can be found on the Companion Website.

Website Highlights—www.prenhall.com/fremgen

CASE STUDY

Put your understanding of medical terms to the test within a real-world scenario. Here you'll be presented with a clinical case followed by a series of questions that quiz your grasp of the situation.

Appendix

Abbreviations

Abbreviation	Meaning	Abbreviation	Meaning
@	at	ARF	acute renal failure
5-FU	5-fluorouracil	ARMD	age-related macular degeneration
^{67}Ga	radioactive gallium	AROM	active range of motion
^{99m}Tc	radioactive technetium	AS	arteriosclerosis, left ear
^{131}I	radioactive iodine	ASA	aspirin
^{133}Xe	radioactive xenon	ASD	atrial septal defect
^{201}Tl	radioactive thallium	ASHD	arteriosclerotic heart disease
α	alpha	ASL	American Sign Language
$\bar{a}$	before	AST	aspartate transaminase
AAROM	active-assisted range of motion	Astigm	astigmatism
AB	abortion	ATN	acute tubulor necrosis
ABGs	arterial blood gases	AU	both ears
ac	before meals	AuD	doctor of audiology
ACTH	adrenocorticotropic hormone	AV, A-V	atrioventricular
AD	right ear, Alzheimer's disease	β	beta
ad lib	as desired	Ba	barium
ADD	attention deficit disorder	BaE	barium enema
ADH	antidiuretic hormone	basos	basophil
ADHD	attention-deficit hyperactivity disorder	BBB	bundle branch block (L for left; R for right)
ADL	activities of daily living	BC	bone conduction
AE	above elbow	BCC	basal cell carcinoma
AF	atrial fibrillation	BDT	bone density testing
AGN	acute glomerulonephritis	BE	barium enema, below elbow
AI	artificial insemination	bid	twice a day
AIDS	acquired immunodeficiency syndrome	BK	below knee
AK	above knee	BM	bowel movement
ALL	acute lymphocytic leukemia	BMD	bone mineral density
ALS	amyotropic lateral sclerosis	BMR	basal metabolic rate
ALT	alanine transaminase	BMT	bone marrow transplant
AMI	acute myocardial infarction	BNO	bladder neck obstruction
AML	acute myelogenous leukemia	BP	blood pressure
Angio	angiography	BPD	bipolar disorder
ANS	autonomic nervous system	BPH	benign prostatic hypertrophy
ante	before	bpm	beats per minute
AP	anteroposterior	Bronch	bronchoscopy
APAP	acetaminophen (Tylenol)	BS	bowel sounds
aq	aqueous (water)	BSE	breast self-examination
ARC	AIDS-related complex	BSN	bachelor of science in nursing
ARDS	adult respiratory distress syndrome	BUN	blood urea nitrogen
		BX, bx	biopsy

Abbreviation	Meaning	Abbreviation	Meaning
c̄	with	CV	cardiovascular
C1, C2, etc.	first cervical vertebra, second cervical vertebra, etc.	CVA	cerebrovascular accident
		CVD	cerebrovascular disease
Ca²⁺	calcium	CVS	chorionic villus biopsy
CA	cancer, chronological age	Cx	cervix
CABG	coronary artery bypass graft	CXR	chest x-ray
CAD	coronary artery disease	cysto	cystoscopic exam
cap(s)	capsule(s)	d	day
CAPD	continuous ambulatory peritoneal dialysis	D	diopter (lens strength)
		D & C	dilation and curettage
CAT	computerized axial tomography	D/C, d/c	discontinue
		dB	decibel
cath	catheterization	DC	doctor of chiropractic
CBC	complete blood count	DDM	doctor of dental medicine
CBD	common bile duct	DDS	doctor of dental surgery
cc	cubic centimeter	DEA	Drug Enforcement Agency
CC	clean catch urine specimen, cardiac catheterization, chief complaint	decub	lying down, decubitus ulcer
		Derm, derm	dermatology
CCS	certified coding specialist	DI	diabetes insipidus, diagnostic imaging
CCU	cardiac care unit, coronary care unit	diff	differential
		dil	dilute
c.gl.	correction with glasses	disc	discontinue
chemo	chemotherapy	disp	dispense
CHF	congestive heart failure	DJD	degenerative joint disease
CIS	carcinoma in situ	DM	diabetes mellitus
Cl⁻	chloride	DO	doctor of osteopathy
CLL	chronic lymphocytic leukemia	DOE	dyspnea on exertion
CLS	clinical laboratory scientist	DPT	diphtheria, pertussis, tetanus; doctor of physical therapy
CLT	clinical laboratory technician		
CMA	certified medical assistant	DRE	digital rectal exam
CML	chronic myelogenous leukemia	DSA	digital subtraction angiography
CNA	certified nurse aide	DSM-IV	*Diagnostic and Statistical Manual for Mental Disorders*, Fourth edition
CNS	central nervous system		
CO₂	carbon dioxide		
CoA	coarctation of the aorta	dtd	give of such a dose
COPD	chronic obstructive pulmonary disease	DTR	deep tendon reflex; dietetic technician, registered
COTA	certified occupational therapy assistant	DVA	distance visual acuity
		DVT	deep vein thrombosis
CP	cerebral palsy, chest pain	Dx	diagnosis
CPK	creatine phosphokinase	DXA	dual-energy absorptiometry
CPR	cardiopulmonary resuscitation	ECC	extracorporeal circulation
CRF	chronic renal failure	ECCE	extracapsular cataract extraction
crit	hematocrit		
CRT	certified respiratory therapist	ECG	electrocardiogram
C & S	culture and sensitivity test	Echo	echocardiogram
CS, CS-section	cesarean section	ECT	electroconvulsive therapy
CSD	congenital septal defect	ED	erectile dysfunction
CSF	cerebrospinal fluid	EDC	estimated date of confinement
CT	computerized tomography, cytotechnologist	EEG	electroencephalogram, electroencephalography
CTA	clear to auscultation		
CTS	carpal tunnel syndrome	EENT	eyes, ears, nose, throat

Abbreviation	Meaning	Abbreviation	Meaning
EGD	esophagogastroduodenoscopy	grav I	first pregnancy
EKG	electrocardiogram	gt	drop
ELISA	enzyme-linked immunosorbent assay	gtt	drops
		GTT	glucose tolerance test
EM	emmetropia	GU	genitourinary
EMB	endometrial biopsy	GVHD	graft vs. host disease
EMG	electromyogram	GYN, gyn	gynecology
EMT-B	emergency medical technician–basic	H_2O	water
		HA	headache
EMT-I	emergency medical technician–intermediate	HAV	hepatitis A virus
		Hb	hemoglobin
EMT-P	emergency medical technician–paramedic	HBV	hepatitis B virus
		HCG, hCG	human chorionic gonadotropin
Endo	endoscopy		
ENT	ear, nose, and throat	HCl	hydrochloric acid
EOM	extraocular movement	HCO_3^-	bicarbonate
eosins, eos	eosinophil	HCT, Hct	hematocrit
ER	emergency room	HCV	hepatitis C virus
ERCP	endoscopic retrograde cholangiopancreatography	HD	Hodgkin's disease, hemodialysis
ERT	estrogen replacement therapy	HDN	hemolytic disease of the newborn
ERV	expiratory reserve volume		
ESR	erythrocyte sedimentation rate	HDV	hepatitis D virus
		HEENT	head, ears, eyes, nose, throat
ESRD	end-stage renal disease	HEV	hepatitis E virus
e-stim	electrical stimulation	Hgb, HGB	hemoglobin
ESWL	extracorporeal shock-wave lithotripsy	HIV	human immunodeficieny virus
		HMD	hyaline membrane disease
et	and	HNP	herniated nucleus pulposus
EU	excretory urography	HPV	human papilloma virus
EUA	exam under anesthesia	HRT	hormone replacement therapy
FBS	fasting blood sugar	hs	at bed time
FDA	Federal Drug Administration	HSG	hysterosalpingography
FEKG	fetal electrocardiogram	HSV	*Herpes simplex* virus
FHR	fetal heart rate	HSV-1	*Herpes simplex* virus type 1
FHT	fetal heart tone	HTN	hypertension
FOBT	fecal occult blood test	Hz	hertz
FRC	functional residual capacity	ī	one
FS	frozen section	IBD	inflammatory bowel disease
FSH	follicle-stimulating hormone	IBS	irritable bowel syndrome
FTND	full-term normal delivery	IC	inspiratory capacity
FVC	forced vital capacity	ICCE	intracapsular cataract cryoextraction
Fx, FX	fracture		
GI	first pregnancy	ICP	intracranial pressure
GA	general anesthesia	ICU	intensive care unit
GB	gallbladder	I & D	incision and drainage
GC	gonorrhea	ID	intradermal
GERD	gastroesophageal reflux disease	IDDM	insulin-dependent diabetes mellitus
GH	growth hormone	Ig	immunoglobins (IgA, IgD, IgE, IgG, IgM)
GI	gastrointestinal		
gm	gram	ī̄	two
GOT	glutamic oxaloacetic transaminase	ī̄ī	three
		IM	intramuscular
gr	grain	inj	injection

Abbreviation	Meaning	Abbreviation	Meaning
I & O	intake and output	mL	milliliter
IOP	intraocular pressure	MLT	medical laboratory technician
IPD	intermittent peritoneal dialysis	MM	malignant melanoma
		mm Hg	millimeters of mercury
IPPB	intermittent positive pressure breathing	MMPI	Minnesota Multiphasic Personality Inventory
IRDS	infant respiratory distress syndrome	mono	mononucleosis
		monos	monocyte
IRV	inspiratory reserve volume	MR	mitral regurgitation
IU	international unit	MRA	magnetic resonance angiography
IUD	intrauterine device		
IV	intravenous	MRI	magnetic resonance imaging
IVC	intravenous cholangiogram	MS	mitral stenosis, multiple sclerosis, musculoskeletal
IVF	in vitro fertilization		
IVP	intravenous pyelogram	MSH	melanocyte-stimulating hormone
JRA	juvenile rheumatoid arthritis		
K^+	potassium	MSN	master of science in nursing
kg	kilogram	MT	medical technologist
KS	Kaposi's sarcoma	MTX	methotrexate
KUB	kidney, ureter, bladder	MUA	manipulation under anesthesia
L	left, liter		
L1, L2, etc.	first lumbar vertebra, second lumbar vertebra, etc.	MVP	mitral valve prolapse
		n & v	nausea and vomiting
LASIK	laser-assisted in-situ keratomileusis	Na^+	sodium
		NB	newborn
LAT, lat	lateral	NG	nasogastric (tube)
LBW	low birth weight	NHL	non-Hodgkin's lymphoma
LDH	lactate dehydrogenase	NIDDM	non–insulin-dependent diabetes mellitus
LE	lower extremity		
LGI	lower gastrointestinal series	NK	natural killer cells
LH	luteinizing hormone	NMR	nuclear magnetic resonance
LL	left lateral	no sub	no substitute
LLE	left lower extremity	noc	night
LLL	left lower lobe	non rep	do not repeat
LLQ	left lower quadrant	NP	nurse practitioner
LMP	last menstrual period	NPH	neutral protamine Hagedorn (insulin)
LP	lumbar puncture		
LPN	licensed practical nurse	NPO	nothing by mouth
LUE	left upper extremity	NS	normal saline, nephrotic syndrome
LUL	left upper lobe		
LUQ	left upper quadrant	NSAID	nonsteroidal anti-inflammatory drug
LVAD	left ventricular assist device		
LVH	left ventricular hypertrophy	O_2	oxygen
lymphs	lymphocyte	OA	osteoarthritis
LVN	licensed vocational nurse	OB	obstetrics
MA	mental age	OCD	obsessive-compulsive disorder
MAO	monoamine oxidase	OCPs	oral contraceptive pills
mcg	microgram	OD	overdose, right eye, doctor of optometry
MD	doctor of medicine, muscular dystrophy		
		oint	ointment
MDI	metered dose inhaler	OM	otitis media
mEq	milliequivalent	O & P	ova and parasites
mets	metastases	Ophth.	ophthalmology
mg	milligram	OR	operating room
MI	myocardial infarction, mitral insufficiency	ORIF	open reduction–internal fixation

Abbreviation	Meaning	Abbreviation	Meaning
Orth, ortho	orthopedics	pro-time	prothrombin time
OS	left eye	PROM	passive range of motion
OT	occupational therapy	prot	protocol
OTC	over the counter	PSA	prostate specific antigen
Oto	otology	pt	patient
OTR	occupational therapist	PT	prothrombin time, physical therapy, physical therapist
OU	each eye		
oz	ounce	PTA	physical therapy assistant
p̄	after	PTC	percutaneous transhepatic cholangiography
P	pulse		
PI	first delivery	PTCA	percutaneous transluminal coronary angioplasty
PA	posteroanterior, physician assistant, pernicious anemia	PTH	parathyroid hormone
PAC	premature atrial contraction	PUD	peptic ulcer disease
PAP	Papanicolaou test, pulmonary arterial pressure	PVC	premature ventricular contraction
para I	first delivery	q	every
PARR	postanesthetic recovery room	qam	every morning
PBI	protein-bound iodine	qd	once a day, every day
pc	after meals	qh	every hour
PCA	patient-controlled administration	qhs	every night
		qid	four times a day
PCP	*Pneumocystis carinii* pneumonia	qod	every other day
		qs	quantity sufficient
PCV	packed cell volume	R	respiration, right, roentgen
PDA	patent ductus arteriosus	Ra	radium
PDR	*Physician's Desk Reference*	RA	rheumatoid arthritis, room air
PE tube	pressure equalizing tube	rad	radiation absorbed dose
PEG	pneumoencephalogram, percutaneous endoscopic gastrostomy	RBC	red blood cell
		RD	registered dietitian
		RDH	registered dental hygienist
per	with	RDS	respiratory distress syndrome
PERRLA	pupils equal, round, react to light and accommodation	REEGT	registered electroencephalography technologist
PET	positron emission tomography	REM	rapid eye movement
PFT	pulmonary function test	REPT	registered evoked potential technologist
pH	acidity or alkalinity of urine		
PharmD	doctor of pharmacy	Rh−	Rh-negative
PID	pelvic inflammatory disease	Rh+	Rh-positive
PMNs	polymorphonuclear neutrophil	RHIA	registered health information administrator
PMS	premenstrual syndrome	RHIT	registered health information technician
PNS	peripheral nervous system		
PO, po	by mouth	RIA	radioimmunoassay
polys	polymorphonuclear neutrophil	RL	right lateral
		RLE	right lower extremity
PORP	partial ossicular replacement prosthesis	RLL	right lower lobe
		RLQ	right lower quadrant
pp	postprandial	RML	right mediolateral, right middle lobe
PPD	purified protein derivative (tuberculin test)		
		RN	registered nurse
preop, pre-op	preoperative	ROM	range of motion
prep	preparation, prepared	RP	retrograde pyelogram
PRK	photo refractive keratectomy	RPh	registered pharmacist
PRL	prolactin	RPR	rapid plasma reagin (test for syphilis)
prn	as needed		

Abbreviation	Meaning	Abbreviation	Meaning
RPSGT	registered polysomnographic technologist	susp	suspension
RRT	registered radiologic technologist, registered respiratory therapist	syr	syrup
		T	tablespoon
		t	teaspoon
		T & A	tonsillectomy and adenoidectomy
RUE	right upper extremity		
RUL	right upper lobe	T1, T2, etc.	first thoracic vertebra, second thoracic vertebra, etc.
RUQ	right upper quadrant		
RV	reserve volume	T_3	triiodothyronine
Rx	take	T_4	thyroxine
s̄	without	tab	tablet
S1	first heart sound	TAH	total abdominal hysterectomy
S2	second heart sound	TAH-BSO	total abdominal hysterectomy–bilateral salpingo-oophorectomy
SA, S-A	sinoatrial		
SAD	seasonal affective disorder		
SARS	severe acute respiratory syndrome	TB	tuberculosis
		tbsp	tablespoon
SC, sc	subcutaneous	TENS	transcutaneous electrical nerve stimulation
SCC	squamous cell carcinoma		
SCI	spinal cord injury	TFT	thyroid function test
SCIDS	severe combined immunodeficiency syndrome	THA	total hip arthroplasty
		THR	total hip replacement
sed-rate	erythrocyte sedimentation rate	TIA	transient ischemic attack
		tid	three times a day
segs	segmented neutrophils	TKA	total knee arthroplasty
SG	skin graft, specific gravity	TKR	total knee replacement
s.gl.	without correction or glasses	TLC	total lung capacity
SGOT	serum glutamic oxaloacetic transaminase	TNM	tumor, nodes, metastases
		TO	telephone order
SIDS	sudden infant death syndrome	top	apply topically
Sig	label as follows/directions	TORP	total ossicular replacement prosthesis
SK	streptokinase		
sl	under the tongue	tPA	tissue-type plasminogen activator
SLE	systemic lupus erythematosus		
SMAC	sequential multiple analyzer computer	TPN	total parenteral nutrition
		TPR	temperature, pulse, and respiration
SMD	senile macular degeneration		
SOB	shortness of breath	TSH	thyroid-stimulating hormone
sol	solution	tsp	teaspoon
SOM	serous otitis media	TSS	toxic shock syndrome
sp. gr.	specific gravity	TUR	transurethral resection
SPP	suprapubic prostatectomy	TURP	transurethral resection of prostate
SR	erythrocyte sedimentation rate		
		TV	tidal volume
s̄s̄	one-half	TX, Tx	traction, treatment
st	stage	u	unit
ST	esotropia	U/A, UA	urinalysis
stat, STAT	at once, immediately	UC	uterine contractions, urine culture
STD	skin test done, sexually transmitted disease		
		UE	upper extremity
STSG	split-thickness skin graft	UGI	upper gastrointestinal series
subcu	subcutaneous	ung	ointment
subq	subcutaneous	URI	upper respiratory infection
supp.	suppository	US	ultrasound
suppos	suppository	UTI	urinary tract infection

Abbreviation	Meaning	Abbreviation	Meaning
UV	ultraviolet	VS	vital signs
VA	visual acuity	VSD	ventricular septal defect
VC	vital capacity	VT	ventricular tachycardia
VCUG	voiding cystourethrography	WBC	white blood cell
VD	venereal disease	wt	weight
VF	visual field	x	times
VFib	ventricular fibrillation	XT	exotropia
VO	verbal order		

Appendix

Appendix

Combining Forms

Combining Form	Meaning	Combining Form	Meaning
abdomin/o	abdomen	carcin/o	cancer
acous/o	hearing	cardi/o	heart
acr/o	extremities	carp/o	wrist
aden/o	gland	caud/o	tail
adenoid/o	adenoids	cec/o	cecum
adip/o	fat	cephal/o	head
adren/o	adrenal glands	cerebell/o	cerebellum
adrenal/o	adrenal glands	cerebr/o	cerebrum
aer/o	air	cerumin/o	cerumen
agglutin/o	clumping	cervic/o	neck, cervix
albin/o	white	chem/o	chemical, drug
alveol/o	alveolus; air sac	chol/e	bile, gall
ambly/o	dull or dim	cholangi/o	bile duct
amni/o	amnion	cholecyst/o	gallbladder
an/o	anus	choledoch/o	common bile duct
andr/o	male	chondr/o	cartilage
angi/o	vessel	chori/o	chorion
ankyl/o	stiff joint	chrom/o	color
anter/o	front	cis/o	to cut
anthrac/o	coal	clavicul/o	clavicle
anxi/o	anxiety	coagul/o	clotting
aort/o	aorta	coccyg/o	coccyx
append/o	appendix	cochle/o	cochlea
appendic/o	appendix	col/o	colon
aque/o	water	colon/o	colon
arteri/o	artery	colp/o	vagina
arthr/o	joint	coni/o	dust
articul/o	joint	conjunctiv/o	conjunctiva
atel/o	incomplete	core/o	pupil
ather/o	fatty substance, plaque	corne/o	cornea
atri/o	atrium	coron/o	heart
audi/o	hearing	cortic/o	outer portion
audit/o	hearing	cost/o	rib
aur/o	ear	crani/o	skull
auricul/o	ear	crin/o	secrete
azot/o	nitrogenous waste	crur/o	leg
bacteri/o	bacteria	cry/o	cold
balan/o	glans penis	crypt/o	hidden
bar/o	weight	culd/o	cul-de-sac
bas/o	base	cutane/o	skin
bi/o	life	cyan/o	blue
blast/o	primitive cell	cycl/o	ciliary muscle
blephar/o	eyelid	cyst/o	urinary bladder
brachi/o	arm	cyt/o	cell
bronch/o	bronchus	dacry/o	tear; tear duct
bronchi/o	bronchiole	dent/o	tooth
bronchiol/o	bronchiole	derm/o	skin
bucc/o	cheek	dermat/o	skin
burs/o	sac	diaphor/o	profuse sweating
calc/o	calcium	diaphragmat/o	diaphragm

Combining Form	Meaning	Combining Form	Meaning
dipl/o	double	ischi/o	ischium
dist/o	away from	jejun/o	jejunum
dors/o	back of body	kal/i	potassium
duoden/o	duodenum	kerat/o	cornea, hard, horny
electr/o	electricity	keton/o	ketone
embry/o	embryo	kinesi/o	movement
encephal/o	brain	kyph/o	hump
enter/o	small intestine	labi/o	lip
eosin/o	rosy red	labyrinth/o	labyrinth
epididym/o	epididymis	lacrim/o	tears
epiglott/o	epiglottis	lact/o	milk
episi/o	vulva	lamin/o	lamina, part of vertebra
epitheli/o	epithelium	lapar/o	abdomen
erg/o	work	laryng/o	larynx, voice box
erythr/o	red	later/o	side
esophag/o	esophagus	leuk/o	white
esthesi/o	feeling, sensation	lingu/o	tongue
estr/o	female	lip/o	fat
fasci/o	fibrous band	lith/o	stone
femor/o	femur	lob/o	lobe
fet/o	fetus	lord/o	bent backwards
fibr/o	fibers	lumb/o	loin
fibrin/o	fibers, fibrous	lymph/o	lymph
fibul/o	fibula	lymphaden/o	lymph node
fluor/o	fluorescence, luminous	lymphangi/o	lymph vessel
gastr/o	stomach	mamm/o	breast
gingiv/o	gums	mandibul/o	mandible
glauc/o	gray	mast/o	breast
gli/o	glue	maxill/o	maxilla
glomerul/o	glomerulus	meat/o	meatus
gloss/o	tongue	medi/o	middle
glute/o	buttock	medull/o	medulla oblongata, inner
glyc/o	sugar		portion
glycos/o	sugar, glucose	melan/o	black
gonad/o	sex glands	men/o	menses, menstruation
granul/o	granules	mening/o	meninges
gynec/o	female	meningi/o	meninges
hem/o	blood	ment/o	mind
hemangi/o	blood vessel	metacarp/o	metacarpals
hemat/o	blood	metatars/o	metatarsals
hepat/o	liver	metr/o	uterus
hidr/o	sweat	morph/o	shape
hist/o	tissue	muscul/o	muscle
home/o	sameness	mut/a	genetic change, mutation
humer/o	humerus	my/o	muscle
hydr/o	water	myc/o	fungus
hymen/o	hymen	myel/o	spinal cord, bone marrow
hyster/o	uterus	myocardi/o	heart muscle
ichthy/o	scaly, dry	myos/o	muscle
ile/o	ileum	myring/o	eardrum
ili/o	ilium	nas/o	nose
immun/o	immune, protection	nat/o	birth
infer/o	below	natr/o	sodium
ir/o	iris	necr/o	death
irid/o	iris	nephr/o	kidney

Appendix

Combining Form	Meaning
neur/o	nerve
neutr/o	neutral
noct/i	night
nyctal/o	night
ocul/o	eye
odont/o	tooth
olig/o	scanty
onc/o	tumor
onych/o	nail
oophor/o	ovary
ophthalm/o	eye
opt/o	eye, vision
optic/o	eye
or/o	mouth
orch/o	testes
orchi/o	testes
orchid/o	testes
organ/o	organ
orth/o	straight, upright
oste/o	bone
ot/o	ear
ov/o	egg
ovari/o	ovary
ox/i	oxygen
ox/o	oxygen
palat/o	palate
pancreat/o	pancreas
papill/o	optic disk
parathyroid/o	parathyroid gland
patell/o	patella
path/o	disease
ped/o	foot, child
pelv/o	pelvis
perine/o	perineum
peritone/o	peritoneum
phac/o	lens
phag/o	eat, swallow
phalang/o	phalanges
pharmac/o	drug
pharyng/o	throat, pharynx
phas/o	speech
phleb/o	vein
phon/o	sound
phot/o	light
phren/o	mind
pil/o	hair
pineal/o	pineal gland
pituitar/o	pituitary gland
plant/o	sole of the foot
pleur/o	pleura
pneum/o	lung, air
pneumon/o	lung, air
pod/o	foot
poli/o	gray matter
pont/o	pons

Combining Form	Meaning
poster/o	back
presby/o	old age
proct/o	anus and rectum
prostat/o	prostate
prosth/o	addition
proxim/o	near to
psych/o	mind
pub/o	pubis, genital region
pulmon/o	lung
pupill/o	pupil
py/o	pus
pyel/o	renal pelvis
pylor/o	pylorus
radi/o	x-ray, radius
radicul/o	nerve root
rect/o	rectum
ren/o	kidney
retin/o	retina
rhin/o	nose
rhytid/o	wrinkle
roentgen/o	X-ray
sacr/o	sacrum
salping/o	fallopian tubes, uterine tubes, eustachian tubes
sanguin/o	blood
scapul/o	scapula
schiz/o	divided
scler/o	hard, sclera
scoli/o	crooked, bent
seb/o	oil
sect/o	cut
sialaden/o	salivary gland
sigmoid/o	sigmoid colon
sinus/o	sinus, cavity
somat/o	body
somn/o	sleep
son/o	sound
spermat/o	sperm
sphygm/o	pulse
spin/o	spine
spir/o	breathing
splen/o	spleen
spondyl/o	vertebrae
staped/o	stapes
stern/o	sternum
steth/o	chest
super/o	above
synovi/o	synovial membrane
synov/o	synovial membrane
system/o	system
tars/o	ankle
ten/o	tendon
tend/o	tendon
tendin/o	tendon
testicul/o	testes

474

Combining Form	Meaning	Combining Form	Meaning
thalam/o	thalamus	urethr/o	urethra
thec/o	sheath (meninges)	urin/o	urine
therm/o	heat	uter/o	uterus
thorac/o	chest	uve/o	vascular
thromb/o	clot	vagin/o	vagina
thym/o	thymus	valv/o	valve
thyr/o	thyroid gland	valvul/o	valve
thyroid/o	thyroid gland	varic/o	varicose veins
tibi/o	tibia	vascul/o	blood vessel
tom/o	to cut	vas/o	vas deferens, vessel, duct
tonsill/o	tonsils	ven/o	vein
tox/o	poison	ventr/o	belly
toxic/o	poison	ventricul/o	ventricle
trache/o	trachea, windpipe	vertebr/o	vertebra
trich/o	hair	vesic/o	bladder
tympan/o	eardrum	vesicul/o	seminal vesicle
uln/o	ulna	viscer/o	internal organ
ungu/o	nail	vitre/o	glassy
ur/o	urine, urinary tract	vulv/o	vulva
ureter/o	ureter	xer/o	dry

Appendix

Appendix

Prefixes

Prefix	Meaning	Prefix	Meaning
a-	without, away from	micro-	small
ab-	away from	mono-	one
ad-	towards	multi-	many
allo-	other, different from usual	neo-	new
an-	without	nulli-	none
ante-	before, in front of	pan-	all
anti-	against	para-	beside, beyond, near
auto-	self	per-	through
bi-	two	peri-	around, about
brady-	slow	poly-	many
circum-	around	post-	behind, after
dys-	painful, difficult	pre-	before, in front of
endo-	within, inner	pseudo-	false
epi-	upon, over, above	quad-	four
eu-	normal, good	retro-	backward, behind
hemi-	half	semi-	partial, half
hetero-	different	sub-	below, under
homo-	same	super-	above, excess
hydro-	water	supra-	above
hyper-	over, above	tachy-	rapid, fast
hypo-	under, below	trans-	through, across
infra-	under, beneath, below	tri-	three
inter-	among, between	ultra-	beyond, excess
intra-	within, inside	uni-	one
macro-	large	xeno-	strange, foreign

Appendix

Suffixes

Suffix	Meaning	Suffix	Meaning
-ac	pertaining to	-ism	state of
-al	pertaining to	-itis	inflammation
-algesia	pain, sensitivity	-kinesia	movement
-algia	pain	-listhesis	slipping
-an	pertaining to	-lith	stone
-apheresis	removal, carry away	-lithiasis	condition of stones
-ar	pertaining to	-logist	one who studies
-arche	beginning	-logy	study of
-ary	pertaining to	-lucent	to shine through
-asthenia	weakness	-lysis	destruction
-blast	immature, embryonic	-malacia	abnormal softening
-capnia	carbon dioxide	-mania	excessive excitement
-cele	hernia, protrusion	-manometer	instrument to measure pressure
-centesis	puncture to withdraw fluid	-megaly	enlargement, large
-cise	cut	-meter	instrument for measuring
-clasia	to surgically break	-metrist	one who measures
-crine	to secrete	-metry	process of measuring
-cusis	hearing	-ole	small
-cyesis	state of pregnancy	-oma	tumor, mass
-cyte	cell	-opaque	nontransparent
-cytosis	more than the normal number of cells	-opia	vision
		-opsy	view of
-derma	skin	-orexia	appetite
-desis	stabilize, fuse	-ory	pertaining to
-dipsia	thirst	-ose	pertaining to
-dynia	pain	-osis	abnormal condition
-eal	pertaining to	-osmia	smell
-ectasia	dilation	-ostomy	surgically create an opening
-ectasis	dilation, expansion	-otia	ear condition
-ectomy	surgical removal, excision	-otomy	cutting into, incision
-emesis	vomit	-ous	pertaining to
-emia	blood condition	-para	to bear (offspring)
-esthesia	feeling, sensation	-paresis	weakness
-gen	that which produces	-partum	childbirth
-genesis	produces, generates	-pathy	disease
-genic	producing, produced by	-penia	abnormal decrease, too few
-globin	protein	-pepsia	digestion
-globulin	protein	-pexy	surgical fixation
-gram	record, picture	-phage	eat, swallow
-graph	instrument for recording	-phagia	eat, swallow
-graphy	process of recording	-phasia	speech
-gravida	pregnancy	-phil	attracted to
-ia	state, condition	-philia	to have an attraction for
-iac	pertaining to	-phobia	irrational fear
-iasis	abnormal condition	-phonia	voice
-iatrist	physician	-phoresis	carrying
-ic	pertaining to	-plasia	growth, formation, development
-ical	pertaining to		
-ile	pertaining to	-plasm	growth, formation, development
-ior	pertaining to		

Suffix	Meaning	Suffix	Meaning
-plasty	surgical repair	-stasis	standing still
-plegia	paralysis	-stenosis	narrowing
-pnea	breathing	-taxia	muscular coordination
-poiesis	formation	-tension	pressure
-porosis	porous	-therapy	treatment
-prandial	pertaining to a meal	-thorax	chest
-ptosis	drooping	-tic	pertaining to
-ptysis	spitting	-tocia	labor, childbirth
-rrhage	excessive, abnormal flow	-tome	instrument used to cut
-rrhaphy	suture	-tonia	tone
-rrhea	discharge, flow	-tripsy	surgical crushing
-rrhexis	rupture	-trophy	nourishment, development
-salpinx	fallopian tube	-tropia	to turn
-sclerosis	hardening	-tropin	stimulate
-scope	instrument for viewing	-ule	small
-scopy	process of visually examining	-uria	condition of the urine
-spermia	condition of sperm		

Glossary

A

abdominal, pertaining to the abdomen

Abdominal cavity, the superior portion of the abdominopelvic cavity

Abdominopelvic cavity, a ventral cavity consisting of the abdominal and pelvic cavities. It contains digestive, urinary, and reproductive organs

Abduction, directional term meaning to move away from the median or middle line of the body

Abnormal psychology, the study and treatment of behaviors that are outside of normal and are detrimental to the person or society. These maladaptive behaviors range from occasional difficulty coping with stress, to bizarre actions and beliefs, to total withdrawal

ABO system, the major system of blood typing

Abortifacient, Medication that terminates a pregnancy

Abrasion, scraping away a portion of the surface of the skin. Performed to remove acne scars, tattoos, and scar tissue

Abruptio placentae, emergency condition in which the placenta tears away from the uterine wall before the twentieth week of pregnancy. Requires immediate delivery of the baby

Abscess, a collection of pus in the skin

Absence seizure, type of epileptic seizure that lasts only a few seconds to half a minute, characterized by a loss of awareness and an absence of activity. It is also called a *petit mal seizure*

Acapnia, lack of carbon dioxide

Accessory organs, the accessory organs to the digestive system consist of the organs that are part of the system, but not part of the continuous tube from mouth to anus. The accessory organs are the liver, pancreas, gallbladder, and salivary glands

ACE inhibitor drugs, medication that produces vasodilation and decreases blood pressure

Achromatopsia, condition of color blindness; more common in males

Acidosis, excessive acidity of body fluids due to the accumulation of acids, as in diabetic acidosis

Acne, inflammatory disease of the sebaceous glands and hair follicles that results in papules and pustules

Acne rosacea, hypertrophy of sebaceous glands causing thickened skin generally on the nose, forehead, and cheeks

Acne vulgaris, a common form of acne occurring in adolescence from an oversecretion of the oil glands. It is characterized by papules, pustules, blackheads, and whiteheads

Acoustic, pertaining to hearing

Acoustic neuroma, benign tumor of the eighth cranial nerve sheath, which can cause symptoms from pressure being exerted on tissues

Acquired immunity, the protective response of the body to a specific pathogen

Acquired immunodeficiency syndrome (AIDS), disease that involves a defect in the cell-mediated immunity system. A syndrome of opportunistic infections that occur in the final stages of infection with the human immunodeficiency virus (HIV). This virus attacks T_4 lymphocytes and destroys them, which reduces the person's ability to fight infection

Acromegaly, chronic disease of adults that results in an elongation and enlargement of the bones of the head and extremities

Action, the type of movement a muscle produces

Active acquired immunity, immunity developing after direct exposure to a pathogen

Active exercises, exercises that a patient performs without assistance

Active range of motion (AROM), range of motion for joints that a patient is able to perform without the assistance of someone else

Active-resistive exercises, exercises in which the patient will work against an artificial resistance applied to a muscle, such as a weight. Used to increase strength

Activities of daily living (ADL), the activities usually performed in the course of a normal day, such as eating, dressing, and washing

Acute care hospitals, hospitals that typically provide services to diagnose (laboratory, diagnostic imaging) and treat (surgery, medications, therapy) diseases for a short period of time. In addition, they usually provide emergency and obstetrical care. Also called general hospital

Acute tubular necrosis (ATN), damage to the renal tubules due to presence of toxins in the urine or to ischemia; results in oliguria

Adaptive equipment, equipment that has been structured to aid in mobility, eating, and managing the other activities of daily living. This equipment includes special walkers and spoons for the stroke patient

Addiction, acquired dependence on a drug

Addison's disease, disease that results from a deficiency in adrenocortical hormones. There may be an increased pigmentation of the skin, generalized weakness, and weight loss

Additive, the sum of the action of two (or more) drugs given; in this case, the total strength of the medications is equal to the sum of the strength of each individual drug

Adduction, directional term meaning to move toward the median or middle line of the body

Adenocarcinoma, malignant adenoma in a glandular organ

Adenoidectomy, excision of the adenoids

Adenoiditis, inflammation of the adenoid tissue

Adenoids, another term for pharyngeal tonsils. The tonsils are a collection of lymphatic tissue found in the nasopharynx to combat microorganisms entering the body through the nose or mouth

Adhesion, scar tissue forming in the fascia surrounding a muscle making it difficult to stretch the muscle

Adipose, a type of connective tissue. Also called fat. It stores energy and provides protective padding for underlying structures

Adrenal, pertaining to the adrenal gland

Adrenal cortex, the outer portion of the adrenal glands; secretes several families of hormones: mineralocorticoids, glucocorticoids, and steroid sex hormones

Adrenal feminization, development of female secondary sexual characteristics (such as breasts) in a male; often as a result of increased estrogen secretion by the adrenal cortex

Adrenal glands, a pair of glands in the endocrine system located just above each kidney. These glands are composed of two sections, the cortex and the medulla, that function independently of each other. The cortex secretes steroids, such as aldosterone, cortisol, androgens, estrogens, and progestins. The medulla secretes epinephrine and norepinephrine. The adrenal glands are regulated by adrenocorticotropin hormone, which is secreted by the pituitary gland

Adrenal medulla, the inner portion of the adrenal gland. It secretes epinephrine and norepinephrine

Adrenal virilism, development of male secondary sexual characteristics (such as deeper voice and facial hair) in a female; often as a result of increased androgen secretion by the adrenal cortex

Adrenalectomy, excision of the adrenal gland

Adrenaline, a hormone produced by the adrenal medulla. Also known as epinephrine. Some of its actions include increasing heart rate and force of contraction, bronchodilation, and relaxation of intestinal muscles

Adrenalitis, inflammation of an adrenal gland

Adrenocorticotropin hormone (ACTH), a hormone secreted by anterior pituitary. It regulates function of the adrenal gland cortex

Adrenomegaly, enlarged adrenal gland

Adrenopathy, adrenal gland disease

Adult respiratory distress syndrome (ARDS), acute respiratory failure in adults characterized by tachypnea, dyspnea, cyanosis, tachycardia, and hypoxemia

Aerosol, drugs inhaled directly into the nose and mouth

Aerosol therapy, medication suspended in a mist that is intended to be inhaled. Delivered by a *nebulizer,* which delivers the mist for a period of time while the patient breathes, or a *metered dose inhaler* (MDI), which delivers a single puff of mist

Afferent arteriole, arteriole that carries blood into the glomerulus

Afferent neurons, nerve that carries impulses to the brain and spinal cord from the skin and sense organs. Also called sensory neurons

Agglutinate, clumping together to form small clusters. Platelets agglutinate to start the clotting process

Agranulocytes, nongranular leukocyte. This is one of the two types of leukocytes found in plasma that are classified as either monocytes or lymphocytes

AIDS-related complex (ARC), early stage of AIDS. There is a positive test for the virus but only mild symptoms of weight loss, fatigue, skin rash, and anorexia

Alanine transaminase (ALT), an enzyme normally present in the blood. Blood levels are increased in persons with liver disease

Albinism, a condition in which the person is not able to produce melanin. An albino person has white hair and skin and the pupils of the eye are red

Albumin, a protein that is normally found circulating in the bloodstream. It is abnormal for albumin to be in the urine

Aldosterone, a hormone produced by the adrenal cortex. It regulates the levels of sodium and potassium in the body and as a side effect the volume of water lost in urine

Alimentary canal, also known as the gastrointestinal system or digestive system. This system covers the area between the mouth and the anus and includes 30 feet of intestinal tubing. It has a wide range of functions. This system serves to store and digest food, absorb nutrients, and eliminate waste. The major organs of this system are the mouth, pharynx, esophagus, stomach, small intestine, colon, rectum, and anus

Allergen, antigen capable of causing a hypersensitivity or allergy in the body

Allergist, a physician who specializes in testing for and treating allergies

Allergy, hypersensitivity to a substance in the environment or a medication

Allograft, skin graft from one person to another; donor is usually a cadaver

Alopecia, absence or loss of hair, especially of the head

Alveoli, the tiny air sacs at the end of each bronchiole. The alveoli are surrounded by a capillary network. Gas exchange takes place as oxygen and carbon dioxide diffuse across the alveolar and capillary walls

Alzheimer's disease, chronic, organic mental disorder consisting of dementia that is more prevalent in adults between 40 and 60. Involves progressive disorientation, apathy, speech and gait disturbances, and loss of memory

Amblyopia, loss of vision not as a result of eye pathology; usually occurs in patients who see two images. In order to see only one image, the brain will no longer recognize the image being sent to it by one of the eyes; may occur if strabismus is not corrected; commonly referred to as lazy eye

Ambulatory care center, a facility that provides services that do not require overnight hospitalization. The services range from simple surgeries, to diagnostic testing, to therapy. Also called a surgical center or an outpatient clinic

Amenorrhea, absence of menstruation, which can be the result of many factors, including pregnancy, menopause, and dieting

American Sign Language (ASL), nonverbal method of communicating in which the hands and fingers are used to indicate words and concepts. Used by people who are deaf and speech impaired

Amino acids, organic substances found in plasma, used by cells to build proteins

Amnesia, loss of memory in which people forget their identity as a result of a head injury or disorder, such as epilepsy, senility, and alcoholism. Can be either temporary or permanent

Amniocentesis, puncturing of the amniotic sac using a needle and syringe for the purpose of withdrawing amniotic fluid for testing. Can assist in determining fetal maturity, development, and genetic disorders

Amnion, the inner of two membranous sacs surrouding the fetus. The amniotic sac contains amniotic fluid in which the baby floats

Amniorrhea, discharge of amniotic fluid

Amniotic, pertaining to the amnion

Amniotic fluid, the fluid inside the amniotic sac

Amniotomy, incision into the amniotic sac

Amputation, partial or complete removal of a limb for a variety of reasons, including tumors, gangrene, intractable pain, crushing injury, or uncontrollable infection

Amylase, digestive enzyme found in saliva that begins the digestion of carbohydrates

Amyotrophic lateral sclerosis (ALS), disease with muscular weakness and atrophy due to degeneration of motor neurons of the spinal cord. Also called *Lou Gehrig's disease,* after the New York Yankees' baseball player who died from the disease

Anacusis, total absence of hearing; unable to perceive sound. Also called *deafness*

Anal, pertaining to the anus

Anal fistula, abnormal tubelike passage from the surface around the anal opening directly into the rectum

Anal sphincter, ring of muscle that controls anal opening

Analgesia, a reduction in the perception of pain or sensation due to a neurological condition or medication

Analgesic, substance that relieves pain without the loss of consciousness. May be either narcotic or non-narcotic. Narcotic drugs are derived from the opium poppy and act on the brain to cause pain relief and drowsiness

Anaphylactic shock, life-threatening condition resulting from the ingestion of food or medications that produce a severe allergic response. Circulatory and respiratory problems occur, including respiratory distress, hypotension, edema, tachycardia, and convulsions

Anaphylaxis, severe reaction to an antigen

Anastomosis, creating a passageway or opening between two organs or vessels

Anatomical position, used to describe the positions and relationships of a structure in the human body. For descriptive purposes the assumption is always that the person is in the anatomical position. The body is standing erect with the arms at the side of the body, the palms of the hands facing forward, and the eyes looking straight ahead. The legs are parallel with the feet and toes pointing forward

Ancillary reports, report in a patient's medical record from various treatments and therapies the patient has received, such as rehabilitation, social services, respiratory therapy, or from the dietician

Androgen, a class of steroid hormones secreted by the adrenal cortex. These hormones, such as testosterone, produce a masculinizing effect

Androgen therapy, replacement male hormones to treat patients who produce insufficient hormone naturally

Andropathy, male disease

Anemia, reduction in the number of red blood cells (RBCs) or amount of hemoglobin in the blood; results in less oxygen reaching the tissues

Anesthesia, partial or complete loss of sensation with or without a loss of consciousness as a result of a drug, disease, or injury

Anesthesiologist, a physician who has a specialization in the practice of administering anesthetics

Anesthesiologist's report, a medical record document that relates the details regarding the drugs given to a patient and the patient's re-

sponse to anesthesia and vital signs during surgery

Anesthesiology, branch of medicine specializing in all aspects of anesthesia, including for surgical procedures, resuscitation measures, and the management of acute and chronic pain. Physician is an *anesthesiologist*

Anesthetic, substance that produces a lack of feeling that may be of local or general effect, depending on the type of administration

Anesthetic ophthalmic solution, eyedrops for pain relief associated with eye infections and corneal abrasions

Aneurysm, weakness in the wall of an artery that results in localized widening of the artery

Aneurysmectomy, surgical removal of an aneurysm

Angiitis, inflammation of vessels

Angina pectoris, severe chest pain with a sensation of constriction around the heart. Caused by a deficiency of oxygen to the heart muscle

Angiogram, record of a vessel

Angiography, process of taking an X-ray of blood or lymphatic vessels after injection of a radiopaque substance

Angioplasty, surgical repair of blood vessels

Angiospasm, involuntary muscle contraction of a vessel

Angiostenosis, narrowing of a vessel

Anhidrosis, abnormal condition of no sweat

Ankylosing spondylitis, inflammatory spinal condition that resembles rheumatoid arthritis; results in gradual stiffening and fusion of the vertebrae; more common in men than women

Anorchism, congenital absence of one or both testes

Anorexia, loss of appetite that can accompany other conditions such as a gastrointestinal (GI) upset

Anorexia nervosa, a type of eating disorder characterized by severe disturbance in body image and marked refusal to eat

Anorexiant, substance that treats obesity by suppressing appetite

Anosmia, loss of the sense of smell

Anoxia, lack of oxygen

Antacid, substance that neutralizes acid in the stomach

Antagonistic pairs, pair of muscles arranged around a joint that produce opposite actions

Anteflexion, while the uterus is normally in this position, an exaggeration of the forward bend of the uterus is abnormal. The forward bend is near the neck of the uterus. The position of cervix, or opening of the uterus, remains normal

Antepartum, before birth

Anterior, directional term meaning near or on the front or belly side of the body

Anterior lobe, the anterior portion of the pituitary gland. It secretes adrenocorticotropin hormone, follicle-stimulating hormone, growth hormone, luteinizing hormone, melanocyte-stimulating hormone, prolactin, and thyroid-stimulating hormone

Anteroposterior view (AP), positioning the patient so that the X-rays pass through the body from the anterior side to the posterior side

Anthracosis, A type of pneumoconiosis that develops from the collection of coal dust in the lung. Also called black lung or miner's lung

Anti-inflammatory otic solution, reduces inflammation, itching, and edema associated with otitis externa

Anti-virals, substance that weakens a viral infection in the body, often by interfering with the virus's ability to replicate

Antiarrhythmic, controls cardiac arrhythmias by altering nerve impulses within the heart

Antibiotic, substance that destroys or prohibits the growth of microorganisms. Used to treat bacterial infections. Not found effective in treating viral infections. To be effective, it must be taken regularly for a specified period

Antibiotic ophthalmic solution, eyedrops for the treatment of bacterial eye infections

Antibiotic otic solution, Eardrops to treat otitis externa

Antibody, protein material produced in the body as a response to the invasion of a foreign substance

Antibody-mediated immunity, the production of antibodies by B cells in response to an antigen. Also called *humoral immunity*

Anticoagulant, substance that prevents or delays the clotting or coagulation of blood

Anticonvulsant, prevents or relieves convulsions. Drugs such as phenobarbital reduce excessive stimulation in the brain to control seizures and other symptoms of epilepsy

Antidepressant drugs, medications classified as stimulants that alter the patient's mood by affecting levels of neurotransmitters in the brain

Antidiarrheal, prevents or relieves diarrhea

Antidiuretic hormone (ADH), a hormone secreted by the posterior pituitary. It promotes water reabsorption by the kidney tubules

Antidote, substance that will neutralize poisons or their side effects

Antiemetic, substance that controls nausea and vomiting

Antifungal, substance that kills fungi infecting the skin

Antigen, substance that is capable of inducing the formation of an antibody. The antibody then intereacts with the antigen in the antigen–antibody reaction

Antigen-antibody complex, combination of the antigen with its specific antibody; increases susceptibility to phagocytosis and immunity

Antiglaucoma medications, a group of drugs that reduce intraocular pressure by lowering the amount of aqueous humor in the eyeball; may achieve this by either reducing the production of aqueous humor or increasing its outflow

Antihemorrhagic, substance that prevents or stops hemorrhaging

Antihistamine, substance that acts to control allergic symptoms by counteracting histamine, which exists naturally in the body, and which is released in allergic reactions

Antilipidemic, substance that reduces amount of cholesterol and lipids in the bloodstream; treats hyperlipidemia

Antiparasitic, substance that kills mites or lice

Antiplatelet agent, substance that interferes with the action of platelets; prolongs bleeding time; commonly referred to as blood thinner. Used to prevent heart attacks and strokes

Antiprostatic agents, medications to treat early cases of benign prostatic hypertrophy; may prevent surgery for mild cases

Antipruritic, substance that reduces severe itching

Antipsychotic drugs, major tranquilizer drugs that have transformed the treatment of patients with psychoses and schizophrenia by reducing patient agitation and panic and shortening schizophrenic episodes

Antiseptic, substance used to kill bacteria in skin cuts and wounds or at a surgical site

Antisocial personality disorder, a personality disorder in which the patient engages in behaviors that are illegal or outside of social norms

Antispasmodic, medication to prevent or reduce bladder muscle spasms

Antithyroid agents, medication given to block production of thyroid hormones in patients with hypersecretion disorders

Antitussive, substance that controls or relieves coughing. Codeine is an ingredient in many prescription cough medicines that acts upon the brain to control coughing

Antrum, the tapered distal end of the stomach

Anuria, complete suppression of urine formed by the kidneys and a complete lack of urine excretion

Anus, the terminal opening of the digestive tube

Anxiety, a feeling of apprehension or worry

Anxiety disorders, Characterized by persistent worry and apprehension; includes panic attacks, anxiety, phobias, and obsessive-compulsive disorder

Aorta, the largest artery in the body. It is located in the mediastinum and carries oxygenated blood away from the left side of the heart

Aortic, pertaining to the aorta

Aortic valve, the semilunar valve between the left ventricle of the heart and the aorta in the heart. It prevents blood from flowing backwards into the ventricle

Apex, directional term meaning tip or summit. An area of the lungs and heart

Apgar score, evaluation of a neonate's adjustment to the outside world; observes color, heart rate, muscle tone, respiratory rate, and response to stimulus

Aphagia, not eating

Aphasia, inability to communicate through speech. Often an after effect of a stroke (CVA)

Aphonia, no voice

Aphthous ulcers, painful ulcers in the mouth of unknown cause. Commonly called *canker sores*

Aplastic anemia, severe form of anemia that develops as a consequence of loss of functioning red bone marrow; results in a decrease in the number of all the formed elements; treatment may eventually require a bone marrow transplant

Apnea, the condition of not breathing

Apocrine gland, type of sweat gland that opens into hair follicles located in the pubic, anal, and mammary areas. These glands secrete a substance that can produce an odor when it comes into contact with bacteria on the skin causing what is commonly referred to as body odor

Appendectomy, surgical removal of the appendix

Appendicitis, inflammation of the appendix

Appendicular skeleton, the appendicular skeleton consists of the bones of the upper and lower extremities, shoulder, and pelvis

Aqueous humor, a watery fluid filling the spaces between the cornea and lens

Arachnoid layer, the delicate middle layer of the meninges

Areola, the pigmented area around the nipple of the breast

Arrector pili, a small slip of smooth muscle attached to hairs; when this muscle contracts the hair shaft stands up and results in "goose bumps."

Arrhythmia, irregularity in the heartbeat or action

Arterial, pertaining to the artery

Arterial anastomosis, surgical joining together of two arteries; performed if an artery is severed or if a damaged section of an artery is removed

Arterial blood gases (ABG), lab test that measures the amount of oxygen, carbon dioxide, and nitrogen in the blood, and the pH

Arteries, the blood vessels that carry blood away from the heart

Arterioles, the smallest branches of the arteries. They carry blood to the capillaries

Arteriorrhexis, a ruptured artery

Arteriosclerosis, condition with thickening, hardening, and loss of elasticity of the walls of the arteries

Arthralgia, pain in a joint

Arthritis, inflammation of a joint that is usually accompanied by pain and swelling. A chronic disease

Arthrocentesis, removal of synovial fluid with a needle from a joint space, such as in the knee, for examination

Arthroclasia, surgically breaking loose a stiffened joint

Arthrodesis, surgical fusion or stiffening of a joint to provide stability. This is sometimes done to relieve the pain of arthritis

Arthrogram, record of a joint

Arthrography, visualization of a joint by radiographic study after injection of a contrast medium into the joint space

Arthroscope, instrument to view inside a joint

Arthroscopic surgery, use of an arthroscope to facilitate performing surgery on a joint

Arthroscopy, examination of the interior of a joint by entering the joint with an arthroscope. The arthroscope contains a small television camera that allows the physician to view the interior of the joint on a monitor during the procedure

Arthrotomy, surgically cutting into a joint

Articular cartilage, layer of cartilage covering the ends of bones forming a synovial joint

Articulation, another term for a joint, the point where two bones meet

Artificial tears, medications, many of them over the counter, to treat dry eyes

Asbestosis, a type of pneumoconiosis that develops from collection of asbestos fibers in the lungs; may lead to the development of lung cancer

Ascending colon, the section of the colon following the cecum. It ascends the right side of the abdomen

Ascending tracts, nerve tracts carrying sensory information up the spinal cord to the brain

Ascites, collection or accumulation of fluid in the peritoneal cavity

Aspartate transaminase (AST), an enzyme normally present in the blood. Blood levels are increased in persons with liver disease

Aspermia, lack of, or failure to ejaculate, sperm

Asphyxia, lack of oxygen that can lead to unconsciousness and death if not corrected immediately. Some of the common causes are drowning, foreign body in the respiratory tract, poisoning, and electric shock

Aspiration, for respiratory system, refers to inhaling food, liquid, or a foreign object into the airways; term also refers to withdrawing fluid from a body cavity using suction

Aspirator, a surgical instrument used to suction fluids

Asthma, disease caused by various conditions, such as allergens, and resulting in constriction of the bronchial airways and labored respirations. Can cause violent spasms of the bronchi (bronchospasms) but is generally not a life-threatening condition. Medication can be very effective

Astigmatism (Astigm), a condition in which light rays are focused unevenly on the eye, which causes a distorted image due to an abnormal curvature of the cornea

Astrocytoma, tumor of the brain or spinal cord that is composed of astrocytes

Ataxia, having a lack of muscle coordination as a result of a disorder or disease

Atelectasis, condition in which lung tissue collapses, which prevents the respiratory exchange of oxygen and carbon dioxide. Can be caused by a variety of conditions, including pressure upon the lung from a tumor or other object

Atherectomy, excision of fatty substance

Atheroma, tumor-like collection of fatty substances

Atherosclerosis, the most common form of arteriosclerosis. Caused by the formation of yellowish plaques of cholesterol buildup on the inner walls of the arteries

Atonia, lack of tone

Atresia, congenital lack of a normal body opening

Atria, the two upper chambers of the heart. The left atrium receives blood returning from the lungs, and the right atrium receives blood returning from the body

Atrial, pertaining to the atrium

Atrioventricular bundle, in the heart, conducts the electrical impulse from the atrioventricular node into the ventricles

Atrioventricular node, this area at the junction of the right atrium and ventricle receives the stimulus from the sinoatrial node and sends the impulse to the ventricles through the bundle of His

Atrioventricular valve (AV), the heart valves located between an atrium and a ventricle. Includes the tricuspid valve in the right side of the heart and the bicuspid or mitral valve in the left side of the heart

Atrophy, lack or loss of normal development

Attention deficit-hyperactivity disorder (ADHD), a type of mental disorder diagnosed in childhood characterized by poor attention and inability to control behavior. The child may or may not be hyperactive

Audiogram, chart that shows the faintest sounds a patient can hear during audiometry testing

Audiologist, provides a comprehensive array of services related to prevention, diagnosis, and treatment of hearing impairment and its associated communication disorders

Audiology, study of hearing

Audiometer, instrument to measure hearing

Audiometry, process of measuring hearing

Auditory, pertaining to hearing

Auditory canal, the canal that leads from the external opening of the ear to the eardrum

Auditory tube, another name for the eustachian tube connecting the middle ear and pharynx

Aura, sensations, such as seeing colors or smelling an unusual odor, that occur just prior to an epileptic seizure or a migraine headache

Aural, pertaining to the ear

Auricle, also called the pinna. The external ear. It functions to capture sound waves as they go past the outer ear

Auricular, pertaining to the ear

Auscultation, listening to the sounds within the body by using a stethoscope

Autism, a type of mental disorder diagnosed in childhood in which the child exhibits an extreme degree of withdrawal from all social contacts

Autograft, skin graft from a person's own body

Autoimmune disease, a disease that results from the body's immune system attacking its own cells as if they were pathogens; examples include systemic lupus erythematosus, rheumatoid arthritis, and multiple sclerosis

Autologous transfusion, procedure for collecting and storing a patient's own blood several weeks prior to the actual need. It can then be used to replace blood lost during a surgical procedure

Autonomic nervous system, the portion of the nervous system that consists of nerves to the internal organs that function involuntarily. It regulates the functions of glands (especially the salivary, gastric, and sweat glands), the adrenal medulla, heart, and smooth muscle tissue. This system is divided into two parts: sympathetic and parasympathetic

Axial skeleton, the axial skeleton includes the bones in the head, spine, chest, and trunk

Axillary, pertaining to the armpit. There is a collection of lymph nodes in this area that drains each arm

Axon, single projection of a neuron that conducts impulse away from nerve cell body

Azotemia, accumulation of nitrogenous waste in the bloodstream. Occurs when the kidney fails to filter these wastes from the blood

B

B cells, common name for B lymphocytes, responds to foreign antigens by producing protective antibodies

B lymphocytes, the humoral immunity cells, which respond to foreign antigens by producing protective antibodies. Simply referred to as *B cells.*

Babinski's reflex, reflex test to determine lesions and abnormalities in the nervous system. The Babinski reflex is present if the great toe extends instead of flexes when the lateral sole of the foot is stroked. The normal response to this stimulation would be a flexion, or upward movement, of the toe

Bacteria, primitive, single-celled microorganisms that are present everywhere. Some are capable of causing disease in humans

Bacteriuria, bacteria in the urine

Balanitis, inflammation of the skin covering the glans penis

Balanoplasty, surgical repair of the glans penis

Balanorrhea, discharge from the glans penis

Bariatric surgery, a group of surgical procedures such as stomach stapling and restrictive banding to reduce the size of the stomach. A treatment for morbid (extreme) obesity

Barium (Ba), soft metallic element from the earth used as a radiopaque X-ray dye

Barrier contraception, prevention of a pregnancy using a device to prevent sperm from meeting an ovum; examples include condoms, diaphragms, and cervical caps

Bartholin's glands, glands located on either side of the vaginal opening that secrete mucus for vaginal lubrication

Basal cell carcinoma, tumor of the basal cell layer of the epidermis. A frequent type of skin cancer that rarely metastasizes or spreads. These cancers can arise on sun-exposed skin

Basal layer, the deepest layer of the epidermis. This living layer constantly multiplies and divides to supply cells to replace the cells that are sloughed off the skin surface

Base, directional term meaning bottom or lower part

Basophil, a granulocyte white blood cell that releases histamine and heparin in damaged tissues

Bell's palsy, one-sided facial paralysis with an unknown cause. The person cannot control salivation, tearing of the eyes, or expression. The patient will eventually recover

Benign, not cancerous. A benign tumor is generally not progressive or recurring

Benign prostatic hypertrophy (BPH), enlargement of the prostate gland commonly seen in males over

Beta blocker drugs, medication that treats hypertension and angina pectoris by lowering the heart rate

Biceps, an arm muscle named for the number of attachment points. *Bi-* means two and biceps have two heads attached to the bone

Bicuspid valve, a valve between the left atrium and ventricle. It prevents blood from flowing backwards into the atrium. It has two cusps or flaps. It is also called the mitral valve

Bicuspids, premolar permanent teeth having two cusps or projections that assist in grinding food. Humans have eight bicuspids

Bile, substance produced by the liver and stored in the gallbladder. It is added to the chyme in the duodenum and functions to emulsify fats so they can be digested and absorbed. Cholesterol is essential to bile production

Bilirubin, waste product produced from destruction of worn-out red blood cells; disposed of by the liver

Binaural, referring to both ears

Biopsy (Bx, bx), a piece of tissue is removed by syringe and needle, knife, punch, or brush to examine under a microscope. Used to aid in diagnosis

Bipolar disorder (BPD), a mental disorder in which the patient has alternating periods of depression and mania

Bite-wing x-ray, x-ray taken with part of the film holder held between the teeth, and the film held parallel to the teeth

Bladder cancer, cancerous tumor that arises from the cells lining the bladder; major symptom is hematuria

Bladder neck obstruction, blockage of the bladder outlet into the urethra

Blepharectomy, excision of the eyelid

Blepharitis, inflammatory condition of the eyelash follicles and glands of the eyelids that results in swelling, redness, and crusts of dried mucus on the lids. Can be the result of allergy or infection

Blepharoplasty, surgical repair of the eyelid

Blepharoptosis, drooping eyelid

Blood, the major component of the hematic system. It consists of watery plasma, red blood cells, and white blood cells

Blood clot, the hard collection of fibrin, blood cells, and tissue debris that is the end result of hemostasis or the blood clotting process

Blood culture and sensitivity (C&S), sample of blood is incubated in the laboratory to check for bacterial growth; if bacteria are present, they are identified and tested to determine which antibiotics they are sensitive to

Blood pressure (BP), measurement of the pressure that is exerted by blood against the walls of a blood vessel

Blood serum test, blood test to measure the level of substances such as calcium, electrolytes, testosterone, insulin, and glucose. Used to assist in determining the function of various endocrine glands

Blood sinuses, spread-out blood vessels within the spleen that result in slow-moving blood flow

Blood transfusion, artificial transfer of blood into the bloodstream

Blood typing, the blood of one person is different from another's due to the presence of antigens on the surface of the erythrocytes. The major method of typing blood is the ABO system and includes types A, B, O, and AB. The other major method of typing blood is the Rh factor, consisting of the two types, Rh+ and Rh−

Blood urea nitrogen (BUN), blood test to measure kidney function by the level of nitrogenous waste, or urea, that is in the blood

Blood vessels, the closed system of tubes that conducts blood throughout the body. It consists of arteries, veins, and capillaries

Body, (1) A whole, living individual; the sum of all the cells, tissues, organs, and systems working together to sustain life; (2) the main portion of an organ such as the stomach or uterus

Body mechanics, use of good posture and position while performing activities of daily living to prevent injury and stress on body parts

Bolus, chewed up morsel of food ready to be swallowed

Bone, a type of connective tissue and an organ of the musculoskeletal system. They provide support for the body and serve as sites of muscle attachments

Bone graft, piece of bone taken from the patient and used to replace a removed bone or a bony defect at another site

Bone marrow, soft tissue found inside cavities in bones; produces blood cells

Bone marrow aspiration, removing a sample of bone marrow by syringe for microscopic examination. Useful for diagnosing such diseases as leukemia. For example, a proliferation (massive increase) of a white blood cells cloud confirm the diagnosis of acute leukemia

Bone marrow transplant (BMT), patient receives red bone marrow from a donor after the patient's own bone marrow has been destroyed by radiation or chemotherapy

Bone reabsorption inhibitors, conditions that result in weak and fragile bones, such as osteoporosis and Paget's disease, are improved by medications that reduce the reabsorption of bones

Bone scan, patient is given a radioactive dye and then scanning equipment is used to visualize bones. It is especially useful in observing the progress of treatment for osteomyelitis and cancer metastases to the bone

Bowel incontinence, inability to control defecation

Bowman's capsule, also called the glomerular capsule. Part of the renal corpuscle. It is a double-walled cuplike structure that encircles the glomerulus. In the filtration stage of urine production, waste products filtered from the blood enter Bowman's capsule as the glomerular filtrate

Brachial, pertaining to the arm

Brachial region, the arm regions of the body

Bradycardia, abonormally slow heart rate, below 60 bpm

Bradykinesia, slow movement, commonly seen with the rigidity of Parkinson's disease

Bradypepsia, slow digestion rate

Bradypnea, slow breathing

Brain, the brain is one of the largest organs in the body and coordinates most body activities. It is the center for all thought, memory, judgment, and emotion. Each part of the brain is responsible for controlling different body functions, such as temperature regulation and breathing. The four sections to the brain are the cerebrum, cerebellum, diencephalon, and brain stem

Brain scan, injection of radioactive isotopes into the circulation to determine the function and abnormality of the brain

Brain stem, this area of the brain has three components: medulla oblongata, pons, and the midbrain. The brain stem is a pathway for impulses to be conducted between the brain and the spinal cord. It also contains the centers that control respiration, heart rate, and blood pressure. In addition, the twelve pairs of cranial nerves begin in the brain stem

Brain tumor, intracranial mass, either benign or malignant. A benign tumor of the brain can be fatal since it will grow and cause pressure on normal brain tissue. The most malignant brain tumors in children are gliomas

Brand name, the name a pharmaceutical company chooses as the trademark or market name for its drug. Also called *proprietary* or *trade name.*

Breast cancer, malignant tumor of the breast; usually forms in the milk-producing gland tissue or the lining of the milk ducts

Breasts, milk-producing glands to provide nutrition for newborn. Also called *mammary glands*

Breech presentation, placement of the fetus in which the buttocks or feet are presented first for delivery rather than the head

Bridge, dental appliance that is attached to adjacent teeth for support to replace missing teeth

Broad spectrum, ability of a drug to be effective against a wide range of microorganisms

Bronchial, pertaining to the bronchi

Bronchial tube, an organ of the respiratory system that carries air into each lung

Bronchiectasis, results from a dilation of a bronchus or the bronchi that can be the result of infection. This abnormal stretching can be irreversible and result in destruction of the bronchial walls. The major symptom is a large amount of purulent (pus-filled) sputum. Rales (bubbling chest sound) and hemoptysis may be present

Bronchioles, the narrowest air tubes in the lungs. Each bronchiole terminates in tiny air sacs called alveoli

Bronchitis, an acute or chronic inflammation of the lower respiratory tract that often occurs after other childhood infections such as measles

Bronchodilator, dilates or opens the bronchi (airways in the lungs) to improve breathing

Bronchogenic, originating in the bronchi

Bronchogenic carcinoma, malignant lung tumor that originates in the bronchi. Usually associated with a history of cigarette smoking

Bronchogram, an X-ray record of the lungs and bronchial tubes

Bronchography, process of taking an X-ray of the lung after a radiopaque substance has been placed into the trachea or bronchial tree

Bronchoplasty, surgical repair of a bronchial defect

Bronchoscope, an instrument to view inside a bronchus

Bronchoscopy (Broncho), using the bronchoscope to visualize the bronchi. The instrument can also be used to obtain tissue for biopsy and to remove foreign objects

Bronchospasm, an involuntary muscle spasm in the bronchi

Bronchus, the distal end of the trachea splits into a left and right main bronchi as it enters each lung. Each main bronchus is subdivided into smaller branches. The smallest bronchi are the bronchioles. Each bronchiole ends in tiny air sacs called alveoli

Buccal, (1) Pertaining to the cheeks. (2) Drugs that are placed under the lip or between the cheek and gum

Buccolabial, pertaining to cheeks and lips

Buffers, chemicals that neutralize acid, particularly stomach acid

Bulbourethral gland, also called *Cowper's gland.* These two small male reproductive system glands are located on either side of the urethra just distal to the prostate. The secretion from these glands neutralizes the acidity in the urethra and the vagina

Bulimia, eating disorder that is characterized by recurrent binge eating and then purging of the food with laxatives and vomiting

Bundle branch block (BBB), occurs when the electrical impulse is blocked from travelling down the bundle of His or bundle branches. Results in the ventricles beating at a different rate than the atria. Also called a *heart block*

Bundle branches, part of the conduction system of the heart; the electrical signal travels down the interventricular septum

Bundle of His, the bundle of His is located in the interventricular septum. It receives the electrical impulse from the atrioventricular node and distributes it through the ventricular walls, causing them to contract simultaneously

Bunion, inflammation of the bursa of the great toe

Bunionectomy, removal of the bursa at the joint of the great toe

Burn, a full-thickness burn exists when all the layers are burned; also called a *third-degree burn.* A partial-thickness burn exists when the first layer of skin, the epidermis, is burned, and the second layer of skin, dermis, is damaged; also called a *second-degree burn.* A *first-degree burn* damages only the epidermis

Bursa, a saclike connective tissue structure found in some joints. It protects moving parts from friction. Some common bursa locations are the elbow, knee, and shoulder joints

Bursectomy, excision of a bursa

Bursitis, inflammation of a bursa between bony prominences and muscles or tendons. Common in the shoulder and knee

C

Cachexia, loss of weight and generalized wasting that occurs during a chronic disease

Calcitonin, a hormone secreted by the thyroid gland. It stimulates deposition of calcium into bone

Calcium, an inorganic substance found in plasma. It is important for bones, muscles, and nerves

Calcium channel blocker drugs, medication that treats hypertension, angina pectoris, and congestive heart failure by causing the heart to beat less forcefully and less often

Calcium supplements, maintaining high blood levels of calcium in association with vitamin D helps maintain bone density and treats osteomalacia, osteoporosis, and rickets

Calculus, a stone formed within an organ by an accumulation of mineral salts. Found in the kidney, renal pelvis, bladder, or urethra. Plural is *calculi*

Callus, the mass of bone tissue that forms at a fracture site during its healing

Calyx, a duct that connects the renal papilla to the renal pelvis. Urine flows from the collecting tubule through the calyx and into the renal pelvis

Cancellous bone, the bony tissue found inside a bone. It contains cavities that hold red bone marrow. Also called *spongy bone*

Cancerous tumors, malignant growths in the body

Candidiasis, yeastlike infection of the skin and mucous membranes that can result in white plaques on the tongue and vagina

Canines, also called the cuspid teeth or eyeteeth. Permanent teeth located between the incisors and the biscuspids that assist in biting and cutting food. Humans have four canine teeth

Capillaries, the smallest blood or lymphatic vessels. Blood capillaries are very thin to allow gas, nutrient, and waste exchange between the blood and the tissues. Lymph capillaries collect lymph fluid from the tissues and carry it to the larger lymph vessels

Capillary bed, the network of capillaries found in a given tissue or organ

Carbon dioxide, a waste product of cellular energy production. It is removed from the cells by the blood and eliminated from the body by the lungs

Carbuncle, inflammation and infection of the skin and hair follicle that may result from several untreated boils. Most commonly found on neck, upper back, or head

Carcinogen, substance or chemical agent that produces cancer or increases the risk of developing it. For example, cigarette smoke and insecticides are considered to be carcinogens

Carcinoma, new growth or malignant tumor that occurs in epithelial tissue. Can spread to other organs through the blood or direct extension from the organ

Carcinoma in situ (CIS), malignant tumor that has not extended beyond the original site

Cardiac, pertaining to the heart

Cardiac arrest, when the heart stops beating and circulation ceases

Cardiac catheterization, passage of a thin tube (catheter) through an arm vein and the blood vessel leading into the heart. Done to detect abnormalities, to collect cardiac blood samples, and to determine the pressure within the cardiac area

Cardiac enzymes, complex protein molecules found only in heart muscle. Cardiac enzymes are taken by blood sample to determine the amount of the heart disease or damage

Cardiac muscle, the involuntary muscle found in the heart

Cardiac scan, patient is given radioactive thallium intravenously and then scanning equipment is used to visualize the heart; it is especially useful in determining myocardial damage

Cardiac sphincter, also called the *lower esophageal sphincter.* Prevents food and gastric juices from backing up into the esophagus

Cardiologist, a physician specializing in treating diseases and conditions of the cardiovascular system

Cardiology, the branch of medicine specializing in conditions of the cardiovascular system

Cardiomegaly, abnormally enlarged heart

Cardiomyopathy, general term for a disease of the myocardium that may be caused by alcohol abuse, parasites, viral infection, and congestive heart failure

Cardiopulmonary resuscitation (CPR), emergency treatment provided by persons trained in CPR and given to patients when their respirations and heart stop. CPR provides oxygen to the brain, heart, and other vital organs until medical treatment can restore a normal heart and pulmonary function

Cardiorrhexis, ruptured heart

Cardiotonic, substance that strengthens the heart muscle

Cardiovascular system (CV), system that transports blood to all areas of the body. Organs of the cardiovascular system include the heart and blood vessels (arteries, veins, and capillaries). Also called the *circulatory system*

Carotid endarterectomy, surgical procedure for removing an obstruction within the carotid artery, a major artery in the neck that carries oxygenated blood to the brain. Developed to prevent strokes but found to be useful only in severe stenosis with TIA

Carpal, pertaining to the wrist

Carpal tunnel release, surgical cutting of the ligament in the wrist to relieve nerve pressure caused by carpal tunnel disease, which can be caused by repetitive motion such as typing

Carpal tunnel syndrome, a painful disorder of the wrist and hand, induced by compression of the median nerve as it passes under ligaments on the palm side of the wrist. Symptoms include weakness, pain, burning, tingling, and aching in the forearm, wrist, and hand

Carpals, the wrist bones in the upper extremity

Cartilage, strong, flexible connective tissue found in several locations in the body, such as covering the ends of bones in a synovial joint, nasal septum, external ear, eustachian tube, larynx, trachea, bronchi, and the intervertebral discs

Cartilaginous joints, a joint that allows slight movement but holds bones firmly in place by a solid piece of cartilage. The public symphysis is an example of a cartilaginous joint. The fetal skeleton is composed of cartilaginous tissue

Cast, application of a solid material to immobilize an extremity or portion of the body as a result of a fracture, dislocation, or severe injury. It is most often made of plaster of Paris

Castration, excision of the testicles in the male or the ovaries in the female

Cataract, diminished vision resulting from the lens of the eye becoming opaque or cloudy. Treatment is usually surgical removal of the cataract

Catheter, a flexible tube inserted into the body for the purpose of moving fluids into or out of the body. In the cardiovascular system used to place dye into blood vessels so they may be visualized on X-rays. In the urinary system used to drain urine from the bladder

Catheterization, insertion of a tube through the urethra and into the urinary bladder for the purpose of withdrawing urine or inserting dye

Caudal, directional term meaning toward the feet or tail, or below

Cauterization, destruction of tissue using an electric current, a caustic product, or a hot iron, or by freezing

Cecum, first portion of the colon. It is a blind pouch off the beginning of the large intestine. The appendix grows out of the end of the cecum

Cell, the basic unit of all living things. All tissues and organs in the body are composed of cells. They perform survival functions such as reproduction, respiration, metabolism, and excretion. Some cells are also able to carry on specialized functions, such as contraction by muscle cells and electrical impulse transmission by nerve cells

Cell membrane, the outermost boundary of the cell

Cell-mediated immunity, immunity that results from the activation of sensitized T lymphocytes. The immune response causes antigens to be destroyed by the direct action of cells. Also called *cellular immunity*

Cellular immunity, also called cell-mediated immunity. This process results in the production of T cells and natural killer, NK, cells that directly attach to foreign cells. This immune response fights invasion by viruses, bacteria, fungi, and cancer

Cellulitis, inflammation of the cellular or connective tissues

Cementum, anchors the root of a tooth into the socket of the jaw

Central canal, canal that extends down the length of the spinal cord; contains cerebrospinal fluid

Central nervous system, the portion of the nervous system that consists of the brain and spinal cord. It receives impulses from all over the body, processes this information, and then responds with an action. It consists of both gray matter and white matter

Cephalalgia, a headache

Cephalic, Directional term meaning toward the head, or above

Cephalic region, the head region of the body

Cerebellar, pertaining to the cerebellum

Cerebellitis, inflammation of the cerebellum

Cerebellum, the second largest portion of the brain, located beneath the posterior portion of the cerebrum. This part of the brain aids in coordinating voluntary body movements and maintaining balance and equilibrium. It is attached to the brain stem by the pons. The cerebellum refines the muscular movement that is initiated in the cerebrum

Cerebral, pertaining to the cerebrum

Cerebral aneurysm, localized abnormal dilatation of a blood vessel, usually an artery; the result of a congenital defect or weakness in the wall of the vessel; a ruptured aneurysm is a common cause for a hemorrhagic CVA

Cerebral angiography, x-ray of the blood vessels of the brain after the injection of a radiopaque dye

Cerebral contusion, bruising of the brain from a blow or impact; symptoms last longer than 24 hours and include unconsciousness, dizziness, vomiting, unequal pupil size, and shock

Cerebral cortex, the outer layer of the cerebrum. It is composed of folds of gray matter called gyri, which are separated by sulci

Cerebral hemispheres, the division of the cerebrum into right and left halves

Cerebral palsy (CP), a group of disabilities caused by injury to the brain either before or during birth or very early in infancy. This is the most common permanent disability in childhood

Cerebrospinal, pertaining to the cerebrum and spine

Cerebrospinal fluid (CSF), watery, clear fluid found in the ventricles of the brain. It provides protection from shock or sudden motion to the brain

Cerebrospinal fluid analysis, laboratory examination of the clear, watery, colorless fluid from within the brain and spinal cord. Infections and the abnormal presence of blood can be detected in this test

Cerebrospinal fluid shunts, a surgical procedure in which a bypass is created to drain cerebrospinal fluid. It is used to treat hydrocephalus by draining the excess cerebrospinal fluid from the brain and diverting it to the abdominal cavity

Cerebrovascular accident (CVA), also called a *stroke.* The development of an infarct due to loss in the blood supply to an area of the brain. Blood flow can be interrupted by a ruptured blood vessel (hemorrhage), a floating clot (embolus), a stationary clot (thrombosis), or compression. The extent of damage depends on the size and location of the infarct and often includes speech problems and muscle paralysis

Cerebrum, the largest section of the brain. It is located in the upper portion and is the area that possesses our thoughts, judgment, memory, association skills, and the ability to discriminate between items. The outer layer of the cerebrum is the cerebral cortex, which is composed of folds of gray matter. The elevated portions of the cerebrum, or convolutions, are called gyri and are separated by fissures or sulci. The cerebrum has both a left and right division or hemisphere. Each hemisphere has four lobes: frontal, parietal, occipital, and temporal

Cerumen, also called ear wax. A thick, waxy substance produced by oil glands in the auditory canal. This wax helps to protect and lubricate the ear

Ceruminoma, a hard accumulation of ear wax in the ear canal

Cervical, (1) Pertaining to the neck. (2) Pertaining to the cervix

Cervical biopsy, taking a sample of tissue from the cervix to test for the presence of cancer cells

Cervical cancer, malignant growth in the cervix. An especially difficult type of cancer to treat, it causes 5% of the cancer deaths in women. Pap tests have helped to detect early cervical cancer

Cervical region, the neck region of the body

Cervical vertebrae, the seven vertebrae in the neck region

Cervicectomy, excision of the cervix

Cervix, the narrow, distal portion of the uterus that joins to the vagina

Cesarean section (CS, C-section), surgical delivery of a baby through an incision into the abdominal and uterine walls. Legend has it that the Roman emperor Julius Caesar was the first person born by this method

Chancroid, highly infectious nonsyphilitic venereal ulcer

Cheeks, form the lateral walls of the oral cavity

Chemabrasion, abrasion using chemicals; also called a *chemical peel.*

Chemical name, the name for a drug based on its chemical formula or molecular structure

Chemical thyroidectomy, large dose of radioactive iodine is given in order to kill thyroid gland cells without having to actually do surgery

Chemotherapy (chemo), treating disease by using chemicals that have a toxic effect on the body, especially cancerous tissue

Chest x-ray (CXR), taking a radiograhic picture of the lungs and heart from the back and sides

Cheyne-Stokes respiration, abnormal breathing pattern in which there are long periods (10 to 60 seconds) of apnea followed by deeper, more rapid breathing

Chiropractic, healthcare profession concerned with diagnosis and treatment of the spine and musculoskeletal system with the intention of affecting the nervous system and improving health. Healthcare practitioner is a *chiropractor*

Chlamydia, parasitic microorganism causing genital infections in males and females; can lead to pelvic inflammatory disease in females and eventual infertility

Cholecystalgia, gallbladder pain

Cholecystectomy, surgical excision of the gallbladder. Removal of the gallbladder through the laparoscope is a newer procedure with fewer complications than the more invasive abdominal surgery. The laparoscope requires a small incision into the abdominal cavity

Cholecystic, pertaining to the gallbladder

Cholecystitis, inflammation of the gallbladder

Cholecystogram, dye given orally to the patient is absorbed and enters the gallbladder. An X-ray is then taken

Choledocholithotripsy, crushing of a gallstone in the common bile duct

Cholelithiasis, formation or presence of stones or calculi in the gallbladder or common bile duct

Chondrectomy, excision of cartilage

Chondroma, cartilage tumor

Chondromalacia, softening of cartilage

Chondroplasty, surgical repair of cartilage

Chorion, the outer of two membranous sacs surrounding the fetus. It helps to form the placenta

Chorionic, pertaining to the chorion

Chorionic villus sampling (CVS), removal of a small piece of the chorion for genetic analysis; may be done at an earlier stage of pregnancy than amniocentesis

Choroid, the middle layer of the eyeball. This layer provides the blood supply for the eye

Chronic obstructive pulmonary disease (COPD), progressive, chronic, and usually irreversible condition in which the lungs have a diminished capacity for inspiration (inhalation) and expiration (exhalation). The person may have difficulty breathing on exertion (dyspnea) and a cough. Also called *chronic obstructive lung disease (COLD)*

Chyme, semisoft mixture of food and digestive fluids that pass from the stomach into the small intestines

Cicatrix, a scar

Cilia, a term for eyelashes that protect the eye from foreign particles or for nasal hairs that help filter dust and bacteria out of inhaled air

Ciliary body, the intraocular eye muscles that change the shape of the lens

Circadian rhythm, the 24-hour clock that governs our periods of wakefulness and sleepiness

Circulating nurse, nurse who assists the surgeon and scrub nurse by providing needed materials during the procedure and by handling the surgical specimen. This person does not wear sterile clothing and may enter and leave the operating room during the procedure

Circulatory system, system that transports blood to all areas of the body. The organs of the circulatory system include the heart and blood vessels (arteries, veins, and capillaries). Also called the *cardiovascular system*

Circumcision, surgical removal of the end of the prepuce or foreskin of the penis. Generally performed on the newborn male at the request of the parents. The primary reason is for ease of hygiene. Circumcision is also a ritual practice in some religions

Circumduction, movement in a circular direction from a central point

Cirrhosis, chronic disease of the liver

Clamp, a surgical instrument used to grasp tissue and control bleeding

Clavicle, also called the collar bone. A bone of the pectoral girdle

Clavicular, pertaining to the clavicle or collar bone

Clean catch specimen (CC), urine sample obtained after cleaning off the urinary opening and catching or collecting a sample in midstream (halfway through the urination process) to minimize contamination from the genitalia

Cleft lip, congenital anomaly in which the upper lip fails to come together. Often seen along with a cleft palate. Corrected with surgery

Cleft palate, congenital anomaly in which the roof of the mouth has a split or fissure. Corrected with surgery

clinical psychologist (PhD), diagnoses and treats mental disorders; specializes in using individual and group counseling to treat patients with mental and emotional disorders

Clitoris, a small organ containing erectile tissue that is covered by the labia minora. It contains sensitive tissue that is aroused during sexual stimulation and is similar to the penis in the male

Closed fracture, a simple fracture with no open skin or wound

Clubbing, the abnormal widening and thickening of the ends of the fingers and toes associated with chronic oxygen deficiency. Seen in patients with chronic respiratory conditions or circulatory problems

Coagulate, convert liquid to a gel or solid, as in blood coagulation

Coarctation of the aorta (CoA), severe congenital narrowing of the aorta

Coccygeal, pertaining to the coccyx or tailbone

Coccyx, the tailbone, the four small fused vertebrae at the distal end of the vertebral column

Cochlea, a portion of the labyrinth associated with hearing. It is rolled in the shape of a snail shell. The organs of Corti line the cochlea

Cochlear, pertaining to the cochlea

Cochlear implant, mechanical device that is surgically placed under the skin behind the outer ear (pinna). It converts sound signals into magnetic impulses to stimulate the auditory nerve. Can be beneficial for those with profound sensorineural hearing loss

Cochlear nerve, the branch of the vestibulocochlear nerve that carries hearing information to the brain

Cognitive disorders, deterioration of mental functions due to temporary brain or permanent brain dysfunction; includes dementia and Alzheimer's disease; also called *organic mental disease*

Colectomy, surgical removal of the colon

Collagen fibers, fibers made up of an insoluble fibrous protein present in connective tissue that forms a flexible mat to protect the skin and other parts of the body

Collecting tubule, a portion of the renal tubule

Colles' fracture, a specific type of wrist fracture

Colon, also called the *large intestine*. Functions to reabsorb most of the fluid in the digested food. The material that remains after water reabsorption is the feces. The sections of the colon are the cecum, ascending colon, transverse colon, descending colon, and sigmoid colon

Colonic, pertaining to the colon

Colonoscope, instrument to view inside the colon

Colonoscopy, a flexible fiberscope passed through the anus, rectum, and colon is used to examine the upper portion of the colon. Polyps and small growths can be removed during this procedure

Color vision tests, use of polychromic (multicolored) charts to determine the ability of the patient to recognize color

Colorectal, pertaining to the colon and rectum

Colorectal carcinoma, cancerous tumor along the length of the colon and rectum

Colostomy, surgical creation of an opening in some portion of the colon through the abdominal wall to the outside surface. The fecal material (stool) drains into a bag worn on the abdomen

Colostrum, a thin fluid first secreted by the breast after delivery; it does not contain much protein, but is rich in antibodies

Colposcope, instrument to view inside the vagina

Colposcopy, visual examination of the cervix and vagina using a colposcope or instrument with a magnifying lens

Coma, profound unconsciousness resulting from an illness or injury

Combining form, the word root plus the combining vowel. It is always written with a / between the word root and the combining vowel. For example, in the combining form *cardi/o, cardi* is the word root and */o* is the combining vowel

Combining vowel, a vowel inserted between word parts that makes it possible to pronounce long medical terms. It is usually the vowel o

Comedo, medical term for a blackhead. It is an accumulation of sebum in a sebaceous gland that has become blackened

Comminuted fracture, a fracture in which the bone is shattered, splintered, or crushed into many pieces or fragments. The fracture is completely through the bone

Common bile duct, a duct that carries bile from the gallbladder to the duodenum

Compact bone, the hard exterior surface bone. Also called *cortical bone*

Complete blood count (CBC), blood test that consists of five tests; red blood cell count (RBC), white blood count (WBC), hemoglobin (Hg), hematocrit (Hct), and white blood cell differential

Compound fracture, an open fracture in which the skin has been broken through by the fracture

Compression fracture, fracture involving loss of height of a vertebral body

Computed tomography scan (CT scan), an imaging technique that is able to produce a cross-sectional view of the body; X-ray pictures are taken at multiple angles through the body and a computer uses all these images to construct a composite cross-section

Conception, fertilization of an ovum by a sperm

Concussion, injury to the brain that results from a blow or impact from an object. Can result in unconsciousness, dizziness, vomiting, unequal pupil size, and shock

Conductive hearing loss, loss of hearing as a result of the blocking of sound transmission in the middle ear and outer ear

Condyle, refers to the rounded portion at the end of a bone

Cones, the sensory receptors of the retina that are active in bright light and see in color

Congenital septal defect (CSD), defect, present at birth, in the wall separating two chambers of the heart. Results in a mixture of oxygenated and deoxygenated blood being carried to the surrounding tissues. There can be an atrial sep-

tal defect (ASD) and a ventricular septal defect (VSD)

Congestive heart failure (CHF), pathological condition of the heart in which there is a reduced outflow of blood from the left side of the heart. Results in weakness, breathlessness, and edema

Conization, surgical removal of a core of cervical tissue. Also refers to partial removal of the cervix

Conjunctiva, a protective mucous membrane lining on the underside of each eyelid and across the anterior surface of each eyeball

Conjunctival, pertaining to the conjunctiva

Conjunctivitis, also referred to as *pink eye* or an inflammation of the conjunctiva

Conjunctivoplasty, surgical repair of the conjunctiva

Connective tissue, the supporting and protecting tissue in body structures. Examples are fat or adipose tissue, cartilage, and bone

Conscious, condition of being awake and aware of surroundings

Constipation, experiencing difficulty in defecation or infrequent defecation

Consultation reports, document in a patient's medical record. They are the reports given by specialists who the physician has requested to evaluate the patient

Contracture, an abnormal shortening of a muscle, making it difficult to stretch the muscle

Contraindication, condition in which a particular drug should not be used

Contrast studies, a radiopaque substance is injected or swallowed; X-rays are then taken that outline the body structure containing the radiopaque substance

Controlled substances, drugs that have a potential for being addictive (habit forming) or can be abused

Contusion, injury caused by a blow to the body; causes swelling, pain, and bruising; the skin is not broken

Conversion reaction, a somatoform disorder in which the patient unconsciously substitutes physical signs or symptoms for anxiety. The most common physical signs or symptoms are blindness, deafness, and paralysis

Convulsions, severe involuntary muscle contractions and relaxations. These have a variety of causes, such as epilepsy, fever, and toxic conditions

Corium, the living layer of skin located between the epidermis and the subcutaneous tissue. Also referred to as the *dermis,* it contains hair follicles, sweat glands, sebaceous glands, blood vessels, lymph vessels, nerve fibers, and muscle fibers

Cornea, a portion of the sclera that is clear and transparent and allows light to enter the interior of the eye. It also plays a role in bending light rays

Corneal, pertaining to the cornea

Corneal abrasion, scraping injury to the cornea; if it does not heal, it may develop into an ulcer

Coronal plane, a vertical plane that divides the body into front (anterior or ventral) and back (posterior or dorsal) sections. Also called the *frontal plane*

Coronal section, sectional view of the body produced by a cut along the frontal plane; also called a *frontal section.*

Coronary, pertaining to the heart

Coronary arteries, a group of three arteries that branch off the aorta and carry blood to the myocardium

Coronary artery bypass graft (CABG), open-heart surgery in which a blood vessel is grafted to route blood around the point of constriction in a diseased coronary artery

Coronary artery disease (CAD), insufficient blood supply to the heart muscle due to an obstruction of one or more coronary arteries; may be caused by atherosclerosis and may cause angina pectoris and myocardial infarction

Corpus, the body or central portion of the uterus

Cortex, the outer layer of an organ. In the endocrine system, it refers to the outer layer of the adrenal glands; in the urinary system, the outer layer of the kidney

Cortical, pertaining to the cortex

Cortical bone, the hard exterior surface bone. Also called *compact bone*

Corticosteroid cream, a powerful anti-inflammatory cream

Corticosteroids, general term for the group of hormones secreted by the adrenal contex. They include mineralocorticoid hormones, glucocorticoid hormones, and steroid sex hormones. Used as a medication for its strong anti-inflammatory properties

Cortisol, a steroid hormone secreted by the adrenal cortex. It regulates carbohydrate metabolism

Costal, pertaining to the ribs

Cowper's glands, also called *bulbourethral glands.* These two small male reproductive system glands are located on either side of the urethra just distal to the prostate. The secretion from these glands neutralizes the acidity in the urethra and the vagina

Cranial, Pertaining to the skull

Cranial cavity, a dorsal body cavity. It is within the skull and contains the brain

Cranial nerves, nerves that arise from the brain

Craniotomy, incision into the skull

Cranium, the skull; bones that form a protective covering over the brain

Creatine phosphokinase (CPK), a muscle enzyme found in skeletal muscle and cardiac muscle; blood test becomes elevated in disorders such as heart attack, muscular dystrophy, and other skeletal muscle pathologies

Creatinine, a waste product of muscle metabolism

Creatinine clearance, test of kidney function. Creatinine is a waste product cleared from the bloodstream by the kidneys. For this test, urine is collected for 24 hours and the amount of creatinine in the urine is compared to the amount of creatinine that remains in the bloodstream

Crepitation, sound of broken bones rubbing together

Cretinism, congenital condition due to a lack of thyroid that may result in arrested physical and mental development

Crohn's disease, form of chronic inflammatory bowel disease affecting the ileum and/or colon. Also called *regional ileitis*

Cross infection, occurs when a person, either a patient or healthcare worker, acquires a pathogen from another patient or healthcare worker

Cross-section, an internal view of the body produced by a slice perpendicular to the long axis of the structure

Croup, acute viral respiratory infection common in infants and young children and characterized by a hoarse cough

Crown, portion of a tooth that is covered by enamel. Also an artificial covering for the tooth created to replace the original enamel

Crowning, when the head of the baby is visible through the vaginal opening. A sign that birth is imminent

Crural, pertaining to the leg

Crural region, the lower extremity region of the body

Cryoextraction, procedure in which cataract is lifted from the lens with an extremely cold probe

Cryoretinopexy, surgical fixation of the retina by using extreme cold

Cryosurgery, exposing tissues to extreme cold in order to destroy them. Used in treating malignant tumors and to control pain and bleeding

Cryotherapy, using cold for therapeutic purposes

Cryptorchidism, failure of the testes to descend into the scrotal sac before birth. Generally, the testes will descend before the boy is 1 year old. A surgical procedure called orchidopexy may be required to bring the testes down into the scrotum permanently. Failure of the testes to descend could result in sterility in the male

Culdoscopy, examination of the female pelvic cavity by introducing an endoscope through the wall of the vagina

Culture and sensitivity (C&S), a laboratory test in which a colony of pathogens that have been removed from an infected area are grown to identify the pathogen and then determine its sensitivity to a variety of antibiotics

Cumulative action, action that occurs in the body when a drug is allowed to accumulate or stay in the body

Curettage, removal of superficial skin lesions with a curette (surgical instrument shaped like a spoon) or scraper

Curette, a surgical instrument used to scrape and remove tissue

Cushing's syndrome, set of symptoms that result from hypersecretion of the adrenal cortex. This may be the result of a tumor of the adrenal glands. The syndrome may present symptoms of weakness, edema, excess hair growth, skin discoloration, and osteoporosis

Cuspids, permanent teeth located between the incisors and the bicuspids that assist in biting and cutting food. Humans have four cuspids. Also called canine teeth or eyeteeth

Cusps, the leaflets or flaps of a heart valve

Cutaneous membrane, this is another term for the skin

Cuticle, the thin skinlike layer overlapping the base of a nail

Cyanosis, slightly bluish color of the skin due to a deficiency of oxygen and an excess of carbon dioxide in the blood. It is caused by a variety of disorders, ranging from chronic lung disease to congenital and chronic heart problems

Cycloplegia, Paralysis of the ciliary body

Cyst, fluid-filled sac under the skin

Cystalgia, bladder pain

Cystectomy, excision of the bladder

Cystic, pertaining to the bladder

Cystic duct, duct leading from the gallbladder to the common bile duct; carries bile

Cystic fibrosis (CF), hereditary condition causing the exocrine glands to malfunction. The patient produces very thick mucus that causes severe congestion within the lungs and digestive system. Through more advanced treatment, many children are now living into adulthood with this disease

Cystitis, inflammation of the bladder

Cystocele, hernia or outpouching of the bladder that protrudes into the vagina. This may cause urinary frequency and urgency

Cystogram, record of the bladder

Cystography, process of instilling a contrast material or dye into the bladder by catheter to visualize the urinary bladder on X-ray

Cystolith, bladder stone

Cystopexy, surgical fixation of the bladder

Cystoplasty, surgical repair of the bladder

Cystorrhagia, rapid bleeding from the bladder

Cystoscope, instrument used to visually examine the bladder

Cystoscopy (cysto), visual examination of the urinary bladder using an instrument called a cystoscope

Cystostomy, creation of an opening through the body wall and into the bladder

Cystotomy, incision into the bladder

Cytologic testing, examination of cells to determine their structure and origin. Pap smears are considered a form of cytologic testing

Cytology, the study of cells

Cytoplasm, the watery internal environment of a cell

Cytotoxic, pertaining to poisoning cells

D

Dacryocystitis, inflammation of tear sac

Day surgery, a type of outpatient surgery in which the patient is discharged on the same day he or she is admitted; also called ambulatory surgery

Deafness, the inability to hear or having some degree of hearing impairment

Debridement, removal of foreign material and dead or damaged tissue from a wound

Decibel (dB), measures the intensity or loudness of a sound. Zero decibels is the quietest sound measured and 120 dB is the loudest sound commonly measured

Deciduous teeth, the twenty teeth that begin to erupt around the age of 6 months. Eventually pushed out by the permanent teeth

Decongestant, substance that reduces nasal congestion and swelling

Decubitus ulcer, bedsore or pressure sore caused by pressure over bony prominences on the body; caused by a lack of blood flow

Deep, directional term meaning away from the surface of the body

Deep tendon reflex (DTR), muscle contraction in response to a stretch caused by striking the muscle tendon with a reflex hammer; test used to determine if muscles are responding properly

Defecation, evacuation of feces from the rectum

Defibrillation, a procedure that converts serious irregular heartbeats, such as fibrillation, by giving electric shocks to the heart

Delirium, state of mental confusion with a lack of orientation to time and place

Delivery, the emergence of the baby from the birth canal

Delusions, a false belief held with conviction even in the face of strong evidence to the contrary

Dementia, progressive impairment of intellectual function that interferes with performing the activities of daily living. Patients have little awareness of their condition. Found in disorders such as Alzheimer's

Dendrite, branched process off a neuron that receives impulses and carries them to the cell body

Dental, pertaining to teeth

Dental caries, gradual decay and disintegration of teeth caused by bacteria that can result in inflamed tissue and abscessed teeth. Commonly called a *tooth cavity*

Dentalgia, tooth pain

Dentin, the main bulk of the tooth. It is covered by enamel

Dentistry, branch of healthcare involved with the prevention, diagnosis, and treatment of conditions involving the teeth, jaw, and mouth. Dentistry is practiced by a *dentist* or *oral surgeon*

Denture, partial or complete set of artificial teeth that are set in plastic materials. Substitute for the natural teeth and related structures

Deoxygenated, blood in the veins that is low in oxygen content

Depigmentation, loss of normal skin color or pigment

Dermabrasion, abrasion or rubbing using wire brushes or sandpaper

Dermatitis, inflammation of the skin

Dermatologist, a physician specialized in the diagnosis and treatment of diseases of the integumentary system

Dermatology, the branch of medicine specializing in conditions of the integumentary system

Dermatome, instrument for cutting the skin or thin transplants of skin

Dermatopathy, general term for skin disease

Dermatoplasty, the surgical repair of the skin

Dermatosis, abnormal condition of the skin

Dermis, the living layer of skin located between the epidermis and the subcutaneous tissue. It is also referred to as the corium or the *true skin.* It contains hair follicles, sweat glands, sebaceous glands, blood vessels, lymph vessels, nerve fibers, and muscle fibers

Descending colon, the section of the colon that descends the left side of the abdomen

Descending tracts, nerve tracts carrying motor signals down the spinal cord to the muscles

Diabetes insipidus (DI), disorder caused by the inadequate secretion of a hormone by the posterior lobe of the pituitary gland. There may be polyuria and polydipsia. This is more common in the young

Diabetes mellitus (DM), a serious disease in which the pancreas fails to produce insulin or the insulin does not work properly. Consequently, the patient has very high blood sugar. The kidney will attempt to lower the high blood sugar level by excreting excess sugar in the urine

Diabetic nephropathy, accumulation of damage to the glomerulus capillaries due to the chronic high blood sugars of diabetes mellitus

Diabetic retinopathy, secondary complication of diabetes that affects the blood vessels of the retina, resulting in visual changes and even blindness

Diagnostic reports, found in a patient's medical record, it consists of the results of all diagnostic tests performed on the patient, principally from the lab and medical imaging (for example, X-ray and ultrasound)

Diaphoresis, excessive or profuse sweating

Diaphragm, The major muscle of inspiration. It separates the thoracic from the abdominal cavity

Diaphragmatic, pertaining to the diaphragm

Diaphysis, the shaft portion of a long bone

Diarrhea, passing of frequent, watery bowel movements. Usually accompanies gastrointestinal (GI) disorders

Diastole, the period of time during which a heart chamber is relaxed

Diastolic pressure, the lower pressure within blood vessels during the relaxation phase of the heart beat

Diencephalon, the portion of the brain that contains two of the most critical areas of the brain, the thalamus and the hypothalamus

Digestive system, system that digests food and absorbs nutrients. Organs include the mouth, pharynx, esophagus, stomach, small and large intestines, liver, gallbladder, and anus. Also called the gastrointestinal system

Digital rectal exam (DRE), manual examination for an enlarged prostate gland performed by palpating (feeling) the prostate gland through the wall of the rectum

Dilation and curettage (D&C), surgical procedure in which the opening of the cervix is dilated and the uterus is scraped or suctioned of its lining or tissue. Often performed after a spontaneous abortion and to stop excessive bleeding from other causes

Dilation stage, the first stage of labor. It begins with uterine contractions that press the fetus against the cervix causing it to dilate to 10 cm and become thin. The thinning of the cervix is called effacement

Dilator, a surgical instrument used to enlarge an opening by stretching

Diphtheria, a bacterial infection of the respiratory system characterized by severe inflammation that can form a membrane coating in the upper respiratory tract that can cause marked difficulty breathing

Diplopia, double vision

Discharge summary, part of a patient's medical record. It is a comprehensive outline of the patient's entire hospital stay. It includes condition at time of admission, admitting diagnosis, test results, treatments and patient's response, final diagnosis, and follow-up plans

Dislocation, occurs when the bones in a joint are displaced from their normal alignment

Disorders diagnosed in infancy and childhood, mental disorders associated with childhood; include mental retardation, attention deficit disorder, and autism

Dissection, the surgical cutting of parts for separation and study

Dissociative disorders, disorders in which severe emotional conflict is so repressed that a split in the personality occurs; include amnesia and multiple personality disorder

Distal, directional term meaning located farthest from the point of attachment to the body

Distal convoluted tubule, a portion of the renal tubule

Diuresis, abnormal secretion of large amounts of urine

Diuretic, substance that increases the excretion of urine, which promotes the loss of water and salt from the body. Can assist in lowering blood pressure; therefore, these drugs are used to treat hypertension. Potassium in the body may be depleted with continued use of diuretics. Potassium-rich foods such as bananas, kiwi, and orange juice can help correct this deficiency

Diverticulectomy, surgical removal of a diverticulum

Diverticulitis, inflammation of a diverticulum or sac in the intestinal tract, especially in the colon

Diverticulosis, abnormal condition of having diverticula (out pouches off the gut)

Dopaminergic drugs, group of medications to treat Parkinson's disease by either replacing the dopamine that is lacking or increasing the strength of the dopamine that is present

Doppler ultrasonography, measurement of soundwave echos as they bounce off tissues and organs to produce an image. In cardiovascular system, used to measure velocity of blood moving through blood vessels to look for blood clots

Dorsal, directional term meaning near or on the back or spinal cord side of the body

Dorsiflexion, backward bending, as of hand or foot

Dorsum, refers to the posterior region of back of the body

Draping, process of covering the patient with sterile cloths that allow only the operative site to be exposed to the surgeon

Drug Enforcement Agency, the government agency that enforces regulation of controlled substances

Drug interaction, occurs when the effect of one drug is altered because it was taken at the same time as another drug

Drug tolerance, decrease in susceptibility to a drug after continued use of the drug

Dry gangrene, late stages of gangrene characterized by the affected area becoming black and leathery

Dual-energy absorptiometry, measurement of bone density using low dose X-ray for the purpose of detecting osteoporosis

Duodenal, pertaining to the duodenum

Duodenum, the first section of small intestines. Digestion is completed in the duodenum after the chyme mixes with digestive juices from the pancreas and gallbladder

Dura mater, the term means tough mother. It is the fibrous outermost meninges layer that forms a tough protective layer

Dwarfism, condition of being abnormally small. It may be the result of a hereditary condition or an endocrine dysfunction

Dyscrasia, a general term indicating the presence of a disease affecting blood

Dysentery, disease characterized by diarrhea, often with mucus and blood, severe abdominal pain, fever, and dehydration

Dyskinesia, difficult or painful movement

Dysmenorrhea, painful cramping that is associated with menstruation

Dysorexia, abnormal appetite

Dyspepsia, indigestion

Dysphagia, having difficulty eating

Dysphasia, impairment of speech as a result of a brain lesion

Dysphonia, abnormal voice

Dyspnea, difficult, labored breathing

Dystocia, abnormal or difficult labor and childbirth

Dystonia, abnormal tone

Dysuria, painful or difficult urination. This is a symptom in many disorders, such as cystitis, urethritis, enlarged prostate in the male, and prolapsed uterus in the female

E

Eardrops, substance placed directly into the ear canal for the purpose of relieving pain or treating infection

Eating disorders, abnormal behaviors related to eating; include anorexia nervosa and bulimia

Ecchymosis, skin discoloration or bruise caused by blood collecting under the skin

Echocardiography (ECHO), noninvasive diagnostic method using ultrasound to visualize internal cardiac structures; cardiac valve activity can be evaluated using this method

Echoencephalography, recording of the ultrasonic echoes of the brain; useful in determining abnormal patterns of shifting in the brain

Eclampsia, convulsive seizures and coma that can occur in a woman between the twentieth week of pregnancy and the first week of postpartum. Often associated with hypertension

Eczema, superficial dermatitis accompanied by papules, vesicles, and crusting

Edema, condition in which the body tissues contain excessive amounts of fluid

Effacement, the thinning of the cervix during labor

Efferent arteriole, arteriole that carries blood away from the glomerulus

Efferent neurons, nerves that carry impulses away from the brain and spinal cord to the muscles and glands. Also called *motor neurons.*

Ejaculation, the impulse of forcing seminal fluid from the male urethra

Elective abortion, the legal termination of a pregnancy for nonmedical reasons

Electrocardiogram (ECG,EKG), record of the electrical activity of the heart. Useful in the diagnosis of abnormal cardiac rhythm and heart muscle (myocardium) damage

Electrocardiography, process of recording the electrical activity of the heart

Electrocautery, to destroy tissue with an electric current

Electroconvulsive therapy (ECT), a procedure occasionally used for cases of prolonged major depression in which an electrode is placed on one or both sides of the patient's head and current is turned on briefly causing a convulsive seizure. A low level of voltage is used in modern ECT, and the patient is administered a muscle relaxant and an anesthesia. Advocates of this treatment state that it is a more effective way to treat severe depression than with the use of drugs. It is not effective with disorders other than depression, such as schizophrenia and alcoholism

Electroencephalogram (EEG), a record of the brain's electrical activity

Electroencephalography (EEG), recording the electrical activity of the brain by placing electrodes at various positions on the scalp. Also used in sleep studies to determine if there is a normal pattern of activity during sleep

Electrolyte, chemical compound that separates into charged particles, or ionizes, in a solution. Sodium chloride (NaCl) and potassium (K) are examples of electrolytes

Electromyogram (EMG), record of muscle electricity

Electromyography, recording of the electrical patterns of a muscle in order to diagnose diseases

Elephantiasis, inflammation, obstruction, and destruction of the lymph vessels that results in enlarged tissues due to edema

Elevation, a muscle action that raises a body part, as in shrug the shoulders

Embolectomy, surgical removal of an embolus or clot from a blood vessel

Embolus, obstruction of a blood vessel by a blood clot that moves from another area

Embryo, the term to describe the developing infant from fertilization until the end of the eighth week

Embryonic, pertaining to the embryo

Emesis, vomiting, usually with some force

Emetic, substance that induces vomiting

Emmetropia (EM), state of normal vision

Emphysema, pulmonary condition that can occur as a result of long-term heavy smoking. Air pollution also worsens this disease. The patient may not be able to breathe except in a sitting or standing position

Empyema, pus within the pleural space, usually the result of infection

Emulsification, to make fats and lipids more soluble in water

Enamel, the hardest substance in the body. Covers the outer surface of teeth

Encapsulated, growth enclosed in a sheath of tissue that prevents tumor cells from invading surrounding tissue

Encephalitis, inflammation of the brain due to disease factors such as rabies, influenza, measles, or smallpox

Endarterectomy, removal of the inside layer of an artery

Endocarditis, inflammation of the inner lining layer of the heart. May be due to microorganisms or to an abnormal immunological response

Endocardium, the inner layer of the heart, which is very smooth and lines the chambers of the heart

Endocervicitis, inflammation of the inner aspect of the cervix

Endocrine glands, a glandular system that secretes hormones directly into the bloodstream rather than into a duct. Endocrine glands are frequently referred to as ductless glands. The endocrine system includes the thyroid gland, adrenal glands, parathyroid glands, pituitary gland, pancreas (islets of Langerhans), testes, ovaries, and thymus gland

Endocrine system, the body system that consists of glands that secrete hormones directly into the blood stream. The endocrine glands include the adrenal glands, parathyroid glands, pancreas, pituitary gland, testes, ovaries, thymus gland, and thyroid gland

Endocrinologist, physician who specializes in the treatment of endocrine glands, including diabetes

Endocrinology, the branch of medicine specializing in conditions of the endocrine system

Endocrinopathy, a disease of the endocrine system

Endometrial biopsy (EMB), taking a sample of tissue from the lining of the uterus to test for abnormalities

Endometrial cancer, cancer of the endometrial lining of the uterus

Endometriosis, abnormal condition of endometrium tissue appearing throughout the pelvis or on the abdominal wall. This tissue is usually found within the uterus

Endometritis, inflammation of the endometrial lining of the uterus

Endometrium, the inner lining of the uterus. It contains a rich blood supply and reacts to hormonal changes every month, which results in menstruation. During a pregnancy, the lining of the uterus does not leave the body but remains to nourish the unborn child

Endoscopic retrograde cholanglopancreatography (ERCP), using an endoscope to X-ray the bile and pancreatic ducts

Endoscopic surgery, use of a lighted instrument to examine the interior of a cavity

Endotracheal, pertaining to inside the trachea

Endotracheal intubation, placing a tube through the mouth to create an airway

Enteric, pertaining to the small intestines

Enteritis, inflammation of only the small intestine

Enucleated, the loss of a cell's nucleus

Enucleation, surgical removal of an eyeball

Enuresis, involuntary discharge of urine after the age by which bladder control should have been established. This usually occurs by age 5. Also called bedwetting at night

Enzyme-linked immunosorbent assay (ELISA), a blood test for an antibody to the AIDS virus. A positive test means that the person has been exposed to the virus. In the case of a false-positive reading, the Western blot test would be used to verify the results

Eosinophils, granulocyte white blood cells that destroy parasites and increase during allergic reactions

Epicardium, the outer layer of the heart. It forms part of the pericardium

Epicondyle, a projection located above or on a condyle

Epidermal, pertaining to upon the skin

Epidermis, the superficial layer of skin. It is composed of squamous epithelium cells. These are flat scalelike cells that are arranged in layers, called stratified squamous epithelium. The many layers of the epidermis create a barrier to infection. The epidermis does not have a blood supply, so it is dependent on the deeper layers of skin for nourishment. However, the deepest epidermis layer is called the basal layer. These cells are alive and constantly dividing. Older cells are pushed out toward the surface by new cells forming beneath. During this process, they shrink and die, becoming filled with a protein called keratin. The keratin-filled cells are sloughed off as dead cells

Epididymal, pertaining to the epididymis

Epididymectomy, surgical excision of the epididymis

Epididymis, a coiled tubule that lies on top of the testes within the scrotum. This tube stores sperm as they are produced and turns into the vas deferens

Epididymitis, inflammation of the epididymis that causes pain and swelling in the inguinal area

Epidural hematoma, mass of blood in the space outside the dura mater of the brain and spinal cord

Epigastric, pertaining to above the stomach. An anatomical division of the abdomen, the middle section of the upper row

Epiglottis, a flap of cartilage that covers the larynx when a person swallows. This prevents food and drink from entering the larynx and trachea

Epilepsy, recurrent disorder of the brain in which convulsive seizures and loss of consciousness occur

Epinephrine, a hormone produced by the adrenal medulla. Also known as *adrenaline.* Some of its actions include increased heart rate and force of contraction, bronchodilation, and relaxation of intestinal muscles

Epiphysis, the wide ends of a long bone

Episiorrhaphy, suture the perineum

Episiotomy, surgical incision of the perineum to facilitate the delivery process. Can prevent an irregular tearing of tissue during birth

Epispadias, congenital opening of the urethra on the dorsal surface of the penis

Epistaxis, nosebleed

Epithelial tissue, tissue found throughout the body as the skin, the outer covering of organs, and the inner lining for tubular or hollow structures

Epithelium, epithelial tissue composed of close-packed cells that form the covering for and lining of body structures

Equilibrium, The sense of balance

Erectile dysfunction (ED), inability to copulate due to inability to maintain an erection; also called *impotence*

Erectile dysfunction agents, medications that temporarily produce an erection in patients with erectile dysfunction

Erectile tissue, tissue with numerous blood vessels and nerve endings. It becomes filled with blood and enlarges in size in response to sexual stimulation

Ergonomics, the study of human work including how the requirements for performing work and the work environment affect the musculoskeletal and nervous system

Erythema, redness or flushing of the skin

Erythrocyte sedimentation rate (ESR, sed rate), blood test to determine the rate at which mature red blood cells settle out of the blood after the addition of an anticoagulant. An indicator of the presence of an inflammatory disease

Erythrocytes, also called red blood cells or RBCs. Cells that contain hemoglobin, an iron-containing pigment that binds oxygen in order to transport it to the cells of the body

Erythrocytosis, too many red cells

Erythroderma, red skin

Erythropenia, too few red cells

Erythropoiesis, the process of forming erythrocytes

Eschar, a thick layer of dead tissue and tissue fluid that develops over a deep burn area

Esophageal, pertaining to the esophagus

Esophageal varices, enlarged and swollen varicose veins in the lower end of the esophagus; they can rupture and result in serious hemorrhage

Esophagectasis, stretched out or dilated esophagus

Esophagogastroduodenoscopy (EGD), use of a flexible fiberoptic scope to visually examine the esophagus, stomach, and beginning of the duodenum

Esophagus, the tube that carries food from the pharynx to the stomach

Esotropia, inward turning of the eye. An example of a form of strabismus (muscle weakness of the eye)

Estrogen, one of the hormones produced by the ovaries. It works with progesterone to control the menstrual cycle and it is responsible for producing the secondary sexual characteristics

Ethmoid bone, a cranial bone

Eupnea, normal breathing

Eustachian tube, tube or canal that connects the middle ear with the nasopharynx and allows for a balance of pressure between the outer and middle ear. Infection can travel via the mucous membranes of the eustachian tube, resulting in middle ear infections

Eversion, directional term meaning turning outward

Ewing's sarcoma, malignant growth found in the shaft of long bones that spreads through the periosteum. Removal is treatment of choice, as this tumor will metastasize or spread to other organs

Excretory urography (EU), injection of dye into the bloodstream followed by taking an X-ray to trace the action of the kidney as it excretes the dye

Exfoliative cytology, scraping cells from tissue and then examining them under a microscope

Exhalation, to breathe air out of the lungs. Also called expiration

Exocrine glands, glands that secrete substances into a duct. Tears and tear ducts are examples of an exocrine gland

Exophthalmos, condition in which the eyeballs protrude, such as in Graves' disease. This is generally caused by an overproduction of thyroid hormone

Exostosis, a bone spur

Exotropia, outward turning of the eye. Also an example of strabismus (muscle weakness of the eye)

Expectorant, substance that assists in the removal of secretions from the bronchopulmonary membranes

Expiratory reserve volume (ERV), the amount of air that can be forcibly exhaled after a normal quiet respiration. This is also called *supplemental air*

Exploratory laparotomy, abdominal operation for the purpose of examining the abdominal organs and tissues for signs of disease or other abnormalities

Exploratory surgery, surgery performed for the purpose of determining if there is cancer present or if a known cancer has spread. Biopsies are generally performed

Explosive disorder, an impulse control disorder in which the patient is unable to control violent rages

Expulsion stage, stage of labor and delivery during which the baby is delivered

Extension, movement that brings limb into or toward a straight condition

Extensor capri, a muscle named for its action, extension

External auditory meatus, the opening into the external ear canal

External ear, the outermost portion of the ear. It consists of the auricle, auditory canal, and eardrum

External oblique, a muscle named for the direction of its fibers, on an oblique angle

External respiration, the exchange of oxygen and carbon dioxide that takes place in the lungs

External sphincter, ring of voluntary muscle that controls the emptying of urine from the bladder,

Extracorporeal circulation (ECC), during open heart surgery, the routing of blood to a heart-lung machine so it can be oxygenated and pumped to the rest of the body

Extracorporeal shockwave lithotripsy (ESWL), use of ultrasound waves to break up stones. Process does not require surgery

Extraction, removing or pulling teeth

Eye muscles, there are six muscles that connect the eyeball to the orbit cavity. These muscles allow for rotation of the eyeball

Eyeball, the eye by itself, without any appendages such as the eye muscles or tear ducts

Eyedrops, substance placed into the eye to control eye pressure in glaucoma. Also used during eye examinations to dilate the pupil of the eye for better examination of the interior of the eye

Eyelashes, along the upper and lower edges of the eyelids; protect the eye from foreign particles; also called *cilia.*

Eyelids, an upper and lower fold of skin that provides protection from foreign particles, injury from the sun and intense light, and trauma. Both the upper and lower edges of the eyelids have small hairs or cilia. In addition, sebaceous or oil glands are located in the eyelids. These secrete a lubricating oil

F

Facial bones, the skull bones that surround the mouth, nose, and eyes; muscles for chewing are attached to the facial bones

Factitious disorders, intentionally feigning illness symptoms in order to gain attention such as malingering

Falling test, test used to observe balance and equilibrium. The patient is observed balancing on one foot, then with one foot in front of the other, and then walking forward with eyes open. The same test is conducted with the patient's eyes closed. Swaying and falling with the eyes closed can indicate an ear and equilibrium malfunction

Fallopian tubes, organs in the female reproductive system that transport eggs from the ovary to the uterus

Family and group psychotherapy, form of psychological counseling in which the therapist places minimal emphasis on patient past history and strong emphasis on having patient state and discuss goals and then find a way to achieve them

Fascia, connective tissue that wraps muscles. It tapers at each end of a skeletal muscle to form tendons

Fascial, pertaining to fascia

Fasciitis, inflammation of fascia

Fasciotomy, incision into fascia

Fasting blood sugar (FBS), blood test to measure the amount of sugar circulating throughout the body after a 12-hour fast

Fats, lipid molecules transported throughout the body dissolved in the blood

Fecal occult blood test (FOBT), laboratory test on the feces to determine if microscopic amounts of blood are present; also called *hemoccult* or *stool guaiac.*

Feces, food that cannot be digested becomes a waste product and is expelled or defecated as feces

Female reproductive system, system responsible for producing eggs for reproduction and provides place for growing baby. Organs include ovaries, fallopian tubes, uterus, vagina, and mammary glands

Femoral, pertaining to the femur or thigh bone

Femur, also called the *thigh bone.* It is a lower extremity bone

Fertility drug, medication that triggers ovulation. Also called *ovulation stimulant*

Fertilization, also called *impregnation.* The fusion of an ova and sperm to produce an embryo

Fetal, pertaining to the fetus

Fetal monitoring, using electronic equipment placed on the mother's abdomen to check the baby's heart rate and strength during labor

Fetus, the term to describe the developing newborn from the end of the eighth week until birth

Fibrillation, abnormal quivering or contractions of heart fibers. When this occurs within the fibers of the ventricle of the heart, arrest and death can occur. Emergency equipment to defibrillate, or convert the heart to a normal beat, is necessary

Fibrin, whitish protein formed by the action of thrombin and fibrinogen, which is the basis for the clotting of blood

Fibrinogen, blood protein that is essential for clotting to take place

Fibrinolysis, destruction of fibers

Fibrinous, pertaining to being fibrous

Fibrocystic breast disease, benign cysts forming in the breast

Fibroid tumor, benign tumor or growth that contains fiberlike tissue. Uterine fibroid tumors are the most common tumors in women

Fibromyalgia, a condition with widespread aching and pain in the muscles and soft tissue

Fibrous joints, a joint that has almost no movement because the ends of the bones are joined together by thick fibrous tissue. The sutures of the skull are an example of a fibrous joint

Fibula, one of the lower leg bones in the lower extremity

Fibular, pertaining to the fibula, a lower leg bone

Film, thin sheet of cellulose material coated with a light-sensitive substance that is used in taking photographs. There is a special photographic film that is sensitive to X-rays

Film badge, badge containing film that is sensitive to X-rays. This is worn by all personnel in radiology to measure the amount of X-rays to which they are exposed

Filtration, first stage of urine production during which waste products are filtered from the blood

Fimbriae, the fingerlike extensions on the end of the fallopian tubes. The fimbriae drape over each ovary in order to direct the ovum into the fallopian tube after it is expelled by the ovary

Fine motor skills, the use of precise and coordinated movements in such activities as writing, buttoning, and cutting

Fissure, a deep groove or slit-type opening

Fistulectomy, excision of a fistula

Fixation, a procedure to stabilize a fractured bone while it heals. *External fixation* includes casts, splints, and pins inserted through the skin. *Internal fixation* includes pins, plates, rods, screws, and wires that are applied during an *open reduction*

Flat bone, a type of bone with a thin flattened shape. Examples include the scapula, ribs, and pelvic bones

Flexion, act of bending or being bent

Flexor carpi, a muscle named for its action, flexion

Fluorescein angiography, process of injecting a dye (fluorescein) to observe the movement of blood for detecting lesions in the macular area of the retina. Used to determine if there is a detachment of the retina

Fluorescein staining, applying dye eyedrops that are a bright green fluorescent color; used to look for corneal abrasions or ulcers

Fluoroscopy, x-rays strike a glowing screen which can change from minute to minute, therefore able to show movement such as the digestive tract moving

Flutter, an arrhythmia in which the atria beat too rapidly, but in a regular pattern

Focal seizure, a localized epileptic seizure often affecting one limb

Follicle-stimulating hormone (FSH), a hormone secreted by the anterior pituitary gland. It stimulates growth of eggs in females and sperm in males

Foramen, a passage or opening through a bone for nerves and blood vessels

Forceps, a surgical instrument used to grasp tissues

Formed elements, the solid, cellular portion of blood. It consists of erythrocytes, leukocytes, and platelets

Fossa, a shallow cavity or depression within or on the surface of a bone

Fovea centralis, the area of the retina that has the sharpest vision

Fowler position, surgical position in which the patient is sitting with back positioned at a 45° angle

Fracture, an injury to a bone that causes it to break. Fractures are named to describe the type of damage to the bone

Fraternal twins, twins that develop from two different ova fertilized by two different sperm; although twins, these siblings do not have identical DNA

Free edge, the exposed edge of a nail that is trimmed when nails become too long

Frequency, a greater than normal occurrence in the urge to urinate, without an increase in the total daily volume of urine. Frequency is an indication of inflammation of the bladder or urethra

Frontal bone, the forehead bone of the skull

Frontal lobe, one of the four cerebral hemisphere lobes. It controls motor functions

Frontal plane, a vertical plane that divides the body into front (anterior or ventral) and back (posterior or dorsal) sections. Also called the *coronal plane*

Frontal section, sectional view of the body produced by a cut along the frontal plane; also called a *coronal section.*

Frozen section (FS), a thin piece of tissue is cut from a frozen specimen for rapid examination under a microscope

Functional residual capacity (FRC), the air that remains in the lungs after a normal exhalation has taken place

Fundus, the domed upper portion of an organ such as the stomach or uterus

Fungal scrapings, scrapings, taken with a curette or scraper, of tissue from lesions are placed on a growth medium and examined under a microscope to identify fungal growth

Fungi, organisms found in the Kingdom Fungi. Some are capable of causing disease in humans, such as yeast infections or histoplasmosis

Furuncle, staphylococcal skin abscess with redness, pain, and swelling. Also called a *boil*

G

Gait, manner of walking

Gait training, assisting a person to learn to walk again or how to use an assistive device to walk

Gallbladder (GB), small organ located just under the liver. It functions to store the bile produced by the liver. The gallbladder releases bile into the duodenum through the common bile duct

Gametes, the reproductive sex cells—ova and sperm

Gamma globulin, protein component of blood containing antibodies that help to resist infection

Ganglion, knotlike mass of nerve tissue located outside the brain and spinal cord

Ganglion cyst, cyst that forms on tendon sheath, usually on hand, wrist, or ankle

Gangrene, necrosis of the skin usually due to deficient blood supply

Gastralgia, stomach pain

Gastrectomy, surgical removal of the stomach

Gastric, pertaining to the stomach

Gastric carcinoma, cancerous tumor of the stomach

Gastric stapling, procedure that closes off a large section of the stomach with rows of staples. Results in a much smaller stomach to assist very obese patients to lose weight

Gastritis, inflammation of the stomach that can result in pain, tenderness, nausea, and vomiting

Gastroenteritis, inflammation of the stomach and small intestines

Gastroenterologist, a physician specialized in treating diseases and conditions of the gastrointestinal tract

Gastroenterology, branch of medicine specializing in conditions of the gastrointestinal system

Gastroesophageal reflux disease (GERD), acid from the stomach backs up into the esophagus, causing inflammation and pain

Gastrointestinal system (GI), system that digests food and absorbs nutrients. Organs include the mouth, pharynx, esophagus, stomach, small and large intestines, liver, gallbladder, and anus. Also called the digestive system

Gastrointestinal tract, the continuous tube that extends from mouth to anus; also called *gut* or *alimentary canal*

Gastromalacia, softening of the stomach

Gastroscope, instrument to view inside the stomach

Gastroscopy, a flexible gastroscope is passed through the mouth and down the esophagus in order to visualize inside the stomach; used to diagnose peptic ulcers and gastric carcinoma

Gastrostomy, surgical creation of a gastric fistula or opening through the abdominal wall. The opening is used to place food into the stomach when the esophagus is not entirely open (esophageal stricture)

Gavage, using a nasogastric tube to place liquid nourishment directly into the stomach

General anesthesia (GA), general anesthesia produces a loss of consciousness including an absence of pain sensation. It is administered to a patient by either an intravenous or inhalation method. The patient's vital signs are carefully monitored when using a general anesthetic

General hospital, hospitals that typically provide services to diagnose (laboratory, diagnostic imaging) and treat (surgery, medications, therapy) diseases for a short period of time. In addition, they usually provide emergency and obstetrical care. Also called an *acute care hospital*

Generic name, the recognized and accepted official name for a drug. Each drug has only one generic name. This name is not subject to trademark, so any pharmaceutical manufacturer may use it. Also called *nonproprietary name*

Genital herpes, creeping skin disease that can appear like a blister or vesicle, caused by a sexually transmitted virus

Genital warts, growths and elevations of warts on the genitalia of both males and females that can lead to cancer of the cervix in females

Genitalia, the male and female reproductive organs

Genitourinary system (GU), the organs of the urinary system and the female or male sexual organs

Gestation, length of time from conception to birth, generally nine months. Calculated from the first day of the last menstrual period, with a range of from 259 days to 280 days

Gigantism, excessive development of the body due to the overproduction of the growth hormone by the pituitary gland. The opposite of dwarfism

Gingiva, the tissue around the teeth; also called *gums*

Gingival, pertaining to the gums

Gingivitis, inflammation of the gums characterized by swelling, redness, and a tendency to bleed

Glands, the organs of the body that release secretions. Exocrine glands, like sweat glands, release their secretions into ducts. Endocrine glands, such as the thyroid gland, release their hormones directly into the blood stream

Glans penis, the larger and softer tip of the penis. It is protected by a covering called the prepuce or foreskin

Glaucoma, increase in intraocular pressure that, if untreated, may result in atrophy (wasting away) of the optic nerve and blindness. Glaucoma is treated with medication and surgery. There is an increased risk of developing glaucoma in persons over 60 years of age, people of African ancestry, persons who have sustained a serious eye injury, and anyone with a family history of diabetes or glaucoma

Globulins, one type of protein found dissolved in the plasma

Glomerular capsule, also called Bowman's capsule. Part of the renal corpuscle. It is a double-walled cuplike structure that encircles the glomerulus. In the filtration stage of urine production, waste products filtered from the blood enter Bowman's capsule as the glomerular filtrate

Glomerular filtrate, the product of the filtration stage of urine production. Water, electrolytes, nutrients, wastes, and toxins that are filtered from blood passing through the glomerulus. The filtrate enters Bowman's capsule

Glomerulonephritis, inflammation of the kidney (primarily of the glomerulus). Since the glomerular membrane is inflamed, it becomes more permeable and will allow protein and blood cells to enter the filtrate. Results in protein in the urine (proteinuria) and hematuria

Glomerulus, ball of capillaries encased by Bowman's capsule. In the filtration stage of urine production, wastes filtered from the blood leave the glomerulus capillaries and enter Bowman's capsule

Glossal, pertaining to the tongue

Glottis, the opening between the vocal cords. Air passes through the glottis as it moves through the larynx. Changing the tension of the vocal cords changes the size of the opening

Glucagon, a hormone secreted by the pancreas. It stimulates the liver to release glucose into the blood

Glucocorticoids, a group of hormones secreted by the adrenal cortex. They regulate carbohydrate levels in the body. Cortisol is an example of a glucocorticoid

Glucose, the form of sugar used by the cells of the body to make energy. It is transported to the cells in the blood

Glucose tolerance test (GTT), test to determine the blood sugar level. A measured dose of glucose is given to a patient either orally or intravenously. Blood samples are then drawn at certain intervals to determine the ability of the patient to utilize glucose. Used for diabetic patients to determine their insulin response to glucose

Gluteal, pertaining to the buttocks

Gluteal region, refers to the buttock region of the body

Gluteus maximus, a muscle named for its size and location: Gluteus means *rump area* and maximus means *large.*

Glycosuria, presence of an excess of sugar in the urine

Goiter, enlargement of the thyroid gland

Gonadotropins, common name for follicle-stimulating hormone and luteinizing hormone

Gonads, the organs responsible for producing sex cells. The female gonads are the ovaries, and they produce ova. The male gonads are the testes, and they produce sperm

Gonorrhea, sexually transmitted inflammation of the mucous membranes of either sex. Can be passed on to an infant during the birth process

Grade, a tumor can be graded from grade I through grade IV. The grade is based on the microscopic appearance of the tumor cells. A grade I tumor is well differentiated and is easier to treat than the more advanced grades

Graft *versus* host disease (GVHD), serious complication of bone marrow transplant; immune cells from the donor bone marrow (graft) attack the recipient's (host's) tissues.

Granulocytes, granular polymorphonuclear leukocyte. There are three types: neutrophil, eosinophil, and basophil

Graves' disease, condition, named for Robert Graves, an Irish physician, that results in overactivity of the thyroid gland and can result in a crisis situation. Also called *hyperthyroidism*

Gray matter, tissue within the central nervous system. It consists of unsheathed or uncovered nerve cell bodies and dendrites

Greenstick fracture, fracture in which there is an incomplete break; one side of the bone is broken and the other side is bent. This type of fracture is commonly found in children due to their softer and more pliable bone structure

Gross motor skills, the use of large muscle groups that coordinate body movements such as walking, running, jumping, and balance

Growth hormone (GH), a hormone secreted by the anterior pituitary that stimulates growth of the body

Guillain-Barré syndrome, disease of the nervous system in which nerves lose their myelin covering; may be caused by an autoimmune reaction; characterized by loss of sensation and/or muscle control in the arms and legs; symptoms then move toward the trunk and may even result in paralysis of the diaphragm

Gums, the tissue around the teeth; also called *gingiva.*

Gut, name for the continuous muscular tube that stretches between the mouth and anus; also called the *alimentary canal*

Gynecologist, a physician specialized in treating conditions and diseases of the female reproductive system

Gynecology, branch of medicine specializing in conditions of the female reproductive system

Gynecomastia, the development of breast tissue in males; may be a symptom of adrenal feminization

Gyri, the convoluted, elevated portions of the cerebral cortex. They are separated by fissures or sulci. Singular is gyrus

H

H₂-receptor antagonist, blocks the production of stomach acids

Habituation, development of an emotional dependence on a drug due to repeated use

Hair, a structure in the integumentary system

Hair follicle, cavities in the dermis that contain the hair root. Hair grows longer from the root

Hair root, deeper cells that divide to grow a hair longer

Hair shaft, older keratinized cells that form most of the length of a hair

Hallucinations, the perception of an object that is not there or event that has not happened. Hallucinations may be visual, auditory, olfactory, gustatory, or tactile

Hashimoto's disease, chronic form of thyroiditis, named for a Japanese surgeon

Head, the large ball-shaped end of a bone. It may be separated from the shaft of the bone by an area called the neck

Health maintenance organization (HMO), an organization that contracts with a group of physicians and other healthcare workers to provide care exclusively for its members. The HMO pays the healthcare workers a prepaid fixed amount per member, called capitation, whether that member requires medical attention or not

Hearing, one of the special senses; sound waves detected by the ear

Hearing aid, apparatus or mechanical device used by persons with impaired hearing to amplify sound. Same as amplification device

Heart, organ of the cardiovascular system that contracts to pump blood through the blood vessels

Heart transplantation, replacement of a diseased or malfunctioning heart with a donor's heart

Heart valve prolapse, the cusps or flaps of the heart valve are too loose and fail to shut tightly, allowing blood to flow backwards through the valve when the heart chamber contracts. Most commonly occurs in the mitral valve, but may affect any of the heart valves

Heart valve stenosis, the cusps or flaps of the heart valve are too stiff. Therefore, they are unable to open fully, making it difficult for blood to flow through, or to shut tightly, allowing blood to flow backwards. This condition may affect any of the heart valves

Heimlich maneuver, technique for removing a foreign body or food from the trachea or pharynx when it is choking a person. The maneuver consists of applying pressure just under the diaphragm to pop the obstruction out

Hematemesis, to vomit blood from the gastrointestinal tract, often looks like coffee grounds

Hematic, pertaining to blood

Hematic system, the system that consists of plasma and blood cells—erythrocytes, leukocytes, and platelets; responsible for transporting oxygen, protecting against pathogens, and controlling bleeding

Hematinic, substance that increases the number of erythrocytes or the amount of hemoglobin in the blood

Hematochezia, passing bright red blood in the stools

Hematocrit (Hct, Hct, crit), blood test to measure the volume of red blood cells (erythrocytes) within the total volume of blood

Hematologist, a physician who specializes in treating diseases and conditions of the blood

Hematology, branch of medicine specializing in conditions of the hematic system

Hematoma, swelling or mass of blood caused by a break in a vessel in an organ or tissue, or beneath the skin

Hematopoiesis, the process of forming blood

Hematosalpinx, condition of having blood in the fallopian tubes

Hematuria, condition of blood in the urine

Hemianopia, loss of vision in half of the visual field. A stroke patient may suffer from this disorder

Hemiparesis, weakness or loss of motion on one side of the body

Hemiplegia, paralysis on only one side of the body

Hemodialysis (HD), use of an artificial kidney machine that filters the blood of a person to remove waste products. Use of this technique in patients who have defective kidneys is lifesaving

Hemoglobin (Hg), iron-containing pigment of red blood cells that carries oxygen from the lungs to the tissue

Hemolysis, the destruction of blood cells

Hemolytic, destruction of blood

Hemolytic anemia, an anemia that develops as the result of the excessive loss of erythrocytes

Hemolytic disease of the newborn (HDN), condition in which antibodies in the mother's blood enter the fetus's blood and cause anemia, jaundice, edema, and enlargement of the liver and spleen. Also called *erythroblastosis fetalis*

Hemolytic reaction, the destruction of a patient's erythrocytes that occurs when receiving a transfusion of an incompatible blood type. Also called a *transfusion reaction*

Hemophilia, hereditary blood disease in which there is a prolonged blood clotting time. It is transmitted by a sex-linked trait from females to males. It appears almost exclusively in males

Hemoptysis, coughing up blood or blood-stained sputum

Hemorrhage, blood flow, the escape of blood from a blood vessel

Hemorrhoid, varicose veins in the rectum

Hemorrhoidectomy, surgical excision of hemorrhoids from the anorectal area

Hemostasis, to stop bleeding or the stagnation of the circulating blood

Hemostat, a surgical instrument used to grasp blood vessels to control bleeding

Hemothorax, condition of having blood in the chest cavity

Hepatic, pertaining to the liver

Hepatic duct, the duct that leads from the liver to the common bile duct; transports bile

Hepatitis, infectious, inflammatory disease of the liver. Hepatitis B and C types are spread by contact with blood and bodily fluids of an infected person

Hepatoma, liver tumor

Herniated nucleus pulposus (HNP), a rupture of the fibrocartilage disk between two vertebrae. This results in pressure on a spinal nerve and causes pain, weakness, and nerve damage. Also called a slipped disk

Hernioplasty, surgical repair of a hernia; also called herniorrhaphy

Herpes labialis, infection of the lip by the herpes simplex virus type 1 (HSV-1). Also called *fever blisters* or *cold sores*

Hertz (Hz), measurement of the frequency or pitch of sound. The lowest pitch on an audiogram is 250 Hz. The measurement can go as high as 8000 Hz, which is the highest pitch measured

Hesitancy, a decrease in the force of the urine stream, often with difficulty initiating the flow. It is often a symptom of a blockage along the urethra, such as an enlarged prostate gland

Heterograft, skin graft from an animal of another species (usually a pig) to a human; also called a *xenograft*

Hiatal hernia, protrusion of the stomach through the diaphragm and extending into the thoracic cavity; gastroesophageal reflux disease is a common symptom

Hilum, the controlled entry/exit point of an organ such as the kidney or lung

Hirsutism, excessive hair growth over the body

Histology, the study of tissues

Histoplasmosis, pulmonary disease caused by a fungus found in dust in the droppings of pigeons and chickens

History and physical, medical record document written by the admitting physician. It details the patient's history, results of the physician's examination, initial diagnoses, and physician's plan of treatment

Hives, appearance of wheals as part of an allergic reaction

Hodgkin's disease (HD), also called Hodgkin's lymphoma. Cancer of the lymphatic cells found in concentration in the lymph nodes

Holter monitor, portable ECG monitor worn by the patient for a period of a few hours to a few days to assess the heart and pulse activity as the person goes through the activities of daily living

Home health care, agencies that provide nursing, therapy, personal care, or housekeeping services in the patient's own home

Homeostasis, steady state or state of balance within the body. The kidneys assist in maintaining this regulatory, steady state

Homologous transfusion, replacement of blood by transfusion of blood received from another person

Hordeolum, a *stye* (or sty), a small purulent inflammatory infection of a sebaceous gland of the eye, treated with hot compresses and surgical incision

Horizontal plane, a horizontal plane that divides the body into upper (superior) and lower (inferior) sections. Also called the *transverse plane*

Hormonal contraception, use of hormones to block ovulation and prevent contraception. May be in the form of a pill, a patch, an implant under the skin, or injection

Hormone, a chemical substance secreted by an endocrine gland. It enters the blood stream and is carried to target tissue. Hormones work to control the functioning of the target tissue. Given to replace the loss of natural hormones or to treat disease by stimulating hormonal effects

Hormone replacement therapy (HRT), artificial replacement of hormones in a patient who is unable to produce sufficient hormones. Example is estrogen replacement in menopausal women

Hormone therapy, treatment of cancer with natural hormones or with chemicals that produce hormonelike effects

Hospice, an organized group of healthcare workers who provide supportive treatment to dying patients and their families

Human growth hormone therapy, therapy with human growth hormone in order to stimulate skeletal growth; used to treat children with abnormally short stature

Human immunodeficiency virus (HIV), virus that causes AIDS; also known as a retrovirus

Humanistic psychotherapy, form of psychological counseling in which the therapist does not delve into the patients' past; it is believed that patients can learn how to use their own internal resources to deal with their problems

Humeral, pertaining to the humerus or upper arm bone

Humerus, the upper arm bone in the upper extremity

Humoral immunity, immunity that responds to antigens, such as bacteria and foreign agents, by producing antibodies. Also called *antibody-mediated immunity*

Hydrocele, accumulation of fluid within the testes

Hydrocephalus, accumulation of cerebrospinal fluid within the ventricles of the brain, causing the head to be enlarged. It is treated by creating an artificial shunt for the fluid to leave the brain

Hydrochloric acid (HCl), acid secreted by the stomach lining. Aids in digestion

Hydronephrosis, distention of the pelvis due to urine collecting in the kidney resulting from an obstruction

Hydrotherapy, using water for treatment purposes

Hymen, a thin membranous tissue that covers the external vaginal opening or orifice. The membrane is broken during the first sexual encounter of the female. It can also be broken prematurely by the use of tampons or during some sports activities

Hymenectomy, surgical removal of the hymen. Performed when the hymen tissue is particularly tough

Hyoid bone, a single, U-shaped bone suspended in the neck between the mandible and larynx. It is a point of attachment for swallowing and speech muscles

Hypercalcemia, condition of having an excessive amount of calcium in the blood

Hypercapnia, excessive carbon dioxide

Hyperemesis, excessive vomiting

Hyperemia, redness of the skin caused by increased blood flow to the skin

Hyperesthesia, having excessive sensation

Hyperglycemia, having an excessive amount of glucose (sugar) in the blood

Hyperhidrosis, abnormal condition of excessive sweat

Hyperkalemia, condition of having an excessive amount of potassium in the blood

Hyperkinesia, an excessive amount of movement

Hyperlipidemia, condition of having too high a level of lipids such as cholesterol in the bloodstream; a risk factor for developing atherosclerosis and coronary artery disease

Hyperopia, with this condition a person can see things in the distance but has trouble reading material at close vision. Also known as *farsightedness*

Hyperparathyroidism, state of excessive thyroid

Hyperpigmentation, abnormal amount of pigmentation in the skin, which is seen in diseases such as acromegaly and adrenal insufficiency

Hyperpituitarism, state of excessive pituitary gland

Hyperplasia, excessive development of normal cells within an organ

Hyperpnea, excessive deep breathing

Hypersecretion, excessive hormone production by an endocrine gland

Hypertension, high blood pressure

Hyperthyroidism, condition resulting from overactivity of the thyroid gland that can result in a crisis situation. Also called *Graves' disease*

Hypertonia, excessive tone

Hypertrophy, an increase in the bulk or size of a tissue or structure

Hyperventilation, to breathe both fast (tachypnea) and deep (hyperpnea)

Hypnotic, substance used to produce sleep or hypnosis

Glossary

Hypocalcemia, condition of having a low calcium level in the blood

Hypochondria, a somatoform disorder involving a preoccupation with health concerns

Hypochromic anemia, anemia resulting from having insufficient hemoglobin in the erythrocytes; named because the hemoglobin molecule is responsible for the dark red color of the erythrocytes

Hypodermic, pertaining to under the skin

Hypodermis, the deepest layer of skin; composed primarily of adipose

Hypogastric, pertaining to below the stomach. An anatomical division of the abdomen, the middle section of the bottom row

Hypoglossal, pertaining to under the tongue

Hypoglycemia, condition of having a low sugar level in the blood

Hypokinesia, insufficient movement

Hyponatremia, condition of having a low sodium level in the blood

Hypoparathyroidism, state of insufficient thyroid

Hypopituitarism, state of insufficient pituitary gland

Hypopnea, insufficient or shallow breathing

Hyposecretion, deficient hormone production by an endocrine gland

Hypospadias, congenital opening of the male urethra on the underside of the penis

Hypotension, low blood pressure

Hypothalamus, a portion of the diencephalon that lies just below the thalamus. It controls body temperature, appetite, sleep, sexual desire, and emotions such as fear. It also regulates the release of hormones from the pituitary gland and regulates the parasympathetic and sympathetic nervous systems

Hypothyroidism, result of a deficiency in secretion by the thyroid gland. This results in a lowered basal metabolism rate with obesity, dry skin, slow pulse, low blood pressure, sluggishness, and goiter. Treatment is replacement with synthetic thyroid hormone

Hypotonia, insufficient tone

Hypoventilation, to breathe both slow (bradypnea) and shallow (hypopnea)

Hypoxemia, deficiency of oxygen in the blood

Hypoxia, absence of oxygen in the tissues

Hysterectomy, removal of the uterus

Hysteropexy, surgical fixation of the uterus

Hysterorrhexis, rupture of the uterus

Hysterosalpingography, process of taking an X-ray of the uterus and oviducts after a radiopaque material is injected into the organs

I

Iatrogenic, usually an unfavorable response that results from taking a medication

Ichthyoderma, dry and scaly skin condition

Ichthyosis, condition in which the skin becomes dry, scaly, and keratinized

Identical twins, twins that develop from the splitting of one fertilized ovum; these siblings have identical DNA

Idiosyncrasy, unusual or abnormal response to a drug or food

Ileal, pertaining to the ileum

Ileocecal valve, sphincter between the ileum and the cecum

Ileostomy, surgical creation of a passage through the abdominal wall into the ileum

Ileum, the third portion of the small intestines. Joins the colon at the cecum. The ileum and cecum are separated by the ileocecal valve

Ileus, severe abdominal pain, inability to pass stools, vomiting, and abdominal distention as a result of an intestinal blockage; may require surgery to reverse the blockage

Iliac, pertaining to the ilium; one of the pelvic bones

Ilium, one of three bones that form the os coxae or innominate bone of the pelvis

Immune response, ability of lymphocytes to respond to specific antigens

Immunity, the body's ability to defend itself against pathogens

Immunization, providing protection against communicable diseases by stimulating the immune system to produce antibodies against that disease. Children can now be immunized for the following diseases; hepatitis B, diphtheria, tetanus, pertussis, tetanus, *Haemophilus influenzae* type b, polio, measles, mumps, rubella, and chickenpox. Also called *vaccination*

Immunocompromised, having an immune system that is unable to respond properly to pathogens

515

Immunoglobulins (Ig), antibodies secreted by the B cells. All antibodies are immunoglobulins. They assist in protecting the body and its surfaces from the invasion of bacteria. For example, the immunoglobulin IgA in colostrum, the first milk from the mother, helps to protect the newborn from infection

Immunologist, a physician who specializes in treating infectious diseases and other disorders of the immune system

Immunology, branch of medicine specializing in conditions of the lymphatic and immune systems

Immunosuppressants, substances that block certain actions of the immune system; required to prevent rejection of a transplanted organ

Immunotherapy, the production or strengthening of a patient's immune system in order to treat a disease

Impacted fracture, fracture in which bone fragments are pushed into each other

Impetigo, a highly contagious staphylococcal skin infection, most commonly occurring on the faces of children. It begins as blisters that then rupture and dry into a thick, yellow crust

Implant, prosthetic device placed in the jaw to which a tooth or denture may be anchored

Implantable cardiovert-defibrillator, a device implanted in the heart that delivers an electrical shock to restore a normal heart rhythm. Particularly useful for persons who experience ventricular fibrillation

Impulse control disorders, inability to resist an impulse to perform some act that is harmful to the individual or others; includes kleptomania, pyromania, explosive disorder, and pathological gambling

Incision and drainage (I&D), making an incision to create an opening for the drainage of material such as pus

Incisors, biting teeth in the very front of the mouth that function to cut food into smaller pieces. Humans have eight incisors

Incus, one of the three ossicles of the middle ear. Also called the *anvil*

Infant respiratory distress syndrome (IRDS), a lung condition most commonly found in premature infants that is characterized by tachypnea and respiratory grunting. Also called *hyaline membrane disease* (HMD) and *respiratory distress syndrome of the newborn*

Infarct, area of tissue within an organ that undergoes necrosis (death) following the loss of blood supply

Inferior, directional term meaning toward the feet or tail, or below

Inferior vena cava, the branch of the vena cava that drains blood from the abdomen and lower body

Infertility, inability to produce children; generally defined as no pregnancy after properly timed intercourse for one year

Inflammation, the tissue response to injury from pathogens or physical agents; characterized by redness, pain, swelling, and feeling hot to touch

Influenza, viral infection of the respiratory system characterized by chills, fever, body aches, and fatigue. Commonly called the *flu*

Informed consent, a medical record document, voluntarily signed by the patient or a responsible party, that clearly describes the purpose, methods, procedures, benefits, and risks of a diagnostic or treatment procedure

Inguinal, pertaining to the groin area. There is a collection of lymph nodes in this region that drain each leg

Inguinal hernia, hernia or outpouching of intestines into the inguinal region of the body

Inhalation, (1) To breathe air into the lungs. Also called *inspiration*. (2) To introduce drugs into the body by inhaling them

Inner ear, the innermost section of the ear. It contains the cochlea, semicircular canals, saccule, and utricle

Innominate bone, also called the os coxae or hip bone. It is the pelvis portion of the lower extremity. It consists of the ilium, ischium, and pubis and unites with the sacrum and coccyx to form the pelvis

Insertion, the attachment of a skeletal muscle to the more movable bone in the joint

Insomnia, a sleeping disorder characterized by a marked inability to fall asleep

Inspiratory capacity (IC), the volume of air inhaled after a normal exhale

Inspiratory reserve volume (IRV), the air that can be forcibly inhaled after a normal respiration has taken place. Also called *complemental air*

Insulin, the hormone secreted by the pancreas. It regulates the level of sugar in the blood stream. The more insulin present in the blood, the lower the blood sugar will be

Insulin-dependent diabetes mellitus (IDDM), also called type 1 diabetes mellitus; it develops early in life when the pancreas stops insulin production. Persons with IDDM must take daily insulin injections

Insulinoma, tumor of the islets of Langerhans cells of the pancreas that secretes an excessive amount of insulin

Integument, another term for skin

Integumentary system, the skin and its appendages including sweat glands, oil glands, hair, and nails. Sense organs that allow us to respond to changes in temperature, pain, touch, and pressure are located in the skin. It is the largest organ in the body

Interatrial, pertaining to between the atria

Interatrial septum, the wall or septum that divides the left and right atria

Intercostal muscles, muscles between the ribs. When they contract, they raise the ribs, which helps to enlarge the thoracic cavity

Intermittent claudication, attacks of severe pain and lameness caused by ischemia of the muscles, typically the calf muscles; brought on by walking even very short distances

Intermittent positive pressure breathing (IPPB), method for assisting patients to breathe using a mask connected to a machine that produces an increased pressure

Internal medicine, branch of medicine involving the diagnosis and treatment of diseases and conditions of internal organs such as the respiratory system. The physician is an *internist*

Internal respiration, the process of oxygen and carbon dioxide exchange at the cellular level when oxygen leaves the bloodstream and is delivered to the tissues

Internal sphincter, ring of involuntary muscle that keeps urine within the bladder

Internist, a physician specialized in treating diseases and conditions of internal organs such as the respiratory system

Interstitial cystitis, disease of unknown cause in which there is inflammation and irritation of the bladder. Most commonly seen in middle-aged women

Interventricular, pertaining to between the ventricles

Interventricular septum, the wall or septum that divides the left and right ventricles

Intervertebral, pertaining to between vertebrae

Intervertebral disk, fibrous cartilage cushion between vertebrae

Intracavitary, injection into a body cavity such as the peritoneal and chest cavity

Intracoronary artery stent, placing a stent within a coronary artery to treat coronary ischemia due to atherosclerosis

Intracranial, pertaining to inside the skull

Intradermal (ID), (1) Pertaining to within the skin. (2) Injection of medication into the skin

Intramuscular (IM), injection of medication into the muscle

Intraocular, pertaining to within the eye

Intraoperative, period of time during an operation

Intrathecal, (1) Pertaining to within the meninges. (2) Injection into the meninges space surrounding the brain and spinal cord

Intrauterine device (IUD), device that is inserted into the uterus by a physician for the purpose of contraception

Intravenous (IV), injection into the veins. This route can be set up so that there is a continuous administration of medication

Intravenous cholecystography, a dye is administered intravenously to the patient that allows for X-ray visualization of the gallbladder

Intravenous pyelogram (IVP), injecting a contrast medium into a vein and then taking an X-ray to visualize the renal pelvis

Intussusception, an intestinal condition in which one portion of the intestine telescopes into an adjacent portion causing an obstruction and gangrene if untreated

Invasive disease, tendency of a malignant tumor to spread to immediately surrounding tissue and organs

Inversion, directional term meaning turning inward or inside out

Involuntary muscles, muscles under the control of the subconscious regions of the brain. The smooth muscles found in internal organs and cardiac muscles are examples of involuntary muscle tissue

Iodine, a mineral required by the thyroid to produce its hormones

Iridal, pertaining to the iris

Iridectomy, excision of the iris

Iridoplegia, paralysis of the iris

Iridosclerotomy, incision into the iris and sclera

Iris, the colored portion of the eye. It can dilate or constrict to change the size of the pupil and control the amount of light entering the interior of the eye

Iritis, inflammation of the iris

Iron-deficiency anemia, anemia that results from having insufficient iron to manufacture hemoglobin

Irregular bones, a type of bone having an irregular shape. Vertebrae are irregular bones

Irritable bowel syndrome (IBS), disturbance in the functions of the intestine from unknown causes. Symptoms generally include abdominal discomfort and an alteration in bowel activity. Also called *functional bowel syndrome* or *spastic colon*

Ischemia, localized and temporary deficiency of blood supply due to an obstruction of the circulation

Ischial, pertaining to the ischium, one of the pelvic bones

Ischium, one of the three bones that form the os coxae or innominate bone of the pelvis

Islets of Langerhans, the regions within the pancreas that secrete insulin and glucagon

J

Jaundice, yellow cast to the skin, mucous membranes, and the whites of the eyes caused by the deposit of bile pigment from too much bilirubin in the blood. Bilirubin is a waste product produced when worn-out red blood cells are broken down. May be a symptom of disorders such as gallstones blocking the common bile duct or carcinoma of the liver

Jejunal, pertaining to the jejunum

Jejunum, the middle portion of the small intestines. Site of nutrient absorption

Joint, the point at which two bones meet. It provides flexibility

Joint capsule, elastic capsule that encloses synovial joints

K

Kaposi's sarcoma (KS), form of skin cancer frequently seen in acquired immunodeficiency syndrome (AIDS) patients. Consists of brownish-purple papules that spread from the skin and metastasize to internal organs

Keloid, formation of a scar after an injury or surgery that results in a raised, thickened red area

Keratin, a hard protein substance produced by the body. It is found in hair and nails, and filling the inside of epidermal cells

Keratitis, inflammation of the cornea

Keratometer, instrument to measure the cornea

Keratometry, measurement of the curvature of the cornea using an instrument called a keratometer

Keratoplasty, surgical repair of the cornea (corneal transplant)

Keratosis, overgrowth and thickening of the epithelium

Keratotomy, incision into the cornea

Ketoacidosis, acidosis due to an excess of ketone bodies (waste products). A serious condition that requires immediate treatment and can result in death for the diabetic patient if not reversed

Ketonuria, ketones in the urine

Kidneys, the two kidneys are located in the lumbar region of the back behind the parietal peritoneum. They are under the muscles of the back, just a little above the waist. The kidneys have a concave or depressed area that gives them a bean-shaped appearance. The center of this concavity is called the hilum

Kidneys, ureters, bladder (KUD), x-ray taken of the abdomen demonstrating the kidneys, ureters, and bladder without using any contrast dye; also called a flat-plate abdomen

Kinesiology, the study of movement

Kleptomania, an impulse control disorder in which the patient is unable to refrain from stealing. The items are often trivial and unneeded

Kyphosis, abnormal increase in the outward curvature of the thoracic spine. Also known as hunchback or humpback

L

Labia majora, the outer folds of skin that serves as protection for the female external genitalia and urethral meatus

Labia minora, the inner folds of skin that serves as protection for the female external genitalia and urethral meatus

Labor, the period of time beginning with uterine contractions and ending with the birth of the baby. There are three stages: the dilation stage, the expulsion stage, and the placental stage

Labyrinth, the term that refers to the inner ear. It is several fluid-filled cavities within the temporal bone. The labyrinth consists of the cochlea, vestibule, and three semicircular canals. Hair cells called the organs of Corti line the inner ear. These hair cells change the sound vibrations to electrical impulses and send the impulses to the brain via the vestibulocochlear nerve

Labyrinthectomy, excision of the labyrinth

Labyrinthitis, labyrinth inflammation

Labyrinthotomy, incision in the labyrinth

Laceration, a torn or jagged wound; incorrectly used to describe a cut

Lacrimal, pertaining to tears

Lacrimal apparatus, consists of the lacrimal gland, lacrimal ducts, and the nasolacrimal duct

Lacrimal bone, a facial bone

Lacrimal ducts, tear ducts located in the inner corner of the eye socket. They collect the tears and drain them into the lacrimal sac

Lacrimal gland, a gland located in the outer corner of each eyelid. It washes the anterior surface of the eye with fluid called tears

Lactation, the function of secreting milk after childbirth from the breasts or mammary glands

Lacteals, lymphatic vessels in the intestines that serve to absorb fats from the diet

Lactic, pertaining to milk

Lactiferous ducts, carry milk from the milk-producing glands to the nipple

Lactiferous glands, milk-producing glands in the breast

Lactorrhea, discharge of milk

Laminectomy, removal of a portion of a vertebra in order to relieve pressure on the spinal nerve

Laparoscope, instrument to view inside the abdomen

Laparoscopic adrenalectomy, excision of the adrenal gland through a small incision in the abdomen and using endoscopic instruments

Laparoscopic cholecystectomy, excision of the gallbladder using a laparoscope

Laparoscopy, an instrument or scope is passed into the abdominal wall through a small incision. The abdominal cavity is then examined for tumors and other conditions with this lighted instrument. Also called *peritoneoscopy*

Laparotomy, incision into the abdomen

Laryngeal, pertaining to the larynx

Laryngectomy, surgical removal of the larynx. This procedure is most frequently performed for excision of cancer

Laryngitis, inflammation of the larynx causing difficulty in speaking

Laryngopharynx, the inferior section of the pharynx. It lies at the same level in the neck as the larynx. Air has already entered the larynx, therefore the laryngopharynx carries food and drink to the esophagus

Laryngoplasty, surgical repair of the larynx

Laryngoplegia, paralysis of the voice box

Laryngoscope, instrument to view the larynx

Laryngoscopy, examination of the interior of the larynx with a lighted instrument called a *laryngoscope*

Larynx, also called the *voice box*. Respiratory system organ responsible for producing speech. It is located just below the pharynx

Laser photocoagulation, the use of a laser beam to destroy very small precise areas of the retina; may be used to treat retinal detachment or macular degeneration

Laser surgery, use of a controlled beam of light for cutting, hemostasis, or tissue destruction

Laser therapy, removal of skin lesions and birthmarks using a laser beam that emits intense heat and power at a close range. The laser converts frequencies of light into one small, powerful beam

Laser-assisted in-situ keratomileusis (LASIK), correction of myopia using laser surgery to remove corneal tissue

Lateral (lat), directional term meaning to the side

Lateral epicondylitis, inflammation of the muscle attachment to the lateral epicondyle of the elbow; often caused by strongly gripping. Commonly called tennis elbow

Lateral recumbent position, lying on either the left or right side

Lateral view, positioning the patient so that the side of the body faces the X-ray machine

Lavage, using an NG tube to wash out the stomach

Laxative, a mild cathartic

Left hypochondriac, an anatomical division of the abdomen, the left side of the upper row

Left iliac, an anatomical division of the abdomen, the left side of the upper row

Left lower quadrant (LLQ), a clinical division of the abdomen. It contains portions of small and large intestines, left ovary and fallopian tube, and left ureter

Left lumbar, an anatomical division of the abdomen, the left side of the middle row

Left upper quadrant (LUQ), a clinical division of the abdomen. It contains the left lobe of the liver, spleen, stomach, portion of the pancreas, and portion of small and large intestines

Legally blind, describes a person who has severely impaired vision. Usually defined as having visual acuity of 20/200

Legionnaire's disease, severe, often fatal disease characterized by pneumonia and gastrointestinal symptoms. Caused by a gram-negative bacillus and named after people who came down with it at an American Legion convention in 1976

Lens, the transparent structure behind the pupil and iris. It functions to bend light rays so they land on the retina

Lesion, a general term for a wound, injury, or abnormality

Leukemia, cancer of the WBC-forming bone marrow; results in a large number of abnormal WBCs circulating in the blood

Leukocytes, also called *white blood cells* or WBCs. A group of several different types of cells that provide protection against the invasion of bacteria and other foreign material. They are able to leave the bloodstream and search out the foreign invaders (bacteria, virus, and toxins), where they perform phagocytosis

Leukocytosis, too many white cells

Leukoderma, disappearance of pigment from the skin in patches, causing a milk-white appearance. Also called *vitiligo*

Leukopenia, too few white (cells)

Leukopoiesis, white (cell) producing

Ligaments, very strong bands of connective tissue that bind bones together at a joint

Ligation and stripping, surgical treatment for varicose veins; the damaged vein is tied off (ligation) and removed (stripping)

Lingual tonsils, tonsils located on the very posterior section of the tongue as it joins with the pharynx

Lipectomy, surgical removal of fat

Lipocytes, medical term for cells that contain fat molecules

Lipoma, fatty tumor that generally does not metastasize

Liposuction, removal of fat beneath the skin by means of suction

Lips, the anterior opening of the oral cavity

Lithium, special category of drug used successfully to calm patients who suffer from bipolar disorder

Lithotomy, surgical incision to remove kidney stones

Lithotomy position, lying face up with hips and knees bent at 90° angles

Lithotripsy, destroying or crushing kidney stones in the bladder or urethra with a device called a lithotriptor

Liver, a large organ located in the right upper quadrant of the abdomen. It serves many functions in the body. Its digestive system role includes producing bile, processing the absorbed nutrients, and detoxifying harmful substances

Liver transplant, transplant of a liver from a donor

Lobectomy, surgical removal of a lobe from an organ, such as a lung. Often the treatment of choice for lung cancer; may also be the removal of one lobe of the thyroid gland

Lobes, subdivisions of an organ such as the lungs or brain

Local anesthesia, substance that produces a loss of sensation in one localized part of the body. The patient remains conscious when this type of anesthetic is used. It is administered either topically or via a subcutaneous route

Long bone, a type of bone that is longer than it is wide. Examples include the femur, humerus, and phalanges

Long-term care facility, a facility that provides long-term care for patients who need extra time to recover from an illness or accident before they return home or for persons who can no longer care for themselves. Also called a *nursing home*

Longitudinal section, an internal view of the body produced by a lengthwise slice along the long axis of a structure

Loop of Henle, a portion of the renal tubule

Lordosis, abnormal increase in the forward curvature of the lumbar spine. Also known as *swayback*

Lower esophageal sphincter, also called the cardiac sphincter. Prevents food and gastric juices from backing up into the esophagus

Lower extremity (LE), the leg

Lower gastrointestinal series (lower GI series), x-ray image of the colon and rectum is taken after the administration of barium by enema; also called a *barium enema*

Lumbar, pertaining to the five low back vertebrae

Lumbar puncture (LP), puncture with a needle into the lumbar area (usually the fourth intervertebral space) to withdraw fluid for examination and for the injection of anesthesia. Also called *spinal puncture* or *spinal tap*

Lumbar vertebrae, the five vertebrae in the low back region

Lumen, the space, cavity, or channel within a tube or tubular organ or structure in the body

Lumpectomy, excision of only a breast tumor and the tissue immediately surrounding it

Lungs, the major organs of respiration. The lungs consist of air passageways, the bronchi and bronchioles, and the air sacs, alveoli. Gas exchange takes place within the alveoli

Lunula, the lighter-colored, half-moon region at the base of a nail

Luteinizing hormone (LH), a hormone secreted by the anterior pituitary. It regulates function of male and female gonads and plays a role in releasing ova in females

Lymph, clear, transparent, colorless fluid found in the lymphatic vessels and the cisterna chyli

Lymph glands, another name for *lymph nodes;* small organs composed of lymphatic tissue located along the route of the lymphatic vessels; remove impurities from the lymph and manufacture lymphocytes and antibodies

Lymph nodes, small organs in the lymphatic system that filter bacteria and other foreign organisms from the body fluids

Lymphadenectomy, excision of the lymph node. This is usually done to test for malignancy

Lymphadenitis, inflammation of the lympth glands. Referred to as swollen glands

Lymphadenopathy, disease of the lymph nodes

Lymphangiogram, x-ray taken of the lymph vessels after the injection of dye. The lymph flow through the chest is traced

Lymphangiography, process of taking an X-ray of the lymph vessels after the injection of a radiopaque material

Lymphangioma, lymph vessel tumor

Lymphatic, pertaining to lymph

Lymphatic and immune system

Lymphatic capillaries, the smallest lymph vessels; they collect excessive tissue fluid

Lymphatic ducts, the two largest vessels in the lymphatic system, the right lymphatic duct and the thoracic duct

Lymphatic system, system that helps the body fight infection. Organs include the spleen, lymph vessels, and lymph nodes

Lymphatic vessels, extensive network of vessels throughout the entire body; conduct lymph from the tissue toward the thoracic cavity

Lymphedema, edema appearing in the extremities due to an obstruction of the lymph flow through the lymphatic vessels

Lymphocytes, an agranulocyte white blood cell that provides protection through the immune response

Lymphoma, a tumor of lymphatic tissue

M

Macrophage, phagocytic cells that are found in large quantities in the lymph nodes. They engulf foreign particles

Macrotia, abnormally large ears

Macula lutea, images are projected onto the area of the retina

Macular degeneration, deterioration of the macular area of the retina of the eye. May be treated with laser surgery to destroy the blood vessels beneath the macula

Macule, flat, discolored area that is flush with the skin surface. An example would be a freckle or a birthmark

Magnetic resonance imaging (MRI), medical imaging that uses radio-frequency radiation as its source of energy. It does not require the injection of contrast medium or exposure to ionizing radiation. The technique is useful for visualizing large blood vessels, the heart, the brain, and soft tissues

Major depression, a mood disorder characterized by a marked loss of interest in usually enjoyable activities, disturbances in sleep and eating patterns, fatigue, suicidal thoughts, and feelings of hopelessness, worthlessness, and guilt

Male reproductive system, system responsible for producing sperm for reproduction; organs include testes, vas deferens, urethra, prostate gland, and penis

Malignant, a tumor that is cancerous. Malignant tumors are generally progressive and recurring

Malignant melanoma (MM), malignant, darkly pigmented tumor or mole of the skin

Malingering, a type of factitious disorder in which the patient intentionally feigns illness for attention or secondary gain

Malleus, one of the three ossicles of the middle ear. Also called the *hammer*

Mammary, pertaining to the breast

Mammary glands, the breasts; milk-producing glands to provide nutrition for newborn

Mammogram, x-ray record of the breast

Mammography, process of X-raying the breast

Mammoplasty, surgical repair of the breast

Mandible, the lower jawbone

Mandibular, pertaining to the mandible or lower jaw

Mania, a mood disorder characterized by extreme elation and euphoria. The patient displays rapid speech, flight of ideas, decreased sleep, distractibility, grandiosity, and poor judgment

Masochism, a sexual disorder characterized by receiving sexual gratification from being hurt or abused

Massage, kneading or applying pressure by hands to a part of the patient's body to promote muscle relaxation and reduce tension

Mastalgia, breast pain

Mastectomy, excision of the breast

Mastitis, inflammation of the breast, which is common during lactation but can occur at any age

Maxilla, the upper jawbone

Maxillary, pertaining to the maxilla or upper jaw

Meatotomy, surgical enlargement of the urinary opening (meatus)

Meconium, a substance that collects in the intestines of a fetus and becomes the first stool of a newborn

Medial, directional term meaning to the middle or near the middle of the body or the structure

Median plane, plane that runs lengthwise from front to back and divides the body or any of its parts into right and left portions; also called the *sagittal plane*

Mediastinal, there is a collection of lymph nodes located in the mediastinum (central chest area) that drain the chest

Mediastinum, the central region of the chest cavity. It contains the organs between the lungs, including the heart, aorta, esophagus, and trachea

Medical record, documents the details of a patient's hospital stay. Each health care professional that has contact with the patient in any capacity completes the appropriate report of that contact and adds it to the medical chart. This results in a permanent physical record of the patient's day-to-day condition, when and what services he or she receives, and the response to treatment. Also called a chart

Medulla, the central area of an organ. In the endocrine system it refers to the adrenal medulla; in the urinary system, it refers to the inner portion of the kidney

Medulla oblongata, a portion of the brain stem that connects the spinal cord with the brain. It contains the respiratory, cardiac, and blood pressure control centers

Medullary, pertaining to the medulla

Medullary cavity, the large open cavity that extends the length of the shaft of a long bone; contains yellow bone marrow

Melanin, the black color pigment in the skin. It helps to prevent the sun's ultraviolet rays from entering the body

Melanocyte-stimulating hormone (MSH), a hormone secreted by the anterior pituitary. It stimulates pigment production in the skin

Melanocytes, special cells in the basal layer of the epidermis. They contain the black pigment melanin that gives skin its color and protects against the ultraviolet rays of the sun

Melanoma, also called *malignant melanoma.* A dangerous form of skin cancer caused by an overgrowth of melanin in a melanocyte. It may metastasize or spread. Exposure to ultraviolet light is a risk factor for developing melanoma

Melatonin, hormone secreted by the pineal gland; plays a role in regulating the body's circadian rhythm

Melena, passage of dark tarry stools; color is the result of digestive enzymes working on blood in the stool

Menarche, the first menstrual period

Ménière's disease, abnormal condition within the labyrinth of the inner ear that can lead to a progressive loss of hearing. The symptoms are dizziness or vertigo, hearing loss, and tinnitus (ringing in the ears)

Meningeal, pertaining to the meninges

Meninges, three connective tissue membrane layers that surround the brain and spinal cord. The three layers are dura mater, arachnoid layer, and pia mater. The dura mater and arachnoid layer are separated by the subdural space. The arachnoid layer and pia mater are separated by the subarachnoid space

Meningioma, slow-growing tumor in the meninges of the brain

Meningitis, inflammation of the membranes of the spinal cord and brain that is caused by a microorganism

Meningocele, congenital hernia in which the meninges, or membranes, protrude through an opening in the spinal column or brain

Menometrorrhagia, excessive bleeding during the menstrual period and at intervals between menstrual periods

Menopause, cessation or ending of menstrual activity. This is generally between the ages of 40 and 55

Menorrhagia, excessive bleeding during the menstrual period. Can be either in the total number of days or the amount of blood or both

Menstrual cycle, the 28-day fertility cycle in women; includes ovulation and sloughing off the endometrium if a pregnancy does not occur

Menstrual period, another name for the menstrual cycle

Menstruation, the loss of blood and tissue as the endometrium is shed by the uterus. The flow exits the body through the cervix and vagina. The flow occurs approximately every 28 days

Mental retardation, a disorder characterized by a diminished ability to process intellectual functions

Metacarpal, pertaining to the hand bones

Metacarpals, the hand bones in the upper extremity

Metastases (mets), the spreading of a cancerous tumor from its original site to different locations of the body. Singular is metastasis

Metastasis (mets), movement and spread of cancer cells from one part of the body to another. Metastases is plural

Metastasize, when cancerous cells migrate away from a tumor site. They commonly move through the lymphatic system and become trapped in lymph nodes

Metatarsal, pertaining to the foot bones

Metatarsals, the ankle bones in the lower extremity

Metrorrhagia, rapid (menstrual) blood flow from the uterus

Metrorrhea, discharge from the uterus

Microtia, abnormally small ears

Micturition, another term for urination

Midbrain, a portion of the brain stem

Middle ear, the middle section of the ear. It contains the ossicles

Migraine, a specific type of headache characterized by severe head pain, photophobia, vertigo, and nausea

Mineralocorticoids, a group of hormones secreted by the adrenal cortex. They regulate electrolytes and fluid volume in the body. Aldosterone is an example of a mineralocorticoid

Minor tranquilizers, medications that are central nervous system depressants and are prescribed for anxiety

Miotic, substance that causes the pupil to constrict

Mitral valve, a valve between the left atrium and ventricle in the heart. It prevents blood from flowing backwards into the atrium. It is also called the bicuspid valve because it has two cusps or flaps

Mobility, state of having normal movement of all body parts

Mobilization, treatments such as exercise and massage to restore movement to joints and soft tissue

Moist hot packs, applying moist warmth to a body part to produce the slight dilation of blood vessels in the skin; causes muscle relaxation in the deeper regions of the body and increases circulation, which aids healing

Molars, large somewhat flat-topped back teeth. Function to grind food. Humans have up to twelve molars

Monoaural, referring to one ear

Monochromatism, unable to perceive one color

Monocytes (monos), an agranulocyte white blood cell that is important for phagocytosis

Mononucleosis (Mono), acute infectious disease with a large number of atypical lymphocytes. Caused by the Epstein–Barr virus. There may be abnormal liver function

Monoparesis, weakness of one extremity

Monoplegia, paralysis of one extremity

Monospot, test of infectious mononucleosis in which there is a nonspecific antibody called heterophile antibody

Mood disorders, characterized by instability in mood; includes major depression, mania, and bipolar disorder

Morbidity, number that represents the number of sick persons in a particular population

Mortality, number that represents the number of deaths in a particular population

Motor neurons, nerves that carry activity instruction from the CNS to muscles or glands out in the body; also called *efferent neurons.*

Mucolytic, substance that liquefies mucus so it is easier to cough and clear it from the respiratory tract

Mucous membrane, membrane that lines body passages that open directly to the exterior of the body, such as the mouth and reproductive tract, and secretes a thick substance, or mucus

Mucus, sticky fluid secreted by mucous membrane lining of the respiratory tract. Assists in cleansing air by trapping dust and bacteria

Multigravida, woman who has had more than one pregnancy

Multipara, woman who has given birth to more than one child

Multiple personality disorder, a type of dissociative disorder in which the person displays two or more distinct conscious personalities that alternate in controlling the body. The alternate personalities may or may not be aware of each other

Multiple sclerosis (MS), inflammatory disease of the central nervous system. Rare in children. Generally strikes adults between the ages of 20 and 40. There is progressive weakness and numbness

Murmur, an abnormal heart sound as a soft blowing sound or a harsh click. It may be soft and heard only with a stethoscope, or so loud it can be heard several feet away. Also called a *bruit*

Muscle biopsy, removal of muscle tissue for pathological examination

Muscle tissue, tissue that is able to contract and shorten its length, thereby producing movement. Muscle tissue may be under voluntary control (attached to the bones) or involuntary control (heart and digestive organs)

Muscle tissue fibers, the bundles of muscle tissue that form a muscle

Muscles, muscles are bundles of parallel muscle tissue fibers. As the fibers contract (shorten in length) they pull whatever they are attached to closer together. This may move two bones closer together or make an opening more narrow. A muscle contraction occurs when a message is transmitted from the brain through the nervous system to the muscles. *See also* Muscular system

Muscular, pertaining to muscles

Muscular dystrophy (MD), inherited disease causing a progressive muscle weakness and atrophy

Musculoskeletal system. system that provides support for the body and produces movement. Organs of the musculoskeletal system includes muscles, tendons, bones, joints, and cartilage. *See* Muscular system; Skeletal system

Mutation, change or transformation from the original

Myalgia, muscle pain

Myasthenia, lack of muscle strength

Myasthenia gravis, disorder causing loss of muscle strength and paralysis. This is an autoimmune disease

Mycoplasma **pneumonia,** a less severe but longer lasting form of pneumonia caused by the *Mycoplasma pneumoniae* bacteria. Also called *walking pneumonia*

Mydriatic, substance that causes the pupil to dilate

Myelin, tissue that wraps around many of the nerve fibers. It is composed of fatty material and functions as an insulator

Myelinated, nerve fibers covered with a layer of myelin

Myelitis, inflammation of the spinal cord

Myelogram, x-ray record of the spinal cord following injection of meninges with radiopaque dye

Myelography, injection of a radiopaque dye into the spinal canal. An X-ray is then taken to examine the normal and abnormal outlines made by the dye

Myeloma, malignant neoplasm originating in plasma cells in the bone

Myelomeningocele, a hernia composed of meninges and spinal cord

Myocardial, pertaining to heart muscle

Myocardial infarction (MI), condition caused by the partial or complete occlusion or closing of one or more of the coronary arteries. Symptoms include severe chest pain or heavy pressure in the middle of the chest. A delay in treatment could result in death. Also referred to as *MI* or *heart attack*

Myocarditis, inflammation of heart muscle

Myocardium, the middle layer of the muscle. It is thick and composed of cardiac muscle. This layer produces the heart contraction

Myometrium, the middle muscle layer of the uterus

Myoneural junction, the point at which a nerve contacts a muscle fiber

Myopathy, any disease of muscles

Myopia, with this condition a person can see things that are close up but distance vision is blurred. Also known as *nearsightedness*

Myoplasty, surgical repair of muscle

Myorrhaphy, suture a muscle

Myorrhexis, muscle ruptured

Myotonia, muscle tone

Myringectomy, excision of the eardrum

Myringitis, eardrum inflammation

Myringoplasty, surgical reconstruction of the eardrum. Also called *tympanoplasty*

Myringotomy, surgical puncture of the eardrum with removal of fluid and pus from the middle ear, to eliminate a persistent ear infection and excessive pressure on the tympanic membrane. A polyethylene tube is placed in the tympanic membrane to allow for drainage of the middle ear cavity

Myxedema, condition resulting from a hypofunction of the thyroid gland. Symptoms can include anemia, slow speech, enlarged tongue and facial features, edematous skin, drowsiness, and mental apathy

N

Nail bed, connects nail body to connective tissue underneath

Nail body, flat plate of keratin that forms most of the nails

Nail root, base of a nail; nails grow longer from the root

Nails, a structure in the integumentary system

Narcissistic personality, a personality disorder characterized by an abnormal sense of self-importance

Narcotic analgesic, drug used to treat severe pain; has the potential to be habit forming if taken for a prolonged time. Also called opiates

Nares, external openings of the nose that open into the nasal cavity

Nasal bone, a facial bone

Nasal cannula, two-pronged plastic device for delivering oxygen into the nose; one prong is inserted into each naris

Nasal cavity, large cavity just behind the external nose that receives the outside air. It is covered with mucous membrane to cleanse the air. The nasal septum divides the nasal cavity into left and right halves

Nasal septum, a flexible cartilage wall that divides the nasal cavity into left and right halves. It is covered by mucous membrane

Nasogastric, pertaining to the nose and stomach

Nasogastric intubation (NG tube), a flexible catheter is inserted into the nose and down the esophagus to the stomach; may be used for feeding or to suction out stomach fluids

Nasolacrimal duct, duct that collects tears from the inner corner of the eye socket and drains them into the nasal cavity

Nasopharyngitis, inflammation of nasal cavity and throat

Nasopharynx, the superior section of the pharynx that receives air from the nose

Natural immunity, immunity that is not specific to a particular disease and does not require prior exposure to the pathogen. Also called innate immunity

Natural killer (NK) cells, t cells that can kill by entrapping foreign cells, tumor cells, and bacteria. Also called T8 cells

Nausea, a feeling of needing to vomit

Neck, a narrow length of bone that connects the ball of a ball-and-socket joint to the diaphysis of a long bone

Necrosis, dead tissue

Neonate, term used to describe the newborn infant during the first four weeks of life

Neonatologist, specialist in the treatment of the newborn

Neonatology, study of the newborn

Neoplasm, an abnormal growth of tissue that may be benign or malignant. Also called a *tumor*

Nephrectomy, excision of a kidney

Nephritis, inflammation of the kidney

Nephrogram, x-ray of the kidney

Nephrolith, kidney stone

Nephrolithiasis, the presence of calculi in the kidney

Nephrolithotomy, incision into the kidney to remove a stone,

Nephrologist, specialist in the treatment of kidney disorders,

Nephrology, branch of medicine specializing in conditions of the urinary system

Nephroma, kidney tumor

Nephromalacia, softening of the kidney

Nephromegaly, enlarged kidney

Nephron, the functional or working unit of the kidney that filters the blood and produces the urine. There are more than 1 million nephrons in an adult kidney. Each nephron consists of a renal corpuscle and the renal tubules

Nephropathy, kidney disease

Nephropexy, surgical fixation of a kidney

Nephroptosis, drooping kidney

Nephrosclerosis, hardening of the kidney

Nephrosis, abnormal condition (degeneration) of the kidney

Nephrostomy, creating a new opening across the body wall into the kidney

Nephrotic syndrome (NS), damage to the glomerulus resulting in protein appearing in the urine, proteinuria, and the corresponding decrease in protein in the bloodstream

Nephrotomy, incision into a kidney

Nerve block, also referred to as regional anesthesia. This anesthetic interrupts a patient's pain sensation in a particular region of the body. The anesthetic is injected near the nerve that will be blocked from sensation. The patient usually remains conscious

Nerve cell body, the portion of the nerve cell that includes the nucleus*f*

Nerve conduction velocity, a test to determine if nerves have been damaged by recording the rate at which an electrical impulse travels along a nerve. If the nerve is damaged, the velocity will be decreased

Nerve root, the point where a spinal or cranial nerve is attached to the CNS

Nerves, structures in the nervous system that conduct electrical impulses from the brain and spinal cord to muscles and other organs

Nervous system, system that coordinates all the conscious and subconscious activities of the body. Organs include the brain, spinal cord, and nerves

Nervous tissue, nervous tissue conducts electrical impulses to and from the brain and the rest of the body

Neural, pertaining to nerves

Neuralgia, nerve pain

Neurectomy, excision of a nerve

Neurogenic bladder, loss of nervous control that leads to retention; may be caused by spinal cord injury or multiple sclerosis

Neuroglial cells, cells that perform support functions for neurons

Neurologist, physician who specializes in disorders of the nervous system

Neurology, branch of medicine specializing in conditions of the nervous system

Neuroma, nerve tumor

Neuron, the name for an individual nerve cell. Neurons group together to form nerves and other nervous tissue

Neuropathy, disease of the nerves

Neuroplasty, surgical repair of nerves

Neurorrhaphy, suture a nerve

Neurosurgery, branch of medicine specializing in surgery on the nervous system

Neurotransmitter, chemical messenger that carries an electrical impulse across the gap between two neurons

Neutrophils, granulocyte white blood cells that are important for phagocytosis. They are also the most numerous of the leukocytes

Nevus, pigmented (colored) congenital skin blemish, birthmark, or mole. Usually benign but may become cancerous

Nipple, point at which milk is released from the breast

Nitrogenous wastes, waste products that contain nitrogen. These products, such as ammonia and urea, are produced during protein metabolism

Nocturia, excessive urination during the night. May or may not be abnormal

Nodule, solid, raised group of cells

Non-Hodgkins's lymphoma (NHL), cancer of the lymphatic tissues other than Hodgkin's lymphoma

Non-insulin-dependent diabetes mellitus (NIDDM), also called type 2 diabetes mellitus. It develops later in life when the pancreas produces insufficient insulin; persons may take oral hypoglycemics to stimulate insulin secretion, or may eventually have to take insulin

Nonproprietary name, the recognized and accepted official name for a drug. Each drug has only one generic name, which is not subject to trademark, so any pharmaceutical manufacturer may use it. Also called *generic name*

Nonsteroidal antiinflammatory drugs (NSAIDs), a large group of drugs including aspirin and ibuprofen that provide mild pain relief and anti-inflammatory benefits for conditions such as arthritis

Norepinephrine, a hormone secreted by the adrenal medulla. It is a strong vasoconstrictor

Normal psychology, behaviors that include how the personality develops, how people handle stress, and the stages of mental development

Nosocomial infection, an infection acquired as a result of hospital exposure

Nuclear medicine, use of radioactive substances to diagnose diseases. A radioactive substance known to accumulate in certain body tissues is injected or inhaled. After waiting for the substance to travel to the body area of interest the radioactivity level is recorded. Commonly referred to as a *scan*

Nucleus, organelle of the cell that contains the DNA

Nulligravida, woman who has never been pregnant

Nullipara, woman who has never produced a viable baby

Nurse, to breastfeed a baby

Nurse anesthetist, a registered nurse who has received additional training and education in the administration of anesthetic medications

Nurse's notes, medical record document that records the patient's care throughout the day. It includes vital signs, treatment specifics, patient's response to treatment, and patient's condition

Nursing home, a facility that provides long-term care for patients who need extra time to recover from all illness or accident before they return home or for persons who can no longer care for themselves. Also called a *long-term care facility*

Nyctalopia, difficulty seeing in dim light; usually due to damaged rods

Nystagmus, jerky-appearing involuntary eye movement

O

Obesity, having an abnormal amount of fat in the body

Oblique fracture, fracture at an angle to the bone

Oblique muscles, oblique means slanted. Two of the eye muscles are oblique muscles

Oblique view, positioning the patient so that the X-rays pass through the body on an angle

Obsessive-compulsive disorder (OCD), a type of anxiety disorder in which the person performs repetitive rituals in order to reduce anxiety,

Obstetrics (OB), branch of medicine that treats women during pregnancy and childbirth, and immediately after childbirth

Occipital bone, a cranial bone

Occipital lobe, one of the four cerebral hemisphere lobes. It controls eyesight

Occupational Safety and Health Administration (OSHA), federal agency that issued mandatory guidelines to ensure that all employees at risk of exposure to body fluids are provided with personal protective equipment

Occupational therapy (OT), assists patients to regain, develop, and improve skills that are important for independent functioning. Occupational therapy personnel work with people who, because of illness, injury, developmental, or psychological impairments, require specialized training in skills that will enable them to lead independent, productive, and satisfying lives. Occupational therapists instruct patients in the use of adaptive equipment and techniques, body mechanics, and energy conservation. They also employ modalities such as heat, cold, and therapeutic exercise

Ocular, pertaining to the eye

Oculomycosis, condition of eye fungus

Oligomenorrhea, scanty menstrual flow

Oligospermia, condition of having few sperm

Oliguria, condition of scanty amount of urine

Oncogenic, cancer causing

Oncology, the branch of medicine dealing with tumors

Onychectomy, excision of a nail

Onychia, infected nailbed

Onychomalacia, softening of nails

Onychomycosis, abnormal condition of nail fungus

Onychophagia, nail biting

Oophorectomy, removal of an ovary

Oophoritis, inflammation of an ovary

Operative report, a medical record report from the surgeon detailing an operation. It includes a pre- and postprocedure itself, and how the patient tolerated the procedure

Ophthalmalgia, eye pain

Ophthalmic, pertaining to the eyes

Ophthalmic decongestants, over-the-counter medications that constrict the arterioles of the eye, reduce redness and itching of the conjunctiva

Ophthalmologist, a physician specialized in treating conditions and diseases of the eye

Ophthalmology (Ophth), branch of medicine specializing in condition of the eye

Ophthalmoplegia, paralysis of the eye

Ophthalmorrhagia, rapid bleeding from the eye

Ophthalmoscope, instrument to view inside the eye

Ophthalmoscopy, examination of the interior of the eyes using an instrument called an ophthalmoscope. The physician will dilate the pupil in order to see the cornea, lens, and retina. Identifies abnormalities in the blood vessels of the eye and some systemic diseases

Opportunistic infections, infectious diseases that are associated with AIDS since they occur as a result of the lowered immune system and resistance of the body to infections and parasites

Opposition, moves thumb away from palm; the ability to move the thumb into contact with the other fingers

Optic, pertaining to the eye

Optic disk, the area of the retina associated with the optic nerve. Also called the blind spot,

Optic nerve, the second cranial nerve that carries impulses from the retinas to the brain

Optician, grinds and fits prescription lenses and contacts as prescribed by a physician or optometrist,

Optometer, instrument to measure vision

Optometrist (OD), doctor of optometry; provides care for the eyes including examining the eyes for diseases, assessing visual acuity, prescribing corrective lenses and eye treatments, and educating patients

Optometry, process of measuring vision

Oral, (1) Pertaining to the mouth. (2) Administration of medication through the mouth

Oral cavity, the mouth

Oral contraceptive pills (OCPs), birth control medication that uses low doses of female hormones to prevent conception by blocking ovulation

Oral hypoglycemic agents, medication taken by mouth that causes a decrease in blood sugar. This is not used for insulin-dependent patients. There is no proof that this medication will prevent the long-term complications of diabetes mellitus

Orchidectomy, excision of the testes

Orchidopexy, surgical fixation to move undescended testes into the scrotum and attaching to prevent retraction

Orchiectomy, surgical removal of the testes

Orchioplasty, surgical repair of the testes

Orchiotomy, incision into the testes

Organic, pertaining to organs

Organic mental disease, deterioration of mental functions due to temporary brain or permanent brain dysfunction; includes dementia and Alzheimer's disease; also called *cognitive disorders.*

Organs, group of different types of tissue coming together to perform special functions. For example, the heart contains muscular fibers, nerve tissue, and blood vessels

Organs of Corti, the sensory receptor hair cells lining the cochlea. These cells change the sound vibrations to electrical impulses and send the impulses to the brain via the vestibulocochlear nerve

Origin, the attachment of a skeletal muscle to the less movable bone in the joint

Oropharynx, the middle section of the pharynx that receives food and drink from the mouth

Orthodontic, pertaining to straight teeth

Orthodontics, the dental specialty concerned with straightening teeth

Orthopedic surgery, the branch of medicine specializing in surgical treatments of the musculoskeletal system

Orthopedics (Ortho), branch of medicine specializing in the diagnosis and treatment of conditions of the musculoskeletal system

Orthopnea, term to describe a patient who needs to sit up straight in order to breathe comfortably

Orthostatic hypotension, the sudden drop in blood pressure a person experiences when standing up suddenly

Orthotics, the use of equipment, such as splints and braces, to support a paralyzed muscle, promote a specific motion, or correct musculoskeletal deformities

Os coxae, also called the innominate bone or hip bone. It is the pelvis portion of the lower extremity. It consists of the ilium, ischium, and pubis and unites with the sacrum and coccyx to form the pelvis

Osseous tissue, bony tissue. One of the hardest tissues in the body

Ossicles, the three small bones in the middle ear. The bones are the incus, malleus, and stapes. The ossicles amplify and conduct the sound waves to the inner ear

Ossification, the process of bone formation

Ostealgia, bone pain

Osteoarthritis (OA), noninflammatory type of arthritis resulting in degeneration of the bones and joints, especially those bearing weight

Osteoblast, an embryonic bone cell

Osteochondroma, tumor composed of both cartilage and bony substance

Osteoclasia, intentional breaking of a bone in order to correct a deformity

Osteocyte, mature bone cells

Osteogenic sarcoma, the most common type of bone cancer; usually begins in osteocytes found at the ends of long bones

Osteomalacia, softening of the bones caused by a deficiency of phosphorus or calcium. It is thought that in children the cause is insufficient sunlight and vitamin D

Osteomyelitis, inflammation of the bone and bone marrow due to infection; can be difficult to treat

Osteopathy, form of medicine that places great emphasis on the musculoskeletal system and the body system as a whole. Manipulation is also used as part of the treatment

Osteoporosis, decrease in bone mass that results in a thinning and weakening of the bone with resulting fractures. The bone becomes more porous, especially in the spine and pelvis

Osteotome, an instrument to cut bone

Osteotomy, incision into a bone

Otalgia, ear pain

Otic, pertaining to the ear

Otitis, ear inflammation

Otitis externa (OE), external ear infection; most commonly caused by fungus. Also called *otomycosis* and commonly referred to as *swimmer's ear*

Otitis media (OM), commonly referred to as middle ear infection; seen frequently in children. Often preceded by an upper respiratory infection

Otologist, a physician specialized in the diagnosis and treatment of diseases of the ear

Otology (Oto), study of the ear

Otomycosis, fungal infection of the ear, usually in the auditory canal

Otoplasty, corrective surgery to change the size of the external ear or pinna. The surgery can either enlarge or lessen the size of the pinna

Otopyorrhea, pus discharge from the ear

Otorhinolaryngology (ENT), branch of medicine that treats diseases of the ears, nose, and throat. Also referred to as *ENT*

Otorrhagia, bleeding from the ear

Otosclerosis, progressive hearing loss caused by immobility of the stapes bone

Otoscope, instrument to view inside the ear

Otoscopy, examination of the ear canal, eardrum, and outer ear using the otoscope. Foreign material can be removed from the ear canal with this procedure

Outpatient clinic, a facility that provides services that do not require overnight hospitalization. The services range from simple surgeries to diagnostic testing to therapy. Also called an ambulatory care center or a surgical center

Ova, female sex cells or gametes produced in the ovary. An ovum fuses with a sperm to produce an embryo. Singular is ovum

Ova and parasites, laboratory examination of feces with a microscope for the presence of parasites or their eggs

Oval window, the division between the middle and inner ear

Ovarian, pertaining to the ovaries

Ovarian carcinoma, cancer of the ovary

Ovarian cyst, sac that develops within the ovary

Ovaries, the female gonads. These two glands are located on either side of the lower abdominopelvic region of the female. They are responsible for the production of the sex cells, ova, and the hormones estrogen and progesterone

Over-the-counter (OTC), drugs that are accessible in drugstores without a prescription. Also called *nonprescription drugs*

Oviducts, tubes that carry the ovum from the ovary to the uterus; also called fallopian tubes or uterine tubes

Ovulation, the release of an ovum from the ovary

Oximeter, instrument to measure oxygen

Oximetry, process of measuring oxygen

Oxygen (O_2), gaseous element absorbed by the blood from the air sacs in the lungs. It is necessary for cells to make energy

Oxygenated, term for blood with a high oxygen level

Oxytocin, a hormone secreted by the posterior pituitary. It stimulates uterine contractions during labor and delivery

P

Pacemaker, another name for the sinoatrial node of the heart

Pacemaker implantation, electrical device that substitutes for the natural pacemaker of the heart. It controls the beating of the heart by a series of rhythmic electrical impulses. An external pacemaker has the electrodes on the outside of the body; an internal pacemaker has the electrodes surgically implanted within the chest wall

Packed cells, a transfusion of only the formed elements and without plasma

Paget's disease, a fairly common metabolic disease of the bone from unknown causes. It usually attacks middle-aged and elderly people and is characterized by bone destruction and deformity

Pain control, managing pain through the use of a variety of means, including medications, biofeedback, and mechanical devices

Palate, the roof of the mouth. The anterior portion is hard or bony, and the posterior portion is soft or flexible

Palatine bone, a facial bone

Palatine tonsils, tonsils located in the lateral wall of the pharynx close to the mouth

Palatoplasty, surgical repair of the palate

Palliative therapy, treatment designed to reduce the intensity of painful symptoms, but not to produce a cure

Pallor, abnormal paleness of the skin

Palpitations, pounding, racing heartbeat

Palsy, temporary or permanent loss of the ability to control movement

Pancreas, organ in the digestive system that produces digestive enzymes. Also a gland in the endocrine system that produces two hormones, insulin and glucagon

Pancreatic, pertaining to the pancreas

Pancreatic duct, duct carrying pancreatic juices from the pancreas to the duodenum

Pancreatic enzymes, digestive enzymes produced by the pancreas and added to the chyme in the duodenum

Pancreatitis, inflammation of the pancreas

Pancytopenia, too few of all types of blood cells

Panhypopituitarism, deficiency in all the hormones secreted by the pituitary gland; often recognized because of problems with the glands regulated by the pituitary—adrenal cortex, thyroid, ovaries, and testes

Panic attacks, a type of anxiety disorder characterized by a sudden onset of intense apprehension, fear, terror, or impending doom often accompanied by a racing heart rate

Pansinusitis, inflammation of all the sinuses

Pap (Papanicolaou) smear, test for the early detection of cancer of the cervix named after the developer of the test, George Papanicolaou, a Greek physician. A scraping of cells is removed from the cervix for examination under a microscope

Papilledema, swelling of the optic disk, often as a result of increased intraocular pressure. Also called *choked disk*

Papule, small, solid, circular raised spot on the surface of the skin, often as a result of an inflammation in an oil gland

Paracentesis, insertion of a needle into the abdominal cavity to withdraw fluid; tests to diagnose disease may be conducted on the fluid

Paralysis, temporary or permanent loss of function or voluntary movement

Paranasal sinuses, air-filled cavities within the facial bones that open into the nasal cavity; act as an echo chamber during sound production

Paranoid personality disorder, a personality disorder characterized by exaggerated feelings of persecution

Paraplegia, paralysis of the lower portion of the body and both legs

Parasympathetic branch, a branch of the autonomic nervous system. This system serves as a counterbalance for the sympathetic nerves. Therefore, it causes the heart rate to slow down, lower the blood pressure, constrict eye pupils, and increase digestion

Parathyroid glands, four small glands located on the back surface of the thyroid gland. The parathyroid hormone secreted by these glands regulates the amount of calcium in the blood

Parathyroid hormone (PTH), the hormone secreted by the parathyroid glands. The more hormone, the higher the calcium level in the blood and the lower the level stored in bone. A low hormone level will cause tetany

Parenteral, a route for introducing medication other than through the gastrointestinal tract; most commonly involves injection into the body through a needle and syringe

Parathyroidal, pertaining to the parathyroid glands

Parathyroidectomy, excision of one or more of the parathyroid glands. This is performed to halt the progress of hyperparathyroidism

Parenteral administration of drugs

Paresthesia, an abnormal sensation such as burning or tingling

Parietal bone, a cranial bone

Parietal layer, the outer pleural layer around the lungs. It lines the inside of the chest cavity

Parietal lobe, one of the four cerebral hemisphere lobes. It receives and interprets nerve impulses from sensory receptors

Parietal pericardium, the outer layer of the pericardium surrounding the heart

Parietal peritoneum, the outer layer of the serous membrane sac lining the abdominopelvic cavity

Parietal pleura, the outer layer of the serous membrane sac lining the thoracic cavity

Parkinson's disease, chronic disorder of the nervous system with fine tremors, muscular weakness, rigidity, and a shuffling gait

Paronychia, infection around a nail

Parotid glands, a pair of salivary glands located in front of the ears

Passive acquired immunity, immunity that results when a person receives protective substances produced by another human or animal. This may take the form of maternal antibodies crossing the placenta to a baby or an antitoxin injection

Passive aggressive personality, a personality disorder in which the person expresses feelings or anger or hostility through indirect or covert actions

Passive aggressive disorder

Passive range of motion (PROM), therapist putting a patient's joints through a full range of motion without assistance from the patient

Patella, also called the *kneecap.* It is a lower extremity bone

Patellar, pertaining to the patella or kneecap

Patent, open or unblocked, such as a patent airway

Patent ductus arteriosus (PDA), congenital heart anomaly in which the opening between the pulmonary artery and the aorta fails to close at birth. This condition requires surgery

Pathogenic, pertaining to microscopic organisms, such as bacteria, that are capable of causing disease

Pathogens, disease-bearing organisms

Pathologic fracture, fracture caused by diseased or weakened bone

Pathological gambling, an impulse control disorder in which the patient is unable to control the urge to gamble

Pathologist, a physician who specializes in evaluating specimens removed from living or dead patients

Pathologist's report, a medical record report given by a pathologist who studies tissue removed from the patient (for example: bone marrow, blood, or tissue biopsy)

Pathology, the branch of medicine specializing in studying how disease affects the body

Pectoral girdle, consists of the clavicle and scapula; functions to attach the upper extremity to the axial skeleton

Pediculosis, infestation with lice

Pedophilia, a sexual disorder characterized by having sexual interest in children

Pelvic, pertaining to the pelvis

Pelvic cavity, the inferior portion of the abdominopelvic cavity

Pelvic examination, physical examination of the vagina and adjacent organs performed by a physician placing the fingers of one hand into the vagina, A visual examination is performed using a speculum

Pelvic girdle, consists of the ilium, ischium, and pubis; functions to attach the lower extremity to the axial skeleton

Pelvic inflammatory disease (PID), any inflammation of the female reproductive organs, generally bacterial in nature

Pelvic region, lowest anterior region of the trunk

Pelvic ultrasonography, use of ultrasound waves to produce an image or photograph of an organ, such as the uterus, ovaries, or fetus

Penis, the male sex organ. It is composed of erectile tissue that becomes erect during sexual stimulation, allowing it to be placed within the female vagina for ejaculation of semen. The larger, soft tip is referred to as the glans penis

Peptic ulcer disease (PUD), ulcer occurring in the lower portion of the esophagus, stomach, and duodenum and thought to be caused by the acid of gastric juices

Percussion, use of the fingertips to tap the body lightly and sharply. Aids in determining the size, position, and consistency of the underlying body part

Percutaneous diskectomy, a thin catheter tube is inserted into the intervertebral disk through the skin and the herniated or ruptured disk material is sucked out or a laser is used to vaporize it

Percutaneous transhepatic cholangiography (PTC), a contrast medium is injected directly into the liver to visualize the bile ducts. Used to detect obstructions

Percutaneous transluminal coronary angioplasty (PTCA), method for treating localized coronary artery narrowing. A balloon catheter is inserted through the skin into the coronary artery and inflated to dilate the narrow blood vessel

Pericardial cavity, cavity formed by the serous membrane sac surrounding the heart

Pericarditis, inflammatory process or disease of the pericardium

Pericardium, the double-walled outer sac around the heart. The inner layer of the pericardium is called the epicardium, the outer layer is the heart itself. This sac contains pericardial fluid that reduces friction caused by the heart beating

Perimetritis, inflammation around the uterus

Perimetrium, the outer layer of the uterus

Perineum, in the male, the external region between the scrotum and anus. In the female, the external region between the vagina and anus

Periodontal disease, disease of the supporting structures of the teeth, including the gums and bones

Periodontal ligaments, small ligaments that anchor the root of a tooth in the socket of the jaw

Periodontic, pertaining to around the teeth

Periodontics, branch of dentistry concerned with treating conditions involving the gums and tissues surrounding the teeth. A specialist is a *periodontist*

Perioperative, the period of time that includes before, during, and after a surgical procedure

Periosteum, the membrane that covers most bones. It contains numerous nerves and lymphatic vessels

Peripheral nervous system (PNS), the portion of the nervous system that contains the cranial nerves and spinal nerves. These nerves are mainly responsible for voluntary muscle movement, smell, taste, sight, and hearing

Peripheral neuropathy, damage to the nerves in the lower legs and hands as a result of diabetes mellitus; symptoms include either extreme sensitivity or numbness and tingling

Peripheral vascular disease (PVD), any abnormal condition affecting blood vessels outside the heart; symptoms may include pain, pallor, numbness, and loss of circulation and pulses

Peristalsis, the wavelike muscular movements in the wall of the digestive system tube—esophagus, stomach, small intestines, and colon—that function to move food along the tube

Peritoneal, pertaining to the peritoneum

Peritoneal dialysis, removal of toxic waste substances from the body by placing warm chemically balanced solutions into the peritoneal cavity. Used in treating renal failure and certain poisonings

Peritoneum, membranous sac that lines the abdominal cavity and encases the abdominopelvic organs. The kidneys are an exception since they lay outside the peritoneum and alongside the vertebral column

Peritubular capillaries, capillary bed surrounding the renal tubules

Permanent teeth, the thirty-two permanent teeth begin to erupt at about the age of 6. Generally complete by the age of 16

Pernicious anemia, anemia associated with insufficient absorption of vitamin B_{12} by the digestive system

Personality disorders, inflexible or maladaptive behavior patterns that affect a person's ability to function in society. Includes paranoid personality disorder, narcissistic personality disorder, antisocial personality disorder, and passive aggressive personality

Perspiration, another term for sweating

Pertussis, a contagious bacterial infection of the larynx, trachea, and bronchi characterized by coughing attacks that end with a whooping sound. Also called *whooping cough*

Petechiae, flat, pinpoint, purplish spots from bleeding under the skin

Phacoemulsification, use of high-frequency sound waves to emulsify (liquefy) a lens with a cataract, which is then aspirated (removed by suction) with a needle

Phagocyte, neutrophil component of the blood; has the ability to ingest and destroy bacteria

Phagocytosis, the process of engulfing or ingesting material. Several types of white blood cells function by engulfing bacteria

Phalangeal, pertaining to the phalanges or finger and toe bones

Phalanges, the finger bones in the upper extremities and the toe bones in the lower extremities

Pharmaceutical, related to medications or pharmacies

Pharmacist (RPh or PharmD), receives drug requests made by physicians, and gathers pertinent information that would affect the dispensing of certain drugs, reviews patients' medications for drug interactions, provides healthcare workers with information regarding drugs, and educates the public

Pharmacology, study of the origins, nature, properties, and effects of drugs on the living organism

Pharyngeal, pertaining to the pharynx

Pharyngeal tonsils, another term for *adenoids*. The tonsils are a collection of lymphatic tissue found in the nasopharynx to combat microorganisms entering the body through the nose

Pharyngitis, inflammation of the mucous membrane of the pharynx, usually caused by a viral or bacterial infection. Commonly called a *sore throat*

Pharyngoplasty, surgical repair of the pharynx

Pharyngoplegia, paralysis of the pharynx

Pharynx, medical term for the throat. The passageway that conducts air from the nasal cavity to the trachea and also carries food and drink from the mouth to the esophagus. The pharynx is divided into three sections: the nasopharynx, oropharynx, and laryngopharynx

Pheochromocytoma, usually benign tumor of the adrenal medulla that secretes epinephrine; symptoms include anxiety, heart palpitations, dyspnea, profuse sweating, headache, and nausea

Phimosis, narrowing of the foreskin over the glans penis that results in difficulty with hygiene. This condition can lead to infection or difficulty with urination. It is treated with circumcision, the surgical removal of the foreskin

Phlebitis, inflammation of a vein

Phlebogram, record of veins

Phlebotomy, creating an opening into a vein to withdraw blood

Phlegm, thick mucus secreted by the membranes that line the respiratory tract. When phlegm is coughed through the mouth, it is called *sputum*. Phlegm is examined for color, odor, and consistency

Phobias, a type of anxiety disorder in which a person has irrational fears. An example is arachnophobia, the fear of spiders

Phonophoresis, the use of ultrasound waves to introduce medication across the skin into the subcutaneous tissues

Photophobia, strong sensitivity to bright light

Photorefractive keratectomy (PRK), use of a laser to reshape the cornea to correct errors of refraction

Photosensitivity, condition in which the skin reacts abnormally when exposed to light such as the ultraviolet rays of the sun

Physical medicine, use of natural methods, including physical therapy, to cure diseases and disorders

Physical therapy (PT), treating disorders using physical means and methods. Physical therapy personnel assess joint motion, muscle strength and endurance, function of heart and lungs, and performance of activities required in daily living, along with other responsibilities. Physical therapy treatment includes gait training, therapeutic exercise, massage, joint and soft tissue mobilization, thermal and cryotherapy, electrical stimulation, ultrasound, and hydrotherapy. These methods strengthen muscles, improve motion and circulation, reduce pain, and increase function

Physician's offices, individual or groups of physicians providing diagnostic and treatment services in a private office setting rather than a hospital

Physician's orders, medical record document that contains a complete list of the care, medications, tests, and treatments the physician orders for the patient

Physician's progress notes, part of a patient's medical record. It is the physician's daily record of the patient's condition, results of the physician's examinations, summary of test results, updated assessment and diagnoses, and further plans for the patient's care

Pia mater, the term means soft mother. This thin innermost meninges layer is applied directly to the surface of the brain

Pineal gland, a gland in the endocrine system that produces a hormone called melatonin

Pinna, also called the *auricle*. The external ear, which functions to capture sound waves as they go past the outer ear

Pituitary, pertaining to the pituitary gland

Pituitary gland, an endocrine gland located behind the optic nerve in the brain. It is also called the master gland since it controls the functions of many other endocrine glands. It is divided into two lobes: anterior and posterior. The anterior pituitary gland secretes hormones that aid in controlling growth and stimulating the thyroid gland, sexual glands, and adrenal cortex. The posterior pituitary is responsible for the antidiuretic hormone and oxytocin

Placebo, inactive, harmless substance used to satisfy a patient's desire for medication. It is also given to control groups of patients in research studies in which another group receives a drug. The effect of the placebo versus the drug is then observed

Placenta, also called afterbirth. An organ attached to the uterine wall that is composed of maternal and fetal tissues. Oxygen, nutrients, carbon dioxide, and wastes are exchanged between the mother and baby through the placenta. The baby is attached to the placenta by way of the umbilical cord

Placenta previa, occurs when the placenta is in the lower portion of the uterus and thus blocks the birth canal

Placental stage, the third stage of labor, which takes place after delivery of the infant. The uterus resumes strong contractions and the placenta detaches from the uterine wall and is delivered through the vagina

Plantar flexion, bend sole of foot; point toes downward

Plaque, a yellow, fatty deposit of lipids in an artery

Plasma, the liquid portion of blood containing 90% water. The remaining 10% consists of plasma proteins (serum albumin, serum globulin, fibrinogen, and prothrombin), inorganic substances (calcium, potassium, and sodium), organic components (glucose, amino acids, cholesterol), and waste products (urea, uric acid, ammonia, and creatinine)

Plasma proteins, proteins that are found in plasma. Includes serum albumin, serum globulin, fibrinogen, and prothrombin

Plasmapheresis, method of removing plasma from the body without depleting the formed elements; whole blood is removed and the cells and plasma are separated; the cells are returned to the patient along with a donor plasma transfusion

Plastic surgery, surgical specialty involved in repair, reconstruction, or improvement of body structures such as the skin that are damaged, missing, or misshapen. Physician is a plastic surgeon

Platelet count, blood test to determine the number of platelets in a given volume of blood

Platelets, cells responsible for the coagulation of blood. These are also called thrombocytes and contain no hemoglobin

Pleura, a protective double layer of serous membrane around the lungs. The parietal membrane is the outer layer and the visceral layer is the inner membrane. It secretes a thin, watery fluid to reduce friction associated with lung movement

Pleural, pertaining to the pleura

Pleural cavity, cavity formed by the serous membrane sac surrounding the lungs

Pleural effusion, abnormal presence of fluid or gas in the pleural cavity. Physicians can detect the presence of fluid by tapping the chest (percussion) or listening with a stethoscope (auscultation)

Pleural rub, grating sound made when two surfaces, such as the pleural surfaces, rub together during respiration. It is caused when one of the surfaces becomes thicker as a result of inflammation or other disease conditions. This rub can be felt through the fingertips when they are placed on the chest wall or heard through the stethoscope

Pleurectomy, excision of the pleura

Pleurisy, inflammation of the pleura

Pleurocentesis, a puncture of the pleura to withdraw fluid from the thoracic cavity in order to diagnose disease

Pleurodynia, Pleural pain

Pneumoconiosis, condition resulting from inhaling environmental particles that become toxic, such as coal dust (anthracosis) or asbestos (asbestosis)

***Pneumocystis carinii* pneumonia (PCP),** pneumonia with a nonproductive cough, very little fever, and dyspnea. Seen in persons with weakened immune systems, such as patients with AIDS

Pneumonia, inflammatory condition of the lung, which can be caused by bacterial and viral infections, diseases, and chemicals

Pneumothorax, collection of air or gas in the pleural cavity, which can result in the collapse of a lung

Podiatry, healthcare profession specializing in diagnosis and treatment of disorders of the feet and lower legs. Healthcare professional is a *podiatrist*

Poliomyelitis, acute viral disease that causes an inflammation of the gray matter of the spinal cord, resulting in paralysis in some cases. Has been brought under almost total control through vaccinations

Polyarteritis, inflammation of many arteries

Polycystic kidneys, formation of multiple cysts within the kidney tissue; results in the destruction of normal kidney tissue and uremia

Polycythemia vera, production of too many red blood cells in the bone marrow

Polydipsia, condition of having an excessive amount of thirst, such as in diabetes

Polymyositis, disease involving muscle inflammation and weakness from an unknown cause

Polyneuritis, inflammation of many nerves

Polyp, small tumor with a pedicle or stem attachment. Commonly found in vascular organs such as the nose, uterus, and rectum

Polyphagia, to eat excessively

Polyposis, small tumors that contain a pedicle or footlike attachment in the mucous membranes of the large intestine (colon)

Polysomnography, monitoring a patient while sleeping to identify sleep apnea. Also called *sleep apnea study*

Polyuria, condition of having excessive urine production. This can be a symptom of disease conditions such as diabetes

Pons, this portion of the brain stem forms a bridge between the cerebellum and cerebrum. It is also where nerve fibers cross from one side of the brain to control functions and movement on the other side of the brain

Pontine, pertaining to the pons

Positron emission tomography (PET), use of positive radionuclides to reconstruct brain sections. Measurements can be taken of oxygen and glucose uptake, cerebral blood flow, and blood volume

Posterior, directional term meaning near or on the back or spinal cord side of the body

Posterior lobe, the posterior portion of the pituitary gland. It secretes antidiuretic hormone and oxytocin

Posteroanterior (PA) view, positioning patient so that X-rays pass through the body from back to front

Postoperative, the period of time immediately following the surgery

Postpartum, period immediately after delivery or childbirth

Postprandial, pertaining to after a meal

Postural drainage, draining secretions from the bronchi by placing the patient in a position that uses gravity to promote drainage. Used for the treatment of cystic fibrosis and bronchiectasis, and before lobectomy surgery

Postural drainage with clapping, drainage of secretions from the bronchi or a lung cavity by having the patient lie so that gravity allows drainage to occur. Clapping is using the hand in a cupped position to perform percussion on the chest. Assists in loosening secretions and mucus

Potassium (K+), an inorganic substance found in plasma. It is important for bones and muscles

Potentiation, giving a patient a second drug to boost (potentiate) the effect of another drug; the total strength of the drugs is greater than the sum of the strength of the individual drugs

Preeclampsia, toxemia of pregnancy that, if untreated, can result in true eclampsia. Symptoms include hypertension, headaches, albumin in the urine, and edema

Prefix, a word part added in front of the word root. It frequently gives information about the location of the organ, the number of parts or the time (frequency). Not all medical terms have a prefix

Pregnancy, the time from fertilization of an ovum to the birth of the newborn

Pregnancy test, chemical test that can determine a pregnancy during the first few weeks. Can be performed in a physician's office or with a home-testing kit

Premature, infant born prior to thirty-seven weeks of gestation

Premenstrual syndrome (PMS), symptoms that develop just prior to the onset of a menstrual period, which can include irritability, headache, tender breasts, and anxiety

Premolar, another term for the bicuspid teeth

Preoperative (preop, pre-op), the period of time preceding surgery

Prepuce, also called the foreskin. A protective covering over the glans penis. It is this covering of the skin that is removed during circumcision

Presbycusis, loss of hearing that can accompany the aging process

Presbyopia, visual loss due to old age, resulting in difficulty in focusing for near vision (such as reading)

Prescription, a written explanation to the pharmacist regarding the name of the medication, the dosage, and the times of administration

Prescription drug, a drug that can only be ordered by a licensed physician, dentist, or veterinarian

Pressure equalizing tube (PE tube), small tube surgically placed in a child's ear to assist in drainage of infection

Priapism, a persistent and painful erection due to pathological causes, not sexual arousal

Primary site, designates where a malignant tumor first appeared

Primigravida, woman who has been pregnant once

Primipara, woman who has given birth once

Probe, a surgical instrument used to explore tissue

Process, a projection from the surface of a bone

Proctologist, specialist in the rectum

Proctology, branch of medicine specializing in conditions of the lower gastrointestinal system

Proctopexy, surgical fixation of the rectum

Proctoptosis, drooping rectum

Progesterone, one of the hormones produced by the ovaries. It works with estrogen to control the menstrual cycle

Prolactin (PRL), a hormone secreted by the anterior pituitary. It stimulates milk production

Prolapsed umbilical cord, when the umbilical cord of the baby is expelled first during delivery and is squeezed between the baby's head and the vaginal wall. This presents an emergency situation since the baby's circulation is compromised

Prolapsed uterus, fallen uterus that can cause the cervix to protrude through the vaginal opening. Generally caused by weakened muscles from vaginal delivery or as the result of pelvic tumors pressing down

Pronation, to turn downward or backward, as with the hand or foot

Prone, directional term meaning lying horizontally facing downward

Prophylaxis, prevention of disease. For example, an antibiotic can be used to prevent the occurrence of a disease

Proprietary name, the name a pharmaceutical company chooses as the trademark or market

name for its drug. Also called *brand* or *trade name*

Prostate cancer, slow-growing cancer that affects a large number of males after age 50. The PSA (prostate-specific antigen) test is used to assist in early detection of this disease

Prostate gland, a gland in the male reproductive system that produces fluids that nourish the sperm

Prostate-specific antigen (PSA), a blood test to screen for prostate cancer. Elevated blood levels of PSA are associated with prostate cancer

Prostatectomy, surgical removal of the prostate gland

Prostatic, pertaining to the prostate gland

Prostatitis, inflamed condition of the prostate gland that may be a result of an infection

Prosthesis, artificial device used as a substitute for a body part that is either congenitally missing or absent as a result of accident or disease; for instance, an artificial leg or hip prosthesis

Prosthetics, artificial devices, such as limbs and joints, that replace a missing body part

Protease inhibitor drugs, medications that inhibit protease, an enzyme viruses need to reproduce

Protein-bound iodine test (PBI), blood test to measure the concentration of thyroxine (T_4) circulating in the blood stream. The iodine becomes bound to the protein in the blood and can be measured. Useful in establishing thyroid function

Proteinuria, protein in the urine

Prothrombin, protein element within the blood that interacts with calcium salts to form thrombin

Prothrombin time (Pro time), measurement of the time it takes for a sample of blood to coagulate

Protocol (prot), the actual plan of care, including the medications, surgeries, and treatments for the care of a patient. Often, the entire healthcare team, including the physician, oncologist, radiologist, nurse, and patient, will assist in designing the treatment plan

Proton pump inhibitor, blocks the stomach's ability to secrete acid. Used to treat peptic ulcers and gastroesophageal reflux disease

Protozoans, single-celled organisms that can infect the body

Proximal, directional term meaning located closest to the point of attachment to the body

Proximal convoluted tubule, a portion of the renal tubule

Pruritus, severe itching

Pseudocyesis, false pregnancy

Pseudohypertrophic muscular dystrophy, one type of inherited muscular dystrophy in which the muscle tissue is gradually replaced by fatty tissue, making the muscle look strong

Psoriasis, chronic inflammatory condition consisting of crusty papules forming patches with circular borders

Psychiatric nurse, a nurse with additional training in the care of patients with mental, emotional, and behavioral disorders

Psychiatric social work, a social worker with additional training in the care of patients with mental, emotional, or behavioral disorders

Psychiatrist (MD or DO), a physician with specialized training in diagnosing and treating mental disorders; prescribes medication and conducts counseling

Psychiatry, the branch of medicine that deals with the diagnosis, treatment, and prevention of mental disorders

Psychoanalysis, method of obtaining a detailed account of the past and present emotional and mental experiences from the patient to determine the source of the problem and eliminate the effects

Psychology, the study of human behavior and thought process. This behavioral science is primarily concerned with understanding how human beings interact with their physical environment and with each other

Psychopharmacology, the study of the effects of drugs on the mind and particularly the use of drugs in treating mental disorders. The main classes of drugs for the treatment of mental disorders are antipsychotic drugs, antidepressant drugs, minor tranquilizers, and lithium

Psychotherapy, a method of treating mental disorders by mental rather than chemical or physical means. It includes psychoanalysis, humanistic therapies, and family and group therapy

Pterygium, hypertrophied conjunctival tissue in the inner corner of the eye

Puberty, beginning of menstruation and the ability to reproduce. Usually occurs around 16 years of age

Pubic, pertaining to the pubis; one of the pelvic bones

Pubic region, the genital region of the body

Pubis, one of the three bones that form the os coxae or innominate bone

Pulmonary, pertaining to the lung

Pulmonary angiography, injecting dye into a blood vessel for the purpose of taking an X-ray of the arteries and veins of the lungs

Pulmonary artery, the large artery that carries de-oxygenated blood from the right ventricle to the lung

Pulmonary capillaries, network of capillaries in the lungs that tightly encase each alveolus; site of gas exchange

Pulmonary circulation, the pulmonary circulation transports deoxygenated blood from the right side of the heart to the lungs where oxygen and carbon dioxide are exchanged. Then it carries oxygenated blood back to the left side of the heart

Pulmonary edema, condition in which lung tissue retains an excessive amount of fluid. Results in labored breathing

Pulmonary embolism, blood clot or air bubble in the pulmonary artery or one of its branches

Pulmonary fibrosis, formation of fibrous scar tissue in the lungs, which leads to decreased ability to expand the lungs. May be caused by infections, pneumoconiosis, autoimmune diseases, and toxin exposure

Pulmonary function test (PFT), breathing equipment used to determine respiratory function and measure lung volumes and gas exchange

Pulmonary valve, the semilunar valve between the right ventricle and pulmonary artery in the heart. It prevents blood from flowing backwards into the ventricle

Pulmonary vein, large vein that returns oxygenated blood from the lungs to the left atrium

Pulmonologist, a physician specialized in treating diseases and disorders of the respiratory system

Pulmonology, branch of medicine specializing in conditions of the respiratory system

Pulp cavity, the hollow interior of a tooth; contains soft tissue made up of blood vessels, nerves, and lymph vessels

Pulse (P), expansion and contraction produced by blood as it moves through an artery. The pulse can be taken at several pulse points throughout the body where an artery is close to the surface

Pupil, the hole in the center of the iris. The size of the pupil is changed by the iris dilating or constricting

Pupillary, pertaining to the pupil

Purkinje fibers, part of the conduction system of the heart; found in the ventricular myocardium

Purpura, hemorrhages into the skin and mucous membranes

Purulent, pus-filled sputum, which can be the result of infection

Pustule, raised spot on the skin containing pus

Pyelitis, inflammation of the renal pelvis

Pyelogram, x-ray record of the renal pelvis after injection of a radiopaque dye

Pyelonephritis, inflammation of the renal pelvis and the kidney. One of the most common types of kidney disease. It may be the result of a lower urinary tract infection that moved up to the kidney by way of the ureters. There may be large quantities of white blood cells and bacteria in the urine, and blood (hematuria) may even be present in the urine in this condition. Can occur with any untreated or persistent case of cystitis

Pyeloplasty, surgical repair of the renal pelvis

Pyloric, pertaining to the pylorus

Pyloric sphincter, sphincter at the distal end of the stomach. Controls the passage of food into the duodenum

Pyoderma, pus producing skin infection

Pyogenic, pus-forming

Pyosalpinx, condition of having pus in the fallopian tubes

Pyothorax, condition of having pus in the chest cavity

Pyromania, an impulse control disorder in which the patient is unable to control the impulse to start fires

Pyrosis, heartburn

Pyuria, presence of pus in the urine

Q

Quadriplegia, paralysis of all four extremities. Same as tetraplegia

R

Radial, pertaining to the radius; a lower arm bone

Radial keratotomy, spokelike incisions around the cornea that result in it becoming flatter; a surgical treatment for myopia

Radiation therapy, use of X-rays to treat disease, especially cancer

Radical mastectomy, surgical removal of the breast tissue plus chest muscles and axillary lymph nodes

Radical surgery, extensive surgery to remove as much tissue associated with a tumor as possible

Radiculitis, nerve root inflammation

Radiculopathy, disease of the nerve root

Radioactive implant, embedding a radioactive source directly into tissue to provide a highly localized radiation dosage to damage nearby cancerous cells. Also called *brachytherapy.*

Radiography, making of X-ray pictures

Radioimmunoassay (RIA), test used to measure the levels of hormones in the plasma of the blood

Radioisotope, radioactive form of an element

Radiologist, physician who practices diagnosis and treatment by the use of radiant energy. He or she is responsible for interpreting X-ray films

Radiology, the branch of medicine that uses radioactive substances such as X-rays, isotopes, and radiation to prevent, diagnose, and treat diseases

Radiolucent, structures that allow X-rays to pass through and expose the photographic plate, making it appear as a black area on the X-ray, are termed radiolucent

Radiopaque, structures that are impenetrable to X-rays, appearing as a light area on the radiograph (X-ray)

Radius, one of the forearm bones in the upper extermity

Rales, abnormal crackling sound made during inspiration. Usually indicates the presence of moisture and can indicate a pneumonia condition

Range of motion, the range of movement of a joint, from maximum flexion through maximum extension. It is measured as degrees of a circle

Raynaud's phenomenon, periodic ischemic attacks affecting the extremities of the body, especially the fingers, toes, ears, and nose. The affected extremities become cyanotic and very painful. These attacks are brought on by arterial constriction due to extreme cold or emotional stress

Reabsorption, second phase of urine production; substances needed by the body are reabsorbed as the filtrate passes through the kidney tubules

Recklinghausen disease, excessive production of parathyroid hormone, which results in degeneration of the bones

Rectal, (1) Pertaining to the rectum. (2) Substances introduced directly into the rectal cavity in the form of suppositories or solution. Drugs may have to be administered by this route if the patient is unable to take them by mouth due to nausea, vomiting, and surgery

Rectocele, protrusion or herniation of the rectum into the vagina

Rectum, an area at the end of the digestive tube for storage of feces that leads to the anus

Rectus abdominis, a muscle named for its location and the direction of its fibers: rectus means straight and abdominis means abdominal

Rectus muscles, rectus means straight. Four of the eye muscles are rectus muscles

Red blood cell count (RBC), blood test to determine the number of erythrocytes in a volume of blood; a decrease in red blood cells may indicate anemia; an increase may indicate polycythemia

Red blood cell morphology, examination of blood for abnormalities in the shape (morphology) of the erythrocytes. Used to determine diseases like sickle-cell anemia

Red blood cells (RBC), also called erythrocytes or RBCs. Cells that contain hemoglobin and iron-containing pigment that binds oxygen in order to transport it to the cells of the body

Red bone marrow, tissue that manufactures most of the blood cells. It is found in cancellous bone cavities

Reduction, correcting a fracture by realigning the bone fragments. *Closed reduction* is doing this without entering the body. *Open reduction* is making a surgical incision at the site of the fracture to do the reduction, often necessary where there are bony fragments to be removed

Refractive error test, eye examination performed by a physician to determine and correct refractive errors in the eye

Refracts, the bending of light rays as they enter the eye

Regional anesthesia, regional anesthesia is also referred to as a nerve block. This anesthetic interrupts a patient's pain sensation in a particular region of the body. The anesthetic is injected near the nerve that will be blocked

from sensation. The patient usually remains conscious

Regurgitation, to flow backwards. In cardiovascular system refers to blood flowing backwards through valve. In digestive system refers to food flowing backwards from stomach to mouth

Rehabilitation, process of treatment and exercise that can help a person with a disability attain maximum function and well-being

Rehabilitation centers, facilities that provide intensive physical and occupational therapy. They include inpatient and outpatient treatment

Reinfection, an infection that occurs when a person becomes infected again with the same pathogen that originally brought him or her to the hospital

Relapse, return of disease symptoms after period of improvement

Remission, period during which the symptoms of a disease or disorder leave. Can be temporary

Renal, pertaining to the kidney

Renal artery, artery that originates from the abdominal aorta and carries blood to the nephrons of the kidney

Renal cell carcinoma, cancerous tumor that arises from kidney tubule cells

Renal colic, pain caused by a kidney stone, which can be excruciating and generally requires medical treatment

Renal corpuscle, part of a nephron. It is a double-walled cuplike structure called the glomerular capsule or Bowman's capsule and contains a capillary network called the glomerulus. An afferent arteriole carries blood to the glomerulus and an efferent arteriole carries blood away from the glomerulus. The filtration stage of urine production occurs in the renal corpuscle as wastes are filtered from the blood in the glomerulus and enter Bowman's capsule

Renal failure, inability of the kidneys to filter wastes from the blood resulting in uremia; may be acute or chronic; major reason for a patient being placed on dialysis

Renal papilla, tip of a renal pyramid

Renal pelvis, large collecting site for urine within the kidney. Collects urine from each calyx. Urine leaves the renal pelvis via the ureter

Renal pyramid, triangular-shaped region of the renal medulla

Renal transplant, surgical replacement with a donor kidney

Renal tubule, network of tubes found in a nephron. It consists of the proximal convoluted tubule, the loop of Henle, the distal tubule, and the collecting tubule. The reabsorption and secretion stages of urine production occur within the renal tubule. As the glomerular filtrate passes through the renal tubule, most of the water and some of the dissolved substances, such as amino acids and electrolytes, are reabsorbed. At the same time, substances that are too large to filter into Bowman's capsule, such as urea, are secreted directly from the bloodstream into the renal tubule. The filtrate that reaches the collecting tubule becomes urine

Renal vein, vein that carries blood away from the kidneys

Repetitive motion disorder, group of chronic disorders involving the tendon, muscle, joint, and nerve damage, resulting from the tissue being subjected to pressure, vibration, or repetitive movements for prolonged periods

Resection, to surgically cut out; excision

Residual hearing, amount of hearing that is still present after damage has occurred to the auditory mechanism

Residual volume (RV), the air remaining in the lungs after a forced exhalation

Respiratory membrane, formed by the tight association of the walls of alveoli and capillaries; gas exchange between lungs and blood occurs across this membrane

Respiratory system, system that brings oxygen into the lungs and expels carbon dioxide. Organs include the nose, pharynx, larynx, trachea, bronchial tubes, and lungs

Respiratory therapist (RT), allied health professional whose duties include conducting pulmonary function tests, monitoring oxygen and carbon dioxide levels in the blood, and administering breathing treatments

Respiratory therapy, allied health specialty that assists patients with respiratory and cardiopulmonary disorders

Retina, the innermost layer of the eye. It contains the visual receptors called rods and cones. The rods and cones receive the light impulses and transmit them to the brain via the optic nerve

Retinal, pertaining to the retina

Retinal blood vessels, the blood vessels that supply oxygen to the rods and cones of the retina

Retinal detachment, occurs when the retina becomes separated from the choroid layer. This separation seriously damages blood vessels and nerves, resulting in blindness

Retinitis pigmentosa, progressive disease of the eye that results in the retina becoming hard (sclerosed), pigmented (colored), and atrophied (wasting away). There is no known cure for this condition

Retinoblastoma, malignant glioma of the retina

Retinopathy, retinal disease

Retinopexy, surgical fixation of the retina

Retrograde pyelogram (RP), a diagnostic X-ray in which dye is inserted through the urethra to outline the bladder, ureters, and renal pelvis

Retroperitoneal, pertaining to behind the peritoneum. Used to describe the position of the kidneys, which is outside of the peritoneal sac alongside the spine

Retrovirus

Reverse transcriptase inhibitor drugs, medication that inhibits reverse transcriptase, an enzyme needed to viruses to reproduce

Reye's syndrome, a brain inflammation that occurs in children following a viral infection, usually the flu or chickenpox. It is characterized by vomiting and lethargy and may lead to coma and death

Rh factor, an antigen marker found on erythrocytes of persons with Rh+ blood

Rh-negative (Rh-), a person with Rh− blood type. The person's RBCs do not have the Rh marker and will make antibodies against Rh+ blood

Rh-positive (Rh+), a person with Rh+ blood type. The person's RBCs have the Rh marker

Rheumatoid arthritis (RA), chronic form of arthritis with inflammation of the joints, swelling, stiffness, pain, and changes in the cartilage that can result in crippling deformities

Rhinitis, inflammation of the nose

Rhinomycosis, condition of having a fungal infection in the nose

Rhinoplasty, plastic surgery of the nose

Rhinorrhagia, rapid and excessive flow of blood from the nose

Rhinorrhea, watery discharge from the nose, expecially with allergies or a cold, runny nose

Rhonchi, somewhat musical sound during expiration, often found in asthma or infection, and caused by spasms of the bronchial tubes. Also called *wheezing*

Rhytidectomy, surgical removal of excess skin to eliminate wrinkles. Commonly referred to as a *facelift*

Rhytidoplasty, excision of wrinkles

Rib cage, also called the chest cavity. It is the cavity formed by the curved ribs extending from the vertebral column around the sides and attaching to the sternum. The ribs are part of the axial skeleton

Rickets, deficiency in calcium and vitamin D found in early childhood that results in bone deformities, especially bowed legs

Right hypochondriac, an anatomical division of the abdomen; the right upper row

Right iliac, an anatomical division of the abdomen; the right lower row. Also called the *right inguinal*

Right lower quadrant (RLQ), a clinical division of the abdomen. It contains portions of small and large intestines, right ovary and fallopian tube, appendix, right ureter

Right lumbar, an anatomical division of the abdomen, the right middle row

Right lymphatic duct, one of two large lymphatic ducts. It drains right arm and the right side of the neck and chest; empties lymph into the right subclavian vein

Right upper quadrant (RUQ), a clinical division of the abdomen. It contains the right lobe of the liver, the gallbladder, a portion of the pancreas, and portions of small and large intestine

Rinne and Weber tuning-fork tests, the physician holds a tuning fork, an instrument that produces a constant pitch when it is struck against or near the bones on the side of the head. These tests assess both nerve and bone conduction of sound

Rods, the sensory receptors of the retina that are active in dim light and do not perceive color

Roentgen (r), unit for describing an exposure dose of radiation

Roentgenology, X-rays

Root, the portion of a tooth below the gum line

Root canal, dental treatment involving the pulp cavity of the root of a tooth. Procedure is used to save a tooth that is badly infected or abscessed

Rotation, moving around a central axis

Rotator cuff injury, the rotator cuff consists of the joint capsule of the shoulder joint that is reinforced by the tendons from several shoulder muscles; at high risk for strain or tearing injuries

Rubella, contagious viral skin infection; commonly called *German measles.*

Rugae, the prominent folds in the mucosa of the stomach. They smooth out and almost disappear allowing the stomach to expand when it is full of food. Also found in the urinary bladder

S

Saccule, found in the inner ear. It plays a role in equilibrium

Sacral, pertaining to the sacrum

Sacrum, the five fused vertebrae that form a large flat bone in the upper buttock region

Sagittal plane, a vertical plane that divides the body into left and right sections

Sagittal section, sectional view of the body produced by a cut along the sagittal plane

Saliva, watery fluid secreted into the mouth from the salivary glands; contains digestive enzymes that break down carbohydrates and lubricants that make it easier to swallow food

Salivary glands, exocrine glands with ducts that open into the mouth. They produce saliva, which makes the bolus of food easier to swallow and begins the digestive process. There are three pairs of salivary glands: parotid, submandibular, and sublingual

Salpingectomy, excision of the fallopian tubes

Salpingitis, inflammation of the fallopian tube or tubes; also, inflammation of the eustachian tube

Salpingocyesis, tubal pregnancy

Salpingotomy, incision into the fallopian tubes

Sanguinous, pertaining to blood

Sarcoidosis, inflammatory disease of the lymph system in which lesions may appear in the liver, skin, lungs, lymph nodes, spleen, eyes, and small bones of the hands and feet

Scabies, contagious skin disease caused by an egg-laying mite that causes intense itching; often seen in children

Scalpel, a surgical instrument used to cut and separate tissue

Scan, recording the emission of radioactive waves on a photographic plate after a substance has been injected into the body

Scapula, also called the shoulder blade. An upper extremity bone

Scapular, pertaining to the scapula or shoulder blade

Schedule I, drugs with the highest potential for addiction and abuse. They are not accepted for medical use. Examples are heroin and LSD

Schedule II, drugs with a high potential for addiction and abuse accepted for medical use in the United States. Examples are codeine, cocaine, morphine, opium, and secobarbital

Schedule III, drugs with a moderate to low potential for addiction and abuse. Examples are butabarbital, anabolic steroids, and acetaminophen with codeine

Schedule IV, drugs with a lower potential for addiction and abuse than Schedule III drugs. Examples are chloral hydrate, phenobarbital, and diazepam

Schedule V, drugs with a low potential for addiction and abuse. An example is low-strength codeine combined with other drugs to suppress coughing

Schizophrenia, mental disorders characterized by distortions of reality such as delusions and hallucinations

Sclera, the tough protective outer layer of the eyeball. It is commonly referred to as the white of the eye

Scleral, pertaining to the sclera

Scleral buckling, placing a band of silicone around the outside of the sclera to stabilize a detaching retina

Scleritis, inflammation of the sclera

Scleroderma, disorder in which the skin becomes taut, thick, and leatherlike

Scleromalacia, softening of the sclera

Sclerotomy, incision into the sclera

Scoliosis, abnormal lateral curvature of the spine

Scratch test, form of allergy testing in which the body is exposed to an allergen through a light scratch in the skin

Scrotum, a sac that serves as a container for the testes. This sac, which is divided by a septum, supports the testicles and lies between the legs and behind the penis

Scrub nurse, surgical assistant who hands instruments to the surgeon. This person wears sterile clothing and maintains the sterile operative field

Sebaceous cyst, sac under the skin filled with sebum or oil from a sebaceous gland. This can grow to a large size and may need to be excised

Sebaceous glands, also called oil glands. They produce a substance called sebum that lubricates the skin surface

Seborrhea, excessive discharge of sebum

Sebum, thick, oily substance secreted by sebaceous glands that lubricates the skin to prevent drying out. When sebum accumulates, it can cause congestion in the sebaceous glands and whiteheads or pimples may form. When the sebum becomes dark it is referred to as a comedo or blackhead

Secretion, third phase of urine production; additional waste products are added to the filtrate as it passes through the kidney tubules

Sedative, produces relaxation without causing sleep

Seizure, sudden attack of severe muscular contractions associated with a loss of consciousness. This is seen in grand mal epilepsy

Self-innoculation, infection that occurs when a person becomes infected in a different part of the body by a pathogen from another part of his or her own body, such as intestinal bacteria spreading to the urethra

Semen, semen contains sperm and fluids secreted by male reproductive system glands. It leaves the body through the urethra

Semen analysis, this procedure is used when performing a fertility workup to determine if the male is able to produce sperm. Semen is collected by the patient afer abstaining from sexual intercourse for a period of three to five days. The sperm in the semen are analyzed for number, swimming strength, and shape. This is also used to determine if a vasectomy has been successful. After a period of six weeks, no sperm should be present in a sample from the patient

Semicircular canals, a portion of the labyrinth associated with balance and equilibrium

Semilunar valve, the heart valves located between the ventricles and the great arteries leaving the heart. The pulmonary valve is located between the right ventricle, and the pulmonary artery and the aortic valve are located between the left ventricle and the aorta

Seminal vesicles, two male reproductive system glands located at the base of the bladder. They secrete a fluid that nourishes the sperm into the vas deferens. This fluid plus the sperm constitutes much of the semen

Seminiferous tubules, network of coiled tubes that make up the bulk of the testes. Sperm development takes place in the walls of the tubules and the mature sperm are released into the tubule in order to leave the testes

Sensorineural hearing loss, type of hearing loss in which the sound is conducted normally through the external and middle ear but there is a defect in the inner ear or with the cochlear nerve, resulting in the inability to hear. A hearing aid may help

Sensory neurons, nerves that carry sensory information from sensory receptors to the brain; also called *afferent neurons*

Sensory receptors, nerve fibers that are located directly under the surface of the skin. These receptors detect temperature, pain, touch, and pressure. The messages for these sensations are conveyed to the brain and spinal cord from the nerve endings in the skin

Septicemia, having bacteria in the blood stream; commonly referred to as *blood poisoning*

Sequential multiple analyzer computer (SMAC), machine for doing multiple blood chemistry tests automatically

Serous fluid, watery secretion of serous membranes

Serum, clear, sticky fluid that remains after the blood has clotted

Serum bilirubin, blood test to determine the amount of the waste product bilirubin in the bloodstream; elevated levels indicate liver disease

Serum lipoprotein, a laboratory test to measure the amount of cholesterol and triglycerides in the blood

Severe acute respiratory syndrome (SARS), acute viral respiratory infection that begins like the flu but quickly progresses to severe dyspnea; high fatality rate. First appeared in China in 2003

Severe combined immunodeficiency syndrome (SCIDS), disease seen in children born with a nonfunctioning immune system; often forced to live in sealed sterile rooms

Sex hormones, hormones secreted by the gonads and the adrenal cortex; estrogen and progesterone in females and testosterone in males

Sexual disorders, disorders include aberrant sexual activity and sexual dysfunction; includes pedophilia, masochism, voyeurism, low sex drive, and premature ejaculation

Sexually transmitted disease (STD), disease usually acquired as the result of sexual intercourse; formerly more commonly referred to as venereal disease

Shield, protective device used to protect against radiation

Shingles, eruption of vesicles along a nerve, causing a rash and pain. Caused by the same virus as chickenpox

Short bone, a type of bone that is roughly cube shaped. The carpals are short bones

Shortness of breath (SOB), term used to indicate that a patient is having some difficulty breathing. The cause can range from mild SOB after exercise to SOB associated with heart disease

Sialadenitis, inflammation of a salivary gland

Sickle cell anemia, severe, chronic, incurable disorder that results in anemia and causes joint pain, chronic weakness, and infections. It is more common in people of Mediterranean and African heritage. The actual blood cell is crescent shaped

Side effect, response to a drug other than the effect desired

Sigmoid colon, the final section of colon. It follows an S-shaped path and terminates in the rectum

Sigmoidal, pertaining to the sigmoid colon

Sigmoidoscope, instrument to view inside the sigmoid colon

Sigmoidoscopy, using a flexible sigmoidoscope to visually examine the sigmoid colon; commonly done to diagnose cancer and polyps

Silicosis, form of respiratory disease resulting from the inhalation of silica (quartz) dust. Considered an occupational disease

Simple mastectomy, surgical removal of the breast tissue

Sinoatrial node (SA), also called the pacemaker of the heart. It is an area of the right atria that initiates the electrical pulse that causes the heart to contract

Sinus, a hollow cavity within a bone

Skeletal muscle, a voluntary muscle that is attached to bones by a tendon

Skeletal muscle relaxant, produces the relaxation of skeletal muscle

Skeleton, bones forming the framework for the body; site for skeletal muscle attachments

Skin, the major organ of the integumentary system. It forms a barrier between the external and internal environments

Skin graft, the transfer of skin from a normal area to cover another site. Used to treat burn victims and after some surgical procedures

Sleep apnea, condition in which breathing stops repeatedly during sleep long enough to cause a drop in oxygen levels in the blood

Sleeping disorder, any condition that interferes with sleep other than environmental noises. Can include difficulty sleeping (insomnia), nightmares, night terrors, sleepwalking, and apnea

Sleepwalking, a sleeping disorder in which the patient performs complex activities while asleep

Slit lamp microscopy, in ophthalmology, examining the posterior surface of the cornea

Small intestine, the portion of the digestive tube between the stomach and colon, and the major site of nutrient absorption. There are three sections: duodenum, jejunum, and ileum

Smooth muscle, an involuntary muscle found in internal organs such as the digestive organs or blood vessels

Snellen chart, chart used for testing distance vision. It contains letters of varying size and is administered from a distance of 20 feet. A person who can read at 20 feet what the average person can read at that distance is said to have 20/20 vision

Sodium (Na⁺), an inorganic substance found in plasma

Somatic, pertaining to the body

Somatic nerves, nerves that serve the skin and skeletal muscles and are mainly involved with the conscious and voluntary activities of the body

Somatoform disorders, patient has physical symptoms for which no physical disease can be determined; include hypochondria and conversion reaction

Somatotropin, another name for growth hormone; a hormone that promotes growth of the body by stimulating cells to rapidly increase in size and divide

Spasm, a sudden, involuntary, strong muscle contraction

Specialty senses, the special sense organs perceive environmental conditions. The eyes, ears, nose, and tongue contain special sense organs

Specialty care hospitals, hospitals that provide care for very specific types of disease. A good example is a psychiatric hospital

Specific gravity (sp. grav.), characteristic of urine that indicates the amount of dissolved substances in urine

Speculum, a surgical instrument used to spread apart walls of a cavity

Sperm, also called spermatozoon (plural is spermatozoa). The male sex cell. One sperm fuses with the ovum to produce a new being

Spermatic, pertaining to sperm

Spermatic cord, the term for the cordlike collection of structures that include the vas deferens, arteries, veins, nerves, and lymph vessels. The spermatic cord suspends the testes within the scrotum

Spermatocide, substance that kills sperm

Spermatogenesis, formation of mature sperm

Spermatolysis, destruction of sperm

Sphenoid bone, a cranial bone

Sphincter, a ring of muscle around a tubular organ. It can contract to control the opening of the tube

Sphygmomanometer, instrument for measuring blood pressure. Also referred to as a *blood pressure cuff*

Spina bifida, congenital defect in the walls of the spinal canal in which the laminae of the vertebra do not meet or close. Results in membranes of the spinal cord being pushed through the opening. Can also result in other defects, such as hydrocephalus

Spinal, pertaining to the spine

Spinal cavity, a dorsal body cavity within the spinal column that contains the spinal cord

Spinal cord, the spinal cord provides a pathway for impulses traveling to and from the brain. It is a column of nerve fibers that extends from the medulla oblongata of the brain down to the level of the second lumbar vertebra

Spinal cord injury (SCI), bruising or severing of the spinal cord from a blow to the vertebral column resulting in muscle paralysis and sensory impairment below the injury level

Spinal fusion, surgical immobilization of adjacent vertebrae. This may be done for several reasons, including correction for a herniated disk

Spinal nerves, the nerves that arise from the spinal cord

Spinal stenosis, narrowing of the spinal canal causing pressure on the cord and nerves

Spiral fracture, fracture in an S-shaped spiral. It can be caused by a twisting injury

Spirometer, instrument consisting of a container into which a patient can exhale for the purpose of measuring the air capacity of the lungs

Spirometry, using a device to measure the breathing capacity of the lungs

Spleen, organ in the lymphatic system that filters microorganisms and old red blood cells from the blood

Splenectomy, excision of the spleen

Splenomegaly, enlargement of the spleen

Spondylolisthesis, the forward sliding of a lumbar vertebra over the vertebra below it

Spongy bone, the bony tissue found inside a bone. It contains cavities that hold red bone marrow. Also called *cancellous bone*

Spontaneous abortion, loss of a fetus without any artificial aid. Also called a *miscarriage*

Sprain, pain and disability caused by trauma to a joint. A ligament may be torn in severe sprains

Sputum, mucus or phlegm that is coughed up from the lining of the respiratory tract. Tested to determine what type of bacteria of virus is present as an aid in selecting the proper antibiotic treatment

Sputum culture and sensitivity (C&S), testing sputum by placing it on a culture medium and observing any bacterial growth. The specimen is then tested to determine antibiotic effectiveness

Sputum cytology, testing for malignant cells in sputum

Squamous cell carcinoma (SCC), epidermal cancer that may go into deeper tissue but does not generally metastasize

Staging, the process of classifying tumors based on their degree of tissue invasion and the potential response to therapy. The TNM staging system is frequently used. The T refers to the tumor's size and invasion, the N refers to lymph node involvement, and the M refers to the presence of metastases of the tumor cells

Staging laparotomy, surgical procedure in which the abdomen is entered to determine the extent and staging of a tumor

Stapedectomy, removal of the stapes bone to treat otosclerosis (hardening of the bone). A prosthesis or artificial stapes may be implanted

Stapes, one of the three ossicles of the middle ear. It is attached to the oval window leading to the inner ear. Also called the *stirrup*

Stent, a stainless steel tube placed within a blood vessel or a duct to widen the lumen

Sterility, inability to father children due to a problem with spermatogenesis

Sterilization, process of rendering a male or female sterile or unable to conceive children

Sternal, pertaining to the sternum or breast bone

Sternocleidomastoid, muscle named for its attachments, the sternum, clavicle, and mastoid process

Sternum, also called the *breast bone*. It is part of the axial skeleton and the anterior attachment for ribs

Steroid sex hormones, a class of hormones secreted by the adrenal cortex. It includes aldosterone, cortisol, androgens, estrogens, and progestins

Stethoscope, instrument for listening to body sounds, such as the chest, heart, or intestines

Stillbirth, viable-aged fetus dies before or at the time of delivery

Stomach, a J-shaped muscular organ that acts as a sac to collect, churn, digest, and store food. It is composed of three parts: the fundus, body, and antrum. Hydrochloric acid is secreted by glands in the mucous membrane lining of the stomach. Food mixes with other gastric juices and the hydrochloric acid to form a semisoft mixture called chyme, which then passes into the duodenum

Stool culture, a laboratory test of feces to determine if there are any pathogenic bacteria present

Strabismus, an eye muscle weakness resulting in each eye looking in a different direction at the same time. May be corrected with glasses, eye exercises, and/or surgery. Also called *lazy eye* or *crossed eyes*

Strabotomy, incision into the eye muscles in order to correct strabismus

Strain, trauma to muscle from excessive stretching or pulling

Stratified squamous epithelium, the layers of flat or scalelike cells found in the epidermis. *Stratified* means multiple layers and *squamous* means flat

Strawberry hemangioma, congenital collection of dilated blood vessels causing a red birthmark that fades a few months after birth

Stress fracture, a slight fracture caused by repetitive low-impact forces, like running, rather than a single forceful impact

Stress testing, method for evaluating cardiovascular fitness. The patient is placed on a treadmill or a bicycle and then subjected to steadily increasing levels of work. An EKG and oxygen levels are taken while the patient exercises

Striated muscle, another name for skeletal muscle, referring to its striped appearance under the microscope

Stricture, narrowing of a passageway in the urinary system

Stridor, harsh, high-pitched, noisy breathing sound that is made when there is an obstruction of the bronchus or larynx. Found in conditions such as croup in children

Subarachnoid space, the space located between the arachnoid layer and pia mater. It contains cerebrospinal fluid

Subcutaneous (SC, sc, sub-q, subcu), (1) Pertaining to under the skin. (2) Injection of medication under the skin

Subcutaneous layer, this is the deepest layer of the skin where fat is formed. This layer of fatty tissue protects the deeper tissues of the body and acts as an insulation for heat and cold

Subdural hematoma, mass of blood forming beneath the dura mater of the brain

Subdural space, the space located between the dura mater and the arachnoid layer

Sublingual (SL), (1) Pertaining to under the tongue. (2) Administration of medicine by placing it under the tongue

Sublingual glands, a pair of salivary glands in the floor of the mouth

Subluxation, an incomplete dislocation, the joint alignment is disrupted, but the ends of the bones remain in contact

Submandibular glands, a pair of salivary glands in the floor of the mouth

Substance-related disorders, overindulgence or dependence on chemical substances including alcohol, illegal drugs, and prescription drugs

Sudden infant death syndrome (SIDS), the sudden, unexplained death of an infant in which a postmortem examination fails to determine the cause of death

Sudoriferous glands, the typical sweat glands of the skin

Suffix, a word part attached to the end of a word. It frequently indicates a condition, disease, or procedure. Almost all medical terms have a suffix

Sulci, also called *fissures.* The grooves that separate the gyri of the cerebral cortex. Singular is sulcus

Superficial, directional term meaning toward the surface of the body

Superior, directional term meaning toward the head, or above

Superior vena cava, the branch of the vena cava that drains blood from the chest and upper body

Supination, turn the palm or foot upward

Supine, directional term meaning lying horizontally and facing upward

Supplemental oxygen therapy, providing a patient with additional concentration of oxygen to improve oxygen levels in the bloodstream. Oxygen may be provided by a mask or nasal cannula

Suppositories (suppos), a method for administering medication by placing it in a substance that will melt after being placed in a body cavity, usually rectally, and release the medication

Suppurative, containing or producing pus

Surgeon, a physician who has completed additional training of five years or more in a surgical specialty area. The specialty areas include orthopedics; neurosurgery; gynecology; ophthalmology; urology; and thoracic, vascular, cardiac, plastic, and general surgery

Surgery, the branch of medicine dealing with operative procedures to correct deformities and defects, repair injuries, and diagnose and cure diseases

Surgical center, a facility that provides services that range from simple surgeries to diagnostic testing to therapy and do not require overnight hospitalization. Also called an *ambulatory care center* or an *outpatient clinic*

Suture material, used to close a wound or incision. Examples are catgut, silk thread, or staples. They may or may not be removed when the wound heals, depending on the type of material that is used

Sweat duct, duct leading from a sweat gland to the surface of the skin; carries sweat

Sweat glands, glands that produce sweat, which assists the body in maintaining its internal temperature by creating a cooling effect when it evaporates

Sweat pore, the surface opening of a sweat duct

Sweat test, test performed on sweat to determine the level of chloride. There is an increase in skin chloride in the disease cystic fibrosis

Sympathetic branch, a branch of the autonomic nervous system. This system stimulates the body in times of stress and crisis by increasing heart rate, dilating airways to allow for more oxygen, increasing blood pressure, inhibiting digestion, and stimulating the production of adrenaline during a crisis

Synapse, the point at which the axon of one neuron meets the dendrite of the next neuron

Synaptic cleft, the gap between two neurons

Syncope, fainting

Syndrome, group of symptoms and signs that when combined present a clinical picture of a disease or condition

Synovectomy, excision of the synovial membrane

Synovial fluid, the fluid secreted by a synovial membrane in a synovial joint. It lubricates the joint and reduces friction

Synovial joint, a freely moving joint that is lubricated by synovial fluid

Synovial membrane, the membrane that lines a synovial joint. It secretes a lubricating fluid called *synovial fluid*

Synovitis, inflammation of the synovial membrane

Syphilis, infectious, chronic, venereal disease that can involve any organ. May exist for years without symptoms. Treated with the antibiotic pencillin

System, several organs working in a compatible manner to perform a complex function or functions. Examples include the digestive system, the cardiovascular system, and the respiratory system

Systematic, pertaining to a system

Systemic circulation, the systematic circulation transports oxygenated blood from the left side of the heart to the cells of the body and then back to the right side of the heart

Systemic lupus erythematosus (SLE), chronic disease of the connective tissue that injures the skin, joints, kidneys, nervous system, and mucous membranes. May produce a characteristic butterfly rash across the cheeks and nose

Systole, the period of time during which a heart chamber is contracting

Systolic pressure, the maximum pressure within blood vessels during a heart contraction

T

T cells, lymphocytes active in cellular immunity

T lymphocytes, a type of lymphocyte involved with producing cells that physically attack and destroy pathogens

Tachycardia, abnormally fast heart rate, over 100 bpm

Tachypnea, rapid breathing rate

Tagging, attachment of a radioactive material to a chemical and tracing it as it moves through the body

Talipes, congenital deformity of the foot. Also referred to as a *clubfoot*

Target organs, the organs that hormones act on to either increase or decrease the organ's activity level

Tarsal, pertaining to the ankle

Tarsals, the ankle bones in the lower extremity

Taste buds, found on the surface of the tongue; designed to detect bitter, sweet, sour, and salty flavors in our food

Tears, fluid that washes and lubricates the anterior surface of the eyeball

Teeth, structures in mouth that mechanically break up food into smaller pieces during chewing

Temporal bone, a cranial bone

Temporal lobe, one of the four cerebral hemisphere lobes. It controls hearing and smell

Tenaculum, a long-handled clamp surgical instrument

Tendinitis, inflammation of tendon

Tendinous, pertaining to a tendon

Tendons, the strong connective tissue cords that attach skeletal muscles to bones

Tendoplasty, surgical repair of a tendon

Tendotomy, incision into a tendon

Tenodesis, surgical procedure to stabilize a joint by anchoring down the tendons of the muscles that move the joint

Tenodynia, pain in a tendon

Tenoplasty, surgical repair of a tendon

Tenorrhaphy, suture a tendon

Testes, the male gonads. The testes are oval glands located in the scrotum that produce sperm and the male hormone, testosterone

Testicles, also called *testes* (singular is testis). These oval-shaped organs are responsible for the development of sperm within the seminiferous tubules. The testes must be maintained at the proper temperature for the sperm to survive. This lower temperature level is controlled by the placement of the scrotum outside the body. The hormone testosterone, which is responsible for the growth and development of the male reproductive organs, is also produced by the testes

Testicular, pertaining to the testes

Testicular carcinoma, cancer of one or both testicles

Testicular torsion, a twisting of the spermatic cord

Testosterone, male hormone produced in the testes. It is responsible for the growth and development of the male reproductive organs

Tetany, a condition that results from a calcium deficiency in the blood. It is characterized by muscle twitches, cramps, and spasms

Tetralogy of Fallot, combination of four congenital anomalies: pulmonary stenosis, an interventricular septal defect, abnormal blood supply to the aorta, and hypertrophy of the right ventricle. Needs immediate surgery to correct

Thalamic, pertaining to the thalamus

Thalamus, a portion of the diencephalon. It is composed of gray matter and acts as a center for relaying impulses from the eyes, ears, and skin to the cerebrum. Pain perception is also controlled by the thalamus

Thalassemia, a genetic disorder in which the person is unable to make functioning hemoglobin; results in anemia

Therapeutic abortion, the termination of a pregnancy for the health of the mother

Therapeutic exercise, exercise planned and carried out to achieve a specific physical benefit, such as improved range of motion, muscle strength, or cardiovascular function

Thermotherapy, applying heat to the body for therapeutic purposes

Thoracalgia, chest pain

Thoracentesis, surgical puncture of the chest wall for the removal of fluids

Thoracic, pertaining to the chest

Thoracic cavity, a ventral body cavity in the chest area that contains the lungs and heart

Thoracic duct, the largest lymph vessel. It drains the entire body except for the right arm, chest wall, and both lungs. It empties lymph into the left subclavian vein

Thoracic region, the chest region of the body

Thoracic surgeon, a physician specialized in treating conditions and diseases of the respiratory system by surgical teams

Thoracic surgery, branch of medicine specializing in surgery on the respiratory system and thoracic cavity

Thoracic vertebrae, the twelve vertebrae in the chest region

Thoracostomy, insertion of a tube into the chest for the purpose of draining off fluid or air

Thoracotomy, incision into the chest

Thrombin, a clotting enzyme that converts fibrinogen to fibrin

Thrombocytes, also called *platelets*. Platelets play a critical part in the blood-clotting process by agglutinating into small clusters and releasing thrombokinase

Thrombocytosis, too many clotting cells (platelets)

Thrombolytic, able to dissolve existing blood clots

Thrombolytic therapy, drugs, such as streptokinase or tissue-type plasminogen activator, are injected into a blood vessel to dissolve clots and restore blood flow

Thrombopenia, too few clotting (cells)

Thrombophlebitis, inflammation of a vein that results in the formation of blood clots within the vein

Thromboplastin, substance released by platelets; reacts with prothrombin to form thrombin

Thrombopoiesis, producing clotting (cells)

Thrombus, a blood clot

Thymectomy, removal of the thymus gland

Thymic, pertaining to the thymus gland

Thymitis, inflammation of the thymus gland

Thymoma, malignant tumor of the thymus gland

Thymosin, hormone secreted by thymus gland. It causes lymphocytes to change into T lymphocytes

Thymus gland, an endocrine gland located in the upper mediastinum that assists the body with the immune function and the development of antibodies. As part of the immune response it secretes a hormone, thymosin, that changes lymphocytes to T cells

Thyroid cartilage, a piece of cartilage associated with the larynx. It is also commonly called the Adam's apple and is larger in males

Thyroid echogram, ultrasound examination of the thyroid that can assist in distinguishing a thyroid nodule from a cyst

Thyroid function test (TFT), blood tests used to measure the levels of T_3, T_4, and TSH in the blood stream to assist in determining thyroid function

Thyroid gland, this endocrine gland is located on either side of the trachea. Its shape resembles a butterfly with a large left and right lobe connected by a narrow isthmus. This gland produces the hormones thyroxine (also known as T_4) and triiodothyronine (also known as T_3)

Thyroid replacement hormone, given to replace thyroid in patients with hypothyroidism or who have had a thyroidectomy

Thyroid replacement therapy

Thyroid scan, test in which a radioactive element is administered that localizes in the thyroid gland. The gland can then be visualized with a scanning device to detect pathology such as tumors

Thyroid-stimulating hormone (TSH), a hormone secreted by the anterior pituitary. It regulates function of the thyroid gland

Thyroidal, pertaining to the thyroid gland

Thyroidectomy, removal of the entire thyroid or a portion (partial thyroidectomy) to treat a variety of conditions, including nodes, cancer, and hyperthyroidism

Thyromegaly, enlarged thyroid

Thyrotoxicosis, condition that results from overproduction of the thyroid glands. Symptoms include a rapid heart action, tremors, enlarged thyroid gland, exophthalmos, and weight loss

Thyroxine (T_4), a hormone produced by the thyroid gland. It is also known as T_4 and requires iodine for its production. This hormone regulates the level of cell metabolism. The greater the level of hormone in the bloodstream, the higher cell metabolism will be

Tibia, also called the *shin bone.* It is a lower extremity bone

Tibial, pertaining to the tibia or shin bone

Tidal volume (TV), the amount of air that enters the lungs in a single inhalation or leaves the lungs in a single exhalation of quiet breathing

Tinea, fungal skin disease resulting in itching, scaling lesions

Tinea capitis, fungal infection of the scalp; commonly called *ringworm.*

Tinea pedis, fungal infection of the foot; commonly called *athlete's foot.*

Tinnitus, ringing in the ears

Tissues, tissues are formed when cells of the same type are grouped to perform one activity. For example, nerve cells combine to form nerve fibers. There are four types of tissue: nerve, muscle, epithelial, and connective

epithelial, Pertaining to the epithelium

Tolerance, development of a capacity for withstanding a large amount of a substance, such as foods, drugs, or poison, without any adverse effect. A decreased sensitivity to further doses will develop

Tongue, a muscular organ in the floor of the mouth. Works to move food around inside the mouth and is also necessary for speech

Tonic-clonic seizure, type of severe epileptic seizure characterized by a loss of consciousness and convulsions. The seizure alternates between strong continuous muscle spasms (tonic) and rhythmic muscle contraction and relaxation (clonic). It is also called a *grand mal seizure*

Tonometry, measurement of the intraocular pressure of the eye using a tonometer to check for the condition of glaucoma. After a local anesthetic is applied, the physician places the tonometer lightly upon the eyeball and a pressure measurement is taken. Generally part of a normal eye exam for adults

Tonsillar, pertaining to the tonsils

Tonsillectomy, surgical removal of the tonsils

Tonsillitis, inflammation of the tonsils

Tonsils, the collections of lymphatic tissue located in the pharynx to combat microorganisms entering the body through the nose or mouth. The tonsils are the pharyngeal tonsils, the palatine tonsils, and the lingual tonsils

Topical, applied directly to the skin or mucous membranes. They are distributed in ointment, cream, or lotion form. Used to treat skin infections and eruptions

Topical anesthesia, topical anesthesia is applied using either a liquid or gel placed directly onto a specific area. The patient remains conscious. This type of anesthetic is used on the skin, the cornea, and mucous membranes in dental work

Torticollis, severe neck spasms pulling the head to one side; commonly called *wryneck* or a *crick in the neck.*

Total abdominal hysterectomy - bilateral salpingo-oophorectomy (TAH-BSO), removal of the entire uterus, cervix, both ovaries, and both fallopian tubes

Total calcium, blood test to measure the total amount of calcium to assist in detecting parathyroid and bone disorders

Total hip arthroplasty (THA), surgical reconstruction of a hip by implanting a prosthetic or artificial hip joint; also called *total hip replacement.*

Total knee arthroplasty (TKA), surgical reconstruction of a knee joint by implanting a prosthetic knee joint; also called *total knee replacement.*

Total lung capacity (TLC), the volume of air in the lungs after a maximal inhalation

Total parenteral nutrition (TPN), providing 100% of a patient's nutrition intravenously. Used when a patient is unable to eat

Toxic shock syndrome (TSS), rare and sometimes fatal staphylococcus infection that generally occurs in menstruating women

Toxicity, extent or degree to which a substance is poisonous

Toxins, substances poisonous to the body. Many are filtered out of the blood by the kidney

Trachea, also called the *windpipe.* It conducts air from the larynx down to the main bronchi in the chest

Tracheostenosis, narrowing and stenosis of the lumen or opening into the trachea

Tracheostomy, surgical procedure used to make an opening in the trachea to create an airway. A tracheostomy tube can be inserted to keep the opening patent

Tracheotomy, surgical incision into the trachea to provide an airway

Trachoma, chronic infectious disease of the conjunctiva and cornea caused by bacteria. Occurs more commonly in people living in hot, dry climates. Untreated, it may lead to blindness when the scarring invades the cornea. Trachoma can be treated with antibiotics

Tract, a bundle of fibers located within the central nervous system

Traction, process of pulling or drawing, usually with a mechanical device. Used in treating orthopedic (bone and joint) problems and injuries

Tractotomy, incision into a spinal cord tract

Trademark, a pharmaceutical company's brand name for a drug

Transcutaneous electrical nerve stimulation (TENS), application of a mild electrical stimulation to skin via electrodes placed over a painful area, causing interference with the transmission of the painful stimuli. Can be used in pain management to interfere with the normal pain mechanism

Transdermal, route of drug administration; medication coats the underside of a patch that is applied to the skin. The medication is then absorbed across the skin

Transient ischemic attack (TIA), temporary interference with blood supply to the brain, causing neurological symptoms such as dizziness, numbness, and hemiparesis. May lead eventually to a full-blown stroke (CVA)

Transurethral resection of the prostate (TUR), surgical removal of the prostate gland by inserting a device through the urethra and removing prostate tissue

Transverse colon, the section of colon that crosses the upper abdomen from the right side of the body to the left

Transverse fracture, complete fracture that is straight across the bone at right angles to the long axis of the bone

Transverse plane, a horizontal plane that divides the body into upper (superior) and lower (inferior) sections. Also called the *horizontal plane*

Transverse section, sectional view of the body produced by a cut along the transverse plane

Tremor, involuntary quivering movement of a part of the body

Trendelenburg position, a surgical position in which the patient is lying face up and on an incline with the head lower than the legs

Trephine, a surgical saw used to remove a disk-shaped piece of tissue

Trichomoniasis, genitourinary infection that is usually without symptoms (asymptomatic) in both males and females. In women the disease can produce itching and/or burning and a foul-smelling discharge, and can result in vaginitis

Trichomycosis, abnormal condition of hair fungus

Tricuspid valve, a valve between the right atrium and ventricle of the heart. It prevents blood from flowing backwards into the atrium. A tricuspid valve has three cusps or flaps

Triiodothyronine (T$_3$), a hormone produced by the thyroid gland known as T$_3$ that requires iodine for its production. This hormone regulates the level of cell metabolism. The greater the level of hormone in the blood stream, the higher cell metabolism will be

Trochanter, the large blunt process that provides the attachment for tendons and muscles

Trunk, the torso region of the body

Tubal ligation, surgical tying off of the fallopian tubes to prevent conception from taking place. Results in sterilization of the female

Tubercle, a small, rounded process that provides the attachment for tendons and muscles

Tuberculin skin tests (TB test), applying a chemical agent (Tine or Mantoux tests) under the surface of the skin to determine if the patient has been exposed to tuberculosis

Tuberculosis (TB), infectious disease caused by the tubercle bacillus, *Myocobacterium tuberculosis.* Most commonly affects the respiratory system and causes inflammation and calcification of the system. Tuberculosis is again on the uprise and is seen in many patients who have AIDS

Tuberosity, a large, rounded process that provides the attachment to tendons and muscles

Tumor, abnormal growth of tissue that may be benign or malignant. Also called a *neoplasm*

Two-hour postprandial glucose tolerance test, blood test to assist in evaluating glucose metabolism.

The patient eats a high-carbohydrate diet and fasts overnight before the test. A blood sample is then taken two hours after a meal

Tympanectomy, excision of the eardrum

Tympanic, pertaining to the eardrum

Tympanic membrane, also called the eardrum. As sound moves along the auditory canal, it strikes the tympanic membrane causing it to vibrate. This conducts the sound wave into the middle ear

Tympanitis, eardrum inflammation

Tympanometer, instrument to measure the eardrum

Tympanometry, measurement of the movement of the tympanic membrane. Can indicate the presence of pressure in the middle ear

Tympanoplasty, another term for the surgical reconstruction of the eardrum. Also called *myringoplasty*

Tympanorrhexis, ruptured eardrum

Tympanotomy, incision into the eardrum

Type A blood, one of the ABO blood types. A person with type A markers on his or her RBCs. Type A blood will make anti-B antibodies

Type AB blood, one of the ABO blood types. A person with both type A and type B markers on his or her RBCs. Since it has both markers, it will not make antibodies against either A or B blood

Type B blood, one of the ABO blood types. A person with type B markers on his or her RBCs. Type B blood will make anti-A antibodies

Type O blood, one of the ABO blood types. A person with no markers on his or her RBCs. Type O blood will not react with anti-A or anti-B antibodies. Therefore, it is considered the universal donor

Type and crossmatch, lab test performed before a person receives a blood transfusion; double checks the blood type of both the donor's and recipient's blood

U

Ulcer, open sore or lesion in skin or mucous membrane

Ulcerative colitis, ulceration of unknown origin of the mucous membranes of the colon. Also known as *inflammatory bowel disease* (IBD)

Ulna, one of the forearm bones in the upper extremity

Ulnar, pertaining to the ulna, one of the lower arm bones

Ultrasound (US), the use of high-frequency sound waves to create heat in soft tissues under the skin. It is particularly useful for treating injuries to muscles, tendons, and ligaments, as well as muscle spasms. In radiology, ultrasound waves can be used to outline shapes of tissues, organs, and the fetus

Umbilical, an anatomical division of the abdomen; the middle section of the middle row

Umbilical cord, a cord extending from the baby's umbilicus (navel) to the placenta. It contains blood vessels that carry oxygen and nutrients from the mother to the baby and carbon dioxide and wastes from the baby to the mother

Unconscious, condition or state of being unaware of surroundings with the inability to respond to stimuli

Unit dose, drug dosage system that provides prepackaged, prelabeled, individual medications that are ready for immediate use by the patient

Universal donor, type O blood is considered the universal donor. Since it has no markers on the RBC surface, it will not trigger a reaction with anti-A or anti-B antibodies

Universal recipient, a person with type AB blood has no antibodies against the other blood types and therefore, in an emergency, can receive any type of blood

Upper extremity (UE), the arm

Upper gastrointestinal (UGI) series, administering a barium contrast material orally and then taking an X-ray to visualize the esophagus, stomach, and duodenum

Uptake, absorption of radioactive material and medicines into an organ or tissue

Urea, a waste product of protein metabolism. It diffuses through the tissues in lymph and is returned to the circulatory system for transport to the kidneys

Uremia, an excess of urea and other nitrogenous waste in the blood

Ureteral, pertaining to the ureter

Ureterectasis, dilation of the ureter

Ureterolith, a calculus in the ureter

Ureterostenosis, narrowing of the ureter

Ureters, organs in the urinary system that transport urine from the kidney to the bladder

Urethra, the tube that leads from the urinary bladder to the outside of the body. In the male it is also used by the reproductive system to release semen

Urethral, pertaining to the urethra

Urethralgia, urethral pain

Urethritis, inflammation of the urethra

Urethrorrhagia, rapid bleeding from the urethra

Urethroscope, instrument to view inside the urethra

Urethrostenosis, narrowing of the urethra

Urgency, Feeling the need to urinate immediately

Urinalysis (U/A, UA), laboratory test that consists of the physical, chemical, and microscopic examination of urine

Urinary, pertaining to urine

Urinary bladder, organ in the urinary system that stores urine

Urinary incontinence, involuntary release of urine. In some patients an indwelling catheter is inserted into the bladder for continuous urine drainage

Urinary meatus, the external opening of the urethra

Urinary retention, an inability to fully empty the bladder, often indicates a blockage in the urethra

Urinary system, system that filters wastes from the blood and excretes the waste products in the form of urine. Organs include the kidneys, ureters, urinary bladder, and urethra

Urinary tract infection (UTI), infection, usually from bacteria such as *E. coli*, of any organ of the urinary system; most often begins with cystitis and may ascend into the ureters and kidneys; most common in women because of their shorter urethra

Urination, the release of urine from the urinary bladder

Urine, the fluid that remains in the urinary system following the three stages of urine production: filtration, reabsorption, and secretion

Urine culture and sensitivity (C&S), laboratory test of urine for bacterial infection; attempt to grow bacteria on a culture medium in order to identify it and determine which antibiotics it is sensitive to

Urinometer, instrument to measure urine

Urologist, a physician specialized in treating conditions and diseases of the urinary system and male reproductive system

Urology, branch of medicine specializing in conditions of the urinary system and male reproductive system

Urticaria, hives, a skin eruption of pale reddish wheals (circular elevations of the skin) with severe itching. Usually associated with food allergy, stress, or drug reactions

Uterine, pertaining to the uterus

Uterine tubes, tubes that carry the ovum from the ovary to the uterus; also called *fallopian tubes* or *oviducts*

Uterus, also called the *womb*. An internal organ of the female reproductive system. This hollow, pear-shaped organ is located in the lower pelvic cavity between the urinary bladder and rectum. The uterus receives the fertilized ovum and it becomes implanted in the uterine wall, which provides nourishment and protection for the developing fetus. The uterus is divided into three regions: fundus, corpus, and cervix

Utricle, found in the inner ear. It plays a role in equilibrium

Uveitis, inflammation of the uvea of the eye

Uvula, structure that hangs down from the posterior edge of the soft palate, helps in the production of speech, and is the location of the gag reflex

V

Vaccination, providing protection against communicable diseases by stimulating the immune system to produce antibodies against that disease. Children can now be immunized for the following diseases: hepatitis B, diphtheria, tetanus, pertussis, *Haemophilus influenzae* type b, polio, measles, mumps, rubella, and chickenpox. Also called *immunization*

Vagina, organ in the female reproductive system that receives the penis and semen

Vaginal, (1) Pertaining to the vagina. (2) Tablets and suppositories inserted vaginally and used to treat vaginal yeast infections and other irritations

Vaginal hysterectomy, removal of the uterus through the vagina rather than through an abdominal incision

Vaginal orifice, the external vaginal opening. It may be covered by a hymen

Vaginitis, inflammation of the vagina

Valve replacement, excision of a diseased heart valve and replacement with an artificial valve

Valves, flaplike structures found within the tubular organs such as lymph vessels, veins, and the heart. They function to prevent the backflow of fluid

Valvoplasty, surgical repair of a valve

Valvular, pertaining to a valve

Valvulitis, inflammation of a valve

Varicella, contagious viral skin infection; commonly called *chickenpox*

Varicocele, enlargement of the veins of the spermatic cord, which commonly occurs on the left side of adolescent males. Seldom needs treatment

Varicose veins, swollen and distended veins, usually in the legs

Vas deferens, also called ductus deferens. The vas deferens is a long, straight tube that carries sperm from the epididymis up into the pelvic cavity, where it continues around the bladder and empties into the urethra. It is one of the components, along with nerves and blood vessels, of the spermatic cord

Vascular, pertaining to vessels

Vasectomy, removal of a segment or all of the vas deferens to prevent sperm from leaving the male body. Used for contraception purposes

Vasoconstrictor, contracts smooth muscle in walls of blood vessels; raises blood pressure

Vasodilator, produces a relaxation of blood vessels to lower blood pressure

Vasopressin, substance given to control diabetes insipidus and promote reabsorption of water in the kidney tubules

Vasovasostomy, creation of a new opening between two sections of vas deferens. Used to reverse a vasectomy

Veins, blood vessels of the cardiovascular system that carry blood toward the heart

Venography, process of taking an X-ray tracing of a vein

Venous, pertaining to a vein

Ventilation, the movement of air in and out of the lungs

Ventilation-perfusion scan, a nuclear medicine diagnostic test that is especially useful in identifying pulmonary emboli. Radioactive air is inhaled for the ventilation portion to determine if air is filling the entire lung. Radioactive intravenous injection shows whether blood is flowing to all parts of the lung

Ventilator, a machine that provides artificial ventilation for a patient unable to breath on his or her own. Also called a *respirator*

Ventral, directional term meaning near or on the front or belly side of the body

Ventricles, the two lower chambers of the heart that receive blood from the atria and pump it back out of the heart. The left ventricle pumps blood to the body, and the right ventricle pumps blood to the lungs. Also fluid-filled spaces within the cerebrum. These contain cerebrospinal fluid, which is the watery, clear fluid that provides a protection from shock or sudden motion to the brain

Ventricular, pertaining to a ventricle

Ventricular septal defect (VSD)

Venules, the smallest veins. Venules receive deoxygenated blood leaving the capillaries

Vermiform appendix, a small outgrowth at the end of the cecum. Its function or purpose is unknown

Verruca, warts; a benign neoplasm (tumor) caused by a virus. Has a rough surface that is removed by chemicals and/or laser therapy

Vertebral, pertaining to the vertebrae

Vertebral canal, the bony canal through the vertebrae that contains the spinal cord

Vertebral column, part of the axial skeleton. It is a column of twenty-six vertebrae that forms the backbone and protects the spinal cord. It is divided into five sections: cervical, thoracic, and lumbar vertebrae, sacrum, and coccyx. Also called *spinal column*

Vertebral region, the spinal column region of the body

Vertigo, dizziness

Vesicle, small, fluid-filled raised spot on the skin

Vesicular, pertaining to the seminal vesicle

Vestibular nerve, the branch of the vestibulo-cochlear nerve responsible for sending equilibrium information to the brain

Vestibulocochlear nerve, the eighth cranial nerve. It is responsible for hearing and balance

Viruses, a group of infectious particles that cause disease

Viscera, the name for the internal organs of the body, such as the lungs, stomach, and liver

Visceral, pertaining to the viscera or internal organs

Visceral layer, the inner pleural layer. It adheres to the surface of the lung

Visceral muscle, the muscle found in the walls of internal organs such as the stomach

Visceral pericardium, the inner layer of the pericardium surrounding the heart

Visceral peritoneum, the inner layer of the serous membrane sac encasing the abdominopelvic viscera

Visceral pleura, the inner layer of the serous membrane sac encasing the thoracic viscera

Visual acuity (VA) test, measurement of the sharpness of a patient's vision. Usually, a Snellen chart is used for this test and the patient identifies letters from a distance of 20 feet

Vital capacity (VC), the total volume of air that can be exhaled after a maximum inhalation. This amount will be equal to the sum of tidal volume, inspiratory reserve volume, and expiratory reserve volume

Vital signs (VS), respiration, pulse, temperature, skin color, blood pressure, and reaction of pupils. These are signs of the condition of body functions

Vitamin D therapy, maintaining high blood levels of calcium in association with vitamin D helps maintain bone density and treats osteomalacia, osteoporosis, and rickets

Vitiligo, disappearance of pigment from the skin in patches, causing a milk-white appearance. Also called *leukoderma*

Vitreous humor, the transparent jellylike substance inside the eyeball

Vocal cords, the structures within the larynx that vibrate to produce sound and speech

Voiding, another term for urination

Voiding cystourethrography (VCUG), x-ray taken to visualize the urethra while the patient is voiding after a contrast dye has been placed in the bladder

Voluntary muscles, muscles that a person can consciously choose to contract. The skeletal muscles of the arm and leg are examples of this type of muscle

Volvulus, condition in which the bowel twists upon itself and causes a painful obstruction that requires immediate surgery

Vomer bone, a facial bone

von Recklinghausen's disease

Voyeurism, a sexual disorder characterized by receiving sexual gratification from observing others engaged in sexual acts

Vulva, a general term meaning the external female genitalia. It consists of the Bartholin's glands, labia major, labia minora, and clitoris

W

Wax emulsifiers, substances used to soften ear wax to prevent buildup within the external ear canal

Western blot, test used as a backup to the ELISA blood test to detect the presence of the antibody to HIV (AIDS virus) in the blood

Wet gangrene, area of gangrene becoming infected by pus-producing bacteria

Wheal, small, round raised area on the skin that may be accompanied by itching

Whirlpool, bath in which there are continuous jets of hot water reaching the body surfaces

White blood cell count (WBC), blood test to measure the number of leukocytes in a volume of blood. An increase may indicate the presence of infection or a disease such as leukemia. A decrease in WBCs is caused by X-ray therapy and chemotherapy

White blood cell differential (diff), blood test to determine the number of each variety of leukocyte

White blood cells (WBC), blood cells that provide protection against the invasion of bacteria and other foreign material

White matter, tissue in the central nervous system. It consists of myelinated nerve fibers

Whole blood, refers to the mixture of both plasma and formed elements

Wilm's tumor, malignant kidney tumor found most often in children

Word root, the foundation of a medical term that provides the basic meaning of the word. In general, the word root will indicate the body system or part of the body that is being discussed. A word may have more than one word root

X

X-rays, high-energy wave that can penetrate most solid matter and present the image on photographic film

Xenograft, skin graft from an animal of another species (usually pig); also called *heterograft.*

Xeroderma, dry skin

Xerophthalmia, dry eyes

Y

Yellow bone marrow, yellow bone marrow is located mainly in the center of the diaphysis of long bones. It contains mainly fat cells

Z

Zygomatic bone, a facial bone

Index

Non-Hodgkin's lymphoma, 189, 466
Non-Hodgkin's lymphoma (NHL), 189
Noninsulin-dependent diabetes
    mellitus (NIDDM), 369, 527
nonproductive cough, 222, 535
Nonprotein nitrogenous (NPN) compounds
    ammonia, 286, 527
Nonsurgical periodontal therapy, healing after
    prophylaxis, 537
    scaling, 551
Norepinephrine, 358, 482
norgestrel, 329
normal skin, 55, 500
Norpace, 160
Nosebleed, 210, 505
Nosocomial infection
    bacterial, 61, 145, 176, 222-223, 257, 293, 325,
        457, 489
    parasitic, 347
    viral, 62-63, 145, 198, 222, 260, 394, 492
Noun suffixes, listed
    -ism, 6, 479
    -osis, 6, 479
Novocain, 65, 407
NPO, 264, 466
Nucleus, 9, 22, 98-100, 170-171, 390-391, 465, 504
Nulligravida, 5, 323, 458, 527
Nursing care plan
    chronic obstructive pulmonary disease, 464
    glomerulonephritis, 463, 510
    hyperthyroidism, 514
    inflammatory bowel disease, 465
    peptic ulcer disease, 467
Nutrition
    total parenteral, 262, 468, 551
Nyctalopia, 432, 528
Nystagmus, 435, 528

O

O2, 227, 466, 530
OA, 99, 529
Obese patients, 263, 509
Oblique muscles, 428, 528
Obstruction, 143, 188-189, 220, 259, 292, 407, 463,
    489
Occipital bone, 87, 528
Occipital lobe, 392-393, 528
Older adult
    endocrine, 367-372, 504
    influenza, 222, 504
    pneumonia, 216, 525
Olecranon, 84
Oligomenorrhea, 322, 528
Oligospermia, 336, 528
Oliguria, 290-291, 482
omeprazole, 264
Oncologist, 199, 537
Onset, 160, 305, 324, 380, 400, 531
Onychomycosis, 54, 528
Oophorectomy, 322, 528
O&P, 260, 466
Open fracture, 97, 497
open heart surgery, 162, 506
Ophthalmologist, 431-432, 528
Ophthalmology
    lacrimal gland, 449
Ophthalmoscope, 431, 528
Ophthalmoscopy, 435, 528
Opiates, 407, 526
opium, 484
Opportunistic infection, 222
Opportunistic infections
    bone marrow transplant, 178, 486
    spleen, 179-181, 543
Opposition, 109, 529
Optic
    disk, 424, 474, 531-532
Optic disk, 424, 474, 529
Optic nerve, 426-427, 510
Optometrist, 431-432, 529
Optometry, 432, 466, 529
Oral cavity
    lips, 244-245, 520
Oral disease, epidemiology of
    tooth loss, 256
Oral embryology and histology
    enamel, 246-247, 498-500
    pulp, 246-247, 538
    supporting structures, 256, 533

Oral irrigation
    home, 305, 520
Oral surgery procedures
    arthrotomy, 113, 487
    exostosis, 95, 506
    sutures, 508
Orbit, 87, 507
Orchidectomy, 336, 529
Orchiectomy, 336, 529
Organic, 37-38, 400, 483
Organs
    digestive organs, 525
Organs of the body, 200, 358, 510
Origin, 107, 311, 438, 499
Origins of organized hydrotherapy and spas
    Roman, 494
Oropharynx, 211-212, 247, 529
ORTHO, 329
Orthopnea, 218-219, 529
Orthostatic hypotension, 144, 529
Orthotics, 96, 529
Osseous tissue, 82, 529
Ossicles, 442-443, 516
Osteoarthritis, 3, 99, 466, 529
Osteoarthritis (OA), 99, 529
Osteocytes, 82, 529
Osteogenesis, 6
Osteogenic sarcoma, 98, 529
Osteomyelitis, 93, 490
Osteoporosis, 97-98, 369, 490
Otalgia, 444, 530
OTC, 467, 530
Otitis, 444, 466, 485
Otitis externa, 446, 485
Otomycosis, 444, 530
otoplasty, 444, 530
Otopyorrhea, 444, 530
Otorhinolaryngology (ENT), 27, 219, 445, 530
Otosclerosis, 446, 530
Otoscope, 444, 530
Otoscopy, 447, 530
Ounces, 282
Outpatient care, 10
Ova and parasites (O&P), 260
Oval window, 442-443, 530
Ovarian cancer, 349
Ovaries
    female reproductive system, 312-314, 357, 507
    oophorectomy, 329-330
Over-the-counter medications, 438, 528
Over-the-counter (OTC), 530
overweight, 255, 382
Oviducts, 315, 515
Ovulation, 314-316, 507
Ovum, 9, 313-316, 488
Oxidase, 466
Oximeter, 217, 530
Oximetry, 224, 530
Oxycodone, 407
oxygen
    cyanosis, 72, 160, 219, 482
Oxygen levels, 52, 149, 222, 545
Oxygen therapy
    nasal cannula, 72, 219, 526
oxymetazoline, 227

P

PA, 37
Pacemaker
    of heart, 158
Pain
    somatic, 398, 545
    stimuli, 400, 552-553
    visceral, 115, 535
Pain management
    postoperative, 416
    protective response, 51
    transcutaneous electrical nerve stimulation, 552
Palatine bone, 85, 531
Pallor, 56, 148, 531
Palpitation, 157
Palsy
    Bell's, 404, 488
Pancreas
    abscess, 481
    hormones secreted, 355, 510
    insulin production, 369, 517
    islets of Langerhans, 356, 504
    pancreatitis, 253, 531

Pancreatic, 251, 367, 504
Pancreatitis, 253, 531
Pancytopenia, 173, 531
Panhypopituitarism, 370, 531
Pansinusitis, 218, 531
pap, 58, 324, 494
Papanicolaou, George, 327, 531
Papilledema, 432, 531
Papilloma, 324, 465
Papule, 58, 531
Papules, 59, 189, 481
Para, 312, 479
Paracentesis, 262, 531
Paralysis
    paraplegia, 400, 531
    quadriplegia, 6, 399, 539
Paranasal sinuses, 210-211, 531
Paraplegia, 400, 531
Parasitic infections
    scabies, 62, 543
Parasympathetic branch, 396, 531
Parathyroid gland disorders
    hyperparathyroidism, 367, 514
    hypoparathyroidism, 367, 515
Parathyroid glands, 28, 356-359, 504
Parathyroid hormone, 359, 467, 531
Parathyroid hormone (PTH), 359, 531
parathyroidectomy, 367, 531
Parenteral, 262, 468, 531
Paresthesia, 400, 531
Parietal
    pleura, 31, 214, 531
Parietal pericardium, 133-134, 531
Parietal pleura, 31, 214, 531
Parkinson, James, 403
Paronychia, 63, 532
Parotid gland, 251
Partial-thickness burn, 491
Passive range of motion (PROM)
    lower body, 141
    upper body, 141, 548
past history, 74, 124, 162, 201, 237, 275, 307, 351,
    382, 418, 459, 507
Patches, 62-63, 372, 520
Pathogenic, 185-187, 261, 532
Pathologic fracture, 114, 532
Pathological gambling, 516
pathology
    digital, 338
Patient education
    adults, 436, 481
Patient examination positions
    lithotomy, 288, 520
    prone, 36, 447, 537
    supine, 36, 150, 548
Patient history
    family history, 162, 380, 433, 510
    of present illness, 72, 122, 160, 199, 236, 273, 305,
        349, 380, 416, 458
Patient/client management process
    plan of care, 537
PBI, 372-373, 467, 537
PCP, 191, 222, 467, 535
Pedophilia, 532
PEG, 467
Pelvic cavity, 31-33, 314, 499
Pelvic examination, 328, 532
Pelvic inflammatory disease (PID), 325, 532
Pelvis
    renal pelvis, 280, 474, 492
Penicillin, 338
Penis
    glans, 331, 472, 488
    male reproductive system, 331-333, 522
Pepcid, 264
Peptic, 257, 467, 509
Peptic ulcer disease (PUD), 257, 532
peptic ulcers, 262, 509
Percutaneous, 5, 100, 151-152, 261, 467, 532
Percutaneous transhepatic cholangiography (PTC),
    261, 532
Percutaneous transluminal coronary angioplasty
    (PTCA), 151, 532
Perfusion, 224, 555
Pericardial fluid, 186, 533
Pericardial sac, 146
Pericarditis, 3, 134, 532
Pericardium, 3, 40, 133-134, 504
Perimetrium, 316, 533

Pulmonary valve, 134-137, 538
Pulmonary veins, 132
Pulmonology
    oxygen and carbon dioxide levels, 220
Pulp, 246-247, 538
Pulse (heart) rate
    beats per minute (bpm), 133
Pulse rate, 141
Pupil, 396, 424-427, 472, 494
Pupillary, 432, 539
Purging, 491
Purified protein derivative (PPD), 224
Purulent, 57, 221, 434, 491
Purulent drainage, 459
Pus, 48, 218, 290, 323, 444, 474, 491
PVD, 148, 533
Pyelogram, 289, 466-467, 517
Pyloric, 248-249, 539
Pyloric sphincter, 248-249, 539
Pylorus, 242, 474, 539
Pyothorax, 218, 539
Pyromania, 516
Pyrosis, 255, 539
Pyuria, 290, 539

Q
Quadriceps, 104
Quadriceps femoris, 104
Quadriplegia, 6, 399, 539

R
Rabies, 504
Radial artery, 140
Radial keratotomy, 437, 539
Radial keratotomy (RK), 437
Radiation
    controlling, 490
Radiation therapy
    brachytherapy, 539
Radical mastectomy, 329, 539
Radiculopathy, 399, 539
Radioactive, 100, 149, 224, 372-373, 405, 463, 490
Radioimmunoassay (RIA), 372, 539
Radiologic technologist, 468
Radiologist, 120, 537
Radionuclides, 406, 536
Radiopaque, 223, 261, 294, 327, 405, 484
Rales, 220-221, 491
Range of motion (ROM) exercise
    upper extremity, 120, 418, 466, 493
ranitidine, 264
Rash, 43, 62-63, 186, 483
Raynaud's phenomenon, 148, 539
RDS, 227, 467
Reabsorption
    tubular, 287, 555
Receptor, 266, 396, 424, 511
receptor cells, 424
Rectocele, 325, 540
Rectum, 6, 242, 314, 474, 483-484
Rectus abdominis, 104, 540
Red blood cells, 168-172, 255, 326, 484
Red blood cells (RBC), 540
Red blood cells (RBCs)
    abnormal, 6-7, 54-56, 111, 144-145, 168, 214, 254,
        287-288, 322, 368, 399-401, 433,
        479-480, 481
    cast, 113, 255, 426, 518
    clotting process, 168, 482
    hemoglobin in, 175, 484
    hypochromic, 175, 515
    oxygenation, 136
Red bone marrow, 82-83, 170, 486
Reflex
    bite, 489
Reflex hematology procedures
    hemoglobin, 173, 465, 484
Reflexes
    deep tendon, 112-113
Reflux, 256, 465, 509
Reflux esophagitis, 273
Regional anesthesia, 526
Regurgitation, 144, 255, 466, 540
Relapse, 540
Religions, 338, 495
REM, 455
Remission, 540
Renal

colic, 291, 540
corpuscle, 283, 490
Renal artery, 140, 282-283, 540
Renal biopsy, 303
Renal calculi, 290
renal corpuscle, 283, 490
Renal disease, 297, 465
Renal failure, 291-292, 463-464, 533
Renal medulla, 541
renal papilla, 282-283, 492
Renal pelvis, 280, 474, 492
renal pyramids, 282
Renal tubule, 286, 496
Renal tubules, 283, 482
Renal vein, 142, 282-283, 541
Renal veins, 286
Repetitive motion, 111-112, 493
Reproductive issues
    abortion, 318, 550
    contraception, 323-324, 555
Reproductive systems, 32, 311
Residual volume (RV), 215, 541
Respiration
    cough, 227, 495
    gas exchange, 209, 521
    orthopnea, 218-219
    tachypnea, 218-219, 516
Respiration (R)
    Cheyne-Stokes, 495
    volume, 214, 466-468, 506
Respirator, 225, 555
Respiratory acidosis, 287
Respiratory bronchiole, 213
Respiratory disease, 545
Respiratory disorders
    acidosis, 287, 481
    acute respiratory distress syndrome, 221
    alkalosis, 287
    atelectasis, 221, 487
    bronchiectasis, 217, 491
    empyema, 223, 503
    epistaxis, 210
    pertussis, 220, 464, 515
    pleural effusion, 223, 535
    pleuritis, 223
Respiratory distress syndrome, 221-222, 463, 482
Respiratory emergencies
    hyperventilation, 219
Respiratory failure, 221, 482
Respiratory management
    sleep apnea, 222, 545
Respiratory rate, 215, 328, 486
Respiratory system
    bronchitis, 217, 491
    laryngitis, 217, 519
    lung tissue, 222, 487
    nasopharyngitis, 217, 526
    trachea, 27, 92, 208-214, 245, 362, 475, 491
Respiratory therapist, 214, 464, 541
Retina
    nyctalopia, 432
Retinitis
    pigmentosa, 434, 541
Retinopathy, 369, 432, 501
retinopexy, 432, 541
Retrograde, 5, 261, 294, 465, 504
Retrograde pyelogram, 294, 467, 541
Retroperitoneal, 33, 282, 541
Retrovirus, 188, 514
Reverse transcriptase, 191, 541
Reverse transcriptase inhibitor drugs, 191, 541
Reye syndrome, 403
Reye's syndrome, 541
Rh antibodies, 173
Rh factor
    test for, 327, 467
Rheumatoid arthritis, 98-99, 187, 373, 466-467, 484
Rhinitis, 217, 542
rhinoplasty, 4, 217, 542
Rhinorrhea, 7, 218, 542
Rhonchi, 220, 542
Rhythm, 149, 357, 495
rhytidectomy, 54, 542
Rhytidoplasty, 54, 542
Ribs, 34, 81, 214-216, 498
Right atrioventricular valve, 136
Right lower quadrant (RLQ), 34, 542
Right lymphatic duct, 181-183, 521
Right upper quadrant (RUQ), 34, 542

Right ventricle, 132, 538
Rigidity, 403, 490
RLQ, 34, 467, 542
Rods, 101, 427, 508
Roentgenology, 542
Role
    fixation, 451, 499
ROM, 122, 224, 385
Rotator cuff, 111, 542
Round window, 441
Routine hematology procedures
    erythrocyte, 6, 173
Rubella, 62, 515
Rue, 102, 468
Rugae, 248, 284, 542
RV, 215, 468

S
S-A, 138, 468
SAC, 33, 58, 134, 208, 248, 282, 312, 364, 395, 429,
    472, 483
Saccule, 442, 516
Sacrum, 80-81, 406, 474, 516
Saliva, 243-244, 483
Salivary glands and ducts
    parotid gland, 251
    sublingual gland, 251
    submandibular gland, 251
Salpingitis, 323, 444, 543
Sampling, 328, 495
Sarcoma
    sarcoma, 62, 98, 189, 466, 506
Sartorius, 104
Scabies, 62, 543
Scaling, 62, 551
Scan, 100, 149, 224, 349, 372, 401, 490
Scapula, 80-81, 474, 508
Schedule III drugs, 543
Science, 57-58, 99, 188, 246, 290, 315, 369, 391, 427,
    463, 538
Sclera, 424-426, 474, 498
Scleritis, 432, 543
Scleroderma, 55, 543
Scoliosis, 95, 543
Scrotum, 4, 333-334, 499
Scrub nurse, 495
Sebaceous glands, 25, 48, 429, 481
Seborrhea, 54, 543
Second stage of labor, 321
Secondary hypertension, 148
Second-degree burn, 491
Secretions, 186, 225, 251, 358, 506
Segment, 339, 555
Semen, 186, 285, 313, 532
Semicircular canals, 441-442, 516
Semilunar, 135-136, 486
Semilunar valves, 135
Seminal fluid, 503
seminal vesicle, 331, 475, 556
Seminal vesicles, 28, 331-333, 544
Seminiferous tubules, 333-334, 544
Senokot, 264
Sensitivity test, 464
Sensorineural hearing loss, 443, 496
Sensory nerves, 390
Sensory perception
    of pain, 399, 484
Sepsis, 175
Septic, 221
Septicemia, 175, 544
Septum, 87, 134-135, 210, 491
Serevent, 227
Serous, 214, 446, 468, 531-532
Serous membranes, 544
Serous otitis media, 446, 468
Severe acute respiratory syndrome (SARS), 222, 544
Sex hormones, 312, 358, 482
Sexual activity, 544
Sexual intercourse, 317, 544
Sexually transmitted diseases (STDs)
    genital herpes, 337, 510
    pelvic inflammatory disease (PID), 325
    trichomoniasis, 338
Sexually transmitted infections (STIs)
    chlamydia, 337, 495
SGOT, 152, 468
Shaft, 52-53, 82, 486
Shield, 186, 544
Shock

anaphylactic shock, 189, 484
  irreversible, 495
  progressive, 400, 483
  toxic shock syndrome (TSS), 325, 551
Shortness of breath, 216, 468, 544
Shoulder muscles, 111, 396, 542
Shunt, 162, 402, 514
Sialadenitis, 253, 544
Side effect, 483
Sideroblastic anemia (SA)
  sex-linked, 174, 513
Sigmoid colon, 242, 474, 496
sigmoidoscopy, 262, 544
simvastatin, 151
Sinemet, 407
Sinex, 227
Sinoatrial (SA)
  node, 136-138, 487
Sinoatrial (SA) node
  blood supply, 184
Sinus, 83-84, 208, 474, 545
Sinuses, 184, 210-211, 489
skeletal muscle relaxants, 112
Skeletal muscles
  movements of, 212
  relaxants, 112
Skeletal system
  appendicular skeleton, 79, 486
  axial skeleton, 85-86, 488
  hips, 520
  shoulders, 109, 215, 503
Skin
  glands of, 347, 489
  hair and nails, 518
  keratin, 50, 505
  melanocytes, 50-51, 364, 523
  superficial layer, 67, 505
skin absorbing essential oils
  acidity, 368, 467, 481
  molecular structure, 495
Skin cancer
  melanoma, 54, 522-523
Skin disorders
  acne, 53, 481
  dermatitis, 54, 500
  herpes simplex, 65, 256, 465, 513
  pruritus, 57, 538
  viral infections, 485
  warts, 57, 347, 555
Skin grafting
  allograft, 64, 483
  autograft, 5, 64, 488
  xenograft, 64, 513
Skin tests, 224, 552
SLE, 65, 99, 468, 549
Sleep apnea, 222, 536
Small bowel, 248
Small intestine, 4, 25, 242-244, 361, 473, 483
Smallpox, 504
snake bites, 191
Snellen chart, 436, 545
SOB, 160, 216, 468, 544
Sodium chloride, 503
Soft palate, 211, 244-245, 554
Soma, 112
Somatoform disorder, 497
Somatotropin, 363, 545
Spastic colon, 259, 518
Special senses, 29, 423, 512
Specialty care, 11, 545
species, 64, 513
Specimen, 63, 135, 169, 223, 260, 290, 464, 495-496
Specimen types
  genital, 20, 495
  respiratory tract, 534
Sperm, 22, 316-317, 359, 474, 480, 487-488
sperm cells, 334
Spermatic cord, 335-337, 545-546
Spermatogenesis, 333, 546
Sphenoid bone, 85, 546
Spinal
  fusion, 98, 416, 484
Spinal cavity, 31-33, 394, 546
Spinal column, 85, 523
Spinal cord
  directional terms, 33
  radiculopathy, 399
  spinal cord injury (SCI), 404, 546
Spinal cord anatomy

tracts, 392-394, 487
Spinal cord injury
  mechanisms, 185, 430
Spinal cord injury (SCI), 404, 546
Spinal fusion, 100, 416, 546
Spinal nerves
  coccygeal, 94, 394
Spinal tap, 406, 521
Spine
  of bone, 94-95, 518
Spirometer, 224, 546
Spirometry, 224, 546
spironolactone, 296
Spleen
  splenectomy, 187, 546
Splenectomy, 187, 546
Splenomegaly, 16, 187, 546
Splint, 96
Spondylitis, 98, 484
Spondylolisthesis, 98, 546
Spontaneous abortion, 327, 501
Sprain, 99
Sprains, 546
Spur, 95, 506
Sputum culture and sensitivity (C&S), 223, 546
Squamous cell carcinoma, 62, 468, 546
Stapes, 439, 474, 529-530
STD, 338, 468, 544
Steady state, 513
Stenosis, 14, 98, 146, 407, 466, 480, 493
Stent, 144, 517
Sterile, 189, 286, 339, 495
Sterility, 336, 499
Sternal, 94, 546
Sternocleidomastoid, 104, 547
Sternum, 80-82, 133, 474, 542
Steroid hormones, 360, 484
Stethoscope, 143-144, 186, 214, 488
Stillbirth, 327, 547
Stimulation, 112, 138, 317, 406, 465, 485
Stomach
  muscular action of, 134
Stomach disorders
  gastritis, 253, 509
  gastroenteritis, 3, 252, 509
Strabismus, 428, 483
Streptokinase, 150, 178, 468, 550
Stress fracture, 97, 547
Stress test, 149
Stress testing, 149, 547
Striated muscle, 106, 547
Stricture, 291, 509
Stridor, 220, 547
Stroke, 396, 435, 482
STSG, 65, 468
Stupor, 399
Sty, 434, 513
Stye, 434, 513
Subarachnoid hemorrhage, 412
Subarachnoid space, 395, 523
Subdural, 395, 523
Subdural hematoma, 405, 547
Subdural space, 395, 523
Sublingual gland, 251
Sublingual glands, 250, 547
Submandibular gland, 251
Substance use and abuse
  steroids, 236, 482
Sudafed, 227
Sudden infant death syndrome (SIDS), 222, 547
sudoriferous glands, 53, 547
Suffixes, listed adjective
  -algesia, 388, 479
  -blast, 80, 479
  -cyte, 6, 195, 479
  -dipsia, 356, 479
  -genesis, 6, 479
  -logy, 6, 479
  -phil, 168
  -stasis, 168, 480
  -therapy, 7, 480
  -um, 9
  -uria, 280, 377, 480
Suffixes, multiple meanings, listed
  -ectasis, 6, 208, 479
  -genic, 6, 187, 479
  -lysis, 6, 479
  -penia, 168, 479
  -plasm, 6, 479

  -plegia, 388, 480
  -ptosis, 6, 280, 480
  -scopy, 8, 480
  -trophy, 6-7, 480
Suffixes, pathological conditions, listed
  -asthenia, 103, 479
  -cele, 6, 479
  -cusis, 439, 479
  -derma, 48, 479
  -emesis, 242, 479
  -itis, 3, 54, 143, 218, 253, 322-323, 367, 398-399,
        431-432, 479
  -malacia, 6, 54, 432, 479
  -mania, 479
  -megaly, 6, 143, 367, 479
  -oma, 6, 54, 143, 253, 367, 398, 479
  -opia, 424, 479
  -pathy, 6, 54, 367, 398-399, 432, 479
  -pepsia, 242, 479
  -phagia, 54, 242, 479
  -phasia, 388, 479
  -phobia, 479
  -plasia, 6, 479
  -pnea, 208, 480
  -ptysis, 208, 480
Suffixes, surgical and diagnostic procedures, listed
  -desis, 80, 479
  -ectomy, 7-8, 54, 141, 187, 217, 252-253, 288,
        321-323, 367-368, 398, 430-431, 479
  -graphy, 8, 479
  -meter, 8, 217, 431, 479
  -metry, 8, 479
  -opsy, 48, 479
  -pexy, 7, 253, 288-289, 322, 432, 479
  -scope, 3, 444, 480
  -tome, 48, 480
  -tripsy, 242, 280, 480
Sulci, 392, 494
Sunlight, 98, 529
Superior section, 526
Superior vena cava, 133-137, 548
Suppositories
  rectal, 540
  vaginal, 555
Suppurative, 57, 548
Surfactant, 222
Surgeon, 11, 57, 96, 219-220, 249, 282, 327, 495
Surgery
  thoracic surgery, 27, 220, 550
Surgery cancer
  dilation and curettage (D&C), 501
  hysterectomy, 329, 515
  valve replacement, 151, 555
Surgical procedures
  adrenalectomy, 372, 482
  aneurysmectomy, 150, 484
  appendectomy, 252, 486
  balloon angioplasty, 151
  biopsy procedures, 63
  blepharoplasty, 430, 489
  bone graft, 100, 490
  bronchoscopy, 224, 491
  bunionectomy, 100, 491
  carotid endarterectomy, 407, 493
  cholecystectomy, 252, 495
  cochlear implant, 447-449, 496
  colonoscopy, 261, 496
  colostomy, 7, 252, 496
  conization, 328, 497
  coronary artery bypass graft (CABG), 150, 498
  craniotomy, 113, 498
  culdoscopy, 327, 499
  cystectomy, 288, 499
  cystoscopy, 294, 499
  dermatoplasty, 7, 54, 500
  diskectomy, 100, 532
  laser, 57, 100, 434, 519
Suspensory ligament, 315-316, 426
Swallowing
  lungs and, 213
Sweat glands, 23, 48, 358, 488
Swimmer's ear, 446, 530
Sympathetic branch, 410, 548
Symphysis, 92, 284, 314, 493
Symptom, 255-256, 291, 489
Symptoms
  dizziness, 161, 401-403, 445-446, 494
  nausea, 162, 369, 403, 485
  shortness of breath, 220, 544

urinalysis, 279, 468, 554
Urine and urination
    albuminuria, 305
    anuria, 289-290, 486
    bacteriuria, 289, 488
    distal convoluted tubule, 283-284, 502
    dysuria, 290, 502
    electrolytes, 285-286, 358, 489
    filtrate, 285-286, 490
    hematuria, 290, 489
    hesitancy, 291, 513
    nephron loop, 283
    oliguria, 290-291, 482
    pyuria, 290, 539
    reabsorption, 101, 285-286, 485
    urgency, 291, 325, 499
    urinary tract infection (UTI), 293, 554
Urine culture, 293, 468, 554
urine formation, 286
Urine ketones, 290
Urine specimens
    24-hour, 287, 495
    2-hour postprandial, 378
Urine-formed elements
    mucus, 488-489
    sperm, 22, 332, 474, 480, 487-488
    yeast, 509
Urologist, 289, 351, 554
Urticaria, 57, 188, 554
Uterine
    corpus, 314-315, 554
    tubes, 312, 474, 507-508
    tumor, 325-326, 468, 474, 481
    wall, 106, 325-327, 481
Uterine tubes, 312, 474, 530
UTI, 293, 468, 554
Utricle, 442, 516
UV, 57, 469
Uvea, 554
Uveitis, 432, 554
Uvula, 244-245, 554

V
Vaccine, 220, 324, 394
Vaginal hysterectomy, 329, 555
Vaginal yeast infections, 555
Vaginitis, 323, 552
Valacyclovir, 65
Valium, 160
Valtrex, 65
Valves
    aortic, 134-137, 486
    atrioventricular, 135-137, 487
    semilunar, 135-136, 486
    tricuspid, 135-137, 487
Valves, heart
    bicuspid or mitral, 487
    murmur, 144, 524
Valvular heart disease
    mitral regurgitation, 152, 466
    mitral stenosis, 466
    mitral valve prolapse, 152, 466
Varicella, 63, 555
Varices, 256, 505
Varicocele, 337, 555
Vas deferens, 28, 331-335, 365, 475, 505
Vasectomy, 338-339, 544
Vasodilation, 151, 481
Vasopressin, 373, 555
Vasovasostomy, 339, 555
Vastus medialis, 104
VC, 215
Veins
    collapsed, 223
    jugular, 142
    leg, 150, 516
    portal, 142
    pulmonary veins, 132
    renal vein, 142
    saphenous, 142
    varicose, 147-148, 256, 331, 475, 505
Vena cava, 133-137, 360, 516
Venereal, 337-338, 469, 495
Venereal disease (VD), 338
Venogram, 143
Venography, 149, 555
Venous blood, 138
Ventilation, 210, 555
Ventolin, 227

Ventricle, 7, 130, 388, 475, 486-487
Ventricles, 134-135, 392, 487
Ventricular, 7, 138, 466-467, 491
Ventricular diastole, 138
Ventricular fibrillation (VF, V fib)
    fine, 508
Ventricular hypertrophy, 152, 466
Ventricular systole, 138
Venules, 141, 555
Vermiform, 249, 555
Vermiform appendix, 249, 555
Verruca, 57, 555
Vertebral
    column, 85, 282, 394, 496
Vertebral column, 85, 282, 394, 496
Vertigo, 445-446, 523-524
Vesicle, 59, 331, 475, 510
Vesicular, 336, 556
Vesicular, 336, 556
Vestibule, 519
Vestibulocochlear nerve, 441, 496
VF, 438
Viagra, 340
Vibration, 111, 423, 541
Viral agents, sample sites and associated
    eye infections, 437, 484-485
    genital infections, 495
Virilism, 369, 482
Viscera, 106, 396, 556
Visceral, 31, 106, 133-134, 214, 535
Visceral muscle, 106, 556
Visceral pericardium, 133-134, 556
Visceral peritoneum, 31, 556
Visceral pleura, 31, 214, 556
Viscosity, 141
Visual acuity
    color vision, 435, 496
Visual acuity (VA), 436, 556
Vital signs
    body temperature, 393, 442
Vitamin K, 178
Vitreous humor, 427, 556
Vocal cords, 211-212, 510
Void, 284
Voiding, 291, 469, 556
Voiding cystourethrography (VCUG), 294, 556
Voiding disorders
    urinary incontinence, 291
    urinary retention, 291
Volume
    complemental air, 215, 516
    expiratory reserve, 215, 465, 506
    functional residual capacity, 215, 465, 509
    supplemental air, 215, 506
    total lung capacity (TLC), 215, 551
    vital capacity (VC), 215, 556
Voluntary muscles, 556
Volvulus, 259, 556
Vomer, 85, 556
Vomer bone, 85, 556
Vomit, 242, 479, 512
Voyeurism, 544
VS, 189, 215, 465, 556
Vulva, 28, 312-314, 473, 556

W
Walking, 111, 222, 447, 507
Walking pneumonia, 222, 525
water intake, 297
Weight gain, 349
Weight loss, 122, 189, 369, 482-483
Well-being, 540
Wheal, 59, 556
wheals, 57, 187, 513
Whiplash, 98
White blood cell count
    corrected, 218, 256, 305, 433-435, 483
White blood cells (WBC), 556
White blood count (WBC), 497
White matter, 390-392, 493
Whiteheads, 481
Whole blood, 169-170, 535
Whooping cough, 220, 533
Windpipe, 208, 475, 551
word parts, 2-3, 19, 47, 79, 129, 167, 207, 241, 279,
    311, 355, 387, 423, 497
Word structure
    pronunciation, 2-3
Worm, 249
Wound healing

drainage, 525
Wryneck, 111, 551
Wt, 469

X
Xalatan, 437
Xenograft, 64, 513
Xeroderma, 55, 557
Xerophthalmia, 432, 557
XT, 435, 469
Xylocaine, 65, 407

Z
Zidovudine, 191
Zovirax, 65
Zygomatic bone, 85, 557